SPINE SECRETS

Vincent J. Devlin, M.D.

Attending Orthopaedic Surgeon
Southern California Permanente Medical Group
Kaiser Fontana Medical Center
Department of Orthopaedic Surgery—Spine Section
Fontana, California
Assistant Clinical Professor, Department of Orthopaedic Surgery
Loma Linda University Medical Center
Loma Linda, California

HANLEY & BELFUS, INC.

An Affiliate of Elsevier

HANLEY & BELFUS, INC.
An Affiliate of Elsevier

The Curtis Center
Independence Square West
Philadelphia, Pennsylvania 19106

Library of Congress Cataloging-in-Publication Data

Spine secrets / [edited by] Vincent J. Devlin.
    p. ; cm. — (The secrets series)
  Includes bibliographical references and index.
  ISBN 1-56053-358-7 (alk. paper)
    1. Spinal cord—Diseases—Examinations, questions, etc. 2. Spine—Surgery—Examinations, questions, etc. 3. Spine—Wounds and injuries—Examinations, questions, etc. I. Devlin, Vincent J. II. Series.
  [DNLM: 1. Spinal Cord Diseases—Examination Questions. 2. Spinal Injuries—Examination Questions. 3. Spine—surgery—Examination Questions. WE 18.2 S757 2002]
  RC400.S665 2002
  616.8'3—dc21

                                         2001018935

SPINE SECRETS   ISBN 1-56053-358-7

Printed in the United States

Last digit is the print number: 9 8 7 6 5 4 3 2 1

CONTENTS

CONTRIBUTORS

Behrooz A. Akbarnia, M.D.
Clinical Professor, Department of Orthopaedic Surgery, University of California at San Diego; Medical Director, San Diego Center for Spinal Disorders, San Diego, California

Todd J. Albert, M.D.
Professor and Vice-Chairman, Department of Orthopaedics, and The Rothman Institute, Thomas Jefferson University Medical College, Philadelphia, Pennsylvania

D. Greg Anderson, M.D.
Assistant Professor, Department of Orthopaedic Surgery, University of Virginia School of Medicine; University of Virginia Hospital, Charlottesville, Virginia

Paul A. Anderson, M.D.
Associate Professor of Orthopedic Surgery, Department of Orthopedic Surgery and Rehabilitation, University of Wisconsin; University of Wisconsin Hospital and Clinics, Madison, Wisconsin

Ramin Bagheri, M.D.
Spine Fellow, San Diego Center for Spinal Disorders, San Diego, California

Darren L. Bergey, M.D.
Clinical Instructor, Department of Orthopaedic Surgery, Loma Linda University Medical Center, Loma Linda, California

Fabien D. Bitan, M.D.
Assistant Professor of Orthopedic Surgery, Albert Einstein College of Medicine; Spine Surgeon and Associate Director, Spine Institute, Beth Israel Medical Center, New York, New York

Keith H. Bridwell, M.D.
Asa C. and Dorothy W. Jones Professor, Department of Orthopaedic Surgery, Washington University School of Medicine; Barnes Hospital, St. Louis, Missouri

Thomas N. Bryce, M.D.
Assistant Professor, Department of Rehabilitation Medicine, Mount Sinai School of Medicine and Mount Sinai Medical Center, New York, New York

Frank P. Castro, M.D.
Spine Surgery, PSC, Louisville, Kentucky

Jens R. Chapman, M.D.
Professor, Department of Orthopaedics and Sports Medicine, University of Washington at Seattle; Harborview Medical Center, University of Washington Medical Center, Seattle, Washington

Adam C. Crowl, M.D.
Department of Orthopaedic Surgery, University of Virginia School of Medicine; University of Virginia Hospital, Charlottesville, Virginia

Gina Cruz, B.S., RPT
Claremont, California

Mark R. Davies, M.D.
Department of Orthopaedic Surgery, University of California at Los Angeles, Los Angeles, California

Jeffrey E. Deckey, M.D.
Orthopaedic Specialty Institute, Orange, California

Stephen L. Demeter, M.D., M.P.H.
Professor and Head, Pulmonary Medicine and Critical Care Medicine, Northeastern Ohio Universities College of Medicine, Rootstown, Ohio; Head of Preventive Medicine, Akron General Medical Center, Akron, Ohio

Sylvia Devlin, B.S.
Information Systems Consultant, Upland, California

Vincent J. Devlin, M.D.
Attending Orthopaedic Surgeon, Southern California Permanente Medical Group, Kaiser Fontana Medical Center, Department of Orthopaedic Surgery–Spine Section, Fontana, California; Assistant Clinical Professor, Department of Orthopaedic Surgery, Loma Linda University Medical Center, Loma Linda, California

Eric W. Edmonds, M.D.
Resident Physician, Department of Surgery, University of California at Davis Health System, Sacramento, California

Maury Ellenberg, M.D., FACP
Clinical Associate Professor and Residency Program Director, Department of Physical Medicine and Rehabilitation, Wayne State University School of Medicine; Sinai-Grace Hospital, Detroit, Michigan; Providence Hospital, Southfield, Michigan

Paul Enker, M.D., FRCS, FAAOS
Associate Director, Orthopedic and Rehabilitation Institute, North Shore University Hospital at Glen Cove, Glen Cove, New York

Jeffrey R. Erickson, B.S., J.D.
Riverside, California

Avital Fast, M.D.
Professor and Chairman, Department of Rehabilitation Medicine, Montefiore Medical Center/Albert Einstein College of Medicine, Bronx, New York

Robert W. Gaines, Jr., M.D.
Columbia Orthopaedic Group, Columbia, Missouri

Jeffrey J. Gilchrist, B.S., C.P., BOCO
Colton, California

John M. Gorup, M.D.
Lafayette Orthopaedic Clinic and Unity Medical Center, Lafayette, Indiana

Munish C. Gupta, M.D.
Associate Professor, Department of Orthopaedics, University of California at Davis; Adult and Pediatric Spine Surgery, University of California at Davis Medical Center, Shriners Hospital for Children, Sacramento, California

Thomas R. Haher, M.D.
Professor, Department of Orthopaedic Surgery, New York Medical College; Adjunct Professor, Department of Civil Engineering, Cooper Union for the Advancement of Science and Art; Chief, Spinal Surgery, Lutheran Medical Center, New York, New York

Stephen M. Hansen, M.D.
Department of Orthopaedics and Rehabilitation, Creighton University; Department of Orthopaedics and Rehabilitation, University of Nebraska Medical Center, Omaha, Nebraska

Richard T. Holt, M.D.
Clinical Professor, Department of Orthopedic Surgery, Tulane University School of Medicine, New Orleans, Louisiana

Joseph C. Honet, M.D., M.S.
Professor, F.T.A., Department of Physical Medicine and Rehabilitation, Wayne State University School of Medicine; Chief, Department of Physical Medicine and Rehabilitation, Sinai-Grace Hospital, Detroit, Michigan

Mary E. Hurley, M.D.
Clinical Professor, Department of Orthopaedics, Loma Linda University, Loma Linda, California; Good Samaritan Hospital, Los Angeles, California; Kaiser Permanente Medical Group, Fontana Medical Center, Fontana, California

Todd S. Jarosz, M.D.
Department of Orthopaedics and Sports Medicine, University of Washington at Seattle; University of Washington Medical Center, Seattle, Washington

Lawrence Karlin, M.D.
Assistant Professor, Department of Orthopaedic Surgery, Harvard Medical School; Department of Orthopaedic Surgery, Children's Hospital, Boston, Massachusetts

Phillip K. Kay, M.D.
Department of Physical Medicine, Kaiser Permanente Medical Group, Woodland Hills, California

Reginald Q. Knight, M.D.
Associate Professor and Chair, Department of Orthopaedics and Rehabilitation, Creighton University; Creighton University Medical Center, Omaha, Nebraska

Anna Lasak, M.D.
Assistant Professor, Department of Rehabilitation Medicine, Montefiore Medical Center/Albert Einstein College of Medicine; Clinical Director, Rehabilitation Medicine, Montefiore Medical Park, Bronx, New York

Baron S. Lonner, M.D.
Assistant Professor, Department of Orthopaedic Surgery, Albert Einstein College of Medicine, New York, New York

Mohammad E. Majd, M.D.
Spine Surgery, PSC, Louisville, Kentucky

Steven Mardjetko, M.D.
Illinois Bone and Joint Institute, Des Plaines, Illinois

Joseph Y. Margulies, M.D., Ph.D.
Associate Professor, Department of Orthopedic Surgery, Albert Einstein College of Medicine, New York, New York

Sohail K. Mirza, M.D.
Associate Professor, Department of Orthopaedics and Sports Medicine, University of Washington at Seattle; Harborview Medical Center, University of Washington Medical Center, Seattle, Washington

Ronald Moskovich, M.D., FRCS
Assistant Professor, Department of Orthopaedic Surgery, New York University School of Medicine; Associate Chief of Spine Surgery, New York University Hospital for Joint Diseases, New York, New York

Douglas H. Musser, D.O.
Associate Clinical Teaching Staff, Department of Orthopaedic Surgery, Division of Spinal Surgery, Ohio University, Athens, Ohio; Humility of Mary Systems and Forum Health Systems, Youngstown, Ohio; Robinson Memorial Hospital, Ravenna, Ohio; Summa Health Systems and Akron General Hospital, Akron, Ohio

Michael G. Neuwirth, M.D.
Director, Spine Institute, Beth Israel Medical Center; Department of Orthopedics, New York University, New York, New York

Ashit C. Patel, M.D.
Instructor/Spine Fellow, Department of Orthopaedics, Division of Surgery, University of Kentucky; Attending Physician, University of Kentucky Hospital and VA Hospital, Lexington, Kentucky

Kristjan T. Ragnarsson, M.D.
Lucy G. Moses Professor and Chairman, Department of Rehabilitation Medicine, Mount Sinai School of Medicine and Mount Sinai Hospital, New York, New York

John D. Ray, M.D.
Department of Orthopaedic Surgery, University of California at Davis, Sacramento, California

Thomas A. Schildhauer, M.D.
Oberarzt, Chirurgische Klinik und Poliklinik, Ruhr Universität Bochum, Bochum, Germany

Jerome Schofferman, M.D.
Director, Research and Education, San Francisco Spine Institute, Daly City, California

William O. Shaffer, M.D.
Associate Professor of Surgery, Residing Program Director, Department of Orthopaedic Surgery, University of Kentucky; University of Kentucky Hospital and VA Hospital, Lexington, Kentucky

Edward D. Simmons, M.D., M.Sc., FRCS(C)
Associate Clinical Professor, Department of Orthopaedic Surgery, State University of New York at Buffalo; Simmons Orthopaedic and Spine Associates, Buffalo, New York

Kern Singh, M.D.
Resident, Department of Orthopaedic Surgery, Rush-Presbyterian-St. Luke's Medical Center, Chicago, Illinois

Richard Lance Snyder, M.D.
Lawrence Memorial Hospital, Lawrence, Kansas

John Steinmann, D.O.
Clinical Professor, Department of Orthopedics, Western University of Health Sciences, Pomona, California; Assistant Clinical Professor, Department of Orthopedics, Loma Linda University Schoof of Medicine, Loma Linda, California

Mark A. Thomas, M.D.
Associate Professor of Rehabilitation Medicine, Albert Einstein College of Medicine/Montefiore Medical Center; Program Director, Department of Physical Medicine and Rehabilitation, Montefiore Medical Center, Bronx, New York

Alexander R. Vaccaro, M.D.
Professor, Department of Orthopaedic Surgery, Thomas Jefferson University School of Medicine; Co-Chief of Spinal Surgery, Jefferson Health System/Rothman Institute; Co-Director, Delaware Regional Spinal Cord Injury Center, Philadelphia, Pennsylvania

Robin H. Vaughn, Ph.D.
San Diego, California

Theodore A. Wagner, M.D.
Clinical Professor, Department of Orthopaedics, University of Washington at Seattle; Swedish Hospital, Harborview Hospital, and Children's Hospital, Seattle, Washington

Jeffrey C. Wang, M.D.
Assistant Professor, Department of Orthopaedic Surgery, University of California at Los Angeles, Los Angeles, California

Motoko Watanabe, M.D.
Brooklyn, New York

Robert G. Watkins, IV, M.D.
Professor of Clinical Orthopaedic Surgery, Department of Orthopaedics, Los Angeles Spine Surgery Institute; St. Vincent Medical Center, Los Angeles, California

Lytton A. Williams, M.D.
Clinical Associate Professor, Department of Orthopaedics, University of Southern California; St. Vincent Medical Center and Los Angeles Spine Surgery Institute, Los Angeles, California

Lance Winter, D.O.
Department of Orthopedics, Riverside County Regional Medical Center, Riverside, California

Ruijin Yao, M.D., Ph.D.
Assistant Professor, Department of Rehabilitation Medicine, Albert Einstein College of Medicine/Montefiore Medical Center, Bronx, New York

Iris Yaron, M.D.
New York, New York

Edwin E. Yeo, M.D.
Department of Nuclear Medicine, Kaiser Permanente Medical Group, Fontana, California

Christopher A. Yeung, M.D.
Arizona Institute for Minimally Invasive Spine Care, Phoenix, Arizona

Yinggang Zheng, M.D.
Department of Orthopaedic Surgery, State University of New York at Buffalo; Simmons Orthopaedic and Spine Associates, Buffalo, New York

PREFACE

Appropriate diagnosis, management, and treatment of spinal disorders remain a challenge for both patient and physician. Rapid advances in the field of spinal disorders have opened new avenues for diagnosis and treatment. A wide range of medical specialties—orthopedic surgery, neurosurgery, physical medicine, radiology, internal medicine, family practice, pediatrics, neurology, anesthesia, emergency medicine, pathology, and psychiatry—participate in the evaluation and treatment of patients with spinal problems on a daily basis. Knowledge of current concepts relating to spinal disorders is crucial to provide appropriate evaluation, referral, and treatment.

The goal of *Spine Secrets* is to provide broad-based coverage of the diverse field of spinal disorders at an introductory level, using the proven and time-tested question-and-answer format of the Secrets Series®. The book is designed to be a handy reference that covers the common conditions encountered during evaluation and treatment of spinal problems. Topics are arranged to provide the reader with a sound knowledge base in the fundamentals of spinal anatomy, clinical assessment, spinal imaging, and nonoperative and operative treatment of spinal disorders. The full spectrum of disorders affecting the cervical, thoracic, and lumbar spine in pediatric and adult patients is covered, including degenerative disorders, fractures, spinal deformities, tumors, infections, and systemic problems such as osteoporosis and rheumatoid arthritis. The detailed information will benefit the reader during patient rounds as well as in the clinic and operating room. The book is not intended to provide comprehensive coverage of specific topics, which is more appropriately the domain of major textbooks. However, it is hoped that readers will be stimulated to further their knowledge of spinal disorders through additional study, as directed by the reference list at the end of each chapter.

The intended audience is wide-ranging and includes all medical practitioners interested in furthering their knowledge and understanding of spinal disorders: medical students, residents, fellows, and practicing physicians. The book may also be of interest to nurses, physical therapists, chiropractors, and biomedical students as well as patients with spinal problems.

I wish to acknowledge the numerous people who have provided guidance over the years and contributed to my development as a physician and spinal surgeon. I am especially grateful to Dr. Marc A. Asher, Dr. Thomas B. Haher, Dr. Behrooz A. Akbarnia, Dr. Oheneba Boachie-Adjel, Dr. David S. Bradford, Dr. James W. Ogilvie, Dr. Ensor E. Transfeldt, Dr. Paul A. Anderson, Dr. Dale E. Rowe, Professor Jurgen Harms, Dr. Arthur D. Steffee, Dr. Joseph Y. Margulies, and Dr. William O. Shaffer. I also thank the staff at Hanley and Belfus, especially William Lamsback and Stan Ward, for bringing this project to completion. Finally, I thank my colleagues at the Kaiser Permanente Fontana Medical Center for their support and efforts in treating patients with challenging spinal problems.

Vincent J. Devlin, M.D.

I. Regional Spinal Anatomy

1. CLINICALLY RELEVANT ANATOMY OF THE CERVICAL REGION

Vincent J. Devlin, M.D., and Darren L. Bergey, M.D.

OSTEOLOGY

1. Describe the bony landmarks of the occiput.

The occiput forms the posterior osseous covering for the cerebellum. The **foramen magnum** is the opening through which the spinal cord joins the brainstem. The anterior border of the foramen magnum is termed the **basion** (clivus), and the posterior border is termed the **opisthion**. The **inion** or **external occipital protruberance** is the midline region of the occiput where bone is greatest in thickness. The **superior and inferior nuchal lines** extend laterally from the inion. The **transverse sinus** is located in close proximity to the inion (Fig. 1). The occipital area in the midline below the inion is the ideal location for screw insertion for occipitocervical fixation as it is the thickest portion of the occiput.

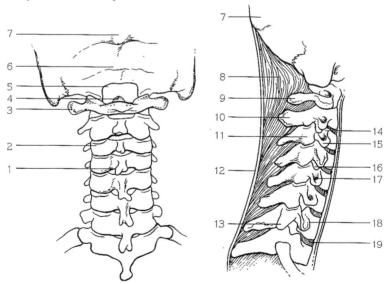

FIGURE 1. Posterior and lateral views of the occiput and cervical spine showing the basic bony anatomy. 1, Spinous process; 2, Lateral articular process or lateral mass; 3, Tranverse process of C1; 4, Odontoid process of C2; 5, Foramen magnum; 6, Inferior nuchal line; 7, Inion; 8, Ligamentum nuchae; 9, Posterior arch of C1; 10, Spinous process of C2; 11, Lateral mass; 12, Supraspinous ligament; 13, Lateral articular process; 14, Uncinate process; 15, Anterior tubercule of transverse process; 16, Neural foramen; 17, Transverse foramen; 18, Carotid tubercle; 19, Intervertebral disc. (From An HS, Simpson JM: Surgery of the Cervical Spine. Baltimore, Williams & Wilkins, 1998, with permission.)

2. What is meant by typical and atypical cervical vertebrae?

C3, C4, C5, and C6 are defined as typical cervical vertebrae because they share common structural characteristics. In contrast, C1 (atlas), C2 (axis), and C7 (vertebra prominens) possess unique structural and functional features and are therefore termed atypical cervical vertebrae.

3. Describe a typical cervical vertebra.

The components of a typical cervical vertebra (C3–C6) include an **anterior body** and a **posterior arch** formed by **lamina** and **pedicles**. The lamina blend into the **lateral mass,** which comprises the bony region between the superior and inferior articular processes. The paired superior and inferior articular processes form the **facet joint.** The **uncovertebral (neurocentral) joints** are bony ridges that extend upward from the lateral margin of the superior surface of the vertebral body. The intervertebral foramina protect the exiting spinal nerves and are located behind the vertebral bodies between the pedicles of adjacent vertebra. The transverse processes of the lower cervical spine are directed anterolaterally and composed of an anterior costal element and a posterior transverse element. The transverse foramen, located at the base of the transverse process, permits passage of the vertebral artery. The spinous process originates in the midsagittal plane at the junction of the lamina and is bifid between C2–C6 (Fig. 2).

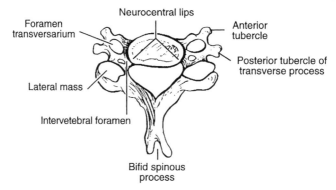

FIGURE 2. Typical cervical vertebra (superior view). (From Raiszadeh K, Spivak JM: Spine. In Spivak JM, DiCasare PE, Feldman DS, et al (eds): Orthopaedics: A Study Guide. New York, McGraw-Hill, 1999, pp 63–72, with permission).

4. What are the distinguishing features of C1 (atlas)?

The ring-like atlas (C1) is unique because during development its body fuses with the axis (C2) to form the odontoid process. Thus, the atlas has no body. It is composed of two thick, load-bearing lateral masses, with concave superior and inferior articular facets. Connecting these facets are a relatively straight, short anterior arch and a longer, curved posterior arch. The anterior ring has an articular facet on its posterior aspect for articulation with the dens. The posterior ring has a grove on its posterior-superior surface for the vertebral artery. The weakest point of the ring is at the narrowed areas where the anterior and posterior arches connect to the lateral masses (location of a Jefferson fracture). The transverse process of the atlas has a single tubercle, which protrudes laterally and can be palpated in the space between the tip of the mastoid process and the ramus of the mandible (Fig. 3).

5. What are the distinguishing features of C2 (axis)?

The axis (C2) receives its name from its odontoid process (dens), which forms the axis of rotation for motion through the atlantoaxial joint. The dens is a bony process extending cranial from the body of C2, formed from the embryologic body of the atlas (C1). The dens has an anterior hyaline articular surface for articulation with the anterior arch of C1 as well as a posterior articular surface for articulation with the transverse ligament. The C2 superior articular processes are

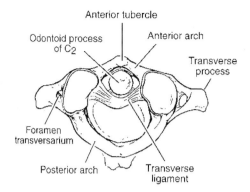

FIGURE 3. Atlas (superior view). (From Raiszadeh K, Spivak JM: Spine. In Spivak JM, DiCasare PE, Feldman DS, et al (eds): Orthopaedics: A Study Guide. New York, McGraw-Hill, 1999, pp 63–72, with permission.)

located anterior and lateral to the spinal canal while the C2 inferior articular processes are located posterior and lateral to the spinal canal. The articular processes are connected by the pars interarticularis. Hyperflexion or hyperextension injuries may subject the axis to shear stresses, resulting in a fracture through the pars region (termed a "hangman's fracture"). The atlantodens interval is the space between the hyaline cartilage surfaces of the anterior tubercle of the atlas and the anterior dens. Normal adult and childhood measurements are 3 mm and 5 mm, respectively.

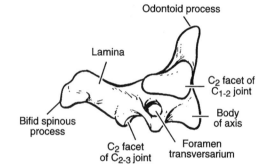

FIGURE 4. Axis (lateral view). (From Raiszadeh K, Spivak JM: Spine. In Spivak JM, DiCasare PE, Feldman DS, et al (eds): Orthopaedics: A Study Guide. New York, McGraw-Hill, 1999, pp 63–72, with permission.)

6. What are the distinguishing features of C7 (vertebra prominens)?

The unique anatomic features of the C7 vertebra reflect its location as the transitional vertebra at the cervicothoracic junction:

- Long non-bifid spinous process which provides a useful landmark
- Its foramen transversarium usually contains vertebral veins but usually does not contain the vertebral artery which generally enters the cervical spine at the C6 level
- The C7 transverse process is large in size and possesses only a posterior tubercle
- The C7 lateral mass is the thinnest lateral mass in the cervical spine
- The inferior articular process of C7 is oriented in a relatively perpendicular direction(like a thoracic facet joint)

ARTICULATIONS, LIGAMENTS, AND DISCS

7. Describe how normal range of motion is distributed across the cervical region.

Facet joint orientation, bony architecture, intervertebral discs, uncovertebral joints and ligaments all play a role in determining range of motion at various levels of the cervical spine. Approximately 50% of cervical flexion-extension occurs at the occiput–C1 level. Approximately 50% of cervical rotation occurs at the C1–C2 level. Lesser amounts of flexion-extension, rotation and lateral bending occur segmentally between C2 and C7.

8. What are the key anatomic features of the atlantooccipital (O–C1) articulation?

The atlantooccipital joints are synovial joints comprised of the convex occipital condyles which articulate with the concave lateral masses of the atlas. Motion at the O–C1 segment is restricted primarily to flexion-extension due to bony and ligamentous constraints and absence of an intervertebral disc. The most important ligaments are the paired alar ligaments(extend from the tip of the dens to the medial aspect of each occipital condyle and restrict rotation of the occiput on the dens). The tectorial membrane is also important(continuous with the posterior longitudinal ligament and extends from the posterior body of C2 to the anterior foramen magnum and occiput). Less important ligaments include the anterior and posterior atlanto-occipital membrane, the O–C1 joint capsules and the apical ligament (see Figure 5).

9. What are the key anatomic features of the atlantoaxial (C1–C2) articulation?

The atlantoaxial articulation is composed of three synovial joints—paired lateral mass articulations and a central articulation between the dens and the anterior C1 arch and transverse ligament (see Figure 5). The primary motion at the atlantoaxial joint is rotation with approximately 50% of rotation of the cervical spine occurring at the C1–C2 joints. The approximation of the odontoid against the anterior arch of C1 resists translation of C1 relative to C2.

The transverse atlantal ligament, the major stabilizer at the C1–C2 level, attaches to the medial aspect of the lateral masses of the atlas (see Figure 5). This ligament has a wide middle portion where it articulates with the posterior surface of the dens. Superior and inferior longitudinal fasciculi extend to insert on the anterior foramen magnum and the posterior body of the axis respectively. These structures are collectively named the cruciform ligament. This ligament holds the dens firmly against the anterior arch of the atlas. Other important ligaments attaching to C2 include:

Anterior atlantoaxial ligament—continuous with the anterior longitudinal ligament in the lower cervical spine

Posterior atlantoaxial ligament—continuous with the ligamentum flavum in the subaxial spine

Apical ligament—extends from the tip of the dens to the foramen magnum

Alar ligaments—extend from the lateral dens and attach to the medial border of the occipital condyles

10. Name the arrangement of ligaments at the craniovertebral junction as the spine is sectioned in an anterior to posterior direction.

1. Anterior atlantooccipital membrane(continuous with anterior longitudinal ligament)
2. Apical ligament (extends from tip of the dens to anterior edge of foramen magnum)
3. Alar ligaments (extend from the tip of the dens to the medial aspect of each occipital condyle)
4. Cruciform liagament
5. Tectorial membrane (continuous with the posterior longitudinal ligament)
6. Posterior atlantooccipital membrane (continuous with the ligamentum flavum)

11. Describe the ligament anatomy of the subaxial spine.

The major ligaments of the subaxial cervical spine are:

Anterior longitudinal ligament (ALL)—this strong ligament extends from the body of the axis to the sacrum binding the anterior aspect of the vertebral bodies and intervertebral discs together. It resists hyperextension of the spine and gives stability to the anterior aspect of the disc space. It is continuous with anterior atlanto-occipital membrane

Posterior longitudinal ligament (PLL)—this is a weaker ligament which extends from the axis to the sacrum It is thicker and wider in the cervical spine than in the thoracolumbar segments. It serves to protect from hyperflexion injury and reinforces the intervertebral discs from herniation. It is continuous with tectorial membrane.

Ligamentum flavum—this structure may be considered to be a segmental ligament which at-

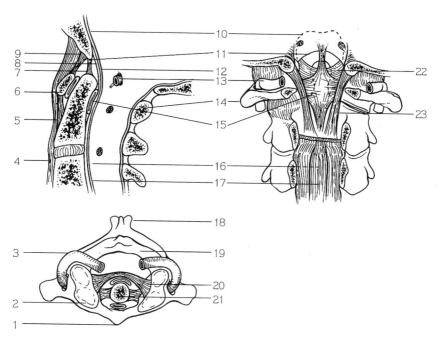

FIGURE 5. Ligamentous and bony anatomy of the upper cervical region. 1, Anterior tubercle; 2, Superior articular facet; 3, Vertebral artery; 4, Anterior longitudinal ligament; 5, Anterior atlas–axis membrane; 6, Anterior arch of atlas; 7, Apical ligament; 8, Vertical cruciform ligament; 9, Anterior atlas–occipital membrane; 10, Attachment of tectorial membrane; 11, Anterior edge of foramen magnum; 12, Tectorial membrane; 13, Vertebral artery; 14, Atlas; 15, Transverse ligament; 16, Origin of tectorial membrane; 17, Posterior longitudinal ligament; 18, Spinous process (axis); 19, Atlas; 20, Transverse ligament; 21, Dens (odontoid process); 22, Alar ligament; 23, Deep tectorial membrane. (From An HS, Simpson JM: Surgery of the Cervical Spine. Baltimore, Williams & Wilkins, 1998, with permission.)

taches to adjacent lamina. This structure attaches to the ventral aspect of the superior lamina and the dorsal aspect of the inferior lamina. Laterally, the ligamentum flavum is in continuity with the facet capsules.

Interspinous and Supraspinous ligaments—these ligaments lie between or dorsal to the spinous processes, respectively. The supraspinous ligament is in continuity with the ligamentum nuchae, which runs from C7 to the occiput and acts as a posterior tension band to maintain an upright neck posture.

12. How are the articulations between vertebrae in the subaxial cervical spine (C3–C7) described in terms of a three-column model?

The anatomy of the lower cervical spine (C3–C7) can be described in terms of a functional spinal unit consisting of two adjacent vertebrae, intervertebral disc, and related ligaments and joint capsules. The functional spinal unit in the subaxial cervical region can be conceptualized in terms of three columns (Fig. 6).

Anterior column: anterior portion of the vertebral body and intervertebral disc (resist compressive forces); anterior longitudinal ligament and anterior annulus fibrosus (resist distraction forces)

Middle column: posterior portion of vertebral body, posterior portion of intervertebral disc and uncovertebral joints (resist compressive force); posterior longitudinal ligament and posterior annulus fibrosus (resist distraction forces)

Posterior column: facet joints and lateral masses (resist compression forces); facet capsules, interspinous ligaments, supraspinous ligaments (resist distraction forces).

This three-column concept is also applicable to the thoracic and lumbar spine.

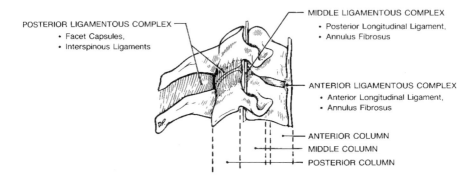

POSTERIOR LIGAMENTOUS COMPLEX
• Facet Capsules,
• Interspinous Ligaments

MIDDLE LIGAMENTOUS COMPLEX
• Posterior Longitudinal Ligament,
• Annulus Fibrosus

ANTERIOR LIGAMENTOUS COMPLEX
• Anterior Longitudinal Ligament,
• Annulus Fibrosus

ANTERIOR COLUMN
MIDDLE COLUMN
POSTERIOR COLUMN

FIGURE 6. Components of the three columns of the cervical spine. (From Stauffer ES, MacMillan M: Fractures and dislocations of the cervical spine. In Rockwood CA, Green DP, Bucholz RW, Heckman JD (eds): Fractures in Adults, vol. 2, 4th ed. Philadelphia, Lippincott-Raven, 1996, pp 1473–1628, with permission.)

13. What are the unique features of the subaxial cervical facet joints?

At each cervical level (C3–C7) there are paired superior and inferior articular processes. The superior articular process is positioned anterior and inferior to the inferior articular process of the adjacent cranial vertebra. These articulations are covered with hyaline cartilage and form synovial zygapophyseal (facet or Z) joints. The orientation of the facet joints is a major factor in the range of motion of the cervical spine. The typical cervical facet joints are oriented 45° in the sagittal plane and 0° in the coronal plane. These are the most horizontally oriented regional facet joints in the spinal column. Laxity of the joint capsule permits sliding motion to occur and explains why unilateral or bilateral dislocation without fracture may occur. The orientation of these facets allows flexion and extension, lateral bending, and rotation of the lower cervical spine. Flexion and extension are greatest at the C5–C6 and C6–C7 levels. This has been postulated to be responsible for the relatively high incidence of degenerative changes noted at these two cervical levels.

14. What are the uncovertebral joints (joints of Luschka)?

When viewed anteriorly, the lateral margin of the superior surface of each subaxial cervical vertebral body extends cranially as a bony process called the uncinate process. These processes articulate with a reciprocal convex area on the inferolateral aspect of the next cranial vertebral body. This articulation is named the uncovertebral joint or neurocentral joint of Luschka. It is believed to form as a degenerative cleft in the lateral part of the annulus fibrosus. The uncinate process, unique to the cervical spine, serves as a "rail" to limit lateral translation or bending and as a guiding mechanism for flexion and extension.

15. What are the components of the intervertebral disc?

Each intervertebral disc is composed of a central gel-like nucleus pulposus surrounded by a peripheral fibrocartilaginous annulus fibrosus. The endplates of the vertebral bodies are lined with hyaline cartilage and bind the disc to the vertebral body. The annulus fibrosus (predominantly type 1 collagen) attaches to the cartilaginous endplates via collagen fibers, which run obliquely at a 30° angle to the surface of the vertebral body and in a direction opposite to the annular fibers of the adjacent layer. The nucleus pulposus is composed primarily of glycosaminoglycans and type 2 collagen, which have the capacity to bind large amounts of water. With aging, less water is bound, viscosity increases, and fissuring of the disc occurs.

NEURAL ANATOMY

16. Describe the cross-sectional anatomy of the spinal cord and the location and function of the major spinal cord tracts.

A cross-sectional view of the spinal cord demonstrates a central butterfly-shaped area of gray matter and peripheral white matter (Fig. 7). The central gray matter contains the neural cell bodies. The peripheral white matter contains the axon tracts. Ascending (afferent tracts) carry impulses toward the brain, whereas the descending (efferent tracts) carry nerve signals away from the brain. The axon tracts may receive and transmit signals to the same side of the body (uncrossed tracts) or may transmit or receive signals from the opposite side (crossed tracts). The major spinal tracts important to the clinician include:

Corticospinal tracts: descending tracts located in lateral portion of the cord that transmit ipsilateral motor function.

Spinothalamic tracts: ascending tracts located in the anterior portion of the cord that transmit sensations of pain and temperature. These tracts cross shortly after entering the spinal cord and therefore transmit sensations from the contralateral side of the body.

Dorsal column tracts: ascending tracts that convey proprioception, vibration, and light touch sensation.

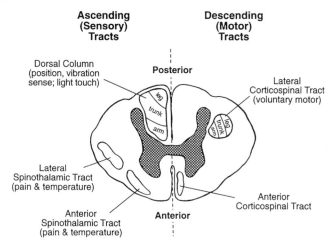

FIGURE 7. Cross-sectional anatomy of the spinal cord. (From Raiszadeh K, Spivak JM: Spine. In Spivak JM, DiCesare PE, Feldman DS, et al: Orthopaedics: A Study Guide. New York, McGraw-Hill, 1999, pp 63–72, with permission.)

17. How many spinal nerves exit from the spinal cord?

The spinal nerves exit from the spinal cord in pairs. There are 31 pairs of spinal nerves: 8 cervical, 12 thoracic, 5 lumbar, 5 sacral, and 1 coccygeal nerve root pairs.

18. What structures contribute to the formation of a spinal nerve? What are the branches of a spinal nerve?

Each spinal nerve (Fig. 8) is composed of both sensory and motor fibers. The collection of sensory fibers is termed the **dorsal root**. The cell bodies for these sensory fibers are located in the **dorsal root ganglion**. The collection of motor fibers is termed the **ventral or anterior root**. A typical spinal nerve is formed by the union of the dorsal and ventral roots, which occurs just distal to the dorsal root ganglion. The spinal nerve becomes covered by a common dural sheath and gives off the following branches:

Dorsal ramus: provides sensation to the medial two-thirds of the back, the facet joint capsules, and the posterior ligaments. The dorsal ramus also innervates the deep spinal musculature.

Ventral ramus: supplies all other skin and muscles of the body. In the cervical and lumbar regions the ventral rami form plexuses (cervical plexus, brachial plexus, lumbar plexus, lumbosacral plexus). In the thoracic levels ventral rami form the intercostal nerve.

Recurrent meningeal branch (sinuvertebral nerve): innervates the periosteum of the posterior aspect of the vertebral body, basivertebral and epidural veins, epidural adipose tissue, posterior annulus and posterior longitudinal ligament, and anterior aspect of the dural sac.

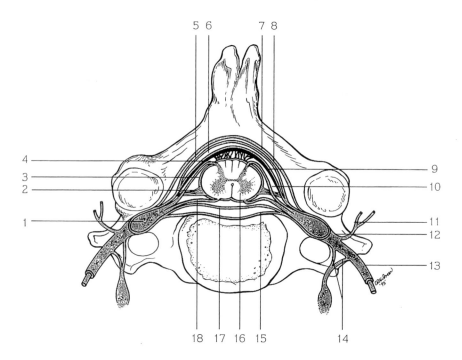

FIGURE 8. Components of a spinal nerve. 1, Spinal ganglion; 2, Dentate ligament; 3, Pia mater; 4, Dorsal root of spinal nerve; 5, Dura mater; 6, Subdural space; 7, Periosteum; 8, Epidural space; 9, Arachnoid membrane; 10, Subarachnoid space; 11, Dorsal ramus; 12, Spinal nerve; 13, Ventral ramus of spinal nerve; 14, Ramus communicans; 15, Periosteum; 16, Medulla spinalis; 17, Dura mater; 18, Ventral root of spinal nerve. (From An HS, Simpson JM: Surgery of the Cervical Spine. Baltimore, Williams & Wilkins, 1998, with permission.)

19. Describe the relationship of the exiting spinal nerve to the numbered vertebral segment for each spinal region.

In the cervical region there are 8 cervical nerve roots and only 7 cervical vertebra. The first 7 cervical nerve roots exit the spinal canal above their numbered vertebra. For example, the C1 root exits the spinal column between the occiput and the atlas (C1). The C5 nerve root passes above the pedicle of the C5 vertebra and occupies the intervertebral foramen between C4 and C5. The C8 nerve root is atypical because it does not have a corresponding vertebral element and exits below the C7 pedicle and occupies the intervertebral foramen between C7 and T1. In the thoracic and lumbar spine, the nerve roots exit the spinal canal by passing below the pedicle of their named vertebra. The T12 nerve passes below the T12 pedicle and exits the interval (neural foramen) between T12 and L1. The L4 nerve root passes beneath the L4 pedicle and exits the neural foramen between L4 and L5.

20. How does the course of the recurrent laryngeal nerve differ from left to right?
The recurrent laryngeal nerve originates from the vagus nerve and enters the tracheoesophageal groove. On the right side it passes around the subclavian artery; on the left side, it passes under the aortic arch. Anterior surgical exposure of the lower cervical spine must be carefully performed in the interval between the tracheoesophageal sheath and carotid sheath to avoid injury to this nerve. The right recurrent laryngeal nerve is at greater risk of injury than the left nerve during surgical exposure because it reaches the tracheoesophageal groove at a higher cervical level and has a less predicatable course

VASCULAR STRUCTURES OF THE CERVICAL REGION

21. Describe the course of vertebral artery
The vertebral artery is the first branch off the subclavian artery and provides the major blood supply to the cervical spinal cord, nerve roots, and vertebrae. It can be divided into four segments. During its first segment, the vertebral artery passes from the subclavian artery anterior to C7 to enter the C6 transverse foramen. In the second segment it continues from the C6 transverse foramina along its course through the cephalad transverse foramina to the level of the atlas. During its course it lies lateral to the vertebral body and in front of the lateral mass. During its upward course between C6 and C2, the vertebral artery gradually shifts to an anterior and medial position, thereby placing the artery at greater risk of injury during anterior decompressive procedures at the upper cervical levels. In its third segment, the artery exits C1 and curves around the C1 lateral mass, running medially along the cranial surface of the posterior arch of C1 in its sulcus, before passing through the atlantooccipital membrane and entering the foramen magnum. The artery stays at least 12 mm lateral from midline of C1, making this a safe zone for dissection. In its fourth segment, the vertebral artery joins the contralateral vertebral artery to form the basilar artery.

22. Describe the blood supply to the spinal cord.
The anterior median spinal artery and the two posterior spinal arteries supply the spinal cord. The anterior spinal artery supplies 85% of the blood supply to the cord throughout its length. Radicular or segmental arteries feed these arteries. In the cervical spine, the majority of radicular arteries arise from the vertebral artery. These arteries enter the spinal canal through the intervertebral foramina and divide into anterior and posterior radicular arteries. The most consistent radicular artery in the cervical spine is located at the C5–C6 level. On average, there are eight radicular feeders to the anterior spinal artery and 12 to the posterior spinal arteries throughout the length of the spinal cord. The basilar artery also anastomoses with the anterior spinal artery, variably supplying the cord to the fourth cervical level.

FASCIA AND MUSCULATURE OF THE CERVICAL SPINE

23. What are the fascial layers of the anterior neck?
The fascial layers of the neck consist of a superficial layer and a deep layer. The superficial layer of the cervical fascia surrounds the platysma muscle. The deep cervical fascia consists of three layers:
1. **Superficial layer:** surrounds the sternocleidomastoid and trapezius muscles.
2. **Middle layer:** consists of the pretracheal fascia, which surrounds the strap muscles, trachea, esophagus, and thyroid gland. This layer is continuous with the lateral margin of the carotid sheath.
3. **Deep layer:** consists of the prevertebral fascia, which surrounds the posterior paracervical and anterior prevertebral musculature.

24. Describe the muscular triangles of the neck.
The anterior aspect of the neck is divided by the sternocleidomastoid into an anterior and posterior triangle. The posterior triangle borders are the trapezius, sternocleidomastoid, and middle

third of the clavicle. The inferior belly of the omohyoid further divides this space into subclavian (lower) and occipital (upper) triangles. The anterior triangle is bounded by the sternocleidomastoid, the anterior median line of the neck, and lower border of the mandible. It is further subdivided into the submandibular, carotid, and muscular triangles. The posterior belly of the digastric separates the carotid from the submandibular triangles. The superior belly of the omohyoid separates the carotid from the muscular triangles (Fig. 9). The standard anterior approach to the mid-cervical spine is done through the muscular triangle.

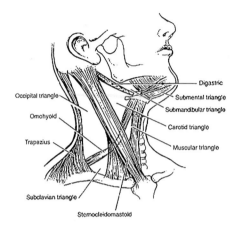

FIGURE 9. Muscular triangles of the neck. (From Raiszadeh K, Spivak JM: Spine. In Spivak JM, DiCesare PE, Feldman DS, et al (eds): Orthopaedics: A Study Guide. New York, McGraw-Hill, 1999, pp 63–72, with permission.)

25. Name the muscles most commonly encountered during anterior and posterior cervical spine procedures.

Anterior muscles: platysma, sternocleidomastoid, strap muscles of the larynx, omohyoid, longus colli

Posterior muscles: superficial layer-trapezius; middle layer-splenius capitis, splenius cervicis; deep layer—semispinalis capitis, longissimus capitis; muscles of the suboccipital triangle—rectus capitis posterior major and minor, obliquus capitis superior and inferior

BIBLIOGRAPHY

1. An HS: Synopsis of Spine Surgery. Baltimore, Williams & Wilkins, 1998.
2. An HS: Principles and Techniques of Spine Surgery. Baltimore, Williams & Wilkins, 1998.
3. An HS, Simpson JM: Surgery of the Cervical Spine. Baltimore, Williams & Wilkins, 1998.
4. Raiszadeh K, Spivak JM: Spine. In Spivak JM, DiCesare PE, Feldman DS, et al (eds): Orthopaedics: A Study Guide. New York, McGraw-Hill, 1999, pp. 3–72.
5. Schneck C: Functional and clinical anatomy of the spine. Phys Med Rehabil State Art Rev 9 (3), 1995.
6. Stauffer ES, MacMillan M: Fractures and dislocations of the cervical spine. In Rockwood CA, Green DP, Bucholz RW, Heckman JD (eds): Fractures in Adults, vol 2, 4th ed. Philadelphia, Lippincott-Raven, 1996, pp 1473–1628.
7. Vaccaro AR: Spine anatomy. In Garfin SR, Vaccaro AR (eds): Orthopaedic Knowledge Update—Spine, vol 1. Rosemont, IL, American Academy of Orthopaedic Surgeons, 1997, pp 3–18.

2. CLINICALLY RELEVANT ANATOMY OF THE THORACIC REGION

Vincent J. Devlin, M.D., and Darren L. Bergey, M.D.

OSTEOLOGY

1. Describe a typical thoracic vertebra.

T1 and T10–T12 possess unique anatomic features due to their transitional location between the cervicothoracic and thoracolumbar spinal regions, respectively. Thoracic vertebra two through nine are termed typical thoracic vertebra because they share common structural features (Fig. 1):

Vertebral body: heart-shaped in cross-section. Posterior vertebral height exceeds anterior vertebral height, resulting in a wedged shape of the vertebral body when viewed in the lateral plane This wedge shape is responsible for the kyphotic alignment in the thoracic region.

Costovertebral articulations: the lateral surface of the vertebral body has both superior and inferior facets for articulation with adjacent ribs.

Costotransverse articulation: rib articulation with the transverse process of vertebra.

Vertebral arch: formed by lamina and two pedicles, which support 7 processes:

Spinous process (1)	Superior facets (2)
Transverse processes (2)	Inferior facets (2)

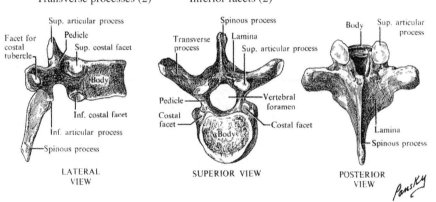

FIGURE 1. Typical thoracic vertebra. (From Pansky B: Review of Gross Anatomy, 4th ed. New York, Macmillan, 1979, with permission.)

2. What are the unique anatomic features of the first thoracic vertebra?

T1 vertebral body dimensions resemble a cervical vertebra more closely than a typical thoracic vertebra. The T1 vertebral body possesses bilateral superior uncinate processes and a well-developed superior vertebral notch. The T1 spinous process is very prominent and may be larger than the C7 spinous process. The first rib articulates with T1 vertebral body via a costal facet

3. What are the unique anatomic features of T10, T11, and T12?

- Lack of costotransverse articulations (T11 and T12)
- Ribs articulate with vertebral bodies and do not overlie the disc space
- Vertebral body dimensions increase and approximate lumbar vertebra dimensions
- Facet morphology transitions from thoracic to lumbar in function and appearance
- T12 transverse process consists of three separate projections

4. What anatomic relationships are useful in determining the level of a thoracic lesion on a thoracic spine radiograph?

The first rib attaches to the T1 vertebral body. The second rib attaches to the T2 vertebral body. The third rib articulates with both the second and third vertebral bodies and overlies the T2–T3 disc space. This pattern continues until the tenth vertebral body. The tenth, eleventh, and twelfth ribs articulate only with the vertebral body of the same number and do not overlie a disc space.

5. Describe the anatomy of the thoracic pedicles.

The paired pedicles arise from the posterior-superior aspect of the vertebral bodies. The superior-inferior pedicle diameter is consistently larger than the medial-lateral pedicle diameter. Pedicle width is narrowest at the T4 level, with medial-lateral pedicle diameter increasing both above (T1–T3) and below this level. The medial pedicle wall is 2–3 times thicker than the lateral pedicle wall across all levels of the thoracic spine. The medial angulation of the pedicle axis decreases from T1 to T12. The site for entry into the thoracic pedicle from a posterior spinal approach is in the region where the facet joint and transverse process intersect and varies slightly, depending on the specific thoracic level.

ARTICULATIONS, LIGAMENTS, AND DISCS

6. What anatomic structures provide articulations between the thoracic vertebral bodies? Between the vertebral arches?

The structures that provide articulations between the thoracic vertebral bodies are (1) the anterior longitudinal ligament, (2) posterior longitudinal ligament, and (3) intervertebral disc.

Five anatomic elements provide articulations between the adjacent vertebral arches:

1. Articular capsules: thin capsules attach to the margins of the articular processes of adjacent vertebra.

2. Ligamentum flavum: yellow elastic tissue that connects laminae of adjacent vertebrae and attaches to the ventral surface of lamina above and to the dorsal surface and superior margin of the lamina below.

3. Supraspinous ligaments: strong fibrous cord that connects the tips of the spinous processes from C7 to sacrum.

4. Interspinous ligaments: interconnect adjoining spinous processes. Attachment extends from base of each spinous process to the tip of the adjacent spinous process.

5. Intertransverse ligaments—interconnect the transverse processes.

The pattern described above continues in the lumbar region as well.

7. What are the two types of articulations between the ribs and the thoracic vertebra?

The two types of articulations between thoracic vertebra and ribs are costovertebral and costotransverse. The **costovertebral articulation** is the articulation between the head of the rib (costa) and the vertebral body. The articular capsule, radiate ligaments, and intraarticular ligaments stabilize this articulation.

The **costotransverse articulation** occurs between the neck and tubercle of the rib (costa) and the transverse process. The ligaments that stabilize this articulation include the superior and lateral costotransverse ligaments (Fig. 2). The T11 and T12 transverse processes do not articulate with their corresponding ribs.

8. Describe the anatomy of the facet joints in the thoracic region.

The facet joints are located at the junction of the vertebral arch and the pedicle. The paired superior articular processes face posterolaterally, and the paired inferior articular processes face anteromedially. The thoracic facets are oriented 60° in the sagittal plane and approximate the coronal plane with a slight medial inclination (20°). Flexion-extension is minimal at T1–T2 and maximal at T12–L1, where facet joint orientation transitions to a lumbar pattern. Axial rotation

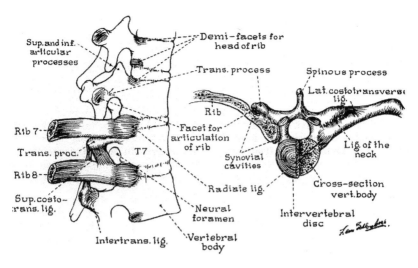

FIGURE 2. Extrinsic ligaments of the thoracic spine. (From Johnson RM, Murphy MJ, Southwick WD: Surgical approaches to the spine. In Herkowitz HN, Garfin SR, Balderston RA, et al (eds): Rothman-Simone—The Spine, 4th ed. Philadelphia, W.B. Saunders, 1999, with permission.)

is maximal at T1–T2 and minimal at the thoracolumbar junction. Lateral bending is more equally distributed across the thoracic region. Motion of the thoracic vertebrae is limited by anatomic constraints, including the rib cage and its attachment to the sternum, ligamentous attachments at the costovertebral and costotransverse joints, narrow intervertebral discs, and overlap of the adjacent lamina and spinous processes.

NEURAL ANATOMY

9. Describe the contents of the spinal canal in relation to the vertebral segments in the thoracic and thoracolumbar spinal regions.

During childhood, the distal end of the spinal cord migrates proximally due to more rapid longitudinal growth of the osseous spinal elements and generally reaches the lower border of L1 by 8 years of age. In the adult, the spinal cord occupies the upper four-fifths of the vertebral canal. It extends from the foramen magnum and ends distally at the level of the L1–L2 disc space (Fig. 3). The inferior region of the spinal cord, named the conus medullaris, is characterized by the presence of both spinal cord and spinal nerve elements within the dural sac. Distal to the termination of the spinal cord (conus), the lumbar, sacral, and coccygeal roots continue as a leash of nerves termed the cauda equina. The filum terminale is a fibrous band extending from the distal tip of the spinal cord and attaching to the first coccygeal segment. Enlargements of the spinal cord between C3 and T2 (cervical enlargement) and between T9 and T12 (lumbar enlargement) correlate with the origin of nerves supplying the upper and lower extremities. The spinal cord posseses a trilayered covering termed meninges and consisting of dura mater, arachnoid mater, and pia mater. The dura mater is the only meningeal layer that extends the entire length of the vertebral column from the foramen magnum to S2. Between the arachnoid and pia mater is the subarachnoid space, a large interval filled with cerebrospinal fluid.

10. Describe the anatomy of thoracic spinal nerves.

Dorsal (sensory) and ventral (motor) roots originate from the spinal cord to form a spinal nerve in the region of the intervertebral foramen. The spinal nerve divides in the region of the foramen into a posterior (dorsal) primary ramus (innervates the posterior aspect of the associated dermatome and myotome) and an anterior (ventral) primary ramus, which continues as the

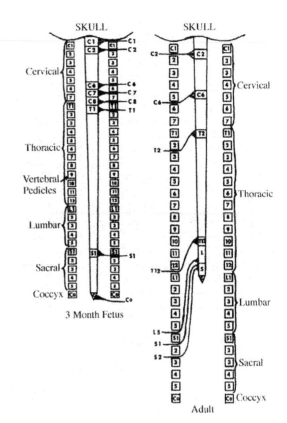

FIGURE 3. Relationships between vertebral levels, spinal nerves, and spinal cord segments in the 3-month fetus and adult (dorsal view). In the fetus, the spinal cord extends the full length of the vertebral column, the spinal cord segments and vertebral levels correspond, and the spinal nerves course horizontally to exit from their intervertebral foramina. However, in adults the spinal cord ends at the L1–L2 vertebral level, only upper cervical cord segments correspond to their vertebral levels with lower cord segments at progressively higher vertebral levels, and lower spinal nerves pursue increasingly more vertical courses. (From Shenk C: Functional and clinical anatomy of the spine. Phys Med Rehabil State Art Rev 9(3):577, 1995.)

intercostal nerve. The thoracic spinal nerves are numbered according to the pedicle of the vertebral body that the nerve contacts. For example, the T6 nerve root passes beneath the pedicle of the T6 vertebra.

11. Describe the contents of a thoracic neurovascular bundle.

Each neurovascular bundle is composed of a posterior intercostal vein, posterior intercostal artery, and anterior primary ramus of a spinal nerve (mnemonic: **VAN** superior to inferior). The neurovascular bundle lies immediately below the inferior edge of each rib in the neurovascular groove.

12. Where is the thoracic portion of the sympathetic trunk located?

The thoracic portion of the sympathetic trunk is located along the anterior surface of the rib head. The sympathetic chain or trunk consists of a series of **ganglia** that extend from the skull to the coccyx. There are two sympathetic chains, located on each of the anterolateral surfaces of the vertebral column. Each consists of approximately 22 ganglia. Each ganglia gives off a **gray ramus communicans** that joins the adjacent spinal nerve just distal to the junction of the anterior and posterior roots.

13. What is the innervation of the diaphragm?

Innervation of the diaphragm is provided by the phrenic nerve, which originates from the C2–C4 segments. Because the diaphragm receives its innervation and blood supply centrally, it can be incised and retracted from its insertion along the thoracic wall to permit surgical exposure of the thoracolumbar vertebral bodies without compromising its neurovascular supply.

VASCULAR STRUCTURES

14. Describe the vascular supply of the thoracic spinal cord.

As in the cervical region, single anterior and paired posterior spinal arteries supply the spinal cord. Radicular (segmental) arteries enter the vertebral canal through the intervertebral foramina and divide into anterior and posterior radicular arteries, which supply the anterior and posterior spinal arteries, respectively. The majority of the vascular supply of the spinal cord is supplied by the anterior spinal artery. In the thoracic spine, the radicular arteries originate from intercostal arteries. The intercostal arteries arise segmentally from the aorta and course along the undersurface of each rib. Segmental arteries supplying the spine branch off of the intercostal arteries at the level of the costotransverse joint and enter the spinal canal via the intervertebral foramen. The number of radicular arteries is variable throughout the thoracic spine. The **radicular artery of Adamkiewicz** is the largest of these segmental arteries and is a major blood supply to the lower spinal cord. It originates from the left side in 80% of people and usually accompanies the ventral root of thoracic nerves 9, 10, or 11. However, it may originate anywhere from T5 to L5. Careful dissection near the intervertebral foramen and costotransverse joints is necessary to prevent injury to this vascular supply.

15. Explain the "watershed region" and "critical supply zone" of the thoracic spinal cord.

The blood supply of the spinal cord is not entirely longitudinal. It is partly transverse and dependent on a series of radicular arteries that feed into the anterior and posterior spinal arteries at various levels. The limited number of radicular arteries supplying the thoracic spinal cord results in a less abundant blood supply in this region compared with the cervical and lumbar regions. Branches of the anterior median spinal artery supply the ventral two-thirds of the spinal cord, whereas branches of the posterior spinal arteries supply the dorsal third of the cord. The region where these two zones meet is relatively poorly vascularized and is termed the **watershed region**. The zone located between the fourth and ninth thoracic vertebrae has the least profuse blood supply and is termed the **critical vascular zone of the spinal cord**. This region corresponds to the narrowest region of the spinal canal. Interference with circulation in this zone during surgery is most likely to result in paraplegia. Surgical dissection in this region of the spine requires added care. Segmental vertebral arteries should be divided as far anteriorly as possible. Dissection in the region of the intervertebral foramen and costotransverse joint should be limited, and electrocautery should not be used in this area.

FASCIA, MUSCULATURE, AND RELATED STRUCTURES

16. Describe the anatomy of the posterior muscles of the thoracic and lumbar spinal regions.

The anatomy of the posterior muscles of the back is confusing because of the multiple overlapping muscle layers and the fact that distinct muscle layers are not seen during posterior surgical dissection. It is helpful to divide the back muscles into three main layers :

Superficial layer: consists of muscles that attach the upper extremity to the spine. The trapezius (innervated by spinal accessory nerve), latissimus dorsi (long thoracic nerve), and levator scapulae (spinal accessory nerve) muscles overlie the deeper rhomboid major and minor muscles (Fig. 4).

Intermediate layer: consists of the serratus posterior superior and inferior. These muscles of accessory respiration are innervated by the anterior primary rami of segmental nerves (Fig. 5).

Deep layer: consists of the intrinsic back muscles, which function in movement of the spinal column. These muscles are innervated by the posterior rami of segmental thoracic and lumbar spinal nerves (Fig. 6). The muscles comprising this deep layer can be subdivided into three layers:

1. Splenius capitis and splenius cervicis.

2. Sacrospinalis (erector spinae), subdivided into spinalis, longissimus, and iliocostalis portions in the thoracic region.

3. Semispinalis, multifidi, rotatores, intertransversari, and interspinales.

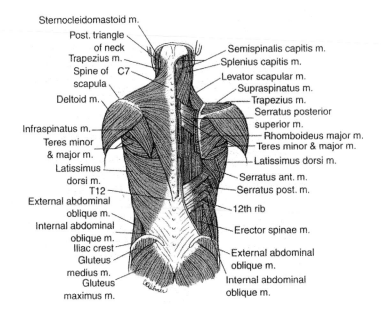

FIGURE 4. Superficial layer of the muscles of the back. (From An HS: Principles and Techniques of Spine Surgery. Baltimore, Williams & Wilkins, 1998, with permission.)

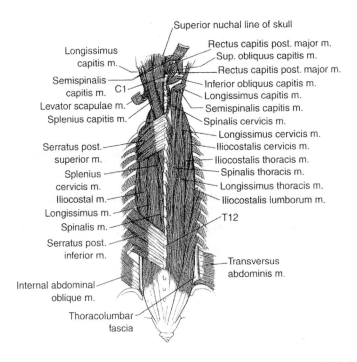

FIGURE 5. Intermediate layer of the muscles of the back. (From An HS: Principles and Techniques of Spine Surgery. Baltimore, Williams & Wilkins, 1998, with permission.)

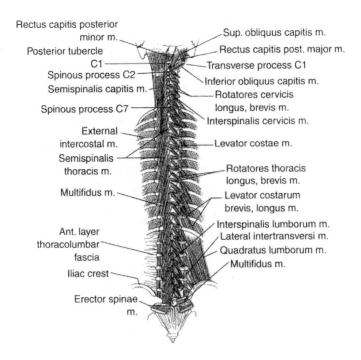

FIGURE 6. Deep layer of the muscles of the back. (From An HS: Principles and Techniques of Spine Surgery. Baltimore, Williams & Wilkins, 1998, with permission.)

17. Why should a spine specialist understand the anatomy of the thoracic cavity?

There are two important reasons why a spine specialist must possess a working knowledge of anatomy and pathology relating to the thoracic cavity. First, extraspinal pathologic processes within the thoracic cavity (e.g., aneurysm, malignancy) may mimic the symptoms of thoracic spinal disorders. Secondly, surgical treatment of many types of spinal problems involves exposure of the anterior aspect of the thoracic spine through a thoracotomy approach.

The thoracic cavity contains the pleural cavities and the mediastinum (Fig. 7). The pleural cavities contain the lungs. The mediastinum is the intrapleural region that separates the pleural cavities and is subdivided into four regions which contain the following structures:

1. Superior mediastinum (thymus gland, aortic arch and great vessels, trachea, bronchi, esophagus)

2. Anterior mediatinum (thymus gland, sternopericardial ligaments)

3. Middle mediastinum (pericardial cavity and related structures)

4. Posterior mediastinum (esophagus, thoracic aorta, inferior vena cava, azygos system, sympathetic chain)

BIBLIOGRAPHY

1. An HS: Principles and Techniques of Spine Surgery. Baltimore, Williams & Wilkins, 1998
2. Herkowitz HN, Garfin SR, Balderston RA, et al (eds): Rothman-Simeone: The Spine, 4th ed. Philadelphia, W.B. Saunders, 1999
3. Hoppenfeld S, deBoer P: Surgical Exposure of the Spine and Extremities. Philadelphia, J.B. Lippincott, 1984.
4. Schneck C: Functional and clinical anatomy of the spine. Phys Med Rehabil State Art Rev 9(3), 1995.
5. Vaccaro AR: Spine anatomy. In Garfin SR, Vaccaro AR (eds): Orthopaedic Knowledge Update—Spine, Vol. 1. Rosemont, IL, American Academy of Orthopaedic Surgeons, 1997, pp 3–18.

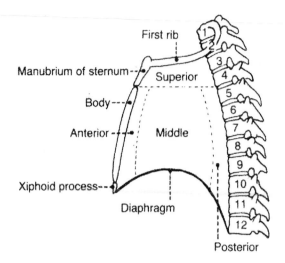

FIGURE 7. Contents of the mediastinum. (From Chung KW: Cross Anatomy, 4th ed. Philadelphia, Lippincott Williams & Wilkins, 2000, with permission.)

3. CLINICALLY RELEVANT ANATOMY THE LUMBAR AND SACRAL REGION

Vincent J. Devlin, M.D., and Darren L. Bergey, M.D.

OSTEOLOGY

1. Describe a typical lumbar vertebra.

The vertebral bodies are kidney-shaped with the transverse diameter exceeding the antero-posterior diameter (Fig. 1). The vertebral body may be divided by an imaginary line passing beneath the pedicles into an upper and lower half. Six posterior elements attach to each lumbar vertebral body. Three structures lie above this imaginary line (superior facet, transverse process, pedicle) and three structures lie below (lamina, inferior facet, spinous process). The pars interarticularis is located along this imaginary dividing line. The transverse processes are long and thin except at L5, where they are thick and broad and possess ligamentous attachments to the pelvis. The five lumbar vertebral bodies increase in size from L1 to L5.

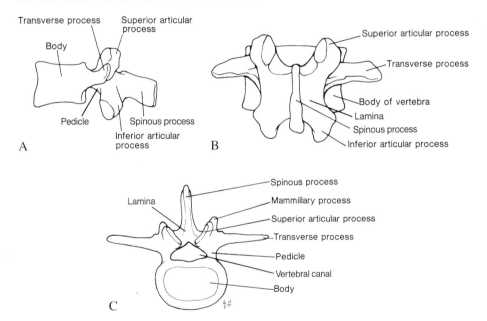

FIGURE 1. Typical lumbar vertebra. Lateral (**A**), posterior (**B**), and cranial (**C**) views, (From Borenstein DG, Wiesel SW, Boden SD: Anatomy and biomechanics of the lumbosacral spine. In Low Back Pain: Medical Diagnosis and Comprehensive Management, 2nd ed. Philadelphia, W.B. Saunders, 1995, with permission.)

2. What region of the posterior elements of the spine is prone to failure when subjected to repetitive stress?

The pars interarticularis is an area of force concentration and is subject to failure with repetitive stress. A defect in the bony arch in this location is termed **spondylolysis**. The pars interarticularis is the concave lateral part of the lamina that connects the superior and inferior articular facets. The medial border of the pedicle is in line with the lateral border of the pars between L1 and L4. At L5 the lateral border of the pars marks the middle of the pedicle.

19

3. Describe the anatomy of the lumbar pedicles.

The pedicle connects the posterior spinal elements (lamina, transverse processes, facets) to the vertebral body. Lumbar pedicle widths are largest at L5 (18mm) and smallest in the upper lumbar region (9 mm at L1). The pedicles in the lumbar spine possess a slight medial inclination, which decreases from distal to proximal levels. The pedicles angle medially 30° at L5 and 12° at L1.

4. What are the key anatomic features of the sacrum?

The sacrum is a triangular structure formed from five fused sacral vertebrae (Fig. 2). The S1 pedicle is the largest pedicle in the body. The sacral promontory is the upper anterior border of the first sacral body. The sacral ala (lateral sacral masses) are bilateral structures formed by the union of vestigial costal elements and the transverse processes of the first sacral vertebra. Four intervertebral foramina give rise to ventral and dorsal sacral foramina. The median sacral crest is formed by the fused spinous processes of the sacral vertebrae. The sacral cornu (horn) is formed by the S5 pedicles and is a landmark for locating the sacral hiatus. The sacral hiatus is an opening in the dorsal aspect of the sacrum due to absence of the 4th and 5th sacral lamina.

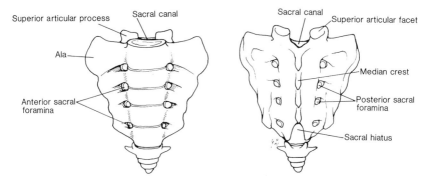

FIGURE 2. Anatomy of the sacrum and coccyx. **Left,** Anterior view. **Right,** Posterior view. (From Borenstein DG, Wiesel SW, Boden SD: Anatomy and biomechanics of the lumbosacral spine. In Low Back Pain: Medical Diagnosis and Comprehensive Management, 2nd ed. Philadelphia, W.B. Saunders, 1995, with permission.)

5. What are the key anatomic features of the coccyx?

The coccyx is a triangular structure that consists of three, four, or five fused coccygeal vertebrae. The coccyx articulates with the inferior aspect of the sacrum.

ARTICULATIONS, LIGAMENTS, AND DISCS

6. Describe the anatomy of the facet joints of the lumbar spine.

The inferior articular process of the cephalad vertebra is located posterior and medial to the superior articular process of the caudad vertebrae. The upper and mid-lumbar facet joints are oriented in the sagittal plane. This orientation allows significant flexion-extension motion in this region but restricts rotation and lateral bending. The facets joints at L5–S1 oriented in the coronal plane, thereby permitting rotation and resisting anterior-posterior translation.

7. What anatomic structures provide articulations between the lumbar vertebral bodies? Between the vertebral arches? Between L5 and the sacrum?

The structures that provide articulations between the lumbar vertebral bodies are the same as in the thoracic region: (1) anterior longitudinal ligament, (2) posterior longitudinal ligament, and (3) intervertebral disc

The anatomic elements that provide articulations between the adjacent lumbar vertebral arches are the same as in the thoracic region: (1)articular capsules, (2) ligamentum flavum, (3) supraspinous ligaments, (4) interspinous ligaments, and (5) intertransverse ligaments.

Specialized ligaments connect L5 and the sacrum: (1) iliolumbar ligament, which arises from the anteroinferior part of the transverse process of the fifth lumbar vertebra and passes inferiorly and laterally to blend with the anterior sacroiliac ligament at the base of the sacrum as well as the inner surface of the ilium, and (2) lumbosacral ligament, which spans from the transverse processes of L5 to the anterosuperior region of the sacral ala and body of S1.

8. Describe the alignment of the normal lumbar spine in reference to the sagittal plane.

The normal lumbar spine is lordotic (sagittal curve with its convexity located anteriorly). Normal lumbar lordosis (L1–S1) ranges from 30° to 80° with a mean lordosis of 50°. Normal lumbar lordosis generally begins at L1–L2 and gradually increases at each distal level toward the sacrum. The apex of lumbar lordosis is normally located at the L3–L4 disc space. Normally two-thirds of lumbar lordosis is located between L4 and S1 and one-third between L1 and L3 (Fig. 3).

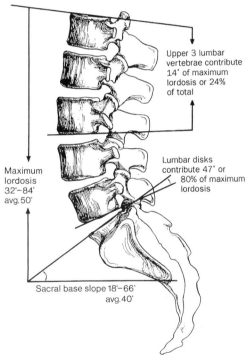

Upper 3 lumbar vertebrae contribute 14° of maximum lordosis or 24% of total

Lumbar disks contribute 47° or 80% of maximum lordosis

Maximum lordosis 32°–84° avg. 50°

Sacral base slope 18°–66° avg. 40°

FIGURE 3. Sagittal alignment of the lumbar spine. Average maximum lordosis as measured from superior L1 to superior S1. (From DeWald RL: Revision surgery for spinal deformity. In Instructional Course Lectures, vol. 41. Park Ridge, IL, American Academy of Orthopaedic Surgeons, 1992, with permission.)

9. Which contributes more significantly to the normal sagittal alignment of the lumbar region—the shape of the intervertebral discs or the shape of the vertebral bodies?

Eighty percent of lumbar lordosis occurs through wedging of the intervertebral discs, and 20% is due to the lordotic shape of the vertebral bodies. The wedge shape of the lowest three discs is responsible for one-half of total lumbar lordosis.

10. Describe the anatomy of the sacroiliac joint.

The sacroiliac joint is a small, auricular-shaped synovial articulation located between the sacrum and ilium (Fig. 4). The complex curvature and strong supporting ligaments of the sacroiliac joint minimzes motion. Ligamentous support is provided by anterior sacroiliac ligaments, interosseous ligaments, and posterior sacroiliac ligaments (most important). Other supporting ligaments in this region include the sacrospinous ligaments (ischial spine to sacrum) and sacrotuberous ligaments (ischial tuberosity to sacrum). Functionally, the sacrum and pelvis can be considered as one vertebra (pelvic vertebra), which functions as an intercalary bone between the trunk and lower extremities.

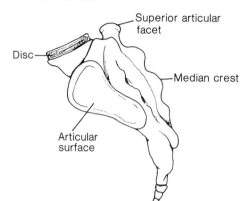

Superior articular facet

Disc

Median crest

Articular surface

FIGURE 4. Lateral view showing the articular surface of the sacrum. (From Borenstein DG, Wiesel SW, Boden SD: Anatomy and biomechanics of the lumbosacral spine. In Low Back Pain: Medical Diagnosis and Comprehensive Management, 2nd ed. Philadelphia, W.B. Saunders, 1995, with permission.)

NEURAL ANATOMY

11. Describe the contents of the spinal canal in the lumbar region.
     The spinal cord terminates as the conus medullaris at the L1–L2 level in adults. Below this level, the **cauda equina,** composed of all lumbar, sacral and coccygeal nerve roots, occupies the thecal sac. The lumbar nerves exit the intervertebral foramen under the pedicle of the same numbered vertebral body.

12. What structures comprise a lumbar anatomic segment?
     The vertebral body, its associated posterior elements, and the disc below comprise an anatomic segment.

13. What is the difference between an exiting nerve root and a traversing nerve root?
     Each lumbar anatomic segment can be considered to possess an exiting nerve root and a traversing nerve root. The **exiting nerve root** passes medial to the pedicle of the anatomic segment. The **traversing nerve root** passes through the anatomic segment to exit beneath the pedicle of the next caudal anatomic segment. For example, the exiting nerve root of the fifth anatomic segment is L5. This nerve passes beneath the L5 pedicle and exits the anatomic segment through the neural foramen of the L5 anatomic segment. The S1 nerve is the traversing nerve root and passes over the L5-S1 disc to exit beneath the pedicle of S1 which is located in the next caudad anatomic segment.

14. What analogy is commonly used to localize spinal pathology from caudad to cephalad within a lumbar anatomic segment?
     The analogy of a house with three floors is most commonly used to localize spinal pathology (Fig. 6). The first story of the anatomical house is the level of the disc space. The second story is the level of the neural foramen and lower vertebral body. The third story is the level of the pedicle and includes the upper vertebral body and transverse process.

15. How is the spinal canal subdivided into zones from medial to lateral to precisely locate compressive spinal pathology within a lumbar anatomic segment?
     Neural compression may affect the thecal sac, nerve roots, or both structures. Central spinal stenosis refers to neural compression in the region of the spinal canal occupied by the thecal sac. Lateral stenosis involves the nerve root and its location is described in terms of three zones (see

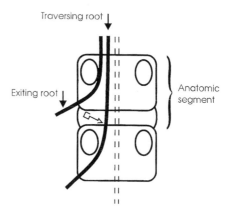

FIGURE 5. The exiting nerve root and traversing root(s) of an unnumbered spinal segment. At the open arrow, the traversing nerve root becomes the exiting root of the anatomic segment below. (From McCulloch JA, Young PH: Musculoskeletal and neuroanatomy of the lumbar spine. In McCulloch JA, Young PH (eds): Essentials of Spinal Microsurgery. Philadelphia, Lippincott-Raven, 1998, pp 249–327, with permission.)

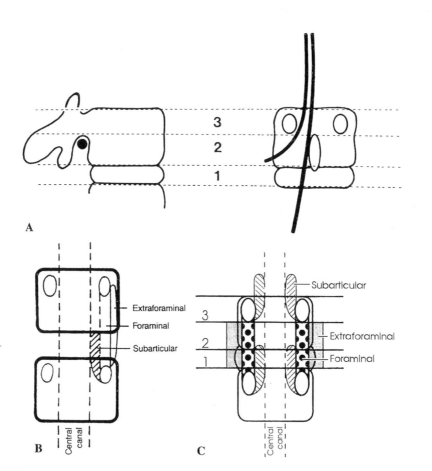

FIGURE 6. A and **B,** Conceptualization of the lumbar anatomic segment as a house. **C,** Zone concept of the lumbar spinal canal. (From McCullough JA: Microdiscectomy: The gold standard for minimally invasive disc surgery. Spine State Art Rev 11(2):382, 1997.)

Fig. 6) using the pedicle as a reference point. Zone 1 (also called the subarticular zone, entrance zone, or lateral recess) includes the area of the spinal canal medial to the pedicle and under the superior articular process. Zone 2 (also called the foraminal or midzone) includes the portion of the nerve root canal located below the pedicle. Zone 3 (also called the extraforaminal or exit zone) refers to the nerve root in the area lateral to the pedicle.

16. An L4–L5 posterolateral disc protrusion located entirely within zone 1 results in compression of which nerve?
   The most common location for a disc protrusion is posterolateral. This type of disc herniation impinges on the traversing nerve root of the L4 anatomic segment. This nerve is the L5 nerve root.

17. An L4–L5 lateral disc protrusion located entirely within zone 3 results in compression of which nerve root?
   This describes the so-called "far lateral" disc protrusion. This type of disc protrusion impinges on the exiting nerve of the L4 anatomic segment. This nerve is the L4 nerve root.

18. Describe the location and significance of the superior hypogastric plexus. What can happen if it is injured during exposure of the anterior aspect of the spine?
   The superior hypogastric plexus is the sympathetic plexus located along the anterior prevertebral tissues in the region of the L5 vertebral body and anterior L5–S1 disc. This sympathetic plexus is at risk during anterior exposure of the L5–S1 disc space. Disruption of this plexus in men may cause retrograde ejaculation and sterility. Erection would not be affected because it is a parasympathetically mediated function.

VASCULAR STRUCTURES

19. Describe the blood supply to the lumbar vertebral bodies.
   Each lumbar vertebra is supplied by a lumbar segmental artery. The segmental arteries for L1–L4 arise from the aorta, whereas the segmental arteries for L5 arise from the iliolumbar artery. As the segmental artery courses toward the intervertebral foramen it divides into three branches: (1) the anterior branch (supplies the abdominal wall), (2) the posterior branch (supplies paraspinous muscles and facets), and (3) the foraminal branch (supplies the spinal canal and its contents). The venous supply of the lumbar region parallels the arterial supply. It consists of a anterior and posterior ladder-like configuration of valveless veins that communicate with the inferior vena cava.

20. What is Batson's plexus?
   Batson's plexus is a system of valveless veins located within the spinal canal and around the vertebral body. It is an alternate route for venous drainage to the inferior vena cava system. Because it is a valveless system, any increase in abdominal pressure (e.g., secondary to positioning during spine surgery) can cause blood to flow preferentially toward the spinal canal and surrounding bony structures. Batson's plexus also serves as a preferential pathway for metastatic tumor and infection spread to the lumbar spine.

21. Where is the bifurcation of the aorta and vena cava located?
   Most commonly, the bifurcation is over the L4–L5 disc or L5 vertebral body.

22. What is the significance of the iliolumbar vein?
   The iliolumbar vein is a branch of the iliac vein that prevents mobilization of the iliac vessels off of the anterior aspect of the spine (Fig. 7). This vein should be carefully isolated and securely ligated before attempting to expose the anterior aspect of the spine at the L4–L5 disc level.

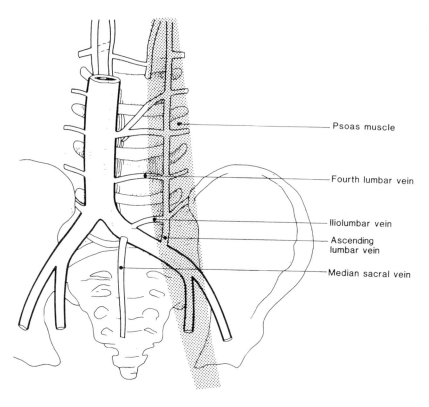

FIGURE 7. Anatomy of the iliolumbar vein and environs. Main veins and branches encountered in anterior lumbar interbody fusion. (From Leong JCY: Anterior lumbar interbody fusion. In Lin PM, Gill K (eds): Lumbar Interbody Fusion. Rockville, MD, Aspen, 1989, pp 133–148, with permission.)

FASCIA, MUSCULATURE, AND RELATED STRUCTURES

23. Why should a spine specialist be knowledgeable about the anatomy of the abdominal and pelvic cavities?

There are many important reasons why a spine specialist must possess a working knowledge of anatomy and pathology relating to the abdominal and pelvic cavity (Fig. 8). Extraspsinal pathologic processes within the abdominal and pelvic cavities (e.g., aneurysm, infection, tumor) may mimic the symptoms of lumbosacral spinal disorders. Surgical treatment of many spinal problems involves exposure of the anterior lumbar spine and/or sacrum through a variety of surgical approaches. Evaluation of complications after spinal procedures requires assessment not only of the vertebral and neural structures but also of vascular and visceral structures (e.g., bladder, intestines, spleen, kidney, ureter).

24. What muscles of the posterior abdominal wall cover the anterolateral aspect of the lumbar spine?

Psoas major and minor. These muscle originate from the lumbar transverse processes, intervertebral discs, and vertebral bodies and insert distally at the lesser trochanter and iliopectineal region, respectively. They must be mobilized during exposure of the anterior lumbar spine, tak-

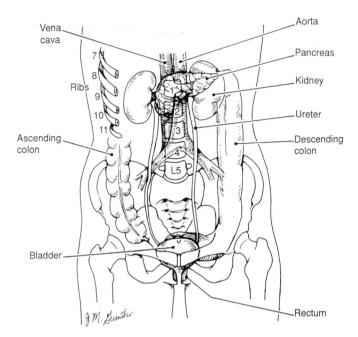

FIGURE 8. Anatomic relationships of visceral organs in the retroperitoneum and the lumbosacral spine. (From Borenstein DG, Wiesel SW, Boden SD: Anatomy and biomechanics of the lumbosacral spine. In Low Back Pain: Medical Diagnosis and Comprehensive Management, 2nd ed. Philadelphia, W.B. Saunders, 1995, with permission.)

ing care to avoid nerves that cross the psoas muscles (genitofemoral nerve, sympathetic trunk) as well as the lumbar plexus, which passes within the substance of these muscles.

BIBLIOGRAPHY

1. Borenstein DG, Wiesel SW, Boden SD: Anatomy and biomechanics of the lumbosacral spine. In Low Back Pain: Medical Diagnosis and Comprehensive Management, 2nd ed. Philadelphia, W.B. Saunders, 1995, pp 1–16.
2. Hanley EN, Delmarter RB, McCulloch JA, Takahashi KA: Surgical indications and techniques. In Wiesel SW, Weinstein JN, Herkowitz H, et al (eds): The Lumbar Spine, 2nd ed. Philadelphia, W.B. Saunders, 1996, pp 492–524.
3. Leong JCY: Anterior lumbar interbody fusion. Chapter 12 p133–148 Lin PM, Gill K(Eds). Lumbar interbody fusion. Aspen Publishers. Rockville, MD,1989
4. McCullough JA: Microdiscectomy: The gold standard for minimally invasive disc surgery. Spine, State Art Rev 11:373–396, 1997.
5. McCulloch JA, Young PH: Musculoskeletal and neuroanatomy of the lumbar spine. In McCulloch JA, Young PH (eds): Essentials of Spinal Microsurgery. Philadelphia, Lippincott-Raven, 1998, pp 249–327.

II. Clinical Examination of the Spine Patient

4. EVALUATION OF CERVICAL SPINE DISORDERS

Mark R. Davies, M.D., and Jeffrey C. Wang, M.D.

1. How does the evaluation of a patient with a spine complaint begin?
As with all patients, a complete history and physical exam are performed. The purpose of the history and physical exam is to make a provisional diagnosis that may be confirmed by subsequent testing.

2. What are some of the key elements to assess in the history of any spine problem?
- Chief complaint: Pain? numbness? weakness? gait difficulty? deformity?
- Symptom onset: Acute vs. insidious.
- Symptom duration: Acute vs. chronic.
- Pain location: Is the pain primarily axial neck pain, arm pain, or a combination of both?
- Pain quality and character: Sharp vs. dull, radiating vs. stabbing.
- Temporal relationship of pain: Night pain, rest pain, or constant unremitting pain suggests systemic problems such as tumor or infection. Morning stiffness that improves throughout the day suggests an arthritic problem or an inflammatory arthropathy.
- Relation of symptoms to neck position: Increased arm pain with neck extension suggests nerve root impingement.
- Aggravating and alleviating factors: Is the pain mechanical or nonmechanical in nature?
- Family history: Inquire about diseases such as ankylosing spondylitis or rheumatoid athritis.
- Concurrent medical illness: Diabetes, peripheral neuropathy, peripheral vascular disease.
- Systemic symptoms: A history of weight loss or fever suggests possibility of tumor or infection.
- Functional impairment: Loss of balance, inability to walk, loss of fine motor skills of hands.
- Prior treatment: Include both nonoperative and operative measures.
- Negative prognostic factor: Pending litigation, workman's compensation claim.

3. What disorders should be considered in the differential diagnosis of neck/arm pain?
- Degenerative spinal disorders: discogenic pain, radiculopathy, myeloradiculopathy, myelopathy.
- Soft tissue disorders: sprains, myofascial pain syndromes, fibromyalgia, whiplash syndrome.
- Inflammatory disorders: rheumatoid arthritis, ankylosing spondylitis.
- Infections: discitis, osteomyelitis.
- Tumors: metastatic vs. primary tumors.
- Intraspinal disorders: tumors, syrinx.
- Systemic disorders with referred pain: angina, apical lung tumors (Pancoast tumor).
- Shoulder and elbow pathology: rotator cuff disorders, medial epicondylitis.
- Peripheral nerve entrapment syndromes: radial, ulnar or median nerve entrapment, suprascapular neuropathy.
- Thoracic outlet syndrome
- Psychogenic pain

4. What are the basic elements of an examination of any spinal region?
- Inspection
- Palpation
- Range of motion (ROM)
- Neurologic exam
- Evaluation of related areas (e.g., shoulder joints)

5. What should the examiner look for during inspection of the cervical region?
During the initial encounter, much can be learned from observing the patient. Assessment of gait and posture of the head and neck is important. Patients should undress to allow inspection of anatomically related areas, including the shoulders, back muscles, and scapulae.

6. What is the purpose of palpation during assessment of the cervical region?
To examine for tenderness and locate bone and soft tissue pathology. Specific areas of palpation correspond to specific levels of the spine:
- Hyoid bone   C3
- Thyroid cartilage   C4–C5
- First cricoid ring   C6

Spinous processes should be palpated and checked for alignment. If tenderness is detected, it should be noted whether the tenderness is focal or diffuse and the area of maximum tenderness should be localized.

7. In which three planes is ROM assessed for the cervical spine?
- Flexion/extension
- Right/left bending
- Right/left rotation

8. What is normal range of motion of the cervical spine?
- Flexion   45°
- Extension   55°
- Right/left bending   40°
- Right/left rotation   70°

Clinical estimates of motion are more commonly used in office practice. Flexion may be reproducibly measured using the distance from the chin to the sternum. For extension, the distance from the occiput to the dorsal spine may be helpful. Distances can be described in terms of fingerbreaths or measured with a ruler. The normal patient, for example, can nearly touch chin to chest in flexion and bring the occiput to within three or four fingerbreaths of the posterior aspect of the cervical spine in extension. Normal rotation permits the chin to align with the shoulder.

9. Describe an overview of the approach to the neurologic exam for cervical disorders.
The goal of examination is to determine the presence or absence of a neurologic deficit. If present, the level of a neurologic deficit is determined through testing of sensory, motor, and reflex function. The neurologic deficit may arise from pathology at the level of the spinal cord, nerve root, brachial plexus, or peripheral nerve. Examination of the cervical region is focused on the C5–T1 nerve roots because they are responsible for supplying the upper extremities. For each nerve root, the examiner tests sensation, strength, and, if one exists, the appropriate reflex.

LEVEL	SENSATION	MOTOR	REFLEX
C5	Lateral arm (axillary patch)	Deltoid	Biceps
C6	Lateral forearm	Wrist extension, biceps	Brachioradialis
C7	Middle finger	Triceps, wrist flexors, finger extension	Triceps
C8	Small finger	Finger flexors	None
T1	Medial arm	Interossei	None

10. How is sensation examined?
Sensation can be assessed using light touch, pin prick, vibration, and two-point discrimination. In assessing light touch, it is helpful to assess both sides of the body simultaneously. In this manner, sensation that is intact but subjectively decreased compared with the contralateral side can be easily documented.

11. What are the pathways tested by light touch, pin prick, and vibration?

- Light touch: corticospinal tract
- Pin prick: spinothalamic tract
- Vibration: posterior columns

12. How is motor strength graded? How are reflexes graded?

MOTOR GRADE	FINDINGS
5	Full range of motion against full resistance
4	Full range of motion against reduced resistance
3	Full range of motion against gravity alone
2	Full range of motion with gravity eliminated
1	Evidence of contractility
0	No contractility

REFLEX GRADE	FINDINGS
4+	Hyperactive
3+	Brisk
2+	Normal
1+	Diminished
0	Absent

13. What is the significance of hyperreflexia? An absent reflex?

Hyperreflexia signifies an upper motor neuron lesion.

An **absent reflex** implies pathology at the nerve root level(s) that transmit the reflex (in the lower motor neuron).

14. What is radiculopathy?

Radiculopathy is a lesion that causes irritation of a nerve root (lower motor neuron). It involves a specific spinal level with sparing of levels immediately above and below. The patient may report pain, burning sensation, or numbness that radiates along the anatomic distribution of the affected nerve root. Other signs include severe atrophy of muscles and loss of the reflex supplied by the nerve. Severe radiculopathy may result in the flaccid paralysis of muscles supplied by the nerve.

15. What symptoms are associated with a C5–C6 disc herniation? Explain.

A disc herniation at the C5–C6 level causes compression of the C6 nerve root. Thus, weakness of biceps and wrist extensors, loss of the brachioradialis reflex, and diminished sensation of the radial forearm into the thumb and index finger are expected. As there are eight nerve roots and seven cervical vertebrae, the C1 nerve root exits above the C1 vertebra, the C2 nerve root below it, and so on. Thus, the C2 nerve root exits through its neuroforamen adjacent to the C1–C2 disc. The nerve root of the inferior vertebra of a given motion segment (e.g., C3 for C2–C3 disc, C7 for C6–C7 disc) is the one usually affected by a herniated disc.

16. Describe testing of the cervical nerve roots.

ROOT LEVEL	DISC LEVEL	SENSATION	REFLEX	MOTOR
C3	C2–C3	Posterior neck to mastoid	None	Nonspecific
C4	C3–C4	Posterior neck to scapula ± anterior chest	None	Nonspecific
C5	C4–C5	Lateral arm (axillary patch) to elbow	± Biceps	Deltoid ± biceps
C6	C5–C6	Radial forearm to thumb	Biceps, brachioradialis	Biceps, wrist extensors
C7	C6–C7	Midradial forearm to middle finger ± index/ring fingers	Triceps	Triceps, wrist flexors, finger extensors
C8	C7–T1	Ulnar forearm to little and ring fingers	None	Finger flexors ± intrinsics
T1	T1–T2	Medial upper arm	None	Hand intrinsics

17. What provocative maneuvers are useful in examining a patient with a suspected radiculopathy? Explain how each is carried out.

Spurling's test (Fig. 1) is used to assess cervical nerve roots for stenosis as they exit the foramen. The patient's neck is extended and rotated *toward* the side of the pathology. Once the patient is in this position, a firm axial load is applied. If radicular symptoms are worsened by this maneuver, the test is said to be positive. It is thought that the extended and rotated position of the neck decreases the size of the foramen through which the nerve roots exit, thereby exacerbating symptoms when an axial load is applied.

Axial cervical compression test: Arm pain that is elicited by axial compressive force on the skull and relieved by distractive force suggests that radicular symptoms are due to neuroforaminal narrowing.

Valsalva maneuver. This manuever may increase radicular symptoms. Increased intraabdominal pressure simultaneously increases cerebrospinal pressure, which, in turn increases pressure about the cervical roots.

Shoulder abduction test. Patients with cervical radiculopathy may obtain relief of radicular symptoms by holding the shoulder in an abducted position, which decreases tension in the nerve root, (Fig. 2).

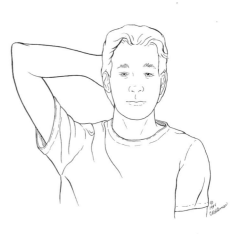

FIGURE 2. Shoulder abduction test.

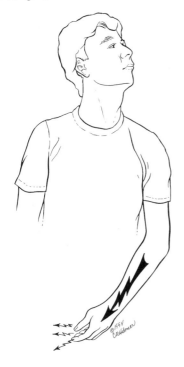

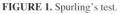

FIGURE 1. Spurling's test.

18. What is Adson's test?

Adson's test helps to distinguish thoracic outlet syndrome from cervical radiculopathy. The affected arm is abducted, extended, and externally rotated at the shoulder while the examiner palpates the radial pulse. The patient turns the head *toward* the affected side and takes a deep breath. In a positive Adson's test, the radial pulse on the affected side is diminished or lost during the maneuver. A positive test suggests thoracic outlet syndrome (compression of the subclavian artery by a cervical rib, scalenus anticus muscle, or other cause).

19. What is cervical myelopathy? How does it present?

Myelopathy is the manifestation of cervical spinal cord compression. Cervical myelopathy arising from spinal cord compression due to cervical degenerative changes is the most common cause of spinal cord dysfunction in patients over 55 years of age. Vague sensory and motor symptoms involving the upper and/or lower extremities are common. Lower motor neuron changes occur at the level of the lesion, with atrophy of upper extremity muscles, especially the intrinsics muscles of the hands. Upper motor neuron findings are noted below the level of the lesion and may involve both the upper and lower extremities. Lower extremity spasticity and hyperreflexia are common. There may be relative hyperreflexia in the legs compared with the arms. Bilateral Hoffman and Babinski signs are frequently present. Additional findings may include neck pain and stiffness, spastic gait, loss of manual dexterity, or problems with sphincter control.

20. What reflexes or signs should be assessed when evaluating a patient with suspected cervical myelopathy? How are they evaluated?

Babinski's test is performed by stroking the lateral plantar surface of the foot from the heel to the ball of the foot and curving medially across the heads of the metatarsals. It is termed positive if there is dorsiflexion of the big toe and fanning of the other toes (Fig. 3).

Hoffmann's sign is performed on the patient's pronated hand while the examiner grasps the patient's middle finger (Fig. 4). The distal phalanx is forcefully and quickly flexed (almost a flicking motion) while the examiner observes the other fingers and thumb. The test is termed positive if flexion is seen in the thumb or index finger, and it specifically refers to upper motor lesions in the cervical spine as it is an upper extremity reflex. In contrast, pathology anywhere along the entire spinal cord can lead to a positive Babinski sign.

Finger escape sign (finger adduction test) is performed by asking the patient to hold all digits of the hand in an extended and adducted position. With myelopathy, the two ulnar digits will fall into flexion and abduction usually within 30 seconds.

Inverted radial reflex is elicited by tapping the distal brachioradialis tendon. The reflex is present when the tapping produces spastic contraction of the finger flexors and suggests cord compression at C5–C6.

Hyperactive scapulohumeral reflex is performed by tapping the tip of the spine of the scapula in a caudad direction. If the scapula elevates or the humerus abducts, it is termed a hyperactive reflex suggesting upper motor neuron dysfunction above the C4 cord level.

Llhermitte's sign is a generalized electric shock sensation that involves the upper and lower extremities as well as the trunk an is associated with extension of the head and neck.

Clonus. Upward thrusting of the ankle joint leads to repetitive motion of the ankle joint.

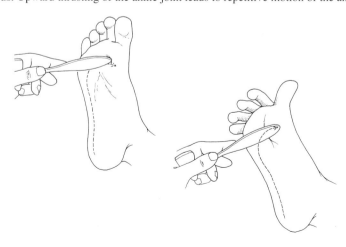

FIGURE 3. Babinski's test.

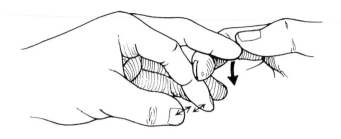

FIGURE 4. Hoffmann's sign.

BIBLIOGRAPHY

1. Hoppenfeld S. Physical Exam of the Spine and Extremities. Appleton-Century-Crofts, New York, 1976.
2. Klein JD, Garfin SR. Clinical evaluation of patients with suspected spine problems. P319–340. The Adult Spine: Principles and Practice. 2nd edition. J.W. Frymoyer, Editor-in-Chief. Lippincott-Raven Publishers, Philadelphia,1997.
3. Macnab I, McCulloch J. Neck Ache and Shoulder pain. William and Wilkins, Baltimore, 1994.
4. Riley LH. History and physical examination of the spine. p91–102. In Principles and Techniques of Spine Surgery. An HS(Ed) Williams & Wikins, Baltimore, 1998.

5. EVALUATION OF THORACIC AND LUMBAR SPINE DISORDERS

Mark R. Davies, M.D., and Jeffrey C. Wang, M.D.

1. What are the most common reasons for referral to evaluate the thoracic spinal region?
Pain and spinal deformity. The differential diagnosis of thoracic pain is extensive and includes both spinal and nonspinal etiologies. Spinal deformities (e.g., scoliosis, kyphosis) are generally painless in children but may become symptomatic in adult life.

2. What are some common spinal causes of thoracic pain?
- Degenerative disorders
  Spondylosis
  Spinal stenosis
  Disc herniation
- Fracture
  Traumatic
  Pathologic
- Neoplasm
- Infection
- Metabolic
  Osteoporosis
  Osteomalacia

- Deformity
  Kyphosis
  Scoliosis
  Trauma
- Neurogenic
  Spinal cord neoplasm
  Arteriovenous malformation
  Inflammatory (e.g., herpes zoster)

3. What are some common nonspinal causes of thoracic pain?

Intrathoracic
- Cardiovascular (angina, aortic aneurysm)
- Pulmonary (pneumonia, carcinoma)
- Mediastinal (mediastinal tumor)

Intra-abdominal
- Hepatobiliary (hepatitis, cholecystitis)
- Gastrointestinal (peptic ulcer, pancreatitis)
- Retroperitoneal (pyelonephritis, aneurysm)

Musculoskeletal
- Postthoracotomy syndrome
- Polymyalgia rheumatica
- Fibromyalgia
- Rib fractures
- Intercostal Neuralgia

4. What should an examiner assess during inspection of the thoracic spinal region?
The patient should be undressed, and posture should be evaluated in both frontal and sagittal planes. Shoulder or rib asymmetry suggests the presence of scoliosis. A forward-bending test should be performed to permit assessment of rib cage and paravertebral muscle symmetry. If increased thoracic kyphosis is noted, it should be determined whether the kyphotic deformity is flexible or rigid. Leg lengths should be assessed. Look for any differences in height of the iliac crests. Note any skin markings such as café-au-lait spots, hairy patches, or birth marks that may suggest occult neurologic or bony pathology.

5. What is the usefulness of palpation during examination of the thoracic spine?
Palpation allows the examiner to locate specific areas of tenderness, which aids in localization of pathology. Tenderness over the paraspinal muscles should be differentiated from tenderness over the spinous processes.

6. How precisely is range of motion assessed in the thoracic region?

Range of motion is limited in the thoracic thoracic region, and precise assessment is not an emphasized component of the thoracic spine exam. Flexion-extension is limited by facet joint orientation, rib cage stability, and small intervertebral disc size. Thoracic rotation is greater than lumbar rotation. Testing of lateral bending is relevant in assessing the flexibility of scoliosis. Asymmetric range of motion, especially in forward-bending, suggests the presence of a lesion that irritates neural structures, such as a tumor or disc herniation.

7. How is the neurologic examination of the thoracic spinal region performed?

Sensory levels are assessed by testing for light touch and pin-prick sensation. The exiting spinal nerves create band-like dermatomes (T4, nipple line; T7, xiphoid process; T10, umbilicus; T12, inguinal crease) (Fig. 1). Motor strength is assessed by having the patient perform a partial sit-up and checking for asymmetry in the segmentally innervated rectus abdominis muscle. Weakness causes the umbilicus to move in the opposite direction and is termed Beevor's sign. Reflex testing consists of evaluation of the superficial abdominal reflex.

8. What is the superfical abdominal reflex? What does it signify?

The superficial abdominal reflex is an upper motor neuron reflex. It is performed by stroking one of the four abdominal quadrants. The umbilicus should move toward the quadrant that was stroked. The reflex should be symmetric from side to side. Asymmetry suggests intraspinal pathology (upper motor neuron lesion) and is assessed with magnetic resonance imaging (MRI) of the spine.

9. What findings in the history and physical exam suggest the presence of a thoracic disc herniation?

Clinically significant thoracic disc herniation is rare. It is difficult to reach an accurate diagnosis from history and physical exam alone. Thoracic disc herniations may cause thoracic axial pain, thoracic radicular pain, myelopathy, or a combination of these symptoms. Neurologic findings may include nonspecific lower extremity weakness, ataxia, spasticity, numbness, hyperreflexia, clonus, and bowel or bladder dysfunction

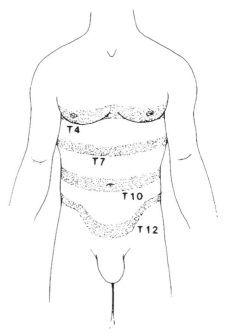

FIGURE 1. Dermatomes of the trunk.

LUMBAR SPINE EXAM

10. What pathologies should be considered in the differential diagnosis of low back pain?
- Spinal disorders (disc herniation, spondylolisthesis, spinal stenosis, osteoarthritis)
- Soft tissue disorders (sprains, myofascial pain syndromes, fibromyalgia, whiplash syndrome)
- Rheumatologic disorders (rheumatoid arthritis, Reiter's syndrome, psoriatic arthrits, ankylosing spondylitis)
- Infection (bacterial, tuberculosis, HIV)
- Tumor
- Trauma (fractures)
- Metabolic disorders (osteoporosis, osteomalacia, Paget's disease)
- Hematologic disorders (sickle-cell disease)
- Systemic disorders with referred pain (peptic ulcers, cholecystitis, pancreatitis, retrocecal appendicitis, dissecting abdominal aortic aneurysm, pelvic inflammatory disease, endometriosis, prostatitis)
- Psychogenic pain

11. Does the age of the patient with low back pain or lower extremity radicular symptoms suggest an etiology?
Yes. In general, disc herniations are more common in patients under 55 years of age, whereas spinal stenosis occurs more frequently in patients over 60.

12. What factors in the patient history should prompt the examiner to consider further diagnostic testing, such as laboratory tests or imaging studies, during evaluation of symptoms of acute low back pain?
Factors that may indicate serious underlying pathology are termed "red flags" and include fever, unexplained weight loss, bowel or bladder dysfunction, cancer history, significant trauma, osteoporosis, age greater than 50 years, failure to improve with standard treatment, and a history of alcohol or drug abuse.

13. What is a simple method for differentiating spinal symptoms due to physical disease from symptoms due to inappropriate illness behavior *before* the patient is examined?
Important clinical information can be obtained by having the patient complete a pain diagram. Pain diagrams completed by patients with physical disease (e.g., disc herniation, spinal stenosis) tend to be localized, anatomic, and proportionate. Pain diagrams completed by patients with magnified or inappropriate illness behavior tend to be regional, nonanatomic, and highly exaggerated.

14. What are the basic elements of a physical examination directed at the lumbar spine?
Examination should address the lumbar region, pelvis, hip joints, lower limbs, gait, and peripheral vascular system. A complete exam should include (1) inspection, (2) palpation, (3) range of motion (lumbar spine, hips, knees), (4) neurologic exam (sensation, muscle testing, reflexes), (5) assessment of nerve root tension signs, and (6) vascular exam.

15. What is looked for during inspection?
During the initial encounter, much can be learned from observing the patient. Abnormalities of gait (e.g., a "drop foot" gait or Trendelenburg gait) and abnormal posturing of the trunk are important clues for the examiner. It is also helpful to watch patients undress to observe how freely and easily they are able to move the trunk and extremities. In addition, the base of the spine should be inspected for a hairy patch or any skin markings that may be associated with spina bifida. The overall alignment and balance of the spine should be assessed by dropping a plumb line from the C7 spinous process to see that it is centered on the sacrum. If it is not, the lateral distance from the gluteal cleft should be noted.

16. What is the purpose of palpation?

To examine for tenderness and localize pathology. Palpation must include the spinous processes as well as the adjacent soft tissues. The area of the sciatic notch should be deeply palpated to look for sciatic irritability. Specific areas of palpation correspond to specific levels of the spine (e.g., iliac crest, L4–L5; posterior superior iliac spine, S2).

17. How is range of motion assessed?

In the spine, motion is assessed in three planes: flexion/extension, right/left bending, and right/left rotation. Range of motion can be estimated in degrees or measured with an inclinometer. It is important to note that a significant portion of lumbar flexion is achieved through the hip joints. The normal range of motion for forward flexion is 40–60°; for extension 20–35°; for lateral bending, 15–20°; and for rotation, 3–18°.

18. What is Schober's test?

Schober's test is a simple clinical test useful to evaluate spinal mobility. This test is based on the principle that the skin over the lumbar spine stretches as a person flexes forward to touch the toes. A tape measure is used to mark the skin at the midpoint between the posterior superior iliac crests and at points 10 cm proximal and 5 cm distal to this mark while the patient is standing. The patient is then asked to bend forward as far as possible, and the distance between the two marked points is measured with the patient in the flexed position. In 90% of asymptomatic persons, there is an increase in length of at least 5 cm. This maneuver eliminates hip flexion and is a true indication of lumbar spine movement.

19. How is the neurologic examination of the lumbar region performed?

Neurologic examination of the lumbar region focuses primarily on a sequential examination of nerve roots. For each nerve root, the examiner tests sensation, motor strength, and, if one exists, the appropriate reflex.

LEVEL	SENSATION	MOTOR	REFLEX
L1	Anterior thigh	Psoas (T12, L1, L2, L3)	None
L2	Anterior thigh, groin	Quadriceps (L2, L3, L4)	None
L3	Anterior and lateral thigh	Quadriceps (L2, L3, L4)	None
L4	Medial leg and foot	Tibialis anterior	Patellar
L5	Lateral leg and dorsal foot	Extensor hallucis longus	None
S1	Lateral and plantar foot	Gastrocnemius, peroneals	Achilles
S2–S4	Perianal	Bladder and foot intrinsics	None

20. What provocative maneuvers are used to assess a patient with a suspected lumbar radiculopathy?

The standard straight-leg raise test and its variants increase tension along the sciatic nerve and are used to assess the L5 and S1 nerve roots. The reverse straight leg raise test increases tension along the femoral nerve and is used to assess the L2, L3, and L4 nerve roots.

21. Describe how the straight leg raise test and the femoral nerve stretch test are performed.

The straight-leg raise test is a tension sign that may be performed with the patient supine (Lasegue's test; Fig. 2) or sitting (flip test; Fig. 3). The leg is elevated with the knee straight to increase tension along the sciatic nerve, specifically the L5 and S1 nerve roots. If the nerve root is compressed, nerve stretch provokes radicular pain. Back pain alone does not consititute a positive test. The most tension is placed on the L5 and S1 nerve roots during a supine straight-leg raise test between 35° and 70° of leg elevation. A variant of this test is the bowstring test, in which the knee is flexed during the standard supine straight-leg raise test to reduce leg pain secondary to sciatic nerve stretch. Finger pressure is then applied over the popliteal space at the terminal aspect of the sciatic nerve in an attempt to reestablish radicular symptoms.

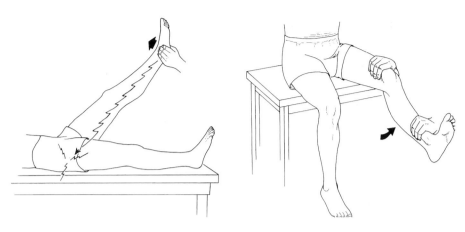

FIGURE 2. Supine straight-leg raise test.   **FIGURE 3.** Seated straight-leg raise test.

The femoral nerve stretch test (or reverse straight-leg raise test) increases tension along the femoral nerve, specifically the L2, L3, and L4 nerve roots (Fig. 4). It may be performed with the patient in the prone position or in the lateral position with the affected side upward. The test is performed by extending the hip and flexing the knee. This is exactly opposite to the standard straight-leg raise test. The femoral nerve stretch test is considered positive if radicular pain in the anterior thigh region occurs.

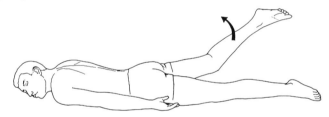

FIGURE 4. Femoral nerve stretch test.

22. What is the contralateral straight-leg raise test? Why is it a significant test?

This test is performed in the same fashion as the standard straight-leg raise test except that the asymptomatic leg is elevated. If this test reproduces the patient's sciatic symptoms in the opposite extremity, it is considered positive. A positive test is strongly suggestive of the a disc herniation medial to the nerve root (in the axilla of the nerve root). The combination of a positive straight-leg raise test on the symptomatic side and a positive contralateral straight-leg raise test is the most specific clinical test for a disc herniation, with accuracy approaching 97%.

23. What nerve root is affected by a posterolateral disc herniation?

The nerve roots of the lumbar spine exit the spinal canal beneath the pedicle of the corresponding numbered vertebra and above the caudad intervertebral disc. The most common location for a lumbar disc herniation is posterolateral. This type of disc herniation compresses the traversing nerve root of the motion segment. For example, a posterolateral disc herniation at the L4–L5 level would compress the traversing nerve root (L5).

24. What nerve root is affected by a disc herniation lateral to the central spinal canal?

A disc herniation lateral to or at the level of the neural foramen compresses the exiting nerve root of the motion segment. For example, a disc herniation at the L4–L5 level located in the region of the neural foramen compresses the exiting L4 nerve root and spares the traversing L5 nerve root.

25. What nerve roots are affected by a central disc herniation?
A central disc herniation can compress one or more of the caudal nerve roots. A large central disc herniation is a common cause of a cauda equina syndrome.

26. What is cauda equina syndrome?
Cauda equina syndrome is a symptoms complex that includes low back pain, unilateral or bilateral sciatica, lower extremity motor weakness, sensory abnormalities, bowel or bladder dysfunction, and saddle anesthesia. Cauda equina syndrome may result from acute or chronic compression of the cauda equina nerve roots. Causes of cauda equina syndrome include massive central lumbar disc protrusion, spinal stenosis, epidural hematoma, spinal tumor, and fracture. The syndrome can result in permanent motor deficit and bowel and bladder incontinence. Once identified, cauda equina syndrome constitutes a true surgical emergency because it can be irreversible if not treated promptly with surgical decompression.

27. What are Waddell's signs?
Waddell described five signs that are useful in evaluating patients with low back pain. These signs do not prove malingering but are useful to highlight the contribution of psychologic and/or socioeconomic factors to spinal symptoms. Presence of three of more of the signs is considered significant. Isolated positive signs are not considred significant. Waddell's signs include:

1. **Superficial tenderness:** nonorganic tenderness with light touch over a wide lumbar area or deeper tenderness in a nonanatomic distribution.

2. **Simulation:** maneuvers that should not be uncomfortable are performed. If pain is reported, nonorganic pathology is suggested. Examples of such tests include production of low back pain with axial loading of the head or when the shoulders and pelvis are passively rotated in the same plane.

3. **Distraction:** The examiner performs a provocative test in the usual manner and rechecks the test when the patient is distracted. For example, a patient with a positive straight-leg raise test in the supine position can be assessed with a straight-leg raise test in the seated position under the guise of examining the foot or another part of the lower extremity. If the distraction test is negative but a formal straight-leg raise test in the supine position is positive, this finding is considered a positive sign.

4. **Regionalization:** Presence of findings that diverge from accepted neuroanatomy. For example, entire muscle groups, which do not have common innervation, may demonstrate "giving way" on strength testing or sensory abnormalities may not follow a dermatomal distribution.

5. **Overreaction:** Disproportionate response to examination may take many forms such a collapsing, inappropriate facial expression, excessive verbalization, or any other type of overreaction to any aspect of the exam.

28. During assessment of a lumbar spine problem, what two nonspinal pathologies should be ruled out during the physical exam?
Degenerative arthritis of the hip joint and vascular disease involving the lower extremities. The presentation of these pathologies and common spinal problems can overlap. Anterior thigh pain may be due to either nerve impingement involving the upper lumbar nerve roots (L2, L3, L4) or hip arthritis. Range-of-motion testing of the hip joints can rule out hip pathology. Lower extremity claudication may be due to either vascular disease or lumbar spinal stenosis (neurogenic claudication). Assessment of peripheral pulses is helpful in diagnosing these problems.

29. How is the sacroiliac joint assessed?
Sacroiliac pain is difficult to confirm on clinical assessment and generally requires a diagnostic joint injection under radiographic control for confirmation. Clinical tests that have been described to assess this joint include:

Patrick's test: With the patient supine, the knee on the affected side is flexed and the foot placed on the opposite patella. The flexed knee is then pushed laterally to stress the sacroiliac joint. This is also called the FABER test (flexion-abduction-external rotation).

Pelvic compression test: With the patient supine, the iliac crests are pushed toward the midline in an attempt to elicit pain in the sacroiliac joint.

BIBLIOGRAPHY

1. Hoppenfeld S: Physical Exam of the Spine and Extremities. New York, Appleton-Century-Crofts, 1976.
2. Klein JD, Garfin SR: Clinical evaluation of patients with suspected spine problems. In Frymoyer JW (ed): The Adult Spine: Principles and Practice, 2nd ed. Philadelphia, Lippincott-Raven, 1997, pp 319–340.
3. Klein JD, Garfin SR: History and physical examination. In Weinstein JM, Rydevik BL, Sonntag VKH (eds): Essentials of the Spine. New York, Raven Press, 1995, pp 71–96.
4. Riley LH: History and physical examination of the spine. In An HS (ed): Principles and Techniques of Spine Surgery. Baltimore, Williams & Wilkins, 1998, pp 91–102.

6. EVALUATION OF THE SPINE TRAUMA PATIENT

John Steinmann, D.O., and Gina Cruz, B.S., RPT

1. What is the incidence of new spinal cord injuries? What are the leading causes?

Eight to ten thousand new cases of spinal cord injuries occur in the United States each year. The male-to-female ratio for spinal cord injury is 5:1, and the average age is 29.7 years. Leading causes of spinal cord injuries are motor vehicle accidents (40–50%), violence (15–30%), falls (10–20%) and sports (10–15%).

2. What are the goals in treating a patient with spinal cord injury?
- Safe extrication and transport
- Prevention of hypoxemia and hypotension
- Accurate identification and classification of the spinal injury
- Rapid reduction of fractures and dislocations
- Steroid therapy when indicated
- Timely stabilization of unstable spinal segments
- Early transfer to appropriate acute spinal cord rehabilitation center

3. Describe important aspects of the prehospital care of the potentially spine-injured patient.

Treatment begins with ensuring an adequate airway, breathing, and circulation. Patients with high-energy mechanisms or altered mental status should be assumed to have suffered a spinal injury and undergo extrication and transport using strict spinal precautions. Prevention of hypoxemia and hypotension through the use of supplemental oxygen, intravenous fluids, and vasopressors helps limit the zone of spinal cord injury. Transport to a facility prepared to manage acute spinal cord injury is essential.

4. Discuss the role of steroids in the treatment of acute spinal cord injury.

Studies have reported enhanced neurologic recovery in patients with incomplete motor lesions when methylprednisolone is administered within 8 hours of injury. A loading dose of 30 mg/kg is followed by 5.4 mg/kg for 23 hours if administered within 3 hours of injury or for 48 hours if administered between 3 and 8 hours after injury.

5. You are called to evaluate a paraplegic patient with a closed C5 fracture. The patient has associated minor closed fractures of the extremities and no evidence of injury to any other organ system. The emergency department physician reports that the patient is hypotensive but bradycardic. What is the etiology of the hypotension?

The scenario is consistent with neurogenic shock. Hypotension in the range of 70–90 mmHg associated with a low or normal pulse (70–90 beats/min) is not uncommon due to a temporary generalized sympathectomy effect. It is important not to confuse this picture with hemorrhagic shock, which presents with hypotension and an increased pulse rate. Increasing fluids will not raise blood pressure in neurogenic shock and instead may cause serious fluid overload and pulmonary edema.

6. In evaluating the conscious patient with spinal injury, what are the important aspects of the history?

The history should establish the mechanism of injury, time of injury, transient or persistent neurologic complaints, loss of consciousness, location of pain, and previous related medical problems.

7. **What is the importance of a transient neurologic deficit?**

A stable spine maintains appropriate alignment and protects the neural elements under physiologic loads. A transient neurologic deficit indicates a moment during the injury when the spine failed to protect the neural elements. Although this may be the result of preexistent stenosis, when associated with a high-energy mechanism it is best to assume that an injury resulting in spinal instability has occurred.

8. **Describe the essential elements of the physical exam in the spine-injured patient.**

A general inspection of the entire body is followed by detailed palpation of the spine. The patient is log-rolled, and the spine is inspected and palpated. One should note localized tenderness, bruising, and interspinous widening or displacement. The neurologic examination should follow the Standard Neurological Classification of Spinal Cord Injury form established by the American Spinal Injury Association (Figs. 1 and 2). A detailed motor, sensory and reflex exam must include a rectal exam to assess for sacral sparing and the bulbocavernosous reflex. Finally, a detailed inspection of all long bones and joints should be completed.

9. **What is sacral sparing? What is its significance in patients with spinal cord injury?**

Sacral sparing refers to the presence of any perianal sensation after an acute spinal cord injury. This finding indicates some degree of transmission of neural impulses across the level of spinal cord injury and that the patient has sustained a partial spinal cord injury, with the potential for some degree of neurologic recovery. Sacral sparing is due to the topographic cross-sectional organization of the spinal cord in which the sensory and motor fibers supplying caudad regions are located laterally and closer to the surface of the spinal cord. Contusion and spinal cord ischemia typically result in greater damage to centrally located tracts than tracts located peripherally in the spinal cord.

10. **What is spinal shock? What is its significance after an acute spinal cord injury?**

Spinal shock refers to the period after spinal cord injury (usually 24 hours) when the reflex activity of the entire spinal cord becomes depressed. During this period the reflex arcs below the level of spinal cord injury are not functioning. The return of reflex activity below the level of a spinal cord injury signifies the end of spinal shock. The significance of spinal shock lies in the determination of whether a patient has sustained a complete vs. incomplete spinal cord injury. This cannot be determined until spinal shock has ended.

11. **What is the bulbocavernosus reflex? What is its significance?**

The bulbocavernosus reflex is a spinal reflex. It is tested by application of digital pressure on the penis or clitoris or gently pulling on the Foley catheter to cause reflex anal sphincter contraction. Absence of this reflex indicates spinal shock. Return of this reflex signifies the end of spinal shock. At this point, the patient with complete loss of motor and sensory function below the level of injury and absence of sacral sparing is considered to have a complete spinal injury.

12. **How should neurologic status be described after a significant spinal injury?**

Practically, patients should be stratified into the following categories:

Neurologically intact. The patient has not sustained a neurologic injury in association with the osteoligamentous spine injury.

Root injury, which signifies a peripheral nerve injury with potential for recovery.

Incomplete spinal cord injury. Partial preservation of neural function is noted below the level of injury. Recovery may vary from minimal to complete, depending on the type of incomplete spinal cord injury. Six incomplete spinal cord injury syndromes have been described: (1) central cord, (2) Brown-Sequard, (3) anterior cord, (4) posterior cord, (5) conus medullaris, and (6) cauda equina.

Complete spinal cord injury: absent sensory and motor function below the level of injury.

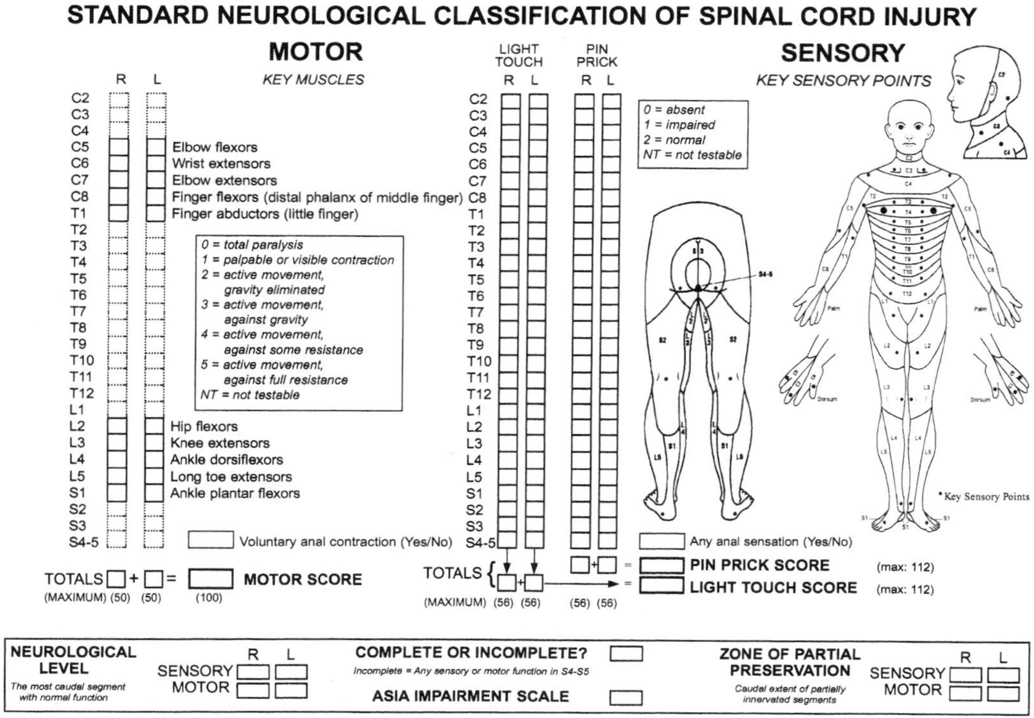
STANDARD NEUROLOGICAL CLASSIFICATION OF SPINAL CORD INJURY
MOTOR
KEY MUSCLES
R L
C2 C3 C4 C5 C6 C7 C8 T1 T2 T3 T4 T5 T6 T7 T8 T9 T10 T11 T12 L1 L2 L3 L4 L5 S1 S2 S3 S4-5
Elbow flexors
Wrist extensors
Elbow extensors
Finger flexors (distal phalanx of middle finger)
Finger abductors (little finger)
0 = total paralysis
1 = palpable or visible contraction
2 = active movement, gravity eliminated
3 = active movement, against gravity
4 = active movement, against some resistance
5 = active movement, against full resistance
NT = not testable
Hip flexors
Knee extensors
Ankle dorsiflexors
Long toe extensors
Ankle plantar flexors
Voluntary anal contraction (Yes/No)
TOTALS + = MOTOR SCORE
(MAXIMUM) (50) (50) (100)
LIGHT TOUCH
PIN PRICK
R L R L
SENSORY
KEY SENSORY POINTS
0 = absent
1 = impaired
2 = normal
NT = not testable
Any anal sensation (Yes/No)
TOTALS
PIN PRICK SCORE (max: 112)
LIGHT TOUCH SCORE (max: 112)
(MAXIMUM) (56) (56) (56) (56)
• Key Sensory Points
Palm
Dorsum
NEUROLOGICAL LEVEL
The most caudal segment with normal function
SENSORY
MOTOR
COMPLETE OR INCOMPLETE?
Incomplete = Any sensory or motor function in S4-S5
ASIA IMPAIRMENT SCALE
ZONE OF PARTIAL PRESERVATION
Caudal extent of partially innervated segments

FIGURE 1. American Spinal Injury Association classification of spinal cord injury.

ASIA IMPAIRMENT SCALE

☐ **A = Complete:** No motor or sensory function is preserved in the sacral segments S4-S5.

☐ **B = Incomplete:** Sensory but not motor function is preserved below the neurological level and includes the sacral segments S4-S5.

☐ **C = Incomplete:** Motor function is preserved below the neurological level, and more than half of key muscles below the neurological level have a muscle grade less than 3.

☐ **D = Incomplete:** Motor function is preserved below the neurological level, and at least half of key muscles below the neurological level have a muscle grade of 3 or more.

☐ **E = Normal:** motor and sensory function are normal

CLINICAL SYNDROMES

☐ Central Cord
☐ Brown-Sequard
☐ Anterior Cord
☐ Conus Medullaris
☐ Cauda Equina

FIGURE 2. American Spinal Injury Association impairment scale.

13. Describe the Frankel classification of spinal cord injury.

The Frankel classification has been used to separate patients with spinal cord injuries into five functional grades:

Grade A: absent motor and sensory function.
Grade B: absent motor function with sensory sparing.
Grade C: very weak motor function (not useful); sensation present.
Grade D: weak but useful motor functions; sensation present.
Grade E: normal motor and sensory function.

14. What is the ASIA Impairment Scale for assessing the spinal cord injured patient?

The American Spinal Injury Association (ASIA) Impairment Scale provides a more detailed method for classifying the neurologic status of patients with spinal injuries:

ASIA A: Complete injury. No motor or sensory function distal to the level of injury including the sacral segments S4–S5.
ASIA B: Incomplete injury. Sensory but not motor function is preserved below the neurologic level and includes the sacral segments S4–S5.
ASIA C: Incomplete injury. Motor function is preserved below the neurologic level, and more than half of key muscles below the neurologic level have a muscle grade < 3.
ASIA D: Incomplete injury. Motor and sensory incomplete (motor functional) with at least half of key muscles below the neurologic level having a muscle grade 3 or 4.
ASIA E: Normal; sensory and motor function intact.

15. Name the location and function of the major spinal cord tracts important in the assessment of the patient with spinal cord injury.

Corticospinal tracts: descending tracts located in the lateral portion of the cord that transmit ipsilateral motor function.

Spinothalamic tracts: ascending tracts located in the anterolateral portion of the cord that transmit sensations of pain and temperature. These tracts cross shortly after entering the spinal cord and therefore transmit sensation from the contralateral side of the body.

Dorsal column tracts: ascending tracts that convey ipsilateral proprioception, vibration, and light touch sensation.

16. Briefly explain the mechanism and clinical presentation of the incomplete spinal cord injury syndromes in the cervical spine.

Central cord syndrome is the most common incomplete spinal cord injury syndrome and results from a hyperextension injury. It is often seen in elderly patients with preexistent cervical stenosis who sustain a hyperextension injury. The clinical presentation includes bilateral sensory and motor deficits with upper extremity weakness greater than lower extremity weakness. Lower extremity hyperreflexia and sacral sparing are noted. The prognosis is good for a partial recovery. Recovery of hand function is generally poor. Decompression of preexistent cervical stenosis can be considered once spinal cord swelling has stabilized or diminished and early recovery has reached a plateau.

Brown-Sequard syndrome is caused by a hemisection of the spinal cord. The clinical presentation includes ipsilateral motor and proprioception loss with contralateral pain and temperature loss distal to the level of injury. The prognosis for recovery is good, with most patients recovering some degree of ambulatory capacity. Common causes include knife wounds and asymmetrically located spinal cord tumors.

Anterior cord syndrome results from vascular ischemia or compression of the anterior spinal artery and anterior spinal cord. Generally, neural function is absent in the anterior two-thirds of the spinal cord. Findings include complete loss of motor function and pain and temperature sensation. Preservation of vibration, proprioception, and light touch is noted. The prognosis for recovery is poor. A common cause is a vertebral body fracture associated with spinal cord injury secondary to retropulsed bone.

Posterior cord syndrome presents with loss of deep pressure, deep pain, and proprioception. However, motor function and pain and temperature sensations are intact. Patients typically ambulate with a foot-slapping gait. This syndrome is extremely rare. Potential causes include vitamin B_{12} deficiency and syphilis.

17. What is SCIWORA?

SCIWORA refers to spinal cord injury without radiographic abnormality. This syndrome is seen in young children and older adults. In children, the elasticity of the immature spine permits neurologic injury without a fracture. In older adults with preexistent central spinal stenosis, an acute central cord syndrome may develop after a fall despite the absence of a spine fracture.

18. What initial radiographs should be obtained in spine-injured patients?

The initial series should include anteroposterior (AP), lateral, and open-mouth views of the cervical spine. The lateral view needs to visualize the occiput to the superior endplate of T1. Inability to visualize T1 necessitates either traction on the arms or a swimmer's view. If adequate assessment of the entire cervical spine cannot be achieved by these means, computerized tomography (CT) with coronal and axial reconstruction is necessary to visualize the cervicothoracic junction and odontoid. If thoracic or lumbar pain exists or if the patient is mentally impaired or unconscious, then AP and lateral x-rays of the thoracic and lumbar spine are indicated.

19. What should be evaluated in looking at the lateral cervical spine in a trauma setting?

Films should be assessed for adequacy and alignment and ensure that the anterior elements (body) and posterior elements remain aligned. When inspecting bony alignment, look for any fractures. Interspinous widening and retropharyngeal swelling may indicate serious injury. This approach is especially helpful in craniovertebral trauma. An increase at the atlantodens interval (normally 3.5 mm in adults and 5 mm in children) indicates rupture of the transverse ligament.

20. What is acceptable retropharyngeal swelling?

Acceptable retropharyngeal swelling is up to 6–7 mm at C2 and 18–21 mm at C6.

21. What are the indications for CT in patients with spinal injury?

In a patient with a high-energy mechanism, CT scanning is indicated to assess all areas of suspected or known injury. CT scanning, therefore, is indicated in all areas of localized tenderness and all areas of fracture or radiographic abnormality.

22. What are the indications for MRI in patients with spinal injury?

- Unexplained neurologic deficit
- Incomplete neurologic deficit
- Neurologic deterioration
- Before reduction of the cervical or thoracic spine in neurologically intact patients or patients with incomplete spinal cord injury
- Preoperatively in neurologically impaired patients if a posterior approach is contemplated
- To assess ligamentous injury

23. When are flexion-extension views indicated?

Flexion-extension views are to be avoided in the acute setting. In a patient who has normal radiographs and spinal tenderness, a hard collar should be used for the first 7–10 days. If tenderness persists, a controlled flexion-extension view under physician supervision may help to rule out a ligamentous injury.

24. What are the criteria necessary to clear the cervical spine?

- Conscious, alert, and oriented patient
- Negative x-rays

- Absence of localized tenderness
- Intact neurologic status

25. What are the indications for emergent surgery in the spine-injured patient?
- Open spine fractures
- Irreducible cervical or thoracic fractures in patients with neurologic deficits
- Neurologic deterioration in the presence of known cord compression

BIBLIOGRAPHY

1. American Spinal Injury Association, International Medical Society of Paraplegia: International Standards for Neurological and Functional Classification of Spinal Cord Injury, Revised 1996. Chicago, American Spinal Injury Association, 1996.
2. Bracken NB, Shepard MJ, Collins WF, et al: A randomized controlled trial of methylprednisolone and naloxone in the treatment of acute spinal cord injury. Results of the Second National Acute Spinal Cord Injury Study. N Engl J Med 322:1405–1411, 1990.
3. Bucholz RW, Hechman JD (eds): Rockwood and Green's Fractures in Adults, 5th ed. Philadelphia, Lippincott Williams & Wilkins, 2001.
4. White AA III, Panjabi MM (eds): Clinical Biomechanics of the Spine, 2nd ed. Philadelphia, J.B. Lippincott, 1990.
5. Zigler JE, Capen DA: Epidemiology of spinal cord injury: A perspective on the problem. In Levine AM, Eismont FJ, Garfin SR, Zigler JE (eds): Spine Trauma. Philadelphia, W.B. Saunders, 1998.

7. EVALUATION OF SPINAL DEFORMITIES

Robert W. Gaines, Jr., M.D., and Vincent J. Devlin, M.D.

1. What are the most common spinal deformities that require recognition by the clinician?
Traditionally spinal deformities have been classified into those that affect predominantly the coronal plane (e.g., idiopathic scoliosis) and those affecting the sagittal plane (e.g., Scheuermann's kyphosis). In reality, spinal deformities are complex and simultaneously affect the sagittal, coronal, and axial plane alignment of the spinal column and its relationship to pelvis and thoracic cage. A spinal deformity may result from a pathologic process at a single vertebra level (e.g., spondylolisthesis), or multiple spinal levels (e.g., Scheuermann's kyphosis), or it may involve the entire spinal column and pelvis due to compromised postural support mechanisms (e.g., neuromuscular scoliosis).

2. Why does the assessment of spinal deformities require a comprehensive assessment of the patient's health status?
Every facet of human disease is associated with spinal deformities. The etiology of spinal deformities is wide ranging and includes congenital disorders, developmental disorders, degenerative disorders, trauma, infection, tumor, metabolic disorders, neuromuscular disorders, and conditions whose precise etiology remains elusive (e.g., idiopathic scoliosis). Clinical examination is critical for detection of spinal deformities and makes subsequent detailed assessment possible. Radiographs and higher-level imaging studies are required to document the severity and extent of a specific spinal deformity. A spinal deformity may be only one manifestation of an underlying systemic disorder that may affect multiple organ systems.

3. What are the potential consequences of untreated spinal deformities?
The consequences depend on many factors, including age, underlying health status, deformity etiology, deformity magnitude, and the potential for future progression of the deformity during the patient's lifespan. Potential consequences of untreated spinal deformity may include cosmetic problems, pain, neurologic deficit, postural difficulty, and impairment in activities of daily living. Severe thoracic deformity may impair respiratory mechanics with resultant hypoxemia, pulmonary hypertension, cor pulmonale, or even death.

4. Describe the basic components of the clinical assessment of a patient with spinal deformity.
1. Detailed history: What is the presenting complaint? (deformity? pain? neurologic symptoms? impaired function in activities of daily living? cardiorespiratory symptoms?) When was the deformity first noticed? Is there a family history of spinal deformity? Were there any abnormalities during development? What is the patient's maturity and growth potential? Has prior treatment been performed? Are there any associated general medical problems?

2. Comprehensive physical exam

Inspection. The patient must be undressed to fully assess the trunk and extremities. Assess for asymmetry of the neck line, shoulder height, rib cage, waist line, flank, pelvis, and lower extremities. The patient should be assessed in the standing position and bent forward to 90°. The patient should be inspected from both anterior and posterior aspects as well as from the side. Note any skin lesions (e.g., midline hair patch, sinus tract, hemangiomas, café-au-lait pigmentation). Observe the patient's gait. Observe body proportions and height.

Palpation. Palpate the spinous processes and paraspinous region for tenderness, deviation in spinous process alignment, or a palpable step-off.

Spinal range of motion. Test flexion-extension, side-bending, and rotation. Any restriction or asymmetry with range of motion is noted.

Neurologic exam. Assess sensory, motor, and reflex function of the upper and lower extremities, including abdominal reflexes.

Spinal alignment and balance in the coronal plane. Normally the head should be centered over the sacrum and pelvis. A plumb line dropped from C7 should fall through the gluteal crease.

Spinal alignment and balance in the sagittal plane. When the patient is observed from the side, assess the four physiologic sagittal curves (cervical and lumbar lordosis, thoracic and sacral kyphosis). When the patient standing with the hips and knees fully extended, the head should be aligned over the sacrum. The ear, shoulder, and greater trochanter of the hip should lie on the same vertical line.

Extremities. Measurement of leg lengths and assessment of joint flexibility is performed. Note any contractures or deformities involving the extremities (e.g., cavus feet).

Examination of related body systems. A detailed medical assessment should be performed. Some spinal deformities are associated with abnormalities in other organ systems, especially the nervous system and renal system. Screening for cardiac disorders, vision problems, hearing problems, and learning disorders may be required.

5. **What are the most common types of scoliosis?**

Scoliosis refers to a spinal deformity in the coronal (frontal) plane. The commonly described causes of scoliosis include:
- Idiopathic
- Neuromuscular (e.g., cerebral palsy, muscular dystrophy, myelomenigocele, Friedreich's ataxia)
- Congenital: failure of formation (e.g., hemivertebra), failure of segmentation (e.g., congenital bar)
- Neurofibromatosis
- Mesenchymal (e.g., Marfan syndrome, Ehlers-Danlos syndrome)
- Trauma
- Secondary to extraspinal contracture (e.g., after empyema)
- Osteochondrodystophies (e.g., Morquio's syndrome, diastrophic dwarfism)
- Infection
- Metabolic (e.g., osteoporosis, rickets)
- Tumor (spinal cord or vertebral column)
- Related to anomalies of the lumbosacral joint (e.g., spondylolisthesis)

6. **Describe the assessment of an adolescent referred for evaluation for possible scoliosis.**

The patient should be examined with the back exposed. First the patient is examined in the standing position. Then the patient is examined as he or she bends forward at the waist with the arms hanging freely, the knees straight, and the feet together. Findings that suggest the presence of scoliosis include:
- Shoulder height asymmetry
- Scapula or rib prominence
- Chest cage asymmetry
- Waist line asymmetry
- Asymmetry of the paraspinous musculature
- Unequal space between the arm and the waist line on side to side comparison.

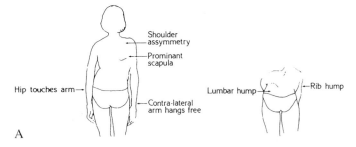

FIGURE 1. A, Physical findings associated with scoliosis. (From Staheli LT (ed): Pediatric Orthopaedic Secrets. Philadelphia, Hanley & Belfus, 1998.) *(continued)*

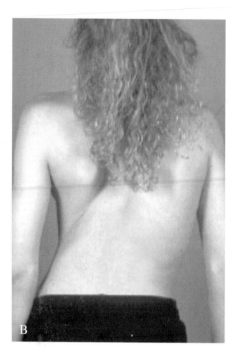
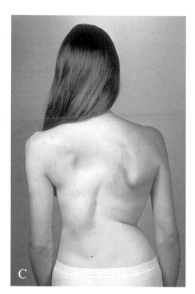

FIGURE 1. (*continued*) **B,** Thoracic scoliosis. **C,** Thoracic and lumbar scoliosis.

7. What is a scoliometer? How is it used?

In North America, it is common for children in the 10- to 14-year age group to undergo a screening assessment at school for detection of scoliosis. The Adams test (assessment for spinal asymmetry with the patient in the forward-bending position) is typically used to assess for possible scoliosis. The use of an inclinometer (scoliometer) has been popularized to quantitate trunk asymmetry and help decide whether radiographs should be obtained to further evaluate a specific patient. The scoliometer is used to determine the angle of trunk rotation (ATR). The ATR is the angle formed between the horizontal plane and the plane across the posterior aspect of the trunk at the point of maximal deformity when a region of the spine is evaluated with the patient in the forward-bending position. According to its developer, an ATR of 5° is correlated with an 11° curve and an ATR of 7° is correlated with a 20° curve.

8. How is scoliosis due to leg length discrepancy distinguished from other types of scoliosis?

Performing the forward-bend test with the patient in the sitting position eliminates the effect of leg length discrepancy on the spine. Alternatively, evaluation of the patient after placing wood blocks beneath the shortened extremity eliminates the contribution of leg length discrepancy to pelvic obliquity and scoliosis. Finally, leg length inequality should be directly quantitated with a tape measure by determining the distance from anteriorsuperior iliac spine to medial malleolus.

9. What is the significance of painful scoliosis in pediatric patients?

The presentation of painful scoliosis is atypical in the pediatric patient. If pain is present in the pediatric patient with idiopathic scoliosis, it is typically mild, nonspecific, intermittent, and nonradiating. It is typically mechanical (improves with rest), does not awaken the patient from sleep, and does not limit activity. Persistent severe back pain should prompt the physician to further investigate the cause of the patient's symptoms. Work-up (e.g., lateral spinal radiograph, magnetic resonance imaging [MRI], bone scan) is needed to rule out etiologies such as spinal tumor, spinal infection, spondylolisthesis, or Scheuermann's disease.

10. What conditions should be considered in the differential diagnosis of neck-line asymmetry or shoulder height asymmetry?

In addition to an upper thoracic curvature secondary to idiopathic scoliosis, other conditions that may be responsible for this clinical finding include torticollis, Klippel-Feil syndrome, and congenital vertebral anomalies.

11. What is Klippel-Feil syndrome?

Klippel-Feil syndrome refers to a congenital fusion of the cervical spine associated with the clinical triad of a short neck, low posterior hairline, and limited neck motion.

12. What condition should be considered in a child with limited lumbar flexion and a fixed lumbar lordosis?

Lumbar lordosis that is rigid and does not correct when the patient is asked to perform a forward-bend test suggests the possibility of an intrathecal mass (tumor). A work-up should be initiated to rule out this possibility, including an MRI of the spine.

13. What should an examiner assess in the evaluation of an adult patient with scoliosis?

In contrast to pediatric patients, it is not uncommon for adult patients with scoliosis to present with back pain. However, the incidence of back pain in the adult population is significant regardless of the presence of a spinal deformity. Thus, it cannot be assumed that symptoms of back pain are necessarily related to the presence of a spinal deformity. Examination of the adult patient should be directed at localizing the painful areas of the spine. Is the pain localized to an area of deformity, or is it localized to the lumbosacral junction? Does the patient have symptoms consistent with spinal stenosis or radiculopathy that warrant further work-up with spinal canal imaging studies (MRI and/or CT-myelography)? Is there evidence of deformity progression or cardiopulmonary dysfunction? There are no short cuts in the evaluation of spinal deformity, and a complete history and physical exam are mandatory.

14. What is sciatic scoliosis?

Pain as a result of lumbar nerve root irritation secondary to a disc herniation or spinal stenosis may lead to a postural abnormality that mimics scoliosis. This condition has been termed sciatic scoliosis.

15. Define gibbus.

The term *gibbus* derives from the Latin word for hump. It refers to a spinal deformity in the sagittal plane characterized by a sharply angulated spinal segment with an apex that points posteriorly.

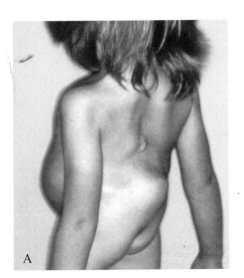

FIGURE 2. A, Congenital kyphosis with gibbus. (*continued*)

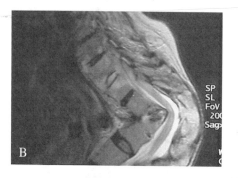

FIGURE 2. (*continued*) **B,** MRI demonstrates sharply angulated kyphotic deformity secondary to congenital kyphosis.

16. What are the common causes of increased thoracic kyphosis?

Thoracic kyphosis is one of the four physiologic sagittal curves in normal people. Many different spinal pathologies can lead to an abnormal increase in thoracic kyphosis. In the pediatric population, increased thoracic kyphosis is commonly associated with Scheuermann's disease or congenital spinal anomalies. In the adult population, a wide range of pathology can manifest as increased thoracic kyphosis. A common cause is osteoporotic compression fractures, which lead to an increased thoracic kyphotic deformity termed "dowager's hump."

Causes of kyphotic spinal deformities
- Postural disorders
- Scheuermann's kyphosis
- Congenital disorders (failure of formation, failure of segmentation)
- Neuromuscular disorders
- Myelomeningocele
- Trauma (acute, chronic)
- Surgery
- Irradiation
- Metabolic (osteoporosis, osteomalacia, ostoeogenesis imperfecta)
- Skeletal dysplasia
- Collagen diseases
- Tumor
- Infection
- Rheumatologic disorders (e.g., ankylosing spondylitis)

17. How are postural kyphosis and kyphosis due to Scheuermann's disease distinguished clinically?

Postural kyphosis (postural roundback) and Scheuermann's kyphosis are common causes of abnormal sagittal plane alignment in teenagers (Fig. 3). They can be distinguished on clinical assessment by performing a forward-bend test and observing the patient from the side. With postural kyphosis, the sagittal contour normalizes because the deformity is flexible. In kyphosis due to Scheuermann's disease, the deformity is rigid (structural) and does not normalize on forward bending.

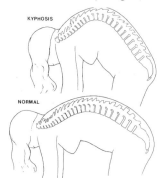

FIGURE 3. Normal and kyphotic sagittal spine profile.

18. What is flatback syndrome? What is the most common cause?

Flatback syndrome is a disabling postural disorder characterized by low back pain, forward inclination of the trunk, and difficulty in maintaining an erect posture (Fig. 4). The patient attempts to compensate for this abnormal posture by either hyperextending the hips or standing with the hips and knees flexed. This syndrome results from decreased lumbar lordosis with subsequent imbalance in the sagittal plane. The disorder is most commonly associated with the surgical treatment of scoliosis, in which a fusion was performed into the lower lumbar spine in association with distraction instrumentation with loss of normal lumbar lordosis. When a patient with a flatback posture attempts to stand with the hips and knees fully extended, the head is no longer aligned over the sacrum. The reference line connecting the ear, shoulder, and greater trochanter of the hip lies anterior to an imaginary line drawn upward from the patient's feet.

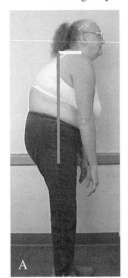 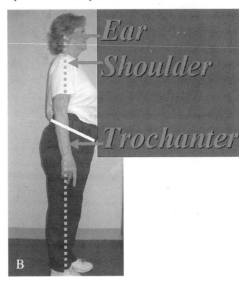

FIGURE 4. A, Flatback syndrome. **B,** Normal sagittal plane alignment.

19. What additional evaluation is indicated for a patient who presents with a congenital spinal deformity?

Congenital spinal deformities are associated with abnormalities in other organ systems in a significant number of patients. Assessment for associated anomalies is part of the work-up of a patient with congenital scoliosis. Associated anomalies of the neural axis (spinal dysraphism) are evaluated with an MRI of the spine. Nonspinal anomalies most frequently involve the renal system and are evaluated with renal ultrasound or intravenous pyelography.

20. Describe the key points to assess during examination of a patient with spinal deformity secondary to neuromuscular disease.

- Assessment of level of function. Can the patient sit independently? Is the patient ambulatory?
- Assessment of general health status. Is there a history of seizures, frequent pneumonia, or poor nutrition?
- Evaluation of head control, trunk control, and motor strength. Does the underlying neuromuscular problem result in a spastic, flaccid, or athetoid picture?
- Assessment of curve flexibility. Curve flexibility can be assessed by grasping the head in the area of the mastoid process and lifting the patient from the sitting or standing position.
- Is pelvic obliquity present? Is it correctable with traction and positioning?
- Evaluation the hip joints for coexistent pathology, including contractures.
- Is the patient's underlying neuromuscular disorder associated with any other organ system problems? For example, Duchenne muscular dystrophy is associated with cardiomyopathy.
- Documentation of pressure sores and areas of skin breakdown.

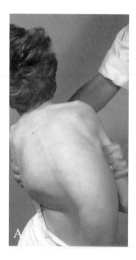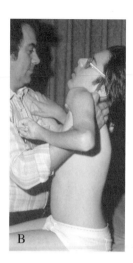

FIGURE 5. Neuromuscular scoliosis. **A,** Long sweeping curve with associated pelvic obliquity and loss of sitting balance. **B,** Assessment of curve flexibility.

21. What findings may be noted in a pediatric patient with spondylolisthesis?

Spondylolisthesis in children may present with a variety of symptoms and physical findings, depending on the degree of slippage and the degree of kyphosis at the level of the slip. Low back pain and buttock pain are the most common presenting symptoms. Physical exam typically reveals localized tenderness with palpation at the level of slippage. Hamstring tightness is a commonly associated finding. In the most severe cases, the patient is unable to stand erect because of sagittal plane decompensation associated with compensatory lumbar hyperlordosis and occasionally neurologic deficit.

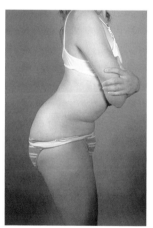

FIGURE 6. Severe spondylolisthesis associated with sagittal plane decompensation.

BIBLIOGRAPHY

1. Drummond DS: Idiopathic scoliosis. In Staheli LT (ed): Pediatric Orthopaedic Secrets. Philadelphia, Hanley & Belfus, 1998, pp 280–282.
2. Lonstein JE: Patient evaluation. In Lonstein JE, Winter RB, Bradford DS, Ogilvie JW (eds): Moe's Textbook of Scoliosis and Other Spinal Deformities, 3rd ed. Philadelphia, W.B. Saunders, 1995, pp 45–86.
3. McCarthy RE: Evaluation of the patient with deformity. In Weinstein SL (ed): The Pediatric Spine Principles and Practice, 2nd ed. Lippincott Williams & Wilkins, Philadelphia, 2001, pp 133–160.
4. Neyt JG, Weinstein SL: Kyphosis and lordosis. In Staheli LT (ed): Pediatric Orthopaedic Secrets. Philadelphia, Hanley & Belfus, 1998, pp 283–288.

III. Spinal Imaging

8. STRATEGIES FOR IMAGING IN SPINAL DISORDERS

Motoko Watanabe, M.D., Josephy Y. Margulies, M.D., Ph.D., and Vincent J. Devlin, M.D.

1. What are the major objectives of spinal imaging?

1. To evaluate spinal morphology in patients presenting with symptoms due to
   - Neural compression
   - Spinal deformity
   - Mechanical insufficiency of the spinal column (spinal instability)
2. To identify the level(s) of a spinal lesion
3. To create a topographic map to guide surgical intervention
4. To evaluate the results of treatment (operative and nonoperative) of spinal disorders

2. What are the most common diagnostic imaging tests used to evaluate spinal disorders?

- Plain radiographs
- Magnetic resonance imaging (MRI)
- Computed tomography (CT)
- CT-myelography
- Bone scan

3. What additional tests may play a role in the diagnosis of spinal disorders?

- **Bone densitometry.** Dual energy x-ray absorptiometry (DEXA) is widely used to assess bone mass.
- **Discography.** This provocative test involves injecting lumbar discs in an attempt to determine whether a degenerated lumbar disc is a pain generator.
- **Facet joint injections.** Local anesthetic or steroid may be injected in the facet region to provide diagnostic information or an anesthetic effect.
- **Selective spinal nerve blocks.** Local anesthetic or steroid may be injected around a segmental spinal nerve to provide diagnostic information or an anesthetic effect.
- **Biopsy.** CT-guided biopsies are commonly used to obtain tissue for diagnostic study in cases of tumor and infection as well as lesions whose diagnosis has yet to be determined.

4. What is the greatest challenge facing both patients and physicians in the use of spinal imaging tests?

Both patients and physicians tend to overestimate the ability of modern imaging tests to detect symptomatic spinal pathology and guide treatment. Each imaging modality—radiographs, CT, MRI, bone scan—is extremely sensitive but relatively nonspecific. Many studies have documented that spinal imaging studies reveal abnormalities in at least one-third of asymptomatic patients. One of the major challenges in utilization of imaging tests is to determine the clinical relevance of abnormal spinal morphology. This determination is especially challenging in attempts to distinguish imaging abnormalities likely to have clinical significance from those that are part of the normal aging process or part of a normal sequence of postoperative healing. In the absence of clinical assessment, imaging tests cannot determine whether a specific spinal structure is responsible for symptoms. Excessive emphasis on imaging tests without clinical correlation is hazardous to both patient and physician and may lead to inappropriate treatment.

5. What steps can the clinician take to minimize the inappropriate use of diagnostic imaging tests?

1. Perform a detailed history and physical exam before ordering any imaging tests.
2. Formulate a working diagnosis to explain symptoms and guide testing.
3. Order the imaging study best suited to evaluate the suspected pathologic process based on the working diagnosis.
4. Order imaging tests only when the information obtained from the test will affect medical decision-making.

6. When should I order a spine radiograph?

Plain radiographs should be the initial imaging study of the spine. Because of the favorable natural history of acute cervical and lumbar pain syndromes, it is not necessary to order spine radiographs for every patient who presents with neck or low back pain. Indications for obtaining spine radiographs in patients presenting with cervical, thoracic, or lumbar pain include:
- Patients younger than 20 years or patients older than 50 years
- Patients who fail to respond to conservative management within 6–8 weeks
- Patients with a history of trauma (to rule out fracture)
- Complaints of pain at rest or night pain, history of cancer, fever, unexplained weight loss (to rule out tumor or infection)

7. What are the major advantages of using plain radiographs to assess spinal disorders?
- Plain radiographs are inexpensive and readily available.
- They provide rapid assessment of a specific spinal region(cervical, thoracic, lumbar) or the entire spinal axis (occiput to sacrum) in orthogonal planes.
- Weight-bearing (standing) and dynamic studies (flexion-extension views, side-bending views) may be obtained.
- Plain radiographs are useful to confirm normal osseous structure, vertebral alignment, and structural integrity of the spine

8. What are the major disadvantages of using plain radiographs to assess spinal disorders?
- Radiographs have a low sensitivity and specificity in identifying symptomatic spinal pathology. Age-related degenerative changes are present equally in symptomatic and asymptomatic populations.
- Radiographs cannot visualize neural structures and other soft tissue lesions (e.g., disc herniation).
- Radiographs cannot diagnose early-stage tumor or infection because significant bone destruction (40–60% of bone mass) must occur before a radiographic abnormality is detectable.

9. When should I order an MRI?

An MRI may be indicated if the clinical history and physical exam suggest a serious spinal problem and initial plain radiographs do not provide sufficient diagnostic information. The clinician should consider how the information obtained from a spinal MRI will affect the decision-making process for a specific patient before ordering this study. The strengths of MRI include its unparalleled ability to visualize pathologic processes involving the disc, thecal sac, epidural space, neural elements, paraspinal soft tissue, and bone marrow.

10. What are the major advantages of using MRI to assess spinal disorders?
- Avoids ionizing radiation
- Provides imaging in orthogonal planes
- Visualizes an entire spinal region and avoids missed pathology at transition zones between adjacent spinal regions

- Provides exquisite soft-tissue detail
- Provides excellent visualization of intrathecal neural elements
- Sensitive to marrow abnormalities

11. What are the major disadvantages of using MRI to assess spinal disorders?

- MRI does not define osseous anatomy as well as CT.
- Implanted devices are contraindications to MRI (e.g., pacemakers, drug pumps, spine stimulators)
- Claustrophobic patients may have difficulty because of the small diameter of the imaging machine.

12. When should I order a CT scan?

CT is most helpful when osseous abnormality is suggested. Common disorders for which CT is helpful include fractures, facet arthrosis, spondylolysis, and spondylolisthesis.

13. What are the major advantages of using CT to assess spinal disorders?

- CT is the best test for assessment of bone anatomy.
- Multiple cross-sectional images can be reconstructed to provide images in orthogonal planes (e.g., coronal, sagittal, and 3-D images are possible).
- CT is useful when MRI is contraindicated (e.g, cardiac pacemaker).

14. What are the major disadvantages of using CT to assess spinal disorders?

- Exposure to ionizing radiation is required.
- CT provides poor delineation of neural elements and adjacent structures. Ligaments, discs, dural sac, and nerve roots appear as different shades of gray.
- Significant pathology can be missed. For example, standard lumbar CT visualizes the L3–S1 region and fails to detect pathology in the upper lumbar region.
- Sagittal images are not routinely reconstructed at many institutions. This omission violates the basic radiologic principle of obtaining orthogonal views.

15. When should I order a myelogram?

Rarely. Myelography is no longer used as a stand-alone test to evaluate spinal pathology. However, myelography has a role in spinal imaging when it is combined with a CT scan. CT-myelography plays an important role in the assessment of complex spine problems such as lumbar spinal stenosis associated with scoliosis and cervical spinal stenosis associated with ossification of the posterior longitudinal ligament (OPLL). CT-myelography plays an important role in the assessment of patients before revision spinal surgery, especially when spinal implant devices are present after prior surgical procedures.

16. What are the main advantages of myelography in the assessment of spinal disorders?

Myelography is the only widely available test that can provide dynamic information about the spine and its relation to the neural elements. Standing weight-bearing views as well as flexion-extension views may be obtained. Such views are especially helpful in assessing patients whose symptoms are exacerbated in the erect position because myelography permits imaging of the spine in the symptomatic position. Other advanced imaging tests such as CT and MRI are generally performed with the patient in the supine position. Standing MRI scanners are currently in development and will represent a major advance in this area.

17. What are the main disadvantages of using myelography as an isolated test to assess spinal disorders?

- Myelography is an invasive test.
- Complications and unpleasant side effects may occur (e.g.,adverse reaction to contrast, spinal fluid leak, spinal headache).
- Myelography is less accurate than CT or MRI in evaluating disc pathology.

- Myelography cannot detect pathology below the level of a complete block to contrast.
- Myelography provides only indirect evidence of neural compression by demonstrating changes in contour of contrast-filled neural structures.
- Myelography cannot differentiate whether extradural compression is due to disc, osteophyte, tumor, or infection.
- Myelography cannot visualize pathology in the lateral zone of the spinal canal because the contrast-filled dural sac ends in the region of the pedicle.
- Pathology may be missed at the L5–S1 level, where the spinal canal is very wide, and a large disc protrusion or osteophyte may not deform the dye column.

18. When should I order a CT-myelogram?

For complex spinal problems, high-quality MRI and CT scans may be used as complementary studies to define the clinical situation more fully. Nevertheless, in certain situations a CT-myelogram remains the test of choice. Some of these situations include:

- Evaluation of the neural elements in a postoperative patient with spinal implants
- Patients with significant symptoms and equivocal MRI findings
- Patients with cervical or lumbar spinal stenosis problems in whom MRI is contraindicated
- Preoperative planning for surgery in patients with spinal stenosis and lumbar scoliosis
- Preoperative planning for revision spinal stenosis surgery, especially if symptoms suggest a relation to postural change
- Preoperative planning for surgical treatment of complex spinal deformities

19. What are the major advantages of CT-myelography to assess spinal disorders?

The use of CT and myelography together exceeds the value of either test performed alone. The addition of contrast to the CT scan improves delineation of neural structures, permitting distinction between disc margin, thecal sac, and ligamentum flavum. As a result, the accuracy of CT-myelography is comparable to MRI for a wide range of spinal disorders. An advantage of CT-myelography is that it can provide useful diagnostic information when MRI is contraindicated.

20. What are the major disadvantages of using CT-myelography to assess spinal disorders?

The disadvantages of CT-myelography include its invasive nature and the fact that it requires ionizing radiation.

21. When should I order a bone scan?

1. To screen the skeletal system for metastatic disease
2. To screen the spinal column for metastatic tumor, primary bone tumor, disc space infection, or vertebral osteomyelitis
3. To assess the relative biologic activity of bone lesions, such as pars interarticularis defects or facet joint degenerative changes
4. To evaluate a spinal fusion for pseudarthrosis
5. To aid in diagnosis of sacroliac joint pathology, such as infection or arthritis
6. To diagnose fractures in areas difficult to visualize with plain radiographs (e.g., sacral insufficiency fractures)

22. What are the major advantages of using a bone scan to assess spinal disorders?

- Bone scans provide an excellent method for rapidly screening the entire skeleton for bony abnormalities; they are especially useful for tumors and infections.
- They are an effective method for determining the relative biologic activity of a bone lesion; for example, they can differentiate between acute vs. chronic vertebral fractures or acute vs. chronic pars defects.
- They provide both planar and cross-sectional images (single-photon emission computed tomography ([SPECT])

23. What are the major disadvantages of using bone scans to assess spinal disorders?
- Bone scans are highly sensitive but not highly specific.
- Bone scans do not have sufficient resolution for surgical planning.
- Certain tumors, such as multiple myeloma or some purely lytic metastases, may not result in increased activity on the bone scan as they do not stimulate a significant osteoblastic response.

24. Into what major etiologic groups can patients presenting with spinal symptomatology be divided?
1. Degenerative disorders
2. Trauma
3. Tumor
4. Infections
5. Spinal deformities
6. Congenital disorders
7. Inflammatory disorders
8. Metabolic disorders
9. Extraspinal conditions that mimic spinal pathology

25. Describe the sequence of ordering spinal imaging studies in terms of an algorithm.
Plain radiographs are the first imaging study obtained in evaluating patients with a spinal problem. If radiographs do not provide sufficient information, MRI is generally the next best study to evaluate most clinical conditions because it provides the greatest amount of information about a single spinal region. CT is generally ordered to complement the information obtained with MRI, especially when additional information is required about osseous anatomy. CT-myelography and radionuclide studies have limited indications but play a crucial role in specific situations.

An exception to this algorithm occurs in the assessment of acute fractures. CT is preferred over MRI as a second-order test because of its superior depiction of bone detail and fracture anatomy. In addition, not all institutions are equipped to provide MRI assessment of unstable multitrauma patients with spine fractures on an emergent basis. In this setting, a CT scan may provide sufficient information to guide initial treatment in most situations.

BIBLIOGRAPHY

1. Bell GR, Ross JS: Imaging studies of the spine. In Garfin SR, Vaccaro AR (eds): Orthopaedic Knowledge Update–Spine. Elk Grove Village, IL, American Academy of Orthopaedic Surgeons, 1997, pp 41–54.
2. Boden SD, Davis DO, Dina TS: Abnormal lumbar spine MRI scans in asymptomatic subjects: A prospective investigation. J Bone Joint Surg 72A 403–408, 1990.
3. Boden SD, McCowin PR, David DO, et al: Abnormal cervical spine MR scans in asymptomatic individuals: A prospective and blinded investigation. J Bone Joint Surg 72A:1178–1184, 1990
4. Boden SD: Diagnostic imaging of the spine. In Weinstein JN, Rydevik BL, Sonntag VKH (eds): Essential of the Spine. New York, Raven Press, 1995, pp 97–110.
5. Herzog RJ: Radiologic imaging of the spine. In Weinstein JN, Rydevik BL, Sonntag VKH (eds): Essential of the Spine. New York, Raven Press, 1995, pp 111–138.
6. Pfirrmann CWA, Resnick DL: Bone imaging: Plain radiography, computed tomography and radionuclide bone scan. In Fardon DF, Garfin SR, et.al (ed): Orthopaedic Knowledge Update 2–Spine. Elk Grove Village, IL, American Academy of Orthopaedic Surgeons, 2002, pp 53–62.
7. Walsh TR, Weinstein JN, Spratt KF, et al: Lumbar discography: A controlled, prospective study. J Bone Joint Surg 72A:1081–1088, 1990.

9. RADIOGRAPHIC ASSESSMENT OF THE SPINE

Vincent J. Devlin, M.D.

CERVICAL SPINE

1. What radiographic views are commonly used to assess the cervical spinal region?

Standard cervical spine views include: anteroposterior (AP) view (Fig. 1), lateral view (Fig. 2), right and left oblique views (Fig. 3), and open-mouth AP odontoid view (Fig. 4).

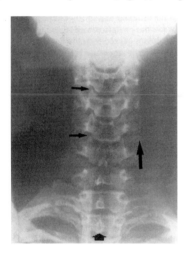

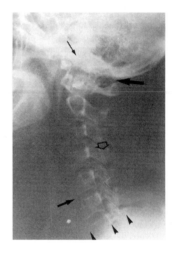

FIGURE 1. Normal anteroposterior cervical radiograph. The joints of Luschka are sharply defined and uniform (*thin arrow*). The spinous processes are midline and aligned (*short thick arrow*). The lateral margins of the articulating masses are smooth and undulating (*long thick arrow*). (From Schwartz AJ: Imaging of degenerative cervical disease. Spine State Art Rev 14:545–569, 2000, with permission.)

FIGURE 2. Normal lateral plain radiograph. The disc and bony margins are well defined (*short thick arrows*). Imaginary lines along the anterior vertebral body surface (*lower arrowhead*), the posterior vertebral body surface (*middle arrowhead*), and the spinal laminar line (*upper arrowhead*) should all reveal a mild lordosis without a sharp step-off. The C1 spinal laminar line is aligned with the posterior rim of the foramen magnum (*long thick arrow*). A line extending off the clivus bisects the dens (*long thin arrow*). The posterior aspect of the articular masses is anterior to the spinal laminar line (*open arrow*). (From Schwartz AJ: Imaging of degenerative cervical disease. Spine State Art Rev 14:545–569, 2000, with permission.)

2. What important parameters require assessment on each cervical radiographic view?

AP view

- Confirm that spinous processes align with each other
- Confirm equal distance between adjacent spinous processes

Lateral view

- Measure the prevertebral soft tissue shadow distance
- Confirm that cervical vertebral body alignment forms an uninterrupted lordotic curve
- Measure the distance from the posterior C1 arch to the anterior aspect of the odontoid

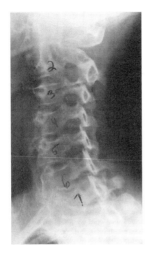

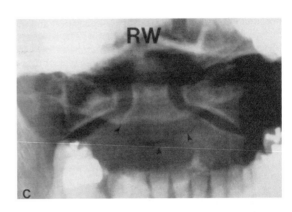

FIGURE 3. Normal 45° oblique cervical radiograph. The foramina are oval spaces and the facet joints are well defined. (From Katz DS, Math KR, Groskin SA (eds): Radiology Secrets. Philadelphia, Hanley & Belfus, 1998).

FIGURE 4. Open-mouth AP view. Note the relationship of the odontoid process and adjacent C1–C2 facet joints. (From Heller JG, Carlson GC: Odontoid fractures. Spine State Art Rev 5:217–234, 1991, with permission.)

- Check that intervertebral disc space heights are equal
- Confirm that the C7–T1 disc space is well visualized

Oblique view
- Assess facet joint alignment
- Assess neural foramina and their bony boundaries

Open-mouth view
- Check symmetry of the odontoid in relation to the lateral masses
- Assess the atlantoaxial joints

3. How is normal cervical alignment assessed on a lateral cervical spine radiograph?

Lines constructed along the anterior and posterior vertebral margins should describe a gentle and uninterrupted curve. An additional line, the spinolaminar line, is drawn by connecting the junction of the spinous process and lamina at each cervical vertebral level (Fig. 5).

4. What radiographic views should be obtained when the C7–T1 level cannot be visualized?

A swimmer's view may be obtained when the C7–T1 level cannot be visualized on a lateral cervical spine radiograph (Fig. 6). In the trauma patient this view is obtained in the supine position by raising the patient's arm overhead and directing the x-ray beam obliquely cephalad through the axilla. An alternative is to obtain a cross-table radiograph with traction applied to the patient's arms. Another option is to obtain bilateral oblique views of the C7–T1 level. When these techniques are unsuccessful in visualizing C7–T1, a computed tomography (CT) scan of the cervical spine with sagittal reconstructions through the C7–T1 spinal level should be obtained.

5. When are flexion-extension views obtained in the cervical spine?
- To assess potential spinal instability due to soft tissue disruption when static radiographs show no significant bony injury or malalignment but clinical findings suggest a significant injury
- To determine healing of a cervical fusion
- To assess integrity of the C1–C2 articulation in patients at high risk for C1–C2 instability (e.g., rheumatoid arthritis, Down syndrome)

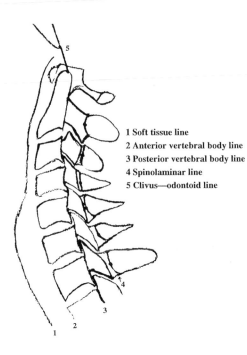

1 Soft tissue line
2 Anterior vertebral body line
3 Posterior vertebral body line
4 Spinolaminar line
5 Clivus—odontoid line

FIGURE 5. Cervical spine alignment. (From Katz DS, Math KR, Groskin SA (eds): Radiology Secrets. Philadelphia, Hanley & Belfus, 1998).

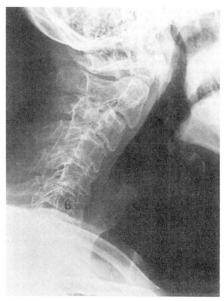
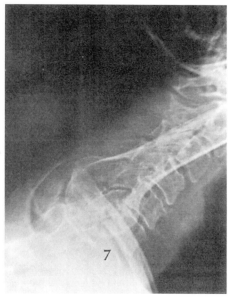

FIGURE 6. Visualizing C7–T1. **Left,** On this lateral view of the cervical spine, the C7 vertebra is obscured by the clavicle. **Right,** The C7 vertebra is readily visualized on this swimmer's view. (From Math E, Math KR: Cervical spine imaging. In Katz DS, Math KR, Groskin SA (eds): Radiology Secrets. Philadelphia, Hanley & Belfus, 1998, pp 335–342, with permission.)

Lateral flexion-extension cervical views should be obtained only in cooperative and alert patients. Neck motion must be voluntary and there is no role for passive or assisted range of motion during these views. Because of protective muscle spasm, flexion-extension views are rarely of value in the acute postinjury period.

6. What is the significance of the prevertebral soft tissue shadow distance?

Increased thickness of the prevertebral soft tissue space may be a tip-off to the presence of a significant soft tissue injury to the bony or ligamentous structures of the anterior cervical spine. This finding is less reliable in infants and children because of the wide normal variation in the pediatric population. The normal prevertebral soft tissue shadow distance in adults is < 7 mm at C2 and < 22 mm at the C6 vertebral level. In general, prevertebral soft tissue thickness should not exceed 50% of the AP diameter of the vertebral body at the same level.

7. Define the anterior and posterior margins of the spinal canal on a lateral cervical radiograph.

The anterior margin of the spinal canal is defined by the posterior vertebral body line. The posterior border of the spinal canal is defined by the spinolaminar line.

8. What is the significance of an abnormal atlantoaxial interval?

Abnormal widening of the space between the posterior aspect of the anterior arch of C1 and the anterior aspect of the odontoid (dens) defines an atlantoaxial subluxation (Fig. 7) and implies laxity of the transverse ligament. This space should not be greater than 3 mm in adults or 5 mm in children. Common causes of atlantoaxial subluxation include trauma, rheumatoid arthritis and Down syndrome.

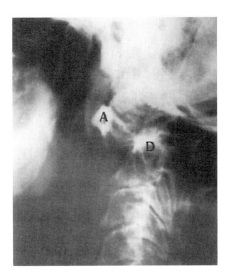

FIGURE 7. Atlantoaxial subluxation in patient with rheumatoid arthritis. Note marked widening of the space between the anterior arch of the atlas (A) and the margin of the dens (D). (From Math KR: Arthritis. In Katz DS, Math KR, Groskin SA (eds): Radiology Secrets. Philadelphia, Hanley & Belfus, 1998, pp 269–281, with permission.)

9. What radiographic criteria are used to define instability of the spine in the region from C2–T1?

Commonly accepted radiographic criteria for diagnosing clinical instability in the middle and lower cervical spine (C2–T1) include sagittal plane translation > 3.5 mm or sagittal plane angulation > 11° in relation to an adjacent vertebra.

THORACIC AND LUMBAR SPINE

10. What radiographic views are used to assess the thoracic spinal region?
Standard thoracic spine views include an AP view and lateral view.

11. What important structures may be examined on AP and lateral thoracic radiographs?
AP view
- Soft tissue shadow
- Spinous process alignment
- Pedicle—check presence bilaterally
- Vertebral body, ribs, transverse processes, costotransverse articulations, laminae

Lateral view
- Soft tissue shadow
- Vertebral body contour and alignment
- Intervertebral disc space height
- Pedicles, spinous processes, superior and inferior articular processes, intervertebral foramina

12. What is the significance of an absent pedicle shadow?
An absent pedicle shadow on the AP view (Fig. 8) is an important radiographic finding because metastatic spinal disease may initially obscure a single pedicle. Pedicle destruction may also result from malignant or primary tumors, histiocytosis, and infection.

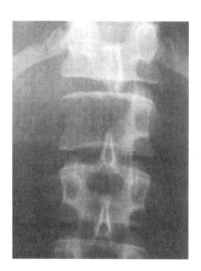

FIGURE 8. Absent pedicle shadow due to vertebral tumor. (From Spine State Art Rev 2:2, 1998, p 178, with permission.)

13. What is a Schmorl's node?
A Schmorl's node (Fig. 9) is an intraosseous herniation of disc material that results in a focal depression in the vertebral endplate. Any condition associated with weakening of the vertebral endplate or subchondral bone may allow disc material to herniate superiorly or inferiorly into the vertebral body. Schmorl's nodes are noted most commonly in the lower thoracic and upper lumbar spinal regions. Spinal pathology associated with Schmorl's nodes include Scheuermann's kyphosis, osteoporosis, and hyperparathyroidism.

14. What radiographic views are commonly used to assess the lumbar spinal region?
Standard lumbar spine views include standing AP and lateral views. Oblique views, lateral flexion-extension views, spot lateral views and Ferguson views are supplementary views that are valuable in specific situations.

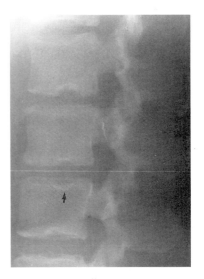

FIGURE 9. Schmorl's nodes. (From Katz DS, Math KR, Groskin SA (eds): Radiology Secrets. Philadelphia, Hanley & Belfus, 1998.)

15. Why should lumbar spine radiographs generally be obtained with the patient in the standing position?

Lumbar spine pathology (e.g., spondylolisthesis) tends to be exacerabated in the upright position and relieved with recumbency. Most other spinal imaging procedures are performed in the supine position (e.g., CT, magnetic resonance imaging). Standing radiographs provide the opportunity to obtain valuable information about spinal alignment in the erect weight-bearing position.

16. What important structures may be assessed on lumbar radiographs?
AP view
- Psoas soft tissue shadow
- Spinous process alignment
- Pedicle—check presence bilaterally
- Vertebral body and disc
- Facet joints
- Sacrum, sacral ala, sacroiliac joints

Lateral view
- Vertebral body contour and alignment
- Intervertebral disc space height
- Pedicles, spinous processes, superior and inferior articular processes, intervertebral foramina
- Sacrum, sacral promontory

Oblique views
- Pars interarticularis
- Facet joints
- Neural foramina

17. When are oblique views of the lumbar spine helpful?
- To diagnose spondylolysis
- To assess healing of lumbar posterolateral fusion

18. What anatomic structures comprise the "Scotty dog" on the oblique lumbar radiograph?

On the oblique lumbar radiograph, the vertebra and its processes can be imagined to outline the shape of a dog (Fig. 10): ear = superior articular process; head = pedicle; collar/neck = pars

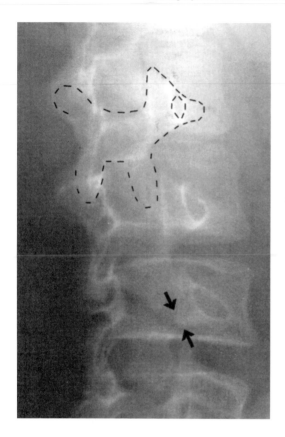

FIGURE 10. Oblique radiographic view of the lumbar spine.

interarticularis; front leg/foot = inferior articular process; body = lamina; hind leg/foot = contralateral inferior articular process; tail = spinous process. **Spondylolysis** refers to a defect in the region of the pars interarticularis. It appears as a radiolucent defect in the region of the neck or collar of the "Scotty dog".

19. What is a Ferguson view and when should it be ordered?

A Ferguson view is an AP view of the lumbosacral junction taken with the x-ray tube angled 30° cephalad in a man and 35° in women. The x-ray beam goes through the plane of the L5–S1 disc, permitting the anatomy of the lumbosacral junction to be well visualized. This view is ordered when it is difficult to visualize the L5–S1 level in patients with severe spondylolisthesis and to assess an intertransverse fusion at the L5–S1 level (Fig. 11).

20. What are coned-down views? When should they be ordered?

Coned down views or spot views limit scatter of the x-ray beam and are useful to define bone detail for a limited area of the spine. For example, a spot lateral view of the lumbosacral junction is helpful to assess the L5–S1 level in cases of severe spondylolisthesis.

21. Explain the major pitfall involved in interpreting flexion-extension lumbar spine radiographs.

No universally accepted definition of radiographic instability of the lumbar spine exists. In asymptomatic subjects, up to 3 mm of translation and 7–14° of angular motion may be present.

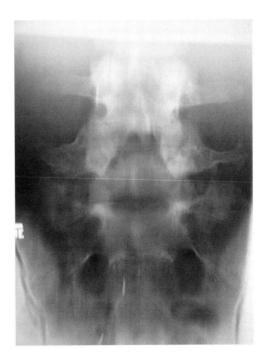

FIGURE 11. Fergusion AP view of the lumbosacral junction. Note the failure of fusion between the transverse processes of L5 and the sacral ala.

22. What radiographic criteria are used to determine instability in the lumbar spine?
On static radiographs
- Sagittal plane displacement > 4.5 mm or 15% in relation to an adjacent vertebra
- Relative sagittal plane angulation > 22° in relation to an adjacent vertebra

On dynamic(flexion-extension) radiographs
- Sagittal plane translation > 4.5 mm or 15% in relation to an adjacent vertebra
- Sagittal plane rotation > 15° at L1–L2, L2–L3, L3–L4
                            > 20° at L4–L5
                            > 25° at L5–S1

23. What is a lumbosacral transitional vertebra?
In the normal spine, the 24th vertebra below the occiput is the last presacral vertebra (L5), and the 25th vertebral segment is the body of S1. In the normal spine, there are five non–rib-bearing lumbar vertebra above the sacrum. People who possess four non–rib-bearing lumbar vertebra are considered to have **sacralization** of the L5 vertebra. People who possess six non–rib-bearing lumbar vertebra are considered to have **lumbarization** of the S1 vertebral body. The term **lumbosacral transitional vertebra** has been adopted because it is difficult to determine whether the transitional vertrebra is the 24th or 25th vertebra below the occiput without obtaining additional spinal radiographs. There are a variety of types of lumbosacral transitional vertebra. Vertebral anomalies ranging from hyperplasia of the transverse processes to large transverse processes that articulate with the sacrum or fusion of the transverse process and vertebral body with the sacrum are noted. These abnormalities may be partial or complete, unilateral or bilateral. Proper identification of lumbar spine segments in relation to the sacrum on plain radiographs is essential in planning lumbar spine procedures to ensure that surgery is carried out at the correct spinal level(s).

24. Define the following terms commonly used to describe abnormal vertebral alignment: spondylolisthesis, retrolisthesis, lateral listhesis, and rotatory subluxation.
Spondylolisthesis is defined as the forward displacement of a vertebra in relation to the vertebra below it. The degree of spondylolisthesis is determined by measuring the percentage of verte-

bral body translation: 0–25% (grade 1); 26–50 % (grade 2); 51–75% (grade 3); and 76–100% (grade 4). Other terms used to describe abnormal alignment between adjacent vertebra include **retrolisthesis** (posterior translation of a vertebra in relation to the vertebra below), **lateral listhesis** (lateral subluxation) and **rotatory subluxation** (abnormal rotation between adjacent vertebrae).

SPINAL DEFORMITY ASSESSMENT

25. What standard radiographs are used to evaluate spinal deformities?

Biplanar deformity radiographs (posteroanterior [PA] and lateral 14 × 36-inch radiographs) are the most frequent imaging studies used to assess spinal deformities (Fig. 12). The techniques for positioning, shielding, and performing this radiographic examination have been standardized. Radiographs are taken with the patient standing if possible. Sitting or supine radiographs may be required for patients who are unable to stand without support, including very young patients, paraplegic patients, and patients with severe neuromuscular disorders.

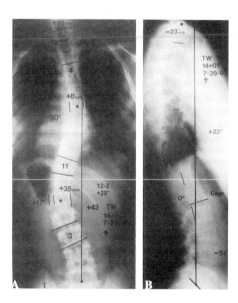

FIGURE 12. PA and lateral spinal deformity radiographs. (From Asher MA: Anterior surgery for thoracolumbar and lumbar idiopathic scoliosis. Spine State Art Rev 12:701–711, 1998, with permission.)

26. When should I order a radiograph of a specific spinal region? When should I order a 36" radiograph that images the entire spine?

Radiographs of a specific spinal region (cervical, thoracic, lumbar) are obtained for diagnosis and initial assessment of spinal pathology involving a specific vertebral or disc level within a spinal region (e.g., spondylolisthesis, fracture, infection, tumor). 14 × 36" spinal radiographs are required for assessment of spinal pathology that involves multiple spinal segments (e.g., scoliosis, kyphosis). 14 × 36" spine radiographs are valuable in planning spinal fusion procedures and in the assessment of postoperative spinal alignment.

27. What specialized radiographs are commonly used to assess flexibility of spinal deformities?

- Supine AP side-bending radiographs (Fig. 13)
- Supine AP traction radiograph
- Lateral hyperextension radiograph
- Lateral hyperflexion radiograph

Specialized radiographs are frequently obtained to assist in surgical planning before surgical correction of spinal deformities. Bending films are used to aid in selection of spinal levels that should be included in a scoliosis fusion. Supine AP bending films have been shown to be supe-

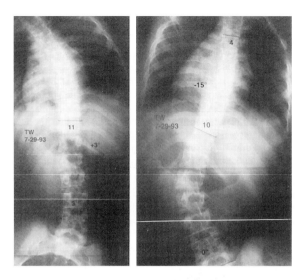

FIGURE 13. Supine 36" long cassette side bending radiographs. (From Asher MA: Anterior surgery for thoracolumbar and lumbar idiopathic scoliosis. Spine State Art Rev 12:701–711, 1998, with permission.)

rior to standing bending films for assessing coronal curve flexibility. Supine AP traction radiographs are helpful in patients with neuromuscular scoliosis to assess curve flexibility and correction of pelvic obliquity. A hyperextension lateral radiographs performed with a bolster placed at the apex of kyphosis may be useful for assessing the flexibility of a kyphotic deformity. A hyperflexion lateral view may be helpful to assess the flexibility of a lordotic spinal deformity.

28. What is the method used to quantify sagittal and coronal plane curvatures?

The **Cobb method** is most commonly used to quantify curvature in the coronal and sagittal planes (Fig. 14). The following steps are involved in this measurement:

1. Identify the end vertebra of the curvature whose measurement is desired.

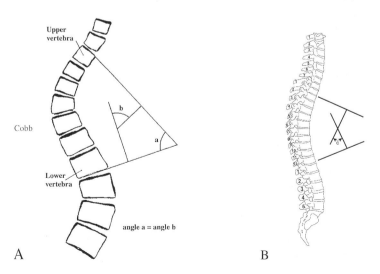

FIGURE 14. A, Measurement of scoliosis. (From Katz DS, Math KR, Groskin SA (eds): Radiology Secrets. Philadelphia, Hanley & Belfus, 1998). **B,** Measurement of kyphosis. (From Spine State Art Rev 12:1, 1998.)

2. Construct lines along the superior aspect of the upper end vertebra and along the inferior aspect of the lower end vertebra

3. Next construct lines perpendicular to the lines previously drawn along the end vertebra . Measure the angle between these two lines with a protractor to determine the Cobb angle.

4. In large curves it is possible to measure the Cobb angle directly from the lines along the end vertebra without the need to construct perpendicular lines.

29. What is spinal balance?

Spinal balance has been defined as stability produced by even distribution of weight on either side of a vertical axis (Fig. 15). From the point of view of the spine, it implies that, in both the frontal and sagittal planes, the head is positioned correctly over the sacrum and pelvis in both a translational and angular sense. Normal coronal balance is present when a plumb line dropped from the center of the C7 vertebral body lies within 1 cm of the middle of the sacrum. Normal sagittal plane balance is present when a plumb line dropped from the center of C7 lies within 2.5 cm of the posterior superior corner of S1. Another term for the plumb line measurement is the sagittal vertical axis (SVA). By convention, when the SVA falls behind the L5–S1 disc space, the SVA is considered negative. When the SVA falls through the L5–S1 disc, the SVA is considered neutral. When the SVA fall in front of the L5–S1 disc, the SVA is considered positive. In normal patients, the SVA is usually neutral or negative. In the normal patient, the SVA passes anterior to the thoracic spine, through the center of the L1 vertebral body, posterior to the lumbar spine, and through the posterior corner of S1.

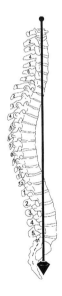

FIGURE 15. Measurement of spinal balance. (From Devlin VJ, Narvaez JC: Imaging strategies for spinal deformities. Spine State Art Rev 12:1, 1998, with permission.)

30. What are normal values for the sagittal curves (Fig. 16) of the different spinal regions?

Cervical region. Cervical lordosis (occiput–C7) averages 40°, with the majority of cervical lordosis occurring at the C1–C2 motion segment.

Thoracic region. Normal kyphosis (T1–T12) in young adults ranges from 20° to 50° with a tendency to increase slightly with age. The kyphosis in the thoracic region usually starts at T1–T2 and gradually increases at each level toward the apex (T6–T7 disc). Below the thoracic apex, segmental kyphosis gradually decreases until the thoracolumbar junction is reached.

Thoracolumbar region. The thoracolumbar junction (T12-L1) is essentially straight with respect to the sagittal plane. It serves as the transition area between the relatively stiff kyphotic thoracic region and the relatively mobile lordotic lumbar region.

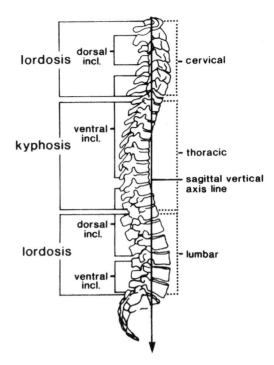

FIGURE 16. The sagittal curves of the spine. (From De Wald RL: Revision surgery for spinal deformity. In Eilert RE (ed): Instructional Course Lectures, vol. 41 Rosemont, IL, American Academy of Orthopaedic Surgeons, 1992, p 241, with permission.)

Lumbar region. Normal lumbar lordosis (L1–S1) ranges from 30° to 80° with a mean lordosis of 60°. Lumbar lordosis generally begins at L1–L2 and gradually increases at each distal level toward the sacrum. The apex of lumbar lordosis is normally located at the L3–L4 disc space.

31. Describe the relationship between thoracic kyphosis and lumbar lordosis in normal patients.

The relationship between these two sagittal curves is such that lumbar lordosis generally exceeds thoracic kyphosis by 20–30° in a normal patient. This relationship allows the body to maintain normal sagittal balance and maintain the sagittal vertical axis(SVA) in a physiologic position. The body attempts to maintain the SVA in its physiologic position through a variety of compensatory mechanisms. Functionally, the sacrum and pelvis can be considered as one vertebra (pelvic vertebra), which functions as an intercalary bone between the trunk and the lower extremities. Motion of the hip joints and lumbar spine can alter sacral inclination and, in this manner, alter the sagittal orientation of the base of the spine. This permits the body to compensate for increased thoracic kyphosis by increasing lumbar lordosis.

32. What radiographic hallmarks indicate a flatback syndrome?

Flatback syndrome is a sagittal malalignment syndrome. Radiographically the hallmarks of flatback syndrome include a markedly positive sagittal vertical axis and decreased lumbar lordosis after a spinal fusion procedure. Classically, it has been reported after use of a straight Harrington distraction rod to correct a lumbar or thoracolumbar curvature. When the thoracic and lumbar spine is fused in a nonphysiologic alignment with loss of lumbar lordosis, the patient cannot assume normal erect posture and assumes instead a stooped forward posture. The patient attempts to compensate for this abnormal posture by hyperextending the hip joints and flexing the knee joints. These compensatory mechanisms are ultimately ineffective in maintaining the SVA in a physiologic position and result in symptoms of back pain, knee pain, and inability to maintain an upright posture.

BIBLIOGRAPHY

1. Bernhardt M, Bridwell KH: Segmental analysis of the sagittal plane alignment of the normal thoracic and lumbar spine and lumbosacral junction. Spine 14: 717–721, 1989.
2. Devlin VJ, Narvaez JC: Imaging strategies for spinal deformities. Spine State Art Rev 12:1, 1998.
3. Katz DS, Math KR, Groskin SA: Radiology Secrets. Philadelphia, Hanley & Belfus, 1998.
4. Kricum ME (ed): Imaging Modalities in Spinal Disorders. Philadelphia, W.B. Saunders, 1988.
5. Lonstein JE: Patient evaluation. In Lonstein JE, Bradford DS, Winter RB, Ogilvie JW (eds): Moe's Textbook of Scoliosis and Other Spinal Deformities, 3rd ed. Philadelphia, W.B. Saunders, 1995, pp 45–86.

10. MAGNETIC RESONANCE IMAGING OF THE SPINE

Vincent J. Devlin, M.D.

1. How is a magnetic resonance (MR) scan produced?

The hydrogen atoms (protons) in the human body are single charged atoms spinning on random axes such that the body's total magnetic field is zero. During an MR scan, the patient is placed in a magnetic field that causes the hydrogen nuclei to align parallel with the magnetic field. Application of radiofrequency(RF) pulses cause the hydrogen nuclei to enter a higher energy state. When the RF pulses are terminated, the excited hydrogen nuclei release energy and return to a lower energy state in a process termed **relaxation**. The energy released during this transition is detected by the MR receiver coil. Signal data are processed in terms of origin within the imaging plane and subseqently displayed on a monitor. The time between RF pulses is termed the **repetition time** (TR). The time between the application of RF pulses and the recording of the MR signal is termed the **echo time** (TE). The process of relaxation is described in terms of two independent time constants called T1 and T2.

2. What is signal intensity?

Signal intensity describes the brightness of tissues on an MR image. Tissues may be described as high-intensity(bright), intermediate-intensity(gray), or low-intensity(dark). When the tissue intensity of a pathologic process is described relative to the intensity of surrounding normal tissue, it may be described as hyperintense, isointense, or hypointense. MR signal intensity depends on the T1, T2, and proton density (number of mobile hydrogen ions) of the tissue under evaluation.

3. Explain the differences between T1-, T2-, and proton density-weighted MR images.

T1 (longitudinal relaxation time) and T2 (horizontal relaxation time) are intrinsic physical properties of tissues. Different tissues have different T1 and T2 properties based on how their hydrogen nuclei respond to radiofrequency pulses during the MR scan. Proton density refers to the number of mobile hydrogen ions in the tissue under evaluation. Image contrast of an MRI is determined by varying the scanning parameters (TE and TR) to emphasize the relative contributions of T1, T2, and proton density.

T1 images are produced with a short TR (< 1000 msec) and a short TE (< 30 msec). T1 images are weighted toward fat. Fat appears bright on T1 images and less bright on T2 images. T1-weighted images are excellent for evaluating structures containing fat, hemorrhage, or proteinaceous fluid, all of which have a short T1 and demonstrate a high signal on T1-weighted images. T1 images demonstrate anatomic structures well because of their high signal-to-noise ratio.

T2 images are produced with a long TR (> 1500 msec) and a long TE (> 45 msec). T2 images are weighted toward water. Water appears bright on T2 images and dark on T1 images (mnemonic: water [H_2O] is bright on T2). Signal intensity on T2 images is related to the state of tissue hydration. Tissue with a high water content (cerebrospinal fluid, cysts, normal intervertebral disc) shows an increased signal on T2 images. T2 images are most useful for contrasting normal and abnormal anatomy. In general, pathologic processes (e.g., neoplasm, infection) are associated with increased water content and appear hyperintense on T2 images and hypointense on T1.

Proton density images or spin density-weighted images are produced with a long TR (> 1500 msec) and short TE (15–30 msec). Signal intensity on proton density images is related to the absolute number of mobile hydrogen ions in the tissue.

4. Describe the signal intensity of common tissue types on T1- and T2-weighted MR images.

Mineralized tissue (e.g., bone) shows low signal intensity on both T1 and T2 images because it contains few mobile hydrogen ions. Gas contains no mobile hydrogen ions and does not generate an MR signal. The relative signal intensities of different tissue types on T1- and T2-weighted images are summarized below.

TISSUE	APPEARANCE ON T1	APPEARANCE ON T2
Fat	Bright	Intermediate
Normal fluid (e.g., CSF)	Low–intermediate	Bright
Cortical bone	Low	Low
Tendon/ligament	Low	Low
Fibrocartilage	Low	Low
Hyaline cartilage	Intermediate	High
Muscle	Intermediate	Intermediate
Fat	High	Intermediate
Red marrow	Low	Intermediate
Yellow marrow	High	Intermediate
Intervertebral disc (central)	Intermediate	Bright
Intervertebral disc (peripheral)	Low	Intermediate
Osteomyelitis	Low	High
Benign neoplasm	Low–intermediate	Low–intermediate (occasionally high)
Malignant neoplasm	Low–intermediate	Intermediate–high (occasionally low)
Marrow edema	Low	High

CSF = cerebrospinal fluid.

5. How do I know whether I am looking at a T1- or T2-weighted image?

One method is to look at the TE (time to echo) and TR (time to repetition) numbers on the scan.

IMAGE TYPE	TE	TR
T1	15–30 ms	400–600ms (< 1000)
T2	60–120 ms	1500–3000 ms (> 1000)
Proton density	15–30 ms	1500–2000 ms

A simpler method is to recall the signal characteristics of water and fat. Locate a fluid-containing structure(e.g., CSF surrounding the spinal cord). If the fluid is bright, the image is probably a T2–weighted image. If the fluid is dark, the image is probably a T1-weighted image. If the fluid looks bright but the remainder of the image does not look T2-weighted and the TE and TR are low, the image is probably a gradient echo image.

The above criteria refer to the most basic pulse sequence, spin echo (SE). In other pulse sequences, contrast phenomenology is somewhat more complex.

6. What are pulse sequences?

The term *pulse sequence* refers to a specific method for collecting MR data. The SE pulse sequence is commonly used and is obtained by varying the TR and TE as described above. New techniques have been developed to decrease scan time and artifact and to improve visualization of specific pathologic processes. Examples include fast-spin echo imaging, gradient echo imaging, and short time inversion recovery (STIR) imaging. Explanation of these sequences is beyond the scope of this chapter and is not required for basic clinical interpretation of spine pathology.

7. What are the contraindications to obtaining an MR scan?

MR scans are contraindicated in patients with implanted devices that may be subject to magnetically induced malfunction or potentially harmful movement. Examples include certain cochlear and ocular implants, cardiac pacemakers, certain prosthetic heart valves, implanted pain pumps or bone growth stimulators, brain aneurysm clips, carotid clips, certain Swan-Ganz catheters, periorbital metal fragments, and certain penile prostheses. Pregnancy is considered by some to be a relative contraindication to MRI during the first trimester

Spinal fixation devices are not a contraindication to MRI. However, if these implants are located near the intended site of imaging, significant image artifacts may result and render the scan useless. It is still possible to obtain useful imaging information at spinal segments above and below the instrumented segments. The type of implant metal is also an important consideration. Useful imaging information can be achieved in certain cases in the presence of titanium implants. Stainless steel implants generally create excessive artifact, and a computed tomography (CT) or CT-myelogram study is required to evaluate patients with stainless steel spinal implants.

8. Describe the normal appearance of critical bone and soft tissue structures on MR scans of the cervical spine.

See Figure 1.

9. Describe the important anatomic structures of the thoracic spine on MR scans.

See Figure 2.

10. What anatomic structures should be routinely assessed on an MR study of the lumbar spine?

See Figure 3.

11. When is a screening MRI study indicated for evaluation of the spine?

A screening MRI visualizes the entire spinal cord and vertebral column from foramen magnum to distal sacrum. A screening MRI is indicated to evaluate patients with spinal deformities known to be associated with abnormalities of the neural axis. Examples include left thoracic scoliosis, juvenile scoliosis, congenital scoliosis, and myelodysplasia. Pathologic conditions that may be detected in such patients include syrinx, Arnold-Chiari malformation, diastematomyelia, spinal cord tumor, tethered spinal cord, and congenital spinal stenosis.

A screening MRI also may be valuable in the assessment of patients with metastatic spinal tumor to rule out multifocal spinal involvement before surgical intervention.

12. A 9-year-old girl presents with a 50° left thoracic scoliosis and complains of pain in the upper thoracic region. The screening MRI is shown below. What is the diagnosis?

See Figure 4.

13. Define the terms used to describe abnormal disc morphology on MR studies.

Annular tear: a disruption of the ligament surrounding the periphery of the disc.

Bulge: extension of disc tissue beyond the disc space with a diffuse, circumferential, nonfocal contour.

Protrusion: displaced disc material extending focally and asymmetrically beyond the disc space. The displaced disc material is in continuity with the disc of origin. The diameter of the base of the displaced portion, where it is continuous with the disc material within the disc space of origin, has a greater diameter than the largest diameter of the disc tissue extending beyond the disc space.

Extrusion: displaced disc material extending focally and asymmetrically beyond the disc space. The displaced disc material has a greater diameter than the disc material maintaining continuity (if any) with the disc of origin.

Sequestration: a fragment of disc that has no continuity with the disc of origin. Another commonly used term is free disc fragment. By definition, all sequestered discs are extruded; however, not all extruded discs are sequestered.

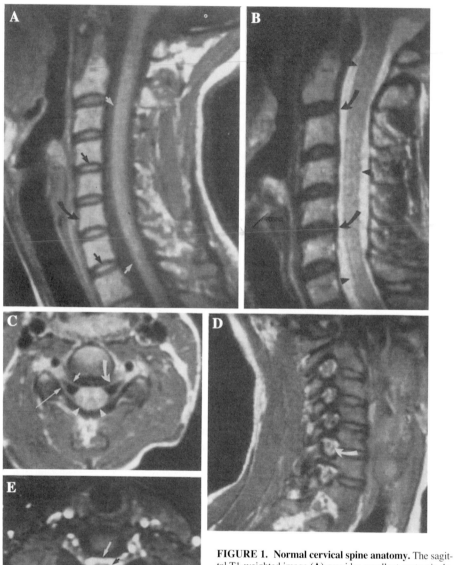

FIGURE 1. Normal cervical spine anatomy. The sagittal T1-weighted image **(A)** provides excellent anatomic delineation of the vertebral bodies *(curved black arrows)*, intervertebral discs *(straight black arrows)*, and spinal cord *(white arrows)*. On the sagittal cardiac gated T2-weighted image **(B)**, a myelographic effect is created by the increased signal intensity in the cerebrospinal fluid (CSF). There is an excellent interface between the posterior margin of the discovertebral joints *(curved black arrows)* and the cerebrospinal fluid as well as excellent delineation of the spinal cord *(black arrowheads)*. The axial T1-weighted image **(C)** provides excellent delineation of the spinal cord *(white arrowheads)*, ventral *(short white arrow)* and dorsal *(long white arrow)* nerve roots, and the intervertebral canals *(curved white arrow)*. On the oblique T1-weighted image **(D)**, the fat in the intervertebral canals outlines the neural *(curved arrow)* and vascular structures. On the axial gradient echo image **(E)**, the high signal intensity of the CSF produces excellent contrast for the delineation of the spinal cord *(black arrow)* and the posterior margin of the discovertebral joint *(white arrow)*. (From Herzog RJ: State of the art imaging of spinal disorders. Phys Med Rehabil State Art Rev 4:230, 1990, with permission.)

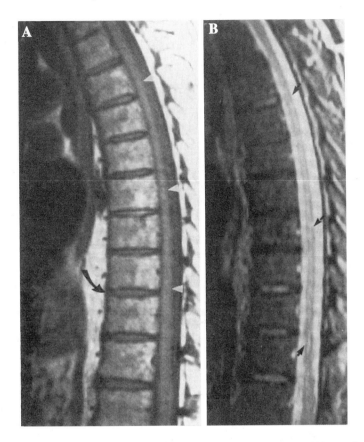

FIGURE 2. Normal thoracic spine anatomy. The sagittal T1-weighted image **(A)** provides excellent anatomic delineation of the vertebral bodies, intervertebral discs *(curved black arrow)*, and spinal cord *(white arrowheads)*. On the sagittal cardiac-gated T2-weighted image **(B)**, the myelographic effect results in an excellent CSF–extradural interface along with delineation of the thoracic spinal cord *(black arrows)*. (From Herzog RJ: State of the art imaging of spinal disorders. Phys Med Rehabil State Art Rev 4:231, 1990, with permission).

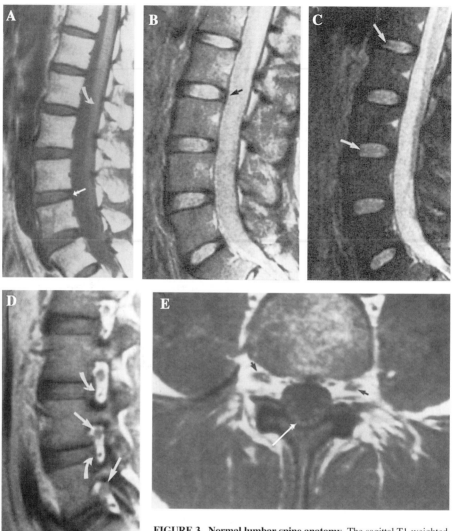

FIGURE 3. Normal lumbar spine anatomy. The sagittal T1-weighted image **(A)** provides excellent delineation of the vertebral bodies, intervertebral discs, thecal sac, lower thoracic cord, and conus medullaris *(curved white arrow)*. The high signal intensity of the vertebral bodies is secondary to the fat in the cancellous marrow. The interface between the posterior outer annular fibers *(straight white arrow)* and the CSF is not well defined. On the sagittal proton-density weighted image **(B)**, increased signal intensity in the disc is identified, along with increased signal intensity of the CSF. This results in improved delineation of the posterior annular–posterior longitudinal ligament complex *(arrow)*. On the sagittal T2-weighted image **(C)**, increased signal intensity in the disc is identified, along with a linear horizontal area of decreased signal intensity in the center of the disc representing the intranclear cleft *(arrows)*. Increased signal intensity in the CSF creates a myelographic effect and provides an excellent CSF–extradural interface. The sagittal T1-weighted image **(D)** through the intervertebral canals provides excellent delineation of the dorsal root ganglia *(straight white arrows)* positioned subjacent to the vertebral pedicles. The posterolateral margin of the discs *(curved white arrows)* is well delineated. The axial T1-weighted image **(E)** provides excellent delineation of the individual nerve roots *(long white arrow)* in the thecal sac. The presence of fat in the epidural space and intervertebral canals provides an excellent soft tissue interface to evaluate nerve roots *(short black arrows)*, ligaments, and osseous elements. (From Herzog RJ: State of the art imaging of spinal disorders. Phys Med Rehabil State Art Rev 4:232–233, 1990, with permission.)

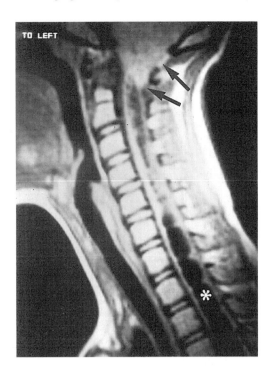

FIGURE 4. Chiari type 1 malformation with an associated syrinx. Chiari type 1 malformation refers to the caudal descent of the cerebellar tonsils below the level of the foramen magnum *(arrow)*. A syrinx is a fluid filled cavity within the spinal cord *(asterisk)*. Symtoms may be due to compression of the medulla at the level of the foramen magnum or to the syrinx. (From Hochhauser L: Miscellaneous conditions of the pediatric central nervous system. In Katz DS, Math KR, Groskin SA (eds): Radiology Secrets. Philadelphia, Hanley & Belfus, 1998, p 429, with permission.)

14. Match each MR image of a disc abnormality with the appropriate description: (1) annular tear, (2) disc bulge, (3) disc protrusion, (4) disc extrusion, and (5) disc sequestration.

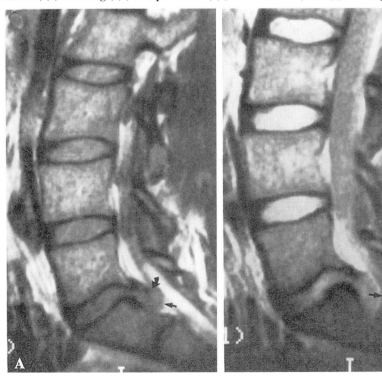

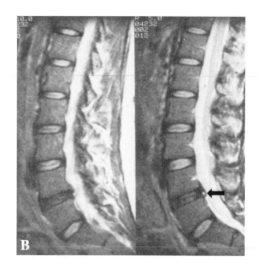

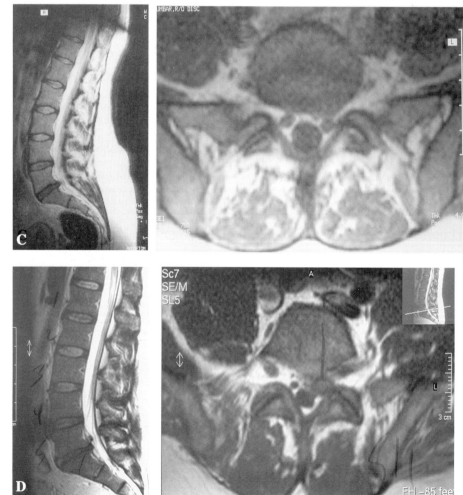

Photograph credits: A, Herzog RJ: State of the art imaging of spinal disorders. Phys Med Rehabil State Art Rev 4:239, 1990. *B,* Gundry CR, Heithoff KB, Pollei SR: Lumbar degenerative disk disease. Spine State Art Rev 9:151, 1995. *C, D,* and *E:* Russo RB: Diagnosis of low back pain: Role of imaging studies. Phys Med Rehabil State Art Rev 13:437–439, 1999.

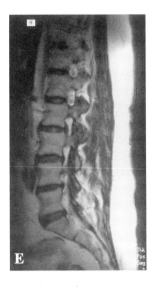

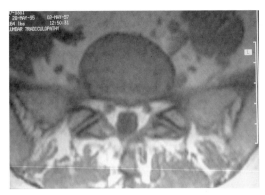

Answers: (1) Annular tear, B; (2) disc bulge, E; (3) disc protrusion, C; (4) disc extrusion, A; (5) disc sequestration, D.

15. Match each cervical MR image with the appropriate description. Each image depicts a patient who presents with symptoms consistent with cervical spinal stenosis.

1. Complex cervical spinal deformity. Cervical kyphosis is associated with posterior spinal cord compression at C2–C4 and anterior spinal cord compression C4–C6.

2. Severe multilevel cervical spinal stenosis due to anterior and posterior cord compression in a patient with severe myelopathy.

3. Single level cervical disc herniation associated with severe spinal cord compression.

4. Multilevel cervical spondylosis superimposed on developmental stenosis. The anteroposterior diameter of the central spinal canal is narrowed on a developmental basis from the C3–C4 level and distally. A cervical disc protrusion is noted at C3–C4, and spondylotic ridges cause mild cord impingement at C4–C5 and C5–C6.

5. Single-level cervical disc protrusion associated with mild spinal cord compression.

6. Congenital stenosis of the cervical spinal canal associated with multilevel disc protrusions and severe multilevel spinal cord compression. Congenital fusion of the C6 and C7 vertebral bodies is noted.

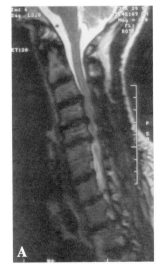

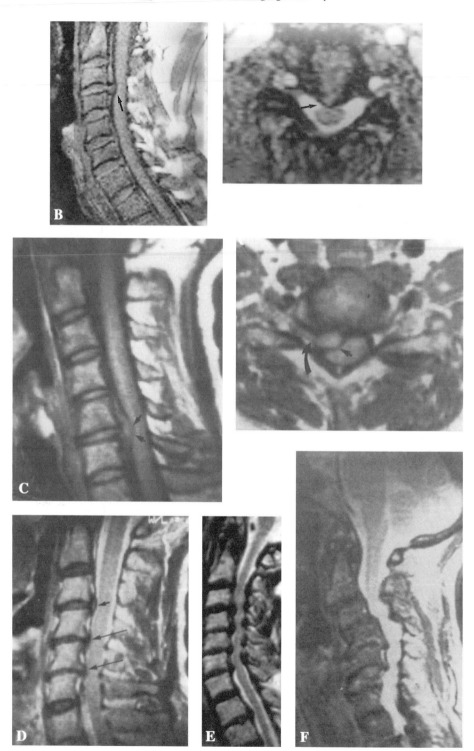

Answers: (1), F; (2), E; (3), C; (4), D; (5), B; (6), A.

16. Match each lumbar MR image with the appropriate description. Each image depicts a patient who presents with symptoms consistent with lumbar spinal stenosis.

1. Ligamentum flavum hypertrophy causing stenosis of the central spinal canal and lateral recess.

2. Hypertrophy of the superior articular process at L5–S1 associated with thickened ligamentum flavum and resulting in front-to-back narrowing of the L5–S1 intervertebral nerve root canal with compression of the L5 ganglion.

3. Synvoial cyst arising from the L4–L5 facet joint, resulting in compression of the left side of the thecal sac and left L5 nerve root.

4. Degenerative spondylolisthesis associated with L4–L5 central spinal stenosis.

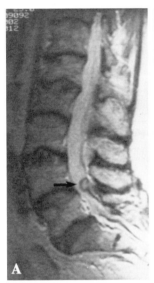
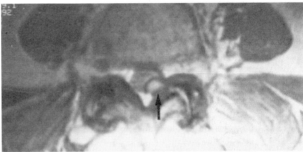

Photograph credits: A and *C,* Gundry CR, Heithoff KB, Pollei SR: Lumbar degenerative disk disease. Spine State Art Rev 9:169, 1995. *B,* Barckhausen RR, Math KR: Lumbar spine diseases. In Katz DS, Math KR, Groskin SA (eds): Radiology Secrets. Philadelphia, Hanley & Belfus, 1998. *D,* Figueroa RE, Stone JA: MR imaging of degenerative spine disease: MR myelography and imaging of the posterior spinal elements. Castillo M (ed): Spinal Imaging: State of the Art. Philadelphia, Hanley & Belfus, 2001.

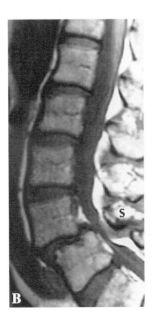
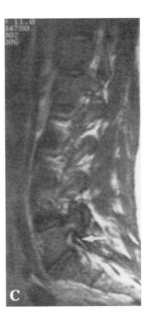

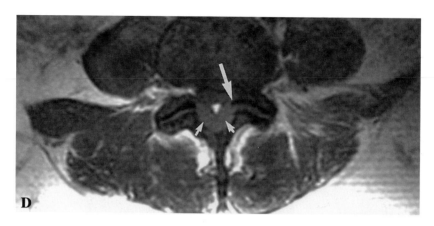

Answers: (1), D; (2), C; (3), A; (4), B.

17. A 50-year-old diabetic man presents with a 2-month history of low back pain refractory to bedrest and analgesics. An MRI (Fig. 8) is obtained by the patient's primary physician, and the patient is referred for consultation. What is the diagnosis?

The imaging findings are classic for a disc space infection. Pyogenic infection typically begins at the vertebral endplates, then involves the disc, and finally spreads to involve the adjacent vertebral bodies. T1-weighted images show decreased signal intensity in the disc and vertebral bodies. T2-weighted images show increased signal intensity in the disc and vertebral bodies. Additional findings that may be present include inflammatory changes in the paravertebral soft tissues and abscess formation in either the epidural space or anterior paravertebral tissues.

18. A 70-year-old woman presents with back pain and a thoracic fracture. She has a history of breast cancer and a documented history of osteoporosis. How can MR scans help determine whether the fracture is the result of osteoporosis or metastatic breast cancer?

Findings on MRI that support a diagnosis of metastatic tumor include abnormal marrow signal in other vertebrae, a convex posterior margin of the vertebral body (i.e., an expanded appearance), and compression of the entire vertebral body, including its posterior third. Additional features supporting a diagnosis of metastatic disease include involvement of the pedicle, presence of an extraosseous soft tissue mass, and diffuse marrow replacement throughout the vertebral body without focal fat preservation (Fig. 9).

Findings on MRI that support a diagnosis of a benign osteoporotic compression fracture include normal or mildly abnormal signal in the fractured vertebral body, a wedge-shaped vertebral body without compression of the posterior third, and a horizontally oriented low signal line paralleling the vertebral body endplate (Fig. 10).

MRI can be useful in determining the age of a vertebral fracture. The presence of marrow edema indicates that the fracture is less than 2 months old. The absence of marrow edema indicates a more chronic fracture.

The MRI findings in acute osteoporotic compression fractures may overlap the findings in cases of malignant collapse. Fracture edema and hemorrhage can surround a vertebral body and give the appearance of a soft tissue mass. Fracture-related edema in acute osteoporotic fractures may cause diffuse vertebral body enhancement similar to the findings in metastatic disease. However, after osteoporotic fractures heal, signal intensities in the collapsed and adjacent normal vertebral bodies are identical. In equivocal cases, a follow-up MR scan can be performed to reassess the bone marrow for resolution of signal abnormalities and reversion to normal fat signal. A CT-guided biopsy is indicated when questions about the cause of a spine fracture remain after imaging studies have been performed.

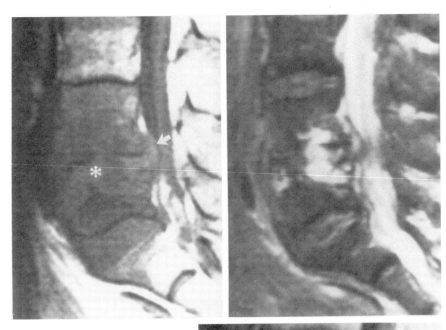

FIGURE 8. MR of *Streptococcus pneumoniae* discitis/osteomyelitis. **Above left,** Sagittal T1-weighted conventional spine-echo (CSE) image reveals an extensive hypointensity involving the L4–L5 disc space (*asterisk*) and the adjacent vertebral bodies. An extradural soft tissue mass compresses the thecal sac (*arrow*). **Above right,** Sagittal T2-weighted CSE image shows mixed hyperintensity and isointensity in the involved L4–L5 intervertebral disc and adjacent vertebrae. **Right,** Sagittal T1-weighted CSE image following gadolinium administration reveals peripheral enhancement of the disc (*straight arrows*) and uniform enhancement of the epidural mass (*curved arrows*), representing discitis and epidural phlegmon. (From Reddy S, Leite CC, Jinkins JRZ: Imaging of infectious disease of the spine. Spine State Art Rev 9:135, 1995, with permission.)

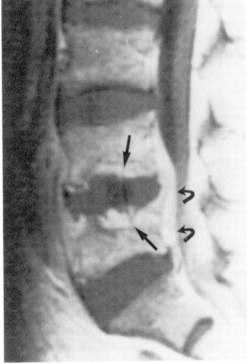

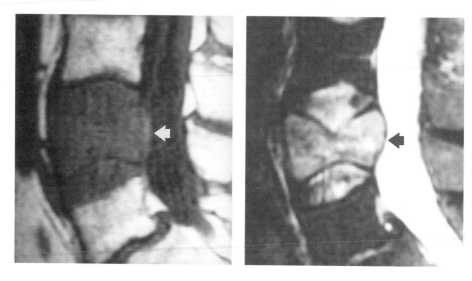

FIGURE 9. Bone metastasis. (From Palmer WE, Suri R: MR differentiation of benign versus malignant collapse. In Castillo M (ed): Spinal Imaging: State of the Art. Philadelphia, Hanley & Belfus, 2001, with permission.)

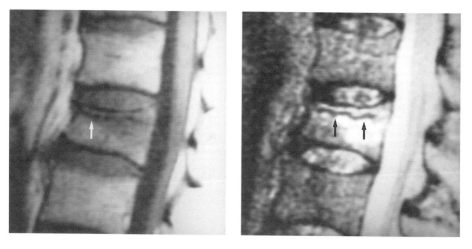

FIGURE 10. Benign osteoporotic compression fracture. (From Palmer WE, Suri R. MR differentiation of benign versus malignant collapse. In Castillo M (ed) Spinal Imaging: State of the Art. Philadelphia, Hanley & Belfus, 2001 with permission.)

BIBLIOGRAPHY

1. Castillo M (ed): Spinal Imaging: State of the Art. Philadelphia, Hanley & Belfus, 2001.
2. Fardon DF, Herzog RJ, Mink JH, et al: Nomenclature of lumbar disc disorders. In Garfin SR, Vaccaro AR (eds): Orthopaedic Knowledge Update–Spine. Oak Ridge, IL, American Academy of Orthopaedic Surgeons, 1997.
3. Fardon DF, Garfin SR, Abitol JJ, et al (eds:) Orthopaedic Knowledge Update–Spine 2. Oak Ridge, IL, American Academy of Orthopaedic Surgeons and North American Spine Society, 2002.
4. Herzog RJ: State of the art imaging of spinal disorders. Phys Med Rehabil State Art Rev 4:221–270, 1990.
5. Katz DS, Math KR, Groskin SA (eds): Radiology Secrets. Philadelphia, Hanley & Belfus, 1998.
6. Weinstein JN, Rydevik BL, Sonntag VKH: Essentials of the Spine. New York, Raven Press, 1995.

11. COMPUTED TOMOGRAPHY AND CT-MYELOGRAPHY

Vincent J. Devlin, M.D.

1. What is computed tomography (CT)?

Computed tomography (CT) is a noninvasive imaging technology that uses x-rays to generate radiographic images in the axial, coronal, or sagittal plane. The x-ray beam passes through the body and interacts with a series of rotating detectors. Cross-sectional images are generated based on mathematical reconstruction of tissue beam attenuation. Images are represented on a gray scale in which the shade of gray is determined by the density of the structure. Dense structures such as bone appear white, less dense structures appear as various shades of gray, and the least dense structures (containing gas) appear black.

2. What are Hounsfield units?

Hounsfield units (HU) measure the relative attenuation or density of a structure imaged on CT. By convention, -1000 is the attenuation for air, 0 for water, and $+1000$ for dense cortical bone. The operator adjusts the level and width of the displayed range of HU (window) to study different tissues optimally.

3. What is a "scout image"?

A scout image (Fig. 1) is the digital radiograph obtained before beginning the formal CT examination. It is used by the operator to select the levels that will be examined with axial CT images. It is also used as a map to guide localization of levels after completion of the scan.

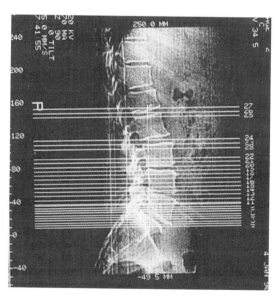

FIGURE 1. CT scout image. (From Gundry CR, Heithoff KB, Pollei SR: Lumbar degenerative disk disease. Spine State Art Rev 9:141–184, 1995, with permission.)

4. Compare the utility of CT and magnetic resonance imaging (MRI) for assessment of cervical radiculopathy.

Cervical radiculopathy typically results from nerve root impingement in the neural foramen by disc material, bone spurs, or a combination of osseous and disc pathology. MRI is the optimal test for visualizing disc material as well as adjacent neural structures and is generally the first test obtained in the evaluation of cervical radiculopathy. CT is the optimal test for visualizing osseous pathology responsible for radiculopathy but does not optimally visualize the spinal cord and nerve roots (Fig. 2). Use of intrathecal contrast can enhance the ability of CT to visualize adjacent soft tissue and neural structures but requires an invasive procedure.

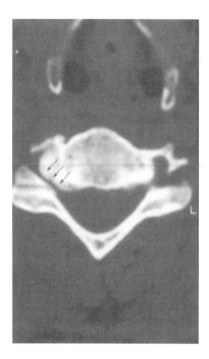 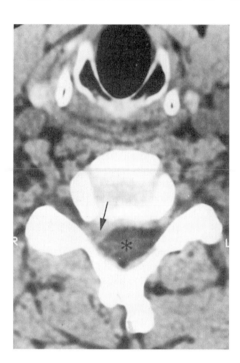

FIGURE 2. CT evaluation of cervical radioculopathy. **Left,** Noncontrast CT demonstrating right-side posterolateral and foraminal disc extrusion compressing the ventral spinal cord and exiting nerve root within the neural foramen. **Right,** Noncontrast CT demonstrating narrowing of the nerve root canal secondary to osteophyte formation. (From Pollei SR, Gundry CR: Cervical and thoracic degenerative disk disease. Spine State Art Rev 9:185–210, 1995, with permission.)

5. Compare the utility of CT-myelography and MRI for assessment of cervical myelopathy.

After plain radiographs are obtained, MRI is usually the next test obtained in the evaluation of cervical myelopathy. MRI provides a noninvasive means of visualizing the entire cervical spine, including the discs, vertebra, spinal cord, and nerve roots, in multiple planes. CT-myelography plays a role when MRI is contraindicated or when osseous pathology contributes to spinal canal encroachment (Fig. 3).

6. Compare the utility of CT and MRI for assessment of lumbar disc pathology.

Both CT (Fig. 4) and MRI are useful techniques for diagnosis of lumbar disc pathology. Both can be used to define disc contour abnormalities (bulge, protrusion, extrusion, sequestration) and guide treatment (see Chapter10, question 13). The most significant difference between these imaging modalities is the ability of MRI to depict changes in disc pathoanatomy and chemistry (e.g., disc dessication, annular tears) before changes in disc contour. For this reason, MRI is the imaging modality of first choice for assessment of lumbar disc pathology.

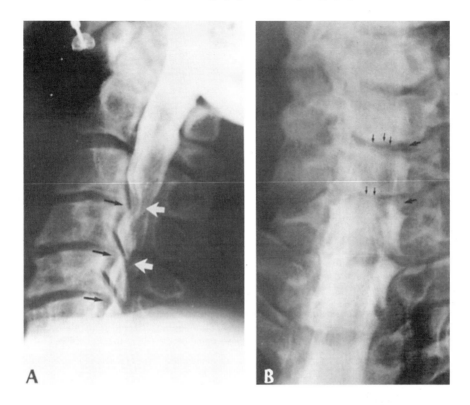

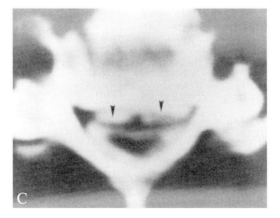

FIGURE 3. Evaluation of cervical myelopathy with CT-myelography. Lateral **(A)** and anteroposterior **(B)** cervical myelogram images. Large osteophytes (*large arrows*) arising posteriorly create severe central stenosis and marked cord compression (*white arrows*) and are best seen on the lateral view. The nerve root sheath cut-off (*medium arrows*) and root compression are better shown on the anteroposterior view. The very small arrows on the AP view mark the location of the large osteophytes on the lateral view. **C,** Axial CT following myelopathy demonstrates posterior osteophytes (*arrowheads*) displacing the contrast-filled thecal sac posteriorly and narrowing the central canal. (From Pollei SR, Gundry CR: Cervical and thoracic degenerative disk disease. Spine State Art Rev 9:185–210, 1995, with permission.)

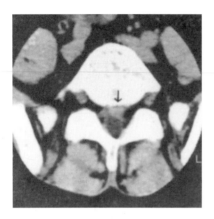 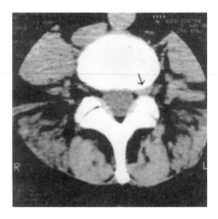

FIGURE 4. CT assessment of lumbar disc pathology. **Left,** CT shows an L5–S1 central and midline disc extrusion (*arrow*). **Right,** CT shows an L4–L5 disc extrusion (*arrow*) extending into the left L4–L5 intervertebral foramen.

7. How is lumbar spinal stenosis defined and described on CT and MRI?

Lumbar spinal stenosis refers to any type of bone or soft tissue pathology that results in narrowing or constriction of the spinal canal, nerve root canal, or both. Central spinal stenosis refers to compression in the region of the spinal canal occupied by the thecal sac. Lateral stenosis involves the nerve root canal and is described in terms of three zones, using the pedicle as a reference point (Fig. 5). Spinal stenosis may involve a single spine segment or multiple spinal segments. It may or may not be associated with instability of the spine.

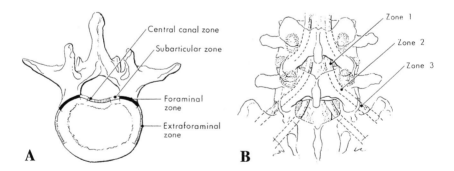

FIGURE 5. Anatomic description of spinal stenosis. Axial **(A)** and sagittal **(B)** views demonstrate the anatomic relationships of the thecal sac and nerve roots to the surrounding osseous structures and intervertebral disc. The nerve root may be compressed along its course through the subarticular zone (zone 1), the foraminal zone (zone 2), and the extraforaminal zone (zone 3). In zone 3, the nerve root may be compressed as it exits the nerve root canal or even further laterally in the so-called far-lateral region. (From Devlin VJ: Degenerative lumbar spinal stenosis and decompression. Spine State Art Rev 11:107–128, 1997, with permission.)

8. A 65-year-old woman presents with symptoms of back pain and neurogenic claudication. Available imaging studies include a lateral myelogram image (Fig. 6A) and an axial CT images (Fig. 6B). What is the patient's diagnosis? Explain what neural structures are compressed.

The clinical and radiographic findings are classic for L4–L5 degenerative spondylolisthesis (grade 1). The lateral myelogram image shows an intact neural arch at the level of spondylolisthesis, leading to the diagnosis of degenerative spondylolisthesis. Disc degeneration and subluxation with subsequent facet joint and ligamentum flavum hypertrophy result in central spinal stenosis (open arrow and opposing arrows) and zone 1 (subarticular) lateral canal stenosis (small arrows). L4–L5 degenerative spondylolisthesis typically results in central spinal stenosis at the L4–L5 level associated with compression of the traversing L5 nerve roots bilaterally. The exiting L4 nerve roots are not typically involved unless there is advanced loss of disc space height, at which time the L4 nerve roots become compressed in the region of the neural foramen. Degenerative spondylolisthesis does not progress past a grade 2 (50%) slip unless prior surgery has been performed at the level of listhesis.

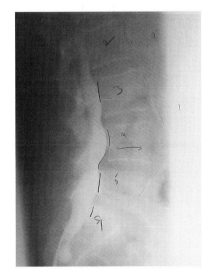

FIGURE 6A. Lateral myelographic view.

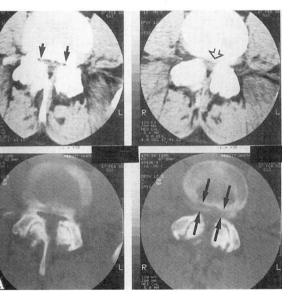

FIGURE 6B. Axial CT scan at the L4–5 level. (From Cole AJ, Herring SA: The Low Back Pain Handbook. Philadelphia, Hanley & Belfus, 1997.)

9. A 45-year-old woman presents with symptoms of back pain and lower extremity radiculopathy. Available imaging studies include a standing lateral radiograph (Fig. 7A) and an axial CT scan (Fig. 7B). What is the patient's diagnosis? Explain what neural structures are compressed.

The diagnosis is L4–L5 isthmic spondylolisthesis (grade 1). A defect in the pars interarticularis is present on the lateral radiograph and axial CT scan. Typically, isthmic spondylolisthesis does not result in central spinal stenosis at the level of listhesis. Isthmic spondylolisthesis is associated with radiculopathy due to irritation of the exiting nerve root (in this case, the L4 root). The exiting nerve root can be irritated by fibrocartilage build-up at the level of the pars, forward traction on the root itself, or compression between a disc bulge and the adjacent pedicle.

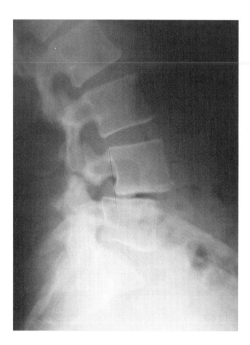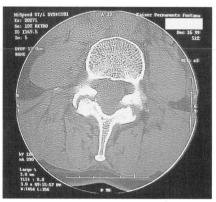

FIGURE 7. Left, Lateral radiograph. **Right,** Axial CT.

10. Compare the use of CT and MRI for assessment of spinal tumors and spinal infections.

MRI is the optimal test for initial evaluation of spinal tumor and infection after plain radiographs have been obtained. MRI provides information about the spinal canal, disc, bone, and surrounding soft tissues that may not be evident on CT. CT plays a role in determining the extent of bone destruction due to infection or tumor (Fig. 8). This determination is important in determining the risk of vertebral fracture and in planning surgical treatment.

11. What is the role of CT in assessment of spinal trauma?

After initial plain radiographs, CT is the next imaging study obtained. The complex osseous anatomy of the spine is not visualized in sufficient detail on plain radiographs and CT scan is required to accurately classify spinal fractures. MRI plays a complementary role to CT in the assessment of ligamentous injury and neurologic compression syndromes in the spine trauma patient.

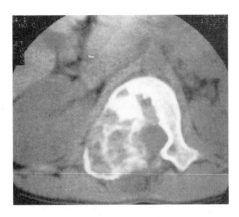

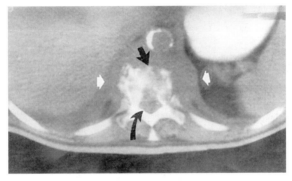

FIGURE 8. Top, Spinal tumor. CT scan at the L1 level in a 9-year-old boy with an aneurysmal bone cyst involving the lamina, pedicle, and vertebral body with expansion of the cortex. **Bottom,** Spinal infection. Axial CT scan of a patient with pyogenic spondylitis shows marked bony fragmentation (*straight arrow*), extension of the paraspinal mass across the complete anterior extent of the vertebral body (*white arrows*), and extension of the process into the spinal canal (*curved arrow*).

12. What problems can be diagnosed with CT after a lumbar decompression and spinal fusion with instrumentation? When should a myelogram be added?

A CT scan can provide critical information after a fusion procedure with spinal implants. A myelogram should be performed in conjunction with the CT scan if it is necessary to assess the spinal canal and nerve root canals at the operative site. Problems that can be diagnosed with CT with or without myelograpy include:

- Incorrect placement of spinal implants such as pedicle screws, interbody grafts, or fusion cages
- Failure of spinal fusion (pseudarthrosis) (see Fig. 9)
- Persistent neural compression

13. A 65-year-old woman underwent an L4–S1 laminectomy and fusion and posterior spinal fixation 7 years ago. The patient did well until the past year when she reported the gradual return of low back, buttock pain and new-onset anterior thigh pain. A myelogram followed by CT scan was obtained (Fig. 10). What is the most likely diagnosis?

The patient's history and imaging findings are consistent with a transition syndrome. After a spinal fusion procedure, increased stress on the adjacent spinal segments can lead to adjacent level degenerative changes with subsequent spinal stenosis and spinal instability. The myelogram shows spondylolisthesis and spinal stenosis at L3–L4 and is consistent with a transition syndrome.

14. What questions should be considered before ordering a CT-myelogram study of the spine?

1. Can the pertinent clinical question be answered with noninvasive diagnostic imaging, such as MRI or a combination of MRI and CT?

2. Are the patient's symptoms sufficiently severe to warrant surgical intervention and is the patient accepting of surgical treatment if it is offered?

3. Does the patient have any history of adverse reaction to iodinated contrast media or any conditions that increase the risk of an adverse reaction to these agents? Some factors considered to increase the risk of a reaction to iodinated contrast include renal insufficiency, diabetic nephropathy, significant cardiac or pulmonary disease, asthma, multiple allergies, and patients at the extremes of age.

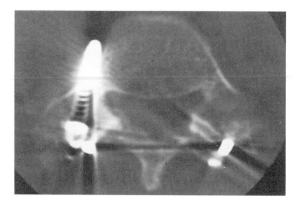

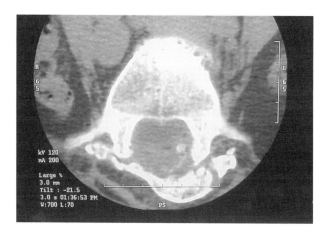

FIGURE 9. Top, Right-sided pedicle screw is improperly placed because it is not contained within bone and impinges on the adjacent nerve root. **Bottom,** Pseudarthrosis following unsuccessful lumbar fusion.

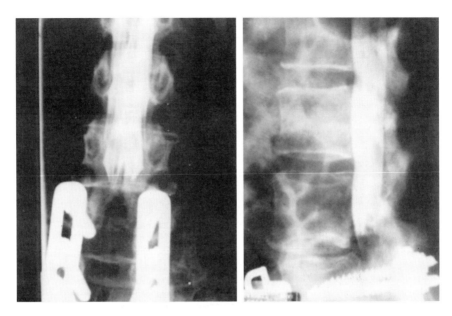

FIGURE 10. Anteroposterior (**left**) and lateral (**right**) myelographic views. (From Gundry CR, Heithoff KB, Pollei SR: Imaging of the preoperative lumbar spine. Spine State Art Rev 9:211–243, 1995, with permission.)

15. What types of adverse reactions can occur during a CT-myelogram- procedure?

Initially patients may experience discomfort during intrathecal injection of the nonionic water soluble contrast agent. After injection, patients may experience an anaphylactoid (idiosyncratic) reaction (urticaria, facial and laryngeal edema, bronchospasm, hypotension) or a nonidiosyncratic reaction due to the adverse effect of contrast on a specific organ system (nephrotoxicity, cardiac arrhythmia, myocardial ischemia, vasovagal reaction). Specific treatment depends on the exact clinical circumstance.

BIBLIOGRAPHY

1. Cole AJ, Herring SA: The Low Back Pain Handbook. Philadelphia, Hanley & Belfus, 1997.
2. Herzog RJ: Radiologic imaging of the spine. In Weinstein JN, Rydevik BL, Sonntag VKH (eds): Essentials of the Spine. New York, Raven Press, 1995, pp 111–138.
3. Katz DS, Math KR, Groskin SA (eds): Radiology Secrets. Philadelphia, Hanley & Belfus, 1998.
4. Lee RR (ed): Spinal Imaging. Spine State Art Rev 9:1, 1995.

12. NUCLEAR IMAGING AND SPINAL DISORDERS

Vincent J. Devlin, M.D., and Edwin Yeo, M.D.

1. What nuclear medicine studies are useful in the evaluation of spinal problems?

Technetium-99m bone scan is the most commonly used study for detection of osseous lesions of the spinal column. Additional studies that are useful in the diagnosis of spinal infections include the gallium-67 scan, which is preferred over the indium-111 white cell scan for this purpose. The role of positron emission tomography (PET) is evolving and has shown utility in diagnosis of spinal metastatic disease.

2. How is a technetium-99m bone scan performed?

A radiopharmaceutical (technetium-99m, typically attached to a diphosphonate derivative) is administered intravenously and rapidly distributed throughout the body. Before excretion through the renal system, the technetium is adsorbed into the hydroxyapatite matrix of bone. A gamma camera is used to record the distribution of radioactivity throughout the body. Areas of increased osteoblastic activity are detected by an increased concentration of radionuclide tracer. A decrease or absence of radionuclide tracer reflects either an interruption of blood flow or decreased osteoblastic activity.

3. For which common spinal disorders does a bone scan provide useful diagnostic information?

- Metastatic bone disease
- Spondylolysis
- Facet joint arthropathy
- Spinal infections (osteomyelitis, discitis)
- Primary spine tumor (e.g., osteoid osteoma)
- Spine fracture

4. What is a three-phase bone scan?

1. **Flow phase study:** assesses vascular spread of the injected radionuclide and obtained immediately after radionuclide injection. It detects perfusion abnormalities in suspect tissue.

2. **Blood pool phase study:** detects hyperemia in bone and soft tissue due to abnormal pooling of the radionuclide.

3. **Delayed static phase study:** obtained usually 2–3 hours after injection. It can detect abnormal increased uptake in areas of active bone remodeling.

5. What is a SPECT scan?

Single-photon emission computed tomography (SPECT) uses a computer-aided gamma camera and the radionuclides of standard nuclear imaging to provide cross-sectional images similar to those of a computed tomography (CT) scan (Fig. 1). A SPECT study is more sensitive than planar scintigraphy in detecting lesions in the spine. It allows precise localization of spinal lesions to the vertebral body, disc space, or vertebral arch. SPECT scans are ideal for localizing spondylolysis and identifying small lesions such as an osteoid osteoma.

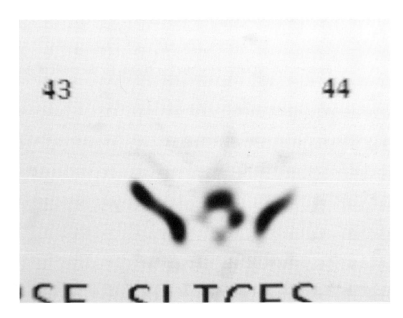

FIGURE 1. Cross-sectional SPECT image at the L5 level showing increased uptake in the left posterior neural arch consistent with spondylolysis.

6. What is the role of nuclear medicine in pediatric patients with back pain?

A bone scan may be considered for patients with normal spinal radiographs and back pain persisting for longer than 6 weeks. A bone scan can diagnose problems such as spinal osteomyelitis and spinal tumor. A bone scan with SPECT images helps to diagnose a stress reaction (impending spondylolysis) or pars fracture in pediatric patients with back pain.

7. What information can a bone scan provide about lumbar spondylolysis?

A bone scan with SPECT images can provide valuable information about lumbar spondylolysis. It can determine whether a spondylolysis detectable by radiography is acute or chronic. In cases in which radiographs are negative, the bone scan can diagnose an impending spondylolysis (stress reaction). In some cases the bone scan may be positive on the side opposite a radiographically detectable pars defect and aids in diagnosis of an impending spondylolysis. Bone scans can also be used to assess healing of an acute spondylolysis.

8. What is the role of nuclear medicine studies in the assessment of adults with back pain?

Serious conditions such as infection or tumor can be identified. Discrete areas of increased uptake in the posterior spinal elements can aid in identification of patients who may benefit from facet injection or other invasive procedures.

9. How does the pattern of radionuclide uptake on a SPECT bone scan aid in the diagnosis of an adult patient with back pain?

Metastatic spine tumors typically involve the posterior portion of the vertebral body as well as the pedicle region. Benign causes of back pain typically spare the pedicle region but involve the posterior elements, disc, or vertebral body

10. What are the advantages of nuclear studies for diagnosis of spinal neoplasms?

A technetium bone scan in association with physical examination and laboratory studies is an effective method for identifying the majority of patients with spinal neoplasms. Technetium bone scans can identify occult lesions and multifocal tumor involvement. In addition, if multiple lesions are detected, a bone scan can help identify the most accessible lesion for biopsy.

11. What pitfalls are associated with the use of nuclear studies for diagnosis of spinal neoplasms?

Technetium bone scans cannot unequivocally distinguish increased uptake due to tumor from increased uptake due to infection or fracture. In addition, certain tumors (e.g., multiple myeloma, hypernephroma) are not likely to demonstrate increased uptake on technetium bone scans because they do not typically stimulate increased osteoblastic activity. PET scanning using FDG (2-deoxy-2-(F18) fluoro-D-glucose) can be useful in symptomatic spinal metastases not identified on radiographs, CT, or technetium bone scan.

12. What is the superscan phenomenon?

The superscan phenomenon occurs when the distribution of disease is so widespread and uniformly distributed that the technetium scan is incorrectly interpreted as negative. Increased radionuclide uptake is noted throughout the skeleton in the presence of diminshed or absent uptake in the kidneys and bladder. This phenomenon can occur with metastatic prostate and breast cancer, renal osteodystrophy, and Paget's disease.

13. What advantages are associated with the use of nuclear studies in the diagnosis of spine infections?

Radionuclide studies can detect a pyogenic infectious process long before plain radiographs demonstrate any abnormality. The combination of a gallium scan and technetium scan has an accuracy greater than 90% in the diagnosis of pyogenic spine infection.

14. What pitfalls are associated with the use of nuclear studies in the diagnosis of spine infections?

Technetium bone scans are flow-dependent studies and may be falsely negative in situations associated with decreased perfusion to target tissues. Gallium scans may be falsely negative in leukopenic patients. Although radionuclide studies are helpful in detection of pyogenic spine infections, a high false-negative rate is associated with their use in the diagnosis of granulomatous infections (e.g., tuberculosis).

15. How can a SPECT bone scan aid in the assessment of patients after lumbar spine surgery?

After lumbar spine surgery, a SPECT bone scan can aid in the diagnosis of pseudarthrosis, facet joint arthrosis, disc space lesions, sacroiliac joint lesions, and vertebral body lesions. For example, a well-healed spinal fusion mass typically has little increased intensity 1 year after surgery. A marked increase in uptake suggests pseudarthosis. Increased uptake adjacent to a fused spinal motion segment suggests facet joint arthrosis and the possibility of a transition syndrome.

16. A 70-year-old women complains of increasing low back and upper sacral pain. A technetium bone scan was obtained (Fig. 2). What is the diagnosis?

The scan shows increased radionuclide activity above the bladder in the sacral area in a H-shaped pattern (Honda sign). Bilateral increased radionuclide uptake in the sacral ala in association with a transverse region of increased radionuclide activity is typical of a sacral insufficiency fracture, most commonly due to osteoporosis.

17. What is the typical pattern on technetium bone scan in a patient with acute vertebral compression fractures secondary to osteoporosis?

The typical appearance of osteoporotic compression fractures on a technetium bone scan (Fig. 3) consists of multiple transverse bands of increased uptake on a posteroanterior image. However, the etiology of the fracture (trauma, tumor, metabolic bone disease) cannot be defini-

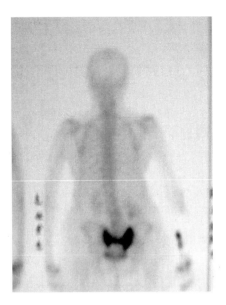

FIGURE 2. Increased radionuclide uptake in sacrum.

tively diagnosed based solely on bone scan. Increased activity can be noted within 72 hours of fracture, and the average time for a bone scan to revert to normal following an osteoporotic vertebral compression fracture is around 7 months.

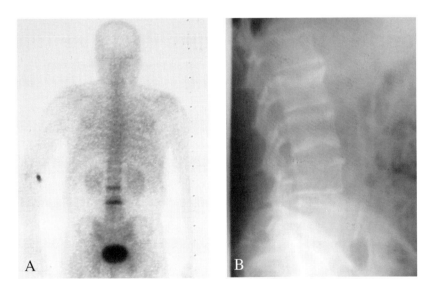

FIGURE 3. Technetium bone scan of multilevel osteoporotic compression fractures.

BIBLIOGRAPHY

1. Henkin RE, Boles MA, Dillehay GL, et al (eds): Nuclear Medicine. St. Louis, Mosby, 1996.
2. Katz DS, Math KR, Groskin SA. Radiology Secrets. Philadelphia, Hanley & Belfus, 1998.
3. Mettler FA, Guiberteau MJ: Essentials of Nuclear Medicine Imaging, 4th ed. Philadelphia, W.B. Saunders, 1998.

IV. Assessment and Nonsurgical Management of Spinal Disorders

13. REHABILITATION MEDICINE APPROACHES TO SPINAL DISORDERS

Anna Lasak, M.D., and Avital Fast, M.D.

1. What is rehabilitation medicine?

Rehabilitation medicine is a medical specialty focused on the prevention, diagnosis, and treatment of acute and chronic diseases of neuromuscular, musculoskeletal, and cardiopulmonary systems. A holistic and comprehensive approach to medical problems is implemented through a coordinated interdisciplinary team. Multiple simultaneous interventions maximize the patient's physical, psychological, social, vocational, and recreational potential, consistent with physiologic or anatomic impairment and environmental limitations. Rehabilitation medicine addresses both the cause and the secondary effects of injury or illness on a person's life. The scope of rehabilitation medicine is broad and includes spinal disorders, musculoskeletal disorders, stroke, cancer, spinal cord injury, cardiac and pulmonary disorders, chronic pain treatment, geriatric rehabilitation, and vocational rehabilitation.

2. List general goals in rehabilitation of patients with spinal disorders.

- Decrease spinal related pain
- Improve strength, flexibility, lifting capacity, and cardiovascular endurance
- Minimize spine-related disability
- Normalize activities of daily living
- Return to work and vocational activities

3. What are "red flags" in the evaluation of spinal pain?

"Red flags" are warning signs of potentially serious conditions. They require special attention and further evaluation (lab tests, imaging studies). A careful history and physical exam are mandatory. Findings such as rest pain, pain at night, extremity numbness or weakness, systemic disease, or bowel or bladder dysfunction should prompt detailed assessment. "Red flags" in evaluation of spinal problems include:

- Fever
- Unexplained weight loss
- Night pain
- Cancer history
- Significant trauma
- Alcohol or drug use
- Age < 20 years
- Age > 50 years
- Osteoporosis
- Failure to improve with treatment

It is also important to recognize patients who are less likely to improve because of psychological or nonmedical problems (e.g., compensation, pending litigation, secondary gain, poor educational level, significant emotional stressors).

4. What components may be included in a nonoperative spine treatment program?

The initial goal of a nonoperative treatment program is pain control. Bedrest for longer than two days is not recommended. Once pain control is achieved, the patient should advance to an exercise program. The ultimate goal of an exercise program is development of adequate dynamic control of the spine to eliminate repetitive injury to pain sensitive structures (e.g., discs, facet joints). Socioeconomic, psychological, and vocational issues are considered during treatment. It is critical to realize that treatment of acute back pain requires a different approach from the treatment of chronic back pain. Components of a nonoperative treatment program for spinal disorders may include:

- Education (optimize biomechanics involved in the activities of daily living)
- Local modalities (heat, ice, ultrasound, transcutaneous electrical nerve stimulation [TENS])
- Medication (analgesics, nonsteroidal anti-inflammatory drugs [NSAIDs], muscle relaxants)
- Injections (trigger point injections, transforaminal and epidural steroid injections)
- Exercise (re-education of range of motion and posture, general strengthening and aerobic exercise, specific spinal exercise [flexion, extension, spinal stabilization], pool therapy)
- Orthoses and assistive devices (braces, canes, walkers, wheelchairs, mobility devices)
- Complementary and alternative therapies (manipulation, myofascial release, accupuncture, prolotherapy)
- Home environment modification (ramps, raised toilet seat, grab bar system for bathroom)
- Ergonomic modifications (chair modification, workstation modification)
- Lifestyle modification (smoking cessation, nutritional counseling, weight reduction)

5. What is the role of therapeutic injections?

Therapeutic injections are used to reduce pain and inflammation and permit initiation of an exercise program.

6. What is the role of physical therapy in treatment of spine disorders?

- Instruction in proper exercise technique
- Advancement of the level of therapy based on the patient's symptoms
- Postural correction
- Administration of modalities
- Spinal manipulation
- Assisting the patient with creation of an individual home exercise program
- Providing supervision, motivation, and goal-setting during a therapy program

7. Discuss the role of physical agents in the treatment of spinal pain.

Physical agents utilize physical forces (e.g., heat, cold, ultrasound, electricity) to speed healing and lessen pain. These agents should not be used in isolation but rather as supplements to a therapy program. Heat and cold provide analgesia and tone reduction. Hydrotherapy uses agitated water to produce convective heating and massage. Immersion in water reduces spinal loads and can be used as an adjunct to an exercise program. Electrical signals (e.g., TENS) can be used to provide analgesia.

8. What is TENS?

Transcutaneous electrical nerve stimulation is the application of small electrical signals to the body via superficial skin electrodes to achieve analgesia. The typical unit consists of a battery, signal generator, and electrode pairs. The exact mechanism of action for TENS is not completely understood. Based on the gate theory of pain, stimulation of large myelinated afferent fibers blocks transmission of pain by small unmyelinated fibers at the level of spinal cord. TENS may also increase endorphin levels in cerebrospinal fluid and enkephalins in the dorsal horn region of the spinal cord. TENS is not a curative modality and should be considered only if other treatment have failed.

9. How is spinal traction used in the treatment of spinal disorders?

The efficacy of traction in treatment of spinal disorders is controversial. Several techniques are available for applying traction to the spine: manual, mechanical (pulley, free weights), gravity (hanging upside down), motorized, and autotraction (a device provides lumbar traction when the patient pulls with the arms). Mechanisms proposed for a positive theraputic effect from traction include distraction of neural foramina and vasa nervorum decompression. Cervical traction can be applied in sitting or supine position with 20–30 lb of traction force. Because approximately 10 lb are required to counteract the weight of the head, cervical traction tends to be more effective in the supine position. Lumbar traction is generally applied in the supine position with 90° of hip and knee flexion. Because of the large forces required to achieve lumbar distraction (50 lb for posterior vertebral separation, 100 lb for anterior vertebral separation), lumbar traction is often poorly tolerated by patients.

10. What are the contraindications to use of traction?

Ligamentous instability, previous spine trauma, osteopenia, pregnancy, spine tumor, and spine infection. Advanced age is a relative contraindication to the use of traction.

11. Which spine patients should be referred for assessment by the psychologist or psychiatrist?

Situations in which referral is indicated include alcohol and drug abuse, depression, noncompliance with treatment, behavioral problems, and traumatic stress syndrome.

12. How can a pain clinic assist in the treatment of spinal disorders?

The pain clinic provides an interdisciplinary program for patients with chronic spinal pain syndromes. The Commission on Accreditation of Rehabilitation Facilities (CARF) pain management guidelines require that the team include a physician, nurse, physical therapist, and psychologist or psychiatrist. Interdisciplinary chronic pain treatment uses the strength of specialists working together. The pain clinic is ideal for the following goals:

- Providing medical management, physical therapy, occupational therapy, vocational therapy, and psychotherapy
- Addressing complex issues related to pain behaviors (e.g., patients being paid for remaining disabled behave differently from patients who are not compensated).
- Identification of psychosocial barriers to treatment (e.g., depression, family distress, anxiety, substance abuse)
- Assessment of the patient's psychological strengths and weaknesses and providing individual or group therapy as indicated.
- Providing disability management with the goal of returning to employment.

13. What are the three levels of nonsurgical care for spinal disorders?

Primary care is applied to patients with acute back and neck pain problems. Symptoms are controlled with medical or surgical management, exercise therapy, medications, modalities, and manual techniques.

Secondary care is applied to patients who did not respond to the initial primary care level of treatment. Such patients require more comprehensive management involving the interdisciplinary care of medical specialists, physical therapists, occupational therapists, psychologists, social workers, and disability managers. During this phase restorative exercise and education are applied to prevent deconditioning and chronic disability. Work-conditioning and work-hardening approaches are included in secondary care.

Tertiary care is indicated for patients who failed primary and secondary conservative care or surgical treatment. Tertiary care or functional restoration involves interdisciplinary team care with all disciplines on site. Functional restoration programs can be provided by some pain clinics. Functional restoration programs include:

- Quantification of physical deconditioning (strength, endurance, aerobic capacity)
- Addressing psychosocial problems (psychopathology, use of narcotics)
- Identification of socioeconomic factors in disability (compensation, psychogenic pain)
- Cognitive behavioral training (relaxation techniques, improve self esteem)
- Restoration of fitness
- Work simulation activities

- Individual, family and group counseling
- Disability and vocational management
- Outcome monitoring

CERVICAL SPINE

14. List the common causes of cervical pain seen in a rehabilitation medicine office practice.
- Myofascial pain
- Cervical spondylosis
- Cervical sprain/strain
- Cervical disc herniation
- Cervical stenosis
- Cervical fractures
- Inflammatory conditions of the spine such as rheumatoid arthritis.

15. Outline a treatment plan for patients with acute neck pain secondary to cervical spondylosis.
Nonoperative options include rest, modalities, isometrics, aerobic conditioning, flexibility exercises, progressive resistance training, disease education, and a home exercise program. Medication (NSAIDs, antidepressants, muscle relaxants) also play a role in treatment.

16. What is the natural history of cervical radiculopathy?
Cervical radiculopathy results from nerve root compression due to a herniated disc and/or cervical spondylosis. In most cases there is no preceding trauma. Patients commonly present with neck pain, headache, and sharp pain radiating to the upper extremity in a dermatomal distribution. Neck movement, cough, and Valsava maneuvers tend to exacerbate pain symptoms. Numbness and paresthesias occur most commonly in the distal part of the involved dermatome. Patients may present with weakness of upper extremity muscles, depending on the specific nerve root that is affected. Other patients present with chronic neck pain, limited neck range of motion, and arm weakness. The majority of patients (70–80%) improve within several weeks. Patients with progressive or persistent neurologic weakness, myelopathy, or intractable pain should be referred for surgical evaluation.

17. Outline a nonsurgical treatment plan for patients with cervical radiculopathy.
- Analgesics, NSAIDs, and possibly a short course of oral steroids
- Soft cervical collar
- Ice, heat
- Massage
- Cervical traction
- Therapeutic injections (cervical epidural injections, trigger point injections)
- Home exercise program
- Ergonomic modifications

18. What is the natural history of cervical spondylotic myelopathy?
Cervical spondylotic myelopathy (CSM) is the most common cause of spinal cord dysfunction in adult patients. Symptoms result from progressive compromise of the spinal cord secondary to degenerative changes in the cervical spine. The first symptoms of CSM are frequently poor balance and lower extremity weakness with resultant gait dysfunction. Patients may also present with gradual weakness and numbness of the hands and fine motor coordination deficits. Some patients may complain of neck pain, although the condition is painless in many patients. Neck flexion may produce a shock-like sensation involving the trunk as well as the upper extremities (Lhermitte's phenomenon). Bowel and bladder function may be affected in later stages of the disease. CSM is a disease with an unpredictable course. Progressive CSM may result in cord ischemia with paralysis due to cervical cord compression. The natural history of CSM has been characterized by long intervals of clinical stability punctuated by short periods of intermittent deterioration in neurologic function.

19. Outline the treatment plan for patients with cervical spondylotic myelopathy.

Nonsurgical management does not alter the natural history of the disease. Surgical intervention is the only treatment that can arrest the progression of CSM and should be considered when feasible. Nonsurgical management may be considered for patients with mild neurologic complaints in the absence of significant disability or patients with advanced CSM whose advanced age and comorbidities significantly increase the risk of surgical intervention. Nonsurgical management may include:

- Immobilization in a cervical collar
- Isometric neck exercises
- Strengthening exercises of upper and lower extremities
- Analgesics, NSAIDs
- Local modalities
- Balance exercises
- Assistive devices (canes, walkers) to minimize risk of falls
- Steroid epidural injections (controversial)
- Education. Patients should be instructed to avoid hyperextension of the cervical spine (e.g., adjust headrest in the car; adjust computer screen and TV set height; avoid using high shelves; avoid painting ceilings; avoid certain sports activities with prolonged neck hyperextension, such as breaststroke swimming). During dental work the dentist should be informed about the neck range-of-motion restrictions; at the hair dresser the patient's face should be positioned toward the sink.

20. What is the treatment of whiplash injury?

Whiplash injury is an acute cervical sprain or strain that results from acceleration and deceleration motion without direct application of force to the head or neck. Whiplash commonly affects the cervical facet joints and related musculature (trapezius, levator scapulae, scalene, sternocleidomastoid, and paraspinals). Although the symptoms of nonradicular neck and shoulder pain are often self-limiting (6–12 months), many people continue to experience chronic symptoms. Treatment options include cervical traction, massage, heat, ice, ultrasound, isometric neck exercises, a soft cervical collar, NSAIDs and/or short-term analgesic use. Patients with persistent pain may have annular tears, coexisting degenerative joint and disc pathology, nerve root entrapment, spinal stenosis, or myelopathy. Neurologic symptoms or intractable pain symptoms that are not responsive to treatment indicate the need for further evaluation.

THORACIC AND LUMBAR SPINE

21. List common causes of thoracic pain seen in a rehabilitation medicine office practice.

- Thoracic sprain/strain
- Myofascial pain
- Compression fracture (usually due to osteoporosis but occasionally due to tumor)
- Thoracic disc pathology (axial pain, radiculopathy, myelopathy)
- Osteoarthritis
- Scheuermann's disease
- Ankylosing spondylitis
- Forrestier's disease (diffuse idiopathic skeletal hyperostosis [DISH])
- Disc space infection
- Scoliosis, kyphosis
- Extraspinal causes (e.g., pancreatitis, peptic ulcer, herpes zoster)

22. Outline a treatment plan for patients with thoracic radiculopathy.

Thoracic radiculopathy may be due to disc herniation or metabolic abnormalities of the nerve root (e.g., diabetes). Patients present with band-like chest pain. Thoracic radiculopathy is not a common diagnosis, and other possible serious pathology should be excluded (malignancy, compression fracture, infection, angina, aortic aneurysm, peptic ulcer disease). Nonsurgical treatment options for thoracic radiculopathy include medication (NSAIDs, narcotics, oral steroids), modalities, TENS, spinal nerve root blocks, spinal stabilization exercises, strengthening of back and abdominal muscles, orthoses, and postural retraining.

23. List some of the common causes of lumbar pain seen in a rehabilitation medicine office practice.

- Lumbar sprain/strain
- Myofascial pain
- Fibromyalgia
- Lumbar spondylosis
- Lumbar radiculopathy
- Lumbar spinal stenosis
- Lumbar spondylolysis and spondylolisthesis
- DISH
- Spondyloarthropathy(ex. ankylosing spondylitis)
- Fracture
- Tumor
- Infection

24. How does the probability of recovery change with time after the onset of low back pain symptoms?

The natural history for recovery after an episode of acute back pain is favorable, with recovery noted in most patients by 6–12 weeks. From the onset of symptoms, 50% of patients recover by 2 weeks, 70% recover by 1 month and 90% recover by 4 months. However, despite the high likelihood of recovery after an episode of acute low back pain, over 50% of patients experience another episode within 1 year. Patients who fail to recover by 4 months frequently progress to long-term chronic disability. Patients with chronic back pain are more difficult to treat than those with acute back pain and require different treatment approaches.

25. Describe a treatment plan for patients with acute low back pain.

The natural history of acute low back pain is improvement over time. Patient reassurance, non-narcotic medication (NSAIDs), and education about back care and exercise are beneficial. Studies suggest that manipulation may decrease pain during the first 3 weeks after onset of symptoms. If pain persists, spinal radiographs should be obtained. Bone scan and/or magnetic resonance imaging (MRI) are indicated if serious underlying pathology is suspected.

26. What is the natural history of a lumbar disc herniation?

The natural history of lumbar disc herniation is quite favorable. Gradual improvement in symptoms over several weeks is noted in the majority of patients. Comparison of nonsurgical and surgical treatment has shown that the major benefit of surgical treatment is quicker relief from sciatic pain symptoms. There is no long-term difference between nonsurgical and surgical treatment.

27. Outline a nonsurgical treatment plan for lumbar radiculopathy due to lumbar disc herniation.

Treatment goals include pain control, reduction of nerve root inflammation, and rapid return to daily activities. Treatment options for achieving these goals include:

- Medication (NSAIDs, analgesics, muscle relaxants, oral steroids)
- Short-term bed rest
- Modalities (ice, TENS, ultrasound, pool therapy)
- McKenzie exercises
- Lumbosacral stabilization program
- Epidural steroid injection, selective nerve root blocks
- Mobilization techniques
- Ergonomic modification
- Patient education (lifting technique, posture, exercise)
- Surgery

28. What is the natural history of lumbar spinal stenosis?

Lumbar spinal stenosis is a potentially disabling condition, caused by compression of the thecal sac (central stenosis) and nerve roots (lateral stenosis). Patients may present with chronic low back pain, leg pain, and/or neurogenic claudication. Pain is characteristically relieved by sitting or flexion of the trunk. In severe cases, patients may develop urinary incontinence from compression of sacral roots. The natural history of lumbar spinal stenosis is generally favorable. In up to two-thirds of patients, lumbar spinal stenosis does not lead to significant deterioration and can be successfully managed with nonsurgical treatment.

29. Outline a treatment plan for a patient with lumbar stenosis.

- Lumbar flexion exercise program (Williams exercises)
- Bicycling
- Uphill treadmill walking
- Physical modalities (heat, cold, electric modalities)
- NSAIDs
- Gabapentin
- Epidural steroid injections

30. What are flexion exercises (Williams exercises)? When they are used?

Examples of flexion exercises include pelvic tilts, knee-to-chest exercises (Fig.1), abdominal crunches, and hip flexor stretches. Flexion exercises are commonly prescribed for facet joint pain, lumbar spinal stenosis, spondylolysis, and spondylolisthesis. Flexion exercises increase intradiscal pressure and are contraindicated in the presence of an acute disc herniation. Flexion exercises are also contraindicated in thoracic and lumbar compression fractures and osteoporotic patients.

Flexion exercises have the following goals:

- Open intervertebral foramina and enlarge the spinal canal
- Stretch back extensors
- Strengthen abdominal and gluteal muscles
- Mobilize the lumbosacral junction

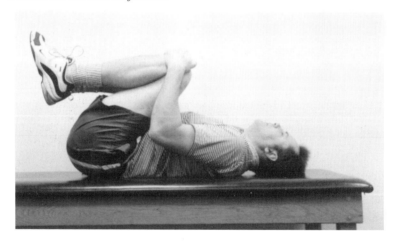

FIGURE 1. Williams exercise: knee to chest.

31. What is the McKenzie exercise approach? How and when is it applied?

McKenzie's exercise philosophy is based on the finding that certain spinal movements may aggravate pain, whereas other movements relieve pain. McKenzie believed that accumulation of flexion forces caused dysfunction of posterior aspect of the disc. Most of McKenzie's exercises are extension-biased. The positions and movement patterns that relieve pain are individually determined for each patient. McKenzie classified lumbar disorders into three syndromes based on posture and response to movement: postural syndrome, dysfunctional syndrome, and derangement syndrome. Each syndrome has a specific treatment and postural correction. Treatment should induce **centralization of the pain** (change in pain location from a distal location in the lower extremity to a proximal or central location). Examples of McKenzie's exercises include:

- Repeat end-range movements while standing: back extension, side gliding (lateral bending with rotation).
- Recumbent end-range movement: passive extension while prone (Fig. 2), prone lateral shifting of hips off midline

McKenzie exercises are most commonly prescribed for disc herniation and lumbar radicular pain.

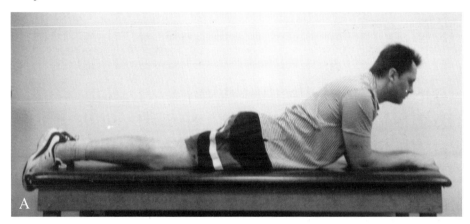

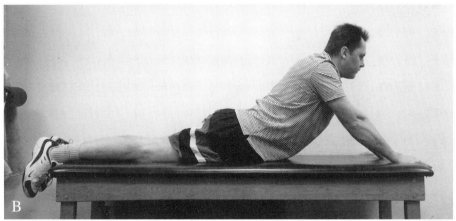

FIGURE 2. A and **B,** McKenzie exercise: passive extension while prone.

32. What are spinal stabilization exercises? When they are used?

Strengthening exercises for a dynamic "corset" of muscle control to maintain a neutral position are known as spinal stabilization exercises. The goal of stabilization exercises is to reduce mechanical stress on the spine. Spinal stabilization exercises can be prescribed for most causes of low back pain. Key concepts of spinal stabilization exercise program include:

- Determination of the functional range (the most stable and asymptomatic position) for all movements
- Strengthening of transversus abdominis (pelvic clock), abdominal obliques (oblique

crunches), rectus abdominis (sagittal plane crunches, supine pelvic bracing with alternating arm and leg raises), gluteus maximus (prone gluteal squeezes, supine pelvic bridging, bridging and marching [Fig. 3]), and gluteus medius (sidestepping),

- Neuromuscular re-education, mobility, and endurance exercises
- Progression of therapy from gross and simple movements to smaller, isolated and complex movements
- Progression to dynamic stabilization exercises (quadriped opposite upper and lower extremity extension [Fig.4], quadriped hip extension and contralateral arm flexion, prone hip extension and contralateral arm flexion, balancing on gymnastic ball, wall slides, squatting, lifting).

33. What is the role of cardiovascular conditioning in low back pain?

Cardiovascular deconditioning develops secondary to inactivity in patients with chronic low back pain. Aerobic training to improve cardiovascular endurance is an extremely important part of rehabilitation of the low back. Heart-rate limitations for patients with known or suspected cardiac disease are based on stress testing. Aerobic training (e.g., treadmill, bike, stepper, arm and leg ergometer, walking, jogging, swimming) has multiple beneficial effects:

- Increases maximal oxygen consumption (VO_2 max)
- Increases cardiac output

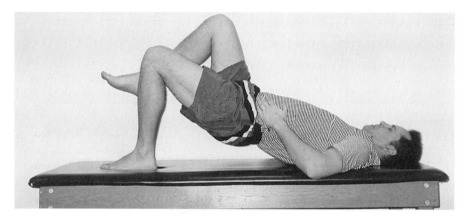

FIGURE 3. Lumbar stabilization exercise: bridging and marching.

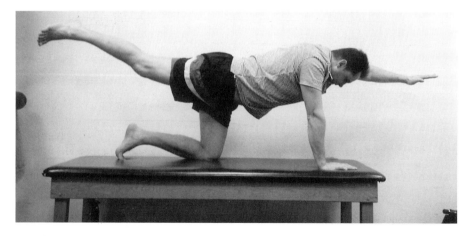

FIGURE 4. Lumbar stabilization exercise: quadriped opposite upper and lower extremity extension.Radiograph

- Increases oxygen extraction
- Improves oxygen utilization by muscle
- Increases endurance, strength and coordination of neuromuscular system
- Increases pain threshold (elevates endorphin levels)
- Decreases depression and anxiety
- Promotes healthy lifestyle
- May prevent work related back injury
- Favorably modifies risk factors for coronary artery disease

34. Define impairment, disability, and handicap.

Impairment is defined as a loss or abnormality of psychological, physical, or anatomic structure or function as determined by medical means. Assessment of impairment is a purely medical determination of deviation from normal health (e.g., weakness of a limb secondary to cervical myelopathy).

Disability is a restriction or inability (resulting from impairment) to perform an activity (e.g., difficulty walking secondary to limb weakness).

Handicap is an inability (resulting from impairment and disability) for a given individual to perform his/her usual interaction with the environment on an appropriate physical, psychological, social, and age level (e.g., inability to climb stairs secondary to limb weakness). A handicap may be overcome by compensating in some way for the impairment (e.g., use of an orthosis or assistive device).

35. How is spinal impairment determined?

Spinal impairment can be evaluated by quantifying spinal range of motion, assessing trunk strength, and determining lifting capacity. Techniques for measuring spinal range of motion include inclinometer, goniometer, modified Schober test, and finger-to-floor distance. There are three basic approaches for testing trunk extensor strength and lifting capacity: isometric (velocity is zero), isokinetic (velocity is constant), and isoinertial (velocity is not constant, but the mass is held constant). Several machines can be used for testing as well as training patients (Cybex trunk extension machine, Biodex, Isostation, LIDO, Kin-Com).

36. What is the normal trunk extensor strength?

Approximately 110–120% of ideal body weight (IBW) for males and 80–95% IBW for females.

37. What deficits in trunk strength are found in patients with chronic low back pain?

The normal average back extensor-to-flexor strength ratio is 1.2–1.5. Patients with chronic low back have deficits in both extensor and flexor strength. The extensor-to-flexor strength ratio is less than 1.0, demonstrating greater deficits in trunk extensor strength. There is approximately a 50% reduction in isometric extension strength in patients with chronic low back pain compared with normal subjects.

38. What impairment in trunk strength is noted after lumbar discectomy? After lumbar fusion?

Postfusion patients typically have a greater deficit in trunk extensor strength than postdiscectomy patients. This weakness is secondary to the atrophy and denervation of the multifidi, iliocostalis, and longissimus muscles that results from disuse as well as injury to the posterior primary rami during posterior fusion surgery. Greater surgical exposure is needed for fusion compared with discectomy, resulting in greater impairment of trunk extensor strength.

39. What is lifting capacity?

Lifting capacity assesses the spinal functional unit (extensor unit/lumbar paraspinals, gluteals, and hamstrings) and its interaction with the body's other functional units in performance of activities of daily living. Patients with chronic low back pain have a 30–50% reduction in lifting capacity. Normal lifting capacity from floor to waist (lumbar lift) is approximately 50% of IBW for men and 35% of IBW for women. Normal lifting capacity from waist to shoulder (cervical lift) is 40% of IBW for men and 25% of IBW for women.

BIBLIOGRAPHY

1. Cailliet R: Neck pain. In O'Young B, Young MA, Stiens SA (eds): PM&R Secrets. Philadelphia. Hanley & Belfus, 1997, pp 302–304.
2. Deschner M, Polatin PB: Interdisciplinary programs: Chronic pain management. In Mayer TG, Gatchel RJ, Polatin PB (eds): Occupational Musculosceletal Disorders: Function, Outcome & Evidence. Philadelphia, Lippincott Williams & Wilkins, 2000, pp 629–637.
3. Fast A, Thomas MA: Cervical myelopathy. Cervical degenerative disease. In Frontera WR, Silver JK (eds): Essentials of Physical Medicine and Rehabilitation, Philadelphia, Hanley & Belfus, 2002, pp 3–9, 12–17.
4. Hinderer SR, Geiringer SR: Traction, manipulation, and massage (the rack, the crack, and the smack). In O'Young B, Young MA, Stiens SA (eds): PM&R Secrets. Philadelphia, Hanley & Belfus, 1997, pp 533–537.
5. Kaelin DL: Thoracic radiculopathy. In Frontera WR, Silver JK (eds): Essentials of Physical Medicine and Rehabilitation. Philadelphia, Hanley & Belfus, 2002, pp 224–227.
6. Leonard JW: Low back pain: Clinical evaluation and treatment. In O'Young B, Young MA, Steins SA (eds): PM&R Secrets. Philadelphia, Hanley & Belfus, 1997, pp 304–309.
7. Pope MH, De Vocht JW, McIntyre DR, et al: The thoracolumbar spine. In Mayer TG, Gatchel RJ, Polatin PB (eds): Occupational Musculoskeletal Disorders: Function, Outcomes & Evidence. Philadelphia, Lippincott Williams & Wilkins, 2000, pp 65–81.
8. Rinke RC, McCarthy TB: Spinal exercise programs. In Placzek JD, Boyce DA (eds): Orthopaedic Physical Therapy Secrets. Philadelphia, Hanley & Belfus 2001, pp 211–215.
9. Weinstein SM, Herring SA, Cole AJ: Rehabilitation of the patient with spinal pain. In DeLisa JA, Gans BM (eds): Rehabilitation Medicine: Principles and Practice, 3rd ed., Philadelphia, Lippincott-Raven, 1998, pp 1423–1451.
10. White AH, Brotzman SB: Low back disorders. In Brotzman SB (ed): Clinical Orthopaedic Rehabilitation. St. Louis, Mosby, 1996, pp 371–387.

14. DIAGNOSTIC AND THERAPEUTIC SPINAL INJECTIONS

Phillip Kay, M.D.

This is an exciting time for interventional pain physicians because of a recent outpouring of new minimally invasive techniques to treat spinal and axial pain. This chapter focuses on basic as well as more recently developed interventional pain procedures .

1. Who are interventional pain physicians?

For many years the majority of interventional pain medicine practitioners were anesthesiologists with a special interest in treating pain. In recent years the field of interventional pain medicine has become a diverse community of physicians from many specialties, including anesthesiologists, physiatrists, interventional radiologists, and neurologists.

2. Where are spinal injections performed?

The preferred setting for both diagnostic and therapeutic spinal injections is the sterile environment of an outpatient/ambulatory surgery center or hospital operating room. Monitoring, including pulse oximetry, blood pressure, and pulse, should be recorded during the procedure and during the recovery period in case of an adverse reaction to the injected local anesthetic or intravenous sedation. Emergency resuscitating equipment, including crash carts, should be available.

3. What instructions should be given to patients prior to a spine injection procedure?

Patients are instructed to continue with their usual medications except those that affect bleeding time. Nonsteroidal anti-inflammatory agents should be discontinued at least 2–3 days before the procedure. Aspirin is discontinued 1 week before injection. Warfarin should be discontinued 4–6 days before injection. If the injection is to occur in the afternoon, a light breakfast in the morning is recommended. A driver is needed to transport the patient to and from the surgery center, especially if conscious sedation is used during the procedure.

4. What are the pain generators of the spine?

Symptoms of axial and radicular pain have been attributed to pathology involving the spinal soft tissues (muscles, ligaments, tendons), intervertebral discs, facet joints, and neurologic structures (spinal cord and nerve roots). The interventional pain physician uses injection techniques in an attempt to identify a specific pain generator responsible for a patient's symptoms and thus to guide subsequent treatment.

Soft tissue sprain or strain (muscle, tendon, ligament) is the most common disorder responsible for low back and neck pain. This diagnosis is generally based on clinical assessment without the need for interventional procedures. Frequently, the diagnosis of soft tissue sprain or strain is made by exclusion of more serious pathology. Normally soft tissue injuries resolve after a few weeks of nonoperative treatment.

In 1934 Mixter and Barr called attention to the **lumbar disc** as a cause of radicular pain due to neural compression. A disc herniation can impinge on a nerve root, resulting in radicular pain that involves the arm or leg. Evidence also suggests that the disc itself can cause pain in the absence of neural compression; *discogenic pain* is the term used to describe such pain. Histologic studies demonstrate the presence of nerve endings throughout the outer third of the annulus fibrosus. These nerve endings are branches of the sinuvertebral nerves, the gray rami communicantes, and the lumbar ventral rami. Annular tears may result from injury or degeneration. These fissures in the outer margins of the annulus can cause pain due to mechanical or chemical irritation.

Facet joints are paired joints in the posterior aspect of the spine. Extension of the spine and prolonged standing aggravate pain originating from the facet joints. Lumbar facet disease can mimic a disc herniation by referring pain to the lower extremity. In the case of lumbar facet disease, the pain usually is not referred distal to the posterior thigh. In the cervical spine, pain of facet origin results from cervical spondylosis or whiplash injury. Symptoms may include neck pain, referred pain to the scapular area, and headaches.

5. List the basic interventional spine procedures.
Epidural and facet injections, medial branch blocks, selective spinal nerve injections.

6. Is fluoroscopy necessary to perform spinal injections?
For many years, epidural injections were performed without the use of radiographic guidance. Success depended on the operator's experience as well as the patient's anatomy. How well the operator could palpate the landmarks of the spine greatly affected the outcome of the injection. Typical patients with low back pain tend to be overweight. Palpation of landmarks is more difficult in this population. One study showed that, even in the hands of an experienced practitioner, needle placement during epidural injection was incorrect in 25% of cases The use of fluoroscopy to guide the needle into the epidural space has greatly enhanced the accuracy of injections. In addition, injection of a small amount of contrast dye can help avoid inadvertent epidural venous injection or intrathecal injection. The use of fluoroscopy is mandatory to perform procedures such as facet injections, medial branch blocks, and transforaminal epidural injections.

7. What are the different approaches for injections into the epidural space?
Epidural steroid injections have been used to treat low back and radicular pain since the early 1900s. The epidural space is a potential space within the spinal canal and outside the dura mater. A mixture of local anesthetic and corticosteroid is injected into the epidural space via various approaches: interlaminar, transforaminal or caudal.

The **interlaminar approach** is the most commonly used approach for cervical, thoracic, and lumbar epidural injections (Fig 1). Epidural needles (Crawford or Tuohy type) are directed midline between the lamina. As the needle penetrates the ligamentum flavum, the epidural space is identified by the loss-of-resistance method. Typically 5–10 ml of corticosteroid and local anesthetic solution is injected in the lumbar and thoracic spine. In the cervical spine 3–5 ml is injected.

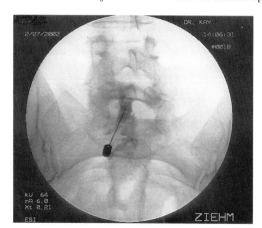

FIGURE 1. Lumbar epidural-interlaminar approach.

The **transforaminal approach** is used to inject the medication directly into the neuroforamen. This is the most direct way to inject an isolated nerve root (Fig. 2 and 3). Transforaminal injection should be performed only under fluoroscopic guidance for accuracy and safety. The needle is directed obliquely to a specific target area in the neuroforamen. Since the needle is placed directly at the target nerve root, less volume is required to achieve pain relief. In the lumbar spine 3–5 ml of corticosteroid and local anesthetic solution is injected. In the cervical spine 1–1.5 ml is required to adequately block the target nerve root.

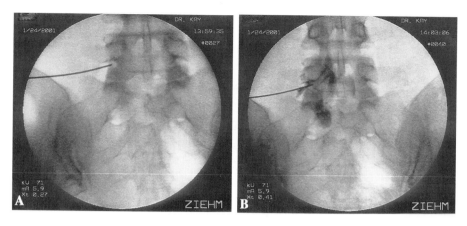

FIGURE 2. A, Lumbar epidural-transforaminal approach. The needle is placed in the left L5 neuroforamen. **B**, Injection of contrast shows epidural dye flow.

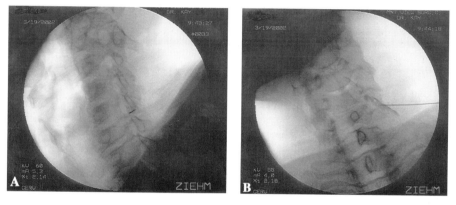

FIGURE 3. A, Cervical epidural-transforaminal approach. The needle is placed in the posterior inferior aspect of the left C6 neuroforamen. **B**, Injection of contrast showing radiculogram.

The **caudal approach** is the safest approach for injection into the lumbar epidural space and has the least risk of dural puncture. The needle is inserted between the sacral cornu into the sacral hiatus, which leads to the caudal epidural space. The drawback of this approach is the large volume of the injection required to reach the target area in the lumbar spine. Frequently, 10–15 ml of corticosteroid and local anesthetic solution is needed to achieve pain relief.

Use of an epidural catheter to deliver the medication to the lumbar spine is helpful in patients with prior history of spine surgery (Fig. 4). Various manufacturers offer epidural catheters specifically designed for pain procedures. An introducer needle is placed caudally, and the flexible epidural catheter is advanced cephalad to the target. These catheters can also be steered to left or right to reach the target area. With the use of a catheter less volume is needed to achieve pain relief if the catheter tip is in close proximity to the target area.

8. What are the indications for epidural injections?

Epidural steroid injections have been highly effective in treatment of radicular symptoms due to disc herniation, central spinal stenosis, and neuroforaminal stenosis. Injections are indicated when pain is refractory to less invasive treatments such as physical therapy and medication. Repeat injections are indicated in patients with partial relief of symptoms after the initial injection.

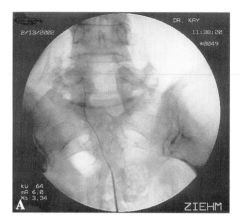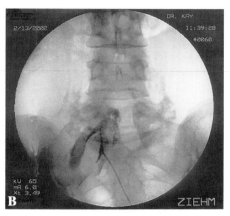

FIGURE 4. A, Lumbar epidural-caudal approach using epidural catheter. Note that the patient had previous decompression and fusion. The catheter tip is in the vicinity of the left L5 neuroforamen. **B,** Injection of contrast showing epidural dye flow as well as left L5 and S1 radiculogram.

Many practitioners limit the number of epidural injections to three per year to minimize the side effects from repeated corticosteroid injections. Each practitioner is advised to weigh the risks and the benefits before proceeding with each injection.

9. What are the contraindications to epidural steroid injections?

Contraindications for epidural steroid injections include local infection at the injection site, systemic infection, bleeding diathesis, uncontrolled diabetes mellitus, and uncontrolled cardiovascular disease. Injections in the presence of local or systemic infection may spread the infection to other areas of the body, including the epidural space. There is a risk of epidural hematoma in patients with bleeding diathesis. Blood sugar may be even more difficult to control after epidural steroid injections in patients with uncontrolled diabetes mellitus. Patients with congestive heart failure, hypertension, or cardiac disease may experience worsening of their condition after corticosteroid injection because of its effects on fluid and electrolyte balance.

10. What are possible complications of epidural injections?

Spinal headache due to spinal fluid leak secondary to inadvertent dural puncture is the most common complication of epidural injections. Frequently, the dural puncture site seals by itself with bedrest. Epidural blood patch is the treatment for persistent spinal headache. Allergic reaction to injected medications or topical antiseptic used to clean the skin may also develop. Improper placement of the needle may lead to nerve injury. Inadvertent intravascular injection of local anesthetic can result in seizures. Epidural abscess, epidural hematoma, and duracutaneous fistula are other possible complications.

11. Discuss the side effects of corticosteroids.

Many adverse effects may be due to corticosteroid injections. Fortunately, the amount of steroid used and the frequency of injection are limited in these procedures. For this reason, fewer complications occur following spinal injections compared with chronic steroid use. Dose-dependent side effects of corticosteroids include nausea, facial flushing, insomnia, low-grade fever (usually < 100°F), and nonpositional headache. Corticosteroids can mask an existing infection or unmask a new one. Peptic ulcer disease can be exacerbated by injection of corticosteroid. Large dose of corticosteroid can result in changes in fluid balance, electrolyte levels, and blood pressure. It is not uncommon to see elevation in blood sugar after steroid injection. With repeated injection, risk of osteoporosis is increased. Avascular necrosis is also a concern with use of corticosteroids. Adrenal suppression can also occur with repeated injection.

12. How long do typical epidural injections last?

The length of time that the effects epidural injection last varies widely depending on the type of spinal pathology. Typically epidural injections using combination of corticosteroid and local anesthetic last between 3 weeks and 3 months. The theraputic effect of corticosteroids is attributed to their anti-inflammatory properties.

13. How do facet joints contribute to spinal pain?

Facet joints (zygapophyseal joints) are a common source of chronic low back and neck pain. Goldthwait first suggested in 1911 that the facet joints might be a source of low back pain. Ghormley described the term *facet syndrome* in 1933 to refer to radiating pain of facet origin.

Lumbar facet disease can cause pain locally in the lumbar area as well as referred pain in the posterior thigh. Lumbar facet pain is generally worse with extension of the spine as well as with prolonged standing (Fig 5).

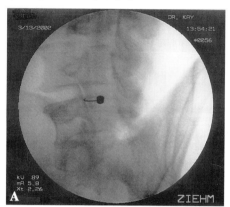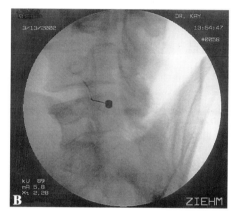

FIGURE 5. A, Lumbar facet injection. The needle is placed in the left L4–L5 facet joint. **B**, Injection of contrast shows dye flow into joint space, confirming the needle placement.

Cervical facet pain frequently results from whiplash-type injuries. Patients with cervical spondylosis may also experience pain of facet origin (Fig 6). Cervical facet pain usually manifests as localized neck pain with pain referred to the trapezius and shoulder blade area. Pain originating from the upper cervical facets may manifest as chronic headache.

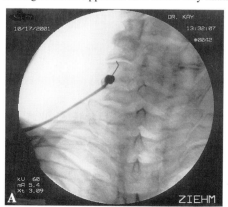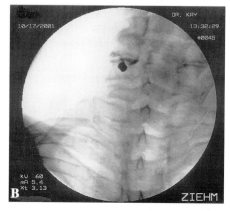

FIGURE 6. A, Cervical facet injection. The needle is placed in the cervical facet joint. **B**, Injection of contrast confirms needle placement.

14. What is the difference between a facet joint injection and a medial branch block?

A painful facet joint can be blocked by injecting into the joint itself or by blocking the nerves that supply the painful joint. The medial branch of the posterior primary ramus of the spinal nerve innervates the facet joint. The medial branch of the adjacent dorsal rami carries the nociceptive fibers supplying the facet joint. Because each facet joint is dually innervated by the medial branch above and below the joint, it can be blocked by injecting the medial branch above and below the joint. For example, the L4–L5 facet is innervated at its upper aspect by branches from L3 and at its lower aspect by branches from L4. Therefore, two injections are necessary to block the innervation of this single facet joint. To block the medial branch, particular attention should be paid to needle placement in order to avoid inadvertent injection into the neuroforamen.

15. How long does a facet joint injection last?

Facet joint injections can be performed purely as a diagnostic block by injecting only local anesthetic or for therapeutic purposes by adding corticosteroid to the local anesthetic. A local anesthetic block lasts only for a few hours. An injection using a corticosteroid and local anesthetic combination may last up to 2 weeks.

16. Explain radiofrequency neurotomy.

Radiofrequency neurotomy is used to denervate a painful facet joint by thermocoagulating the medial branch that supplies its sensation. Each facet joint is innervated by the medial branch above and below the joint. To denervate a particular joint, the medial branch above and below the joint needs to be treated. The insulated probe is inserted percutaneously to the target nerve tissue and connected to the generator, which supplies a radiofrequency current. This current generates heat in the surrounding tissues, creating a lesion that destroys the nerve tissue. Pain relief typically lasts for 6–9 months after a single treatment (Fig. 7).

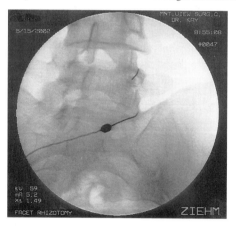

FIGURE 7. Radiofrequency probe in position for lumbar medial branch neurotomy.

17. Describe the pathophysiology of discogenic pain.

Patients with discogenic pain typically present with low back pain that worsens with prolonged sitting. In a normal disc the central portion (nucleus pulposus) is composed of a well-hydrated gelatinous substance. As the disc ages, fine cracks or fissures develop in its outer portion (annulus fibrosus), and fluid leaks out of the disc. The decreased signal intensity noted in the central portion of the disc on T2-weighted magnetic resonance imaging (MRI) is attributed to this loss of fluid content (disc dessication). These changes routinely occur during the normal aging process and are not associated with pain.

In certain patients it is thought that the disc becomes sensitized and generates pain as a result of chemical or mechanical irritation. Histologic studies have demonstrated the presence of nerve endings throughout the outer third of the annulus fibrosus. These nerve endings are branches of the sinuvertebral nerves, the gray rami communicantes, and the lumbar ventral rami. Phospholipase A_2, a known inflammatory mediator, is found in high levels in the intervertebral disc. Chemical irritation is most likely due to leaking of inflammatory mediators such as phospholipase A_2 from the nucleus with subsequent irritation of nerve endings in the annulus.

18. Explain the difference between a degenerated disc and discogenic pain.

Disc degeneration describes the abnormal disc morphology secondary to aging or injury. Discs that exhibit decreased signal intensity in their central region on a T2-weighted MRI are frequently termed *degenerative*. Not all degenerative discs are painful. Provocation discography is a test used to assess whether a disc is a potential pain generator. Positive discographic findings suggest that the target disc is a source of discogenic pain.

19. What is provocation discography?

Provocation discography is a test used to identify painful intervertebral disc. First, a needle is placed percutaneously into the center of the disc in the awake patient. Once the needle placement is confirmed, small amount of fluid (usually contrast dye) is injected. As the contrast is injected, the lateral fluoroscopic projection is used to monitor the contrast pattern. In theory, if the particular disc is a source of pain, the patient will experience the familiar type of back or leg pain as the pressure builds up within the disc on injection of fluid. The volume of fluid injected is recorded for each disc level. The resistance of each disc to injection and the quality of the endpoint with injection are recorded. A disc with an intact annulus will have a high resistance to injection and a firm endpoint. A severely degenerated disc is likely to have reduced resistance to injection and almost no endpoint as the contrast leaks out of the disc without pressurizing the disc. Many practitioners use manometry to monitor pressure as dye is injected and record the opening pressure and pressure at which pain is reproduced. In addition to the suspected disc(s), at least one adjacent disc is tested as a control. Injection of normal discs is not generally associated with pain. Communication must occur between the discographer and patient during the procedure. The patient must report whether the pain experienced during injection is the typical pain for which he or she is seeking relief. The patient should rate the degree of pain on an analog scale for each injected level.

Postdiscography images are recorded as plain x-rays (Fig. 8) or as a computed tomography (CT) scan to document the contrast dye pattern (nucleogram). Nucleograms can be described as cotton ball, lobular, irregular, fissured, or ruptured (Fig. 9). Cottonball and lobular nucleogram patterns are considered normal. As the disc degenerates, nucleograms deteriorate from irregular to fissured and finally to a ruptured pattern.

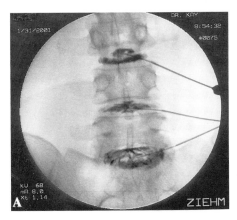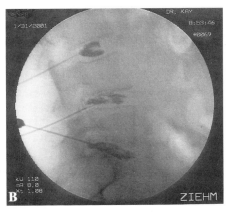

FIGURE 8. A, Lumbar discography, anteroposterior view. B, Lateral view showing normal lobular nucleogram of the top disc and abnormal posterior fissures in the lower two discs.

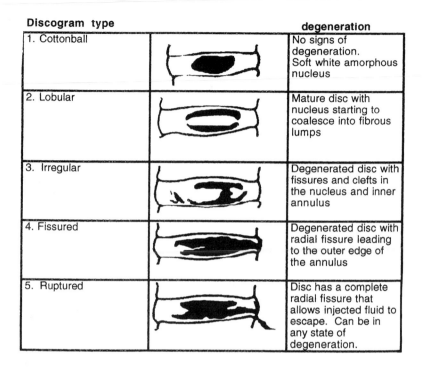

Discogram type		degeneration
1. Cottonball		No signs of degeneration. Soft white amorphous nucleus
2. Lobular		Mature disc with nucleus starting to coalesce into fibrous lumps
3. Irregular		Degenerated disc with fissures and clefts in the nucleus and inner annulus
4. Fissured		Degenerated disc with radial fissure leading to the outer edge of the annulus
5. Ruptured		Disc has a complete radial fissure that allows injected fluid to escape. Can be in any state of degeneration.

FIGURE 9. The five types of discogram and the stages of disc degeneration that they represent.(From Adams M, Dolan P, Hutton W: The stages of disc degeneration as revealed by discograms. J Bone Joint Surg 68B:36–41, 1986, with permission.)

20. What criteria are used to make the diagnosis of discogenic pain based on provocation discography?

To diagnose discogenic pain, one must document evidence of disc degeneration on a nucleogram and concordant pain during injection of the target disc. Injection of adjacent normal control discs should not elicit pain. The sole purpose of discography is to identify painful intervertebral discs. At least one normal-appearing adjacent disc is tested as a control. A valid test requires the absence of pain in the control disc. It has been observed that some discs can be made painful if sufficient pressure is applied. False-positive results can be reduced by using manometry to record pressure during discography. The following criteria for diagnosis of lumbar discogenic pain using manometry are recommended:

1. Stimulation of the suspected disc reproduces concordant or familiar pain.

2. The pain that is reproduced is registered as at least 7 on a 10-point visual analog scale.

3. The pain that is reproduced occurs at a pressure < 50 psi or < 15 psi above the opening pressure. (Opening pressure is defined as the amount of pressure that must be exerted to start the flow into the disc.)

4. Stimulation of adjacent discs provides controls such that when only one adjacent disc can be stimulated, that disc is painless or pain from that disc is not concordant and is produced at a pressure > 15 psi above opening pressure.

21. Discuss the major criticisms of discography.

Discography remains a controversial test. Reasons for lack of universal acceptance include difficulty in performing the test and the high percentage of false-positive results. Further criticisms surround the use of data obtained from testing in the subsequent treatment of patients with discogenic pain. Use of discography to identify candidates for surgical treatment such as a lumbar fusion remains controversial.

22. What are the possible complications of discography?

Discitis is the most common complication with an incidence of 0.7–2.7%. Other complications relate to misplacement of the needle, including nerve injury, dural puncture, and bowel perforation.

23. What are the treatment options for discogenic pain?

There is no consensus about the optimal treatment of discogenic pain. Options include nonsurgical treatment, minimally invasive procedures, fusion, and disc replacement surgery. Nonsurgical treatment options include theraputic exercise, medication, and use of a lumbar support. Intradiscal electrothermal annuloplasty is a minimally invasive procedure specifically designed to treat discogenic pain. Interbody fusion has been advocated as a treatment for discogenic pain. Disc replacement surgery, which at present is not approved by the Food and Drug Administration, is under investigation at multiple centers.

24. What is IDEA?

Intradiscal electrothermal annuloplasty (IDEA) is a minimally invasive outpatient procedure in which a percutaneously placed flexible catheter is threaded inside the painful disc and heated to shrink the collagen in the injured disc annulus. An introducer needle is placed into the target disc in a similar fashion to a discogram. A flexible, navigable catheter is then inserted into the introducer needle and threaded internally around the disc circumference so that the distal 6 cm of the catheter covers the target area (Fig. 10). The catheter is then connected to a generator, and a heating protocol is initiated to a set temperature and time period. Proposed selection criteria for IDEA include chronic low back pain for longer than 3 months, absence of neurologic deficit, negative straight leg-raising test, contained disc protrusions < 5 mm on MRI, loss of disc height no greater than 75%, and a positive provocation discogram.

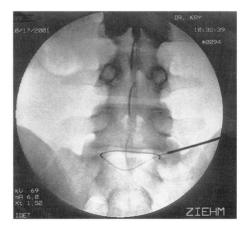

FIGURE 10. SpineCath (Oratec Interventions Inc, Menlo Park, CA), an intradiscal electrothermal catheter fully deployed to cover the entire posterior aspect of the disc.

25. What injection techniques can help differentiate other pain generators that mimic cervical and lumbar pathology?

Shoulder pain can frequently mimic cervical disorders. Careful examination of the shoulder joint should always be performed in a patient presenting with neck pain. Diagnostic injection into the subacromial space and the acromioclavicular joint can differentiate pain originating from the shoulder region from pain originating in the cervical spine.

Pain in the sacroiliac joint can mimic pain originating in the lumbar spine. Sacroiliac joint pain is usually localized to an area in the base of the spine just medial to the posterior superior iliac spine. In most patients one finds a dimple in the area of the sacroiliac joint. SI joint pain can be referred to the anterior groin and mimic hip joint pain. SI joint pain can also mimic pain originating from the lumbar facet joints. Diagnostic injection of the SI joint is helpful in differentiating the source of pain (Fig. 11).

Degenerative arthritis of the hip joint may present with symptoms which mimic an upper lumbar disc herniation or spinal stenosis. Injection of the hip joint with a local anesthetic under fluoroscopic guidance can help differentiate hip and spine pathology.

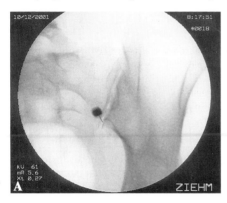 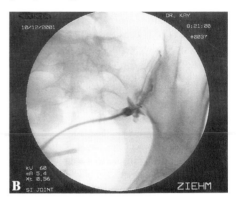

FIGURE 11. A, Sacroiliac joint injection. The needle is placed in the joint space. **B**, Injection of contrast shows dye flow in the joint space, confirming needle placement.

BIBLIOGRAPHY

1. Adams MA, Dolan P, Hutton W: The stages of disc degeneration as revealed by discograms. J Bone Joint Surg 68B:36–41, 1986
2. Bogduk B: Proposed discography standards. ISIS Newslett 2(1):10–13, 1994..
3. Derby R: A second proposal for discography standards. ISIS Newslett 2(2):108–122, 1994.
4. Dreyfuss P, Lagattuta FP, Kaplansky B, Heller B: Zygaphophyseal joint injection techniques in the spinal axis. In Physiatric Procedures in Clinical Practice, Philadelphia, Hanley & Belfus, 1995, pp 206–226.
5. Ghormley RK: Low back pain with special reference to the articular facets, with presentation of an operative procedure. JAMA 101:1773–1777, 1933.
6. Goldthwaith JE: The lumbosacral articulation: An explanation of many cases of lumbago, sciatica and paraplegia. Boston Med Surg J 164:365-372, 1911.
7. Mixter WJ, Barr JS: Rupture of the intervertebral disc with involvement of the spinal canal. N Engl J Med 211:210–215, 1934.
8. Saal JS, Franson RC, Dobrow R, et al: High levels of inflammatory phospholipase A2 activity in lumbar disc herniations. Spine 15:674—678, 1990.
9. Windsor RE, Falco FJ, Dreyer SJ, et al: Lumbar discography. Physical Med Rehabil Clin North America 6:743–770, 1995.
10. Woodward JL, Weinstein S: Epidural injections for the diagnosis and management of axial and radicular pain syndromes. Phys Med Rehabil Clin North Am 6:691–714, 1995.

15. ELECTRODIAGNOSIS IN SPINAL DISORDERS

Mark A. Thomas, M.D., and Ruijin Yao, M.D., Ph.D.

1. List the common reasons for obtaining electrodiagnostic tests (EDX) in the evaluation of patients with spinal disorders.
- To establish and/or confirm a clinical diagnosis. EDX may help differentiate whether neck, low back or extremity symptoms are due to radiculopathy, peripheral entrapment neuropathy, or polyneuropathy.
- To localize nerve lesions. EDX can assist in differentiation between root lesions (radiculopathy), brachial or lumbosacral plexus lesions (plexopathy), and peripheral nerve lesions (entrapment neuropathy). EDX can help distinguish central lesions (e.g, motor neuron disease) from peripheral neuropathy and spinal stenosis.
- To determine the severity and extent of nerve injury. EDX can differentiate a neuropraxic injury (conduction block) from active axonal degeneration. EDX can help to determine whether a lesion is acute or chronic.
- To correlate findings noted on spinal imaging studies. EDX can determine whether an abnormality noted on spinal magnetic resonance imaging (MRI) is the cause of nerve root pathology.
- To provide documentation in medical-legal settings.

2. When should EDX be avoided in the assessment of patients with spinal disorders?
- During the first 2–4 weeks after symptom onset many EDX findings are difficult to detect, and testing is not recommended during this time.
- When the diagnosis of radiculopathy is unequivocal, electromyography (EMG) and nerve conduction studies (NCS) add nothing of value to the plan for treatment and are not required.
- EDX should be avoided when findings will not change medical or surgical management because of extreme illness or patient's refusal of treatment.
- Patients with potential contraindications to EDX testing (e.g., anticoagulated patients, patients with open skin lesions, patients with transmissible diseases, patients with pacemakers and defibrillators).

3. What are the basic components of an electrodiagnostic exam?
EDX is an extension of the history and physical examination. Its goal is to help in distinguishing among the variety of causes for numbness, weakness, and pain. The standard EDX exam consists of two parts, needle EMG and NCS.

EMG or needle electrode exam (NEE) uses a needle "antenna" to detect and record electrical activity directly from a muscle. The four standard components of the exam assess (1) insertional activity, (2) spontaneous activity, (3) motor-unit potentials, and (4) recruitment. The distribution of abnormalities identifies the site of nerve or muscle pathology. EMG is the most useful electrodiagnostic test for the evaluation of radiculopathy

NCS are the recording and analysis of electric waveforms of biologic origin elicited in response to an electric stimulus. NCS are performed to look at the ability of a specific nerve to transmit an impulse down an axon from one area to another. When NCS are abnormal, they give information that a specific nerve is not conducting impulses in the measured area. Both sensory and motor nerve conduction studies can be performed. NCS are most helpful in the diagnosis of entrapment neuropathy and peripheral neuropathy. They are generally expected to be normal in radiculopathy because the lesion is usually preganglionic. Specialized NCS—H-reflex, F-wave, and somatosensory evoked potentials (SEP)—may play a limited role in diagnosis of radiculopathy.

4. What is the anatomic basis for EDX as it relates the assessment of spinal disorders?

The purpose of the EDX is to assess the function of the motor unit, which includes the anterior horn cell, its axon, and all muscle fibers innervated by this axon. Each spinal nerve contains both motor and sensory fibers. The cell bodies for the motor axons are situated within the anterior horn of the spinal cord. The cell bodies for the sensory axons are located within the dorsal root ganglion. The dorsal root ganglion is located along the sensory (dorsal) root near its junction with the ventral root, where it forms the mixed spinal nerve in the region of the intervertebral foramina. After exiting the neural foramen, the spinal nerve root divides into anterior and posterior rami. The anterior rami supply the anterior trunk muscles and, after entering the brachial or lumbosacral plexus, the muscles of the extremities. The posterior rami supply the paraspinal muscles and skin over the neck and trunk (Fig. 1).

Lesions can be classified as either preganglionic (localized to spinal cord or nerve root) or postganglionic (localized to plexus or distal mixed peripheral nerve). Lesions within the spinal canal (myelopathy, radiculopathy) compromise sensory fibers proximal to their cell bodies in the dorsal root ganglion. These lesions do not affect the sensory NCS studies because the injured sensory fibers degenerate centrally as the dorsal root ganglion continues to supply nutrition to the peripheral sensory fiber . In contrast, axon loss lesions located within the plexuses and more peripherally cause sensory fibers to degenerate from that point distally, resulting in abnormal sensory NCS. In contrast, nerve root compression occurs distal to the motor cell bodies in the anterior horn cells, and distal degeneration of motor fibers can be detected on motor NCS and EMG studies.

It is possible for the dorsal root ganglion to be situated slightly more proximal in the foramina and be affected by direct compression or indirectly by vascular insult and edema formation. The dorsal root ganglion can also be damaged in diseases such as diabetes mellitus, herpes zoster, and malignancy. In these conditions, the sensory NCS may be abnormal. However, abnormal sensory NCS rarely occur with discogenic radiculopathies.

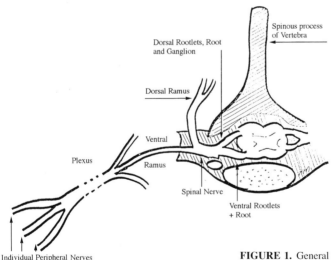

FIGURE 1. General organization of the somatic peripheral system to show the formation of rootlets, spinal nerve rami and plexuses, and individual nerve trunks.

5. Explain how EMG is used to assess patients with spinal disorders for the presence of a radiculopathy.

Specific muscles are selected for EMG assessment. Six upper limb muscles, including paraspinal muscles, consistently identify over 98% of cervical radiculopathies that are confirmable by electrodiagnosis. For upper-limb EMG evaluation, a suggested screen includes deltoid, triceps, pronator teres, abductor pollicis brevis, extensor digitorum communis, and cervical paraspinal muscles. Six lower limb muscles, including paraspinal muscles, consistently identify over 98% of electrodiagnostically confirmable lumbosacral radiculopathies. A suggested lower-limb EMG screen for optimal identification includes the vastus medialis, anterior tibialis, posterior tibialis, short head of biceps femoris, medial gastrocnemius, and lumbar paraspinal muscles. For both lumbosacral and cervical disorders, when paraspinal muscles are not reliable to study, eight distal muscles are needed to achieve optimal identification.

Localization of a nerve injury to a specific root level is achieved by testing a variety of muscles in a multisegmental distribution that are innervated by different peripheral nerves. If the abnormalities are confined to a single myotome but cannot be localized to the distribution of a single peripheral nerve, the diagnosis is consistent with radiculopathy. The paraspinous musculature is generally affected in radiculopathies. However, on occasion, especially in cervical radiculopathies and long-standing radiculopathies, the paraspinous muscles may be normal.

There are four distinct steps in the needle EMG exam of each muscle:

1. Assessment of insertional activity
2. Assessment of spontaneous activity
3. Examination of motor unit potentials
4. Assessment of recruitment

Abnormal resting potentials include fibrillations, positive sharp waves, fasciculations, and high frequency repetitive discharges (see table below). Electrodiagnostic findings must be interpreted in view of the time interval between the onset of the lesion and the performance of the electrical study.

Needle Electromyographic Findings

EMG FINDING	PATHOPHYSIOLOGY	ASSOCIATED DISEASES
Increased insertion activity	Insertion injury of muscle fibers	Acute inflammatory myopathy, acute neuropathy, LMN disease
Fibrillation potentials	Denervation of muscle fibers Membrane instability	Myopathy, neuropathy, anterior horn cell disease, neuromuscular transmission disorders, EMG disease
Positive sharp waves	Denervation of muscle fibers Membrane instability	Myopathy, neuropathy, anterior horn cell disease, neuromuscular transmission disorders, normal inparaspinal and foot musles
Fasciculation	Motor unit irritation	Neuropathy, normal people
Increased duration and amplitude, polyphasics	Reduced motor units Collateral sprouting Reinnervation of muscle fibers	Neurogenic lesions, late stage of myopathy
Decreased duration and amplitude, polyphasics	Necrotic muscle fibers Reinnervation of neurogenic lesions	Early stage of myopathy, late stage of neuropathy
Increased firing rate	Reduced motor units Increased temporal recruitment	Neuropathy, botulism, anterior horn cell disease
Decreased firing rate	Reduced activation from CNS	UMN disease, pain, poor patient effort

EMG = electromyography, LMN = lower motor neuron, CNS = central nervous system, UMN = upper motor neuron.

6. What is the earliest EMG finding in acute radiculopathy?

The earliest EMG finding in acute radiculopathy is a decrease in the number of motor unit potentials (MUPs) seen on recruitment. The recruitment frequency (the rate of firing of the first motor unit recruited at the moment when the second motor unit appears) is increased early in radiculopathy. In other words, the initial motor unit recruited must fire faster before being able to recruit a second unit because there are fewer MUPs to recruit.

7. Describe the temporal sequence of electrophysiologic abnormalities seen in a radiculopathy.

Days after onset	Electrophysiologic abnormalities(radiculopathy)
0+	Reduced numbers of MUPs
	Reduced recruitment interval
	Increased firing rates of MUPs
	Fasciculation potentials may appear
	Prolonged H-reflex latency
	Reduced number of F waves in weak muscles
4+	Compound motor action potential (CMAP) amplitude is reduced unilaterally if axonal degeneration is present
7+	Positive sharp waves in posterior primary ramus innervated muscles (paraspinals)
12+	Positive sharp waves in distal proximal muscles; fibrillations appear in paraspinals
15+	Positive sharp waves in distal limb muscles and fibrillations in proximal limb muscles
18+	Fibrillation potentials occur in most affected muscles

8. What are fibrillation potentials? Why are they important in assessing radiculopathy?

Fibrillation potentials are spontaneous and regularly firing action potentials of individual denervated muscle fibers. Fibrillation potentials are a sensitive indicator of motor axon loss. They can be observed in neuropathy, direct nerve and muscle trauma, myopathy, and some neuromuscular transmission disorders. Fibrillation potentials appear approximately 14 days after nerve fiber injury. However, they appear within 1 week in paraspinal muscles and within 3–6 weeks in the distal limb. Fibrillations can persist for 18–24 months or longer, until muscle fibers are reinnervated.

9. What is the sensitivity of EMG for evaluating radiculopathy?

The sensitivity of needle EMG for lumbosacral radiculopathies has been reported at 50–80%, depending on the diagnostic gold standard used. For cervical radiculopathy, the sensitivity has been reported to range from 60% to 70%. The value of EMG resides in its ability to define, localize, and grade the severity of a radiculopathy with high specificity. This ability makes EMG a complementary test to MRI. If an anatomic lesion, such as a disc herniation, is noted on MRI, the EMG can provide evidence that helps determine whether the lesion is associated with axonal damage. EMG and NCS can exclude other disorders such as polyneuropathy.

10. What are the limitations of needle EMG in the diagnosis of radiculopathy?

1. Needle EMG detects recent motor axon loss but does not detect sensory axon loss, demyelination, or conduction block.

2. False-negative studies can occur in instances of focal demyelination secondary to root compression, when axon loss involves only sensory root fibers, when only a few motor fibers are injured by root compression, during the early postinjury period before denervation potentials appear, or when reinnervation is advanced, several months after the onset of a radiculopathy.

3. False-positive studies are possible when reinnervation is the sole evidence of radiculopathy.

4. A normal EMG of the paraspinal muscles does not rule out the presence of root lesions.

5. Positive sharp waveforms can be found in normal people without low back pain and are not significant.

11. How are NCS obtained? For what diagnoses are NCS most likely to be helpful?

NCS are obtained by stimulating a nerve at one point and measuring the time required for the impulse to travel to a second point at a predetermined distance down the nerve. Sensory responses (SNAP) are picked up over a sensory nerve, whereas motor responses are picked up by recording over a muscle (CMAP). The compound sensory nerve action potential (SNAP) represents the sum of the action potentials of the sensory fibers of individual sensory or mixed nerves. The CMAP is the sum of the action potentials of individual muscle fibers. It is also called the M-wave. The CMAP amplitude reflects the number of muscle fibers activated by nerve stimulation . Special types of nerve conduction studies include F wave, H reflex, somatosensory-evoked potentials (SEPs), and motor-evoked potentials (MEPs).

NCS are most likely to yield positive findings in conditions that may mimic the symptoms of radiculopathy, such as compression neuropathy or peripheral neuropathy. Sensory NCS are expected to be normal in radiculopathy because the pathologic lesion is almost always preganglionic. Motor NCS can be abnormal in severe radiculopathy (i.e., reduced CMAP amplitude).

12. What are H reflexes and F waves?

H reflexes and F waves are special types of conduction studies that give information about nerve conduction in proximal sections of nerves that are difficult to assess by standard NCS techniques. These studies are of limited value in diagnosing radiculopathy, although they are excellent screening tests for polyneuropathy.

13. How is the F wave elicited? What is its value in the assesment of radiculopathy?

The F wave is a compound action potential evoked from a muscle by a supramaximal electric stimulus to its related peripheral nerve. This procedure results in an antidromic activation of the motor neuron. The F wave has variable configuration, latency, and amplitudes. Amplitudes generally range between 1% and 5% of the M wave. F waves are abnormal immediately after nerve root injury, even when the needle EMG is normal. However, an F-wave study has low utility for diagnosing a radiculopathy because a muscle is innervated by multiple roots and any lesion along these multiple neural pathways can render it abnormal. Abnormal F waves are observed only in multiple and severe motor root compromise. Clinically, F waves have been shown to be useful in the diagnosis of multiroot lesions such as Guillain-Barré syndrome and extensive proximal neuropathies such as plexopathies.

14. Describe the H wave and its clinical use.

The H reflex is a monosynaptic spinal reflex first described by Hoffmann in 1918. It is the electrical equivalent of the triceps surae reflex when recorded from the gastrocnemius/soleus muscle. An abnormal H reflex localizes the lesion only to the S1 root or any points along this neural pathway. Prolonged latency and reduced amplitude may indicate an S1 radiculopathy. H-reflex studies are neither highly sensitive nor specific. H reflexes demonstrate approximately a 50% sensitivity for S1 root involvement and may be used to distinguish S1 from L5 radiculopathies. Once abnormal, the H reflex remains so indefinitely, independent of the patient's clinical status. The H reflex is frequently absent bilaterally after lumbar laminectomy and in patients over the age of 60 years.

15. What is SEP testing? What is its value in the investigation of radiculopathy?

SEPs are waveforms recorded over the scalp or spine following electrical stimulation of a mixed or sensory nerve in the periphery. SEPs are carried in the posterior columns of the spinal cord, which represent nerve fibers carrying joint position and vibratory sensation. These nerve fibers usually remain unaffected in radiculopathy. SEPs are used successfully in monitoring spinal cord function during spinal surgery, and prolonged SEP latency can be the earliest sign in extensive multiroot lesions. However, this modality is of limited value for the diagnosis of cervical or lumbar radiculopathy. The range of normal SEP values is broad, and the test has poor sensitivity and specificity for assessing nerve root function.

16. What are the EDX findings in a single-level radiculopathy?
- Abnormal EMG findings in a myotomal distribution
- Normal sensory NCS
- Normal motor NCS or reduced CMAP amplitude with normal conduction velocity when motor root compromise is severe

- Normal F waves
- Abnormal H reflex in most S1 radiculopathies

17. What is the most common root level of cervical radiculopathy?

The C7 root is most commonly involved cervical radiculopathy (31–81%), followed by C6 (19–25%), C8 (4–10%), and C5 (2–10%). Nerve roots C1–C4 have no extremity representation, and lesions affecting these roots cannot be diagnosed on EDX testing.

18. What are the significant EDX findings in a C5 radiculopathy?

Abnormalities are noted on EMG testing of the rhomboids, supraspinatus, infraspinatus, and deltoid muscles. EMG abnormalities may also be seen in the biceps and brachialis, although more distally innervated muscles should be normal.

19. What are the significant EDX findings in a C6 radiculopathy?

EMG abnormalities are commonly seen in the biceps, pronator teres, extensor carpi radialis, and occasionally in the flexor carpi radialis. Rarely are EMG abnormalities detected in the deltoid, supraspinatus, or infraspinatus muscles with C6 radiculopathy. Conditions that may mimic C6 radiculopathy include carpal tunnel syndrome, median nerve entrapment at the elbow, and radial sensory nerve entrapment. These conditions may be differentiated on the basis of abnormal NCS.

20. What are the key muscles to assess for EMG diagnosis of C7 radiculopathy?

The most specific muscles include the anconeus, pronator teres, flexor carpi radialis, triceps, and extensor digitorum communis muscles. NCS may show unilateral abnormalities of the flexor carpi radialis H reflex. Carpal tunnel syndrome may be confused with C7 radiculopathy but can be distinguished with median nerve motor and sensory nerve testing.

21. What are the key muscles to assess for the diagnosis of C8 and T1 radiculopathies?

It is difficult to differentiate C8 from T1 root lesions. The key muscles for the diagnosis of C8–T1 compromise are the flexor digitorium profundus, abductor digiti minimi, first dorsal interosseous, pronator quadratus, abductor pollicis brevis, and opponens pollicis. If abnormalities are found in the extensor indicis proprius and cervical paraspinal muscles but not the pronator teres or extensor carpi radialis muscles, a C8 root lesion may be present since the radial nerve contains very few T1 fibers. The diagnosis of T1 radiculopathy is rare. NCS should be performed to rule out ulnar neuropathy at the elbow or wrist as well as brachial plexopathy and thoracic outlet syndrome.

22. What are the significant EDX findings in L4 radiculopathies?

EMG abnormalities may be seen in the quadriceps, adductors, and occasionally in the tibialis anterior muscle. EMG abnormalities are noted in the paraspinal muscles in radiculopathy and are absent in lumbar plexopathy and femoral neuropathy.

23. What are the significant EDX findings in L5 radiculopathy?

EMG abnormalities are most commonly seen in the peroneal innervated musculature. To differentiate L5 radiculopathy from a peroneal neuropathy, EMG abnormalities should be sought in the flexor digitorum longus and tibialis posterior, as well as in the proximal muscles with L5 innervation(tensor fascia lata, gluteus medius and minimus and lumbar praspinal muscles).

24. What are the significant EDX findings in S1 radiculopathy?

EMG abnormalities are most frequently seen in the gastrocnemius and soleus muscles as well as the lateral hamstring, gluteus maximus, and lumbar paraspinal muscles. EMG abnormalities may also be noted in the intrinsic foot muscles. If EMG abnormalities are limited to the intrinsic foot muscles, the diagnosis of tarsal tunnel syndrome should be suspected.

25. Can needle EMG detect thoracic radiculopathy?

EMG may be useful for the evaluation of possible thoracic radiculopathy. EMG of the anterior abdominal wall muscles (AWMS) may be used to diagnose thoracic radiculopathy. Fibrillations may be noted in the paraspinal musculature in the thoracic region. Seventy-five percent of herniated thoracic discs occur between T8 and T12.

26. What EDX findings are detected in spinal stenosis?

EDX does not reveal abnormalities in mild or early-stage spinal stenosis. In patients with severe stenosis, multilevel and bilateral abnormalities are noted on needle EMG. Sensory NCV is not affected, and motor nerve conduction usually is normal. The F wave may be abnormal, and an abnormal H reflex can be elicited bilaterally. In cervical spinal stenosis, the median nerve SSEP reveals a normal N9 potential (Erb's point potential) and abnormal N13/N14 latencies. The cortical potential may be either prolonged or absent, depending on the severity of neural compromise. Multiply absent or abnormally prolonged SEPs may be helpful in the diagnosis of multiple nerve root compromise that is not evident on needle exam.

27. Why is the EDX evaluation of limited value after a laminectomy?

Postoperative EDX studies are of little value. Abnormalities in the paraspinal muscles are difficult to interpret because denervation potentials can originate from traumatic muscle injury secondary to surgery. Within the first 10–14 postoperative days, the EDX study reveals only preexisting abnormalities. Between 3 weeks and 4 months after surgery, EDX results can reliably investigate a previously unsuspected lesion or be used to assess postoperative weakness. When the EDX exam is performed 4–6 months after cervical laminectomy or 6–12 months after lumbar laminectomy, it is difficult to interpret the significance of findings. Abundant fibrillation potentials found in proximal as well as distal muscles of the myotome may suggest a recurrent or ongoing radiculopathy.

BIBLIOGRAPHY

1. Dillingham TR: Radiculopathies. In O'Young B, Yong MA, Stiens SA (eds): PM&R Secrets. Philadelphia, Hanley & Belfus, 2001, pp 132–137.
2. Dumitru D (ed): Textbook of Electrodiagnostic Medicine, 2nd ed. Philadelphia, Hanley & Belfus, 2001.
3. Gnatz SM, Simpson MJ: Non-surgical evaluation, treatment, and rehabilitation of cervical spine disorders. In An HS, Simpson MJ (eds): Surgery of the Cervical Spine. Baltimore, William & Wilkins, 1994, pp 147–168.
4. Lomen-Hoerth C, Aminoff MJ: Clinical neurophysiologic studies: Which test is useful and when? Neurol Clin North Am 17:65–74, 1999.
5. Nadin RA, Patel MR, Gudas TF, et al: Electromyography and magnetic resonance imaging in the evaluation of radiculopathy. Muscle Nerve 22:151–155, 1999.
6. Oh-Park M, Kim DDJ: General principles of electrodiagnosis. In O'Young B, Yong MA, Stiens SA (eds): PM&R Secrets. Philadelphia, Hanley & Belfus, 2001, pp 125–132.
7. Pezzin LE, Dillingham TR, Lauder TD, et al: Cervical radiculopathies: Relationship between symptom duration and spontaneous EMG activity. Muscle Nerve 22:1412–1418, 1999.
8. Press JM, Young JL: Electrodiagnostic medicine. In Cole AJ, Herring SA (eds): The Low Back Pain Handbook. Philadelphia, Hanley & Belfus,1997, pp 213–226.
9. Robinson LR: Role of neurophysiologic evaluation in diagnosis. J Am Acad Orthop Surg 8:190–199, 2000.
10. Spindler HA, Felsenthal G: Electrodiagnostics and spinal disorders. Spine State Art Rev 9:597–610, 1995.
11. Streib EW, Sun SF, Paustian FF, et al: Diabetic thoracic radiculopathy: Electrodiagnostic study. Muscle Nerve 9:548–553, 1986.

16. SPINAL ORTHOSES

Jeffrey J. Gilchrist, B.S., C.P., BOCO

1. What is a spinal orthosis?

A spinal orthosis is an apparatus that provides support or attempts to improve function of the spine. The device is designed and produced by an orthotist. All orthoses are force systems that act on body segments. The forces that an orthosis may generate are limited by the tolerance of the skin and subcutaneous tissue.

2. What are the most common indications for prescribing a spinal orthosis?

- To prevent or correct a spinal deformity (e.g., scoliosis, kyphosis)
- To immobilize a painful or unstable spinal segment (e.g., spinal fracture, spondylolisthesis)
- To protect internal spinal fixation from potentially dangerous externally applied mechanical loads

3. How are spinal orthoses named?

There are bewildering assortments of names for spinal orthoses. Orthoses are named according to place of origin (e.g., Milwaukee brace, Charleston brace), inventor (e.g., Knight, Williams) or appearance (e.g., halo). The most universally accepted classification system describes spinal orthoses according to the segment of the body controlled by the orthosis:

- Cervical orthosis (CO; e.g., Philadelphia collar)
- Cervicothoracic orthosis (CTO; e.g., SOMI)
- Cervicothoracolumbosacral orthosis (CTLSO; e.g., Milwaukee Brace)
- Thoracolumbosacral orthosis (TLSO; e.g., Jewett)
- Lumbosacral orthosis (LSO; e.g., Knight-Chairback)
- Sacroiliac orthosis (SIO; e.g., Sacroiliac belt)

4. What factors should be considered in prescribing the most appropriate orthosis for a specific spinal problem?

- The patient's body habitus
- Likelihood of patient compliance
- The intended purpose of the orthosis (motion control, deformity correction, pain relief, protection of spinal implants)
- The unique anatomic features of the spinal segment(s) that require immobilization
- The degree of motion control required

5. What orthoses are available for treating cervical disorders?

- Cervical orthoses (CO)
- Cervicothoracic orthoses (CTO)
- Halo skeletal fixator

6. What are the most commonly used types of COs? How do they work? When should they be prescribed?

Cervical orthoses are cylindrical in design and encircle the neck region. They may be anchored to the mandible and/or the occiput to increase stiffness and motion control. Soft collars provide no meaningful motion control. Other COs (e.g., (Philadelphia, Miami-J, Malibu) restrict flexion-extension in the middle and lower cervical region. However, restriction of rotation and lateral bending is less effective, and control of flexion-extension in the occiput-C2 region is limited.

Soft collar (Fig. 1)   *Design:* nonrigid; made of firm foam covered by cotton and fastened posteriorly with Velcro. Provides minimal restriction of cervical movement.

	Indications: Cervical spondylosis, cervical strains. Allows soft tissues to rest, provides warmth to muscles, and reminds the patient to avoid extremes of neck motion. Contraindicated in conditions in which cervical motion must be restricted (e.g., ligamentous injuries, fractures).
Rigid Collar (Fig. 2)	*Design:* vinyl-covered, foam-padded collar with adjustable height, and ventilated; uses a hook-and-pile closure. This semi-rigid support provides mild restriction of sagittal plane motion without restriction of rotation and side bending.
	Indications: used for stable soft tissue injury, whiplash, osteoarthritis.
Philadelphia collar (Fig. 3)	*Design:* Two-piece plastazote foam collar with Velcro fasteners. Includes ventilation, molded chin support, and occipital support. Tracheostomy style available.
	Indications: stable cervical spine injuries, emergent mobilization of cervical injuries, postsurgical immobilization. Not indicated if the patient cannot tolerate pressure over the chin, occiput, or upper sternum.
Miami-J collar (Fig. 4)	*Design:* ventilated, two-piece polyethylene collar. Adjustable mandible and occiptal components. Reported by patients to be more comfortable than Philadelphia collar. Design results in greater limitation of cervical motion than Philadelphia collar.
	Indications: similar to Philadelphia collar. More appropriate for use in patients with altered mental status because collar-skin contact pressures generated by this brace are well below maximal capillary skin pressure.
Malibu collar (Fig. 5)	*Design:* two-piece rigid collar(soft plastazote and kydex) with anterior and posterior openings. Available with a thoracic extension for increased stability.
	Indications: similar to Philadelphia collar.

7. What are the most commonly used types of CTOs? How do they work? When should they be prescribed?

CTOs use chin and occiput fixation attached to the trunk via straps or rigid circumferential supports. Rigid uprights are used to increase stiffness and improve motion control.

These designs provide motion control equal to or slightly greater than the rigid cervical collar designs but are generally reported to be more uncomfortable by patients.

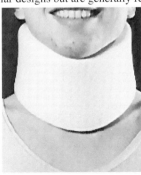

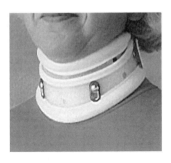

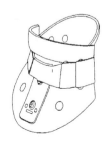

FIGURE 1. Soft collar.   **FIGURE 2.** Rigid collar.   **FIGURE 3.** Philadelphia collar.

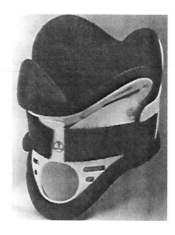

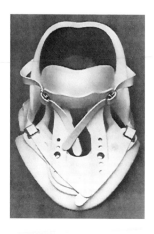

FIGURE 4. Miami-J collar.   **FIGURE 5.** Malibu collar.

SOMI CTO (Fig. 6)

Design: the sternal occipital mandibular immobilizer(SOMI) derives its name from its points of attachment. It consists of a sternal plate with shoulder components, a waist belt, and occipital and mandibular pads connected by uprights to create a three-post design. A head band may be added and is useful if the chin piece must be temporarily removed due to skin irritation. This orthosis can be more easily fitted to the supine patient than poster type CTOs. It is not MRI-compatible. *Indications:* provision of additional support after cervical fusion procedures, immobilization of stable cervical fractures (especially in the lower cervcial region), and as a transition brace after treatment with a halo orthosis.

Two-poster (Fig. 7)

Design: a metal orthosis consisting of an anterior and posterior upright. Occipital, mandibular, sternal, and thoracic pads are attached. Difficult to use if the patient cannot sit upright. *Indications:* similar to SOMI.

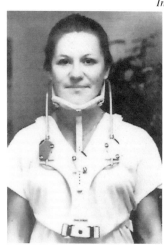

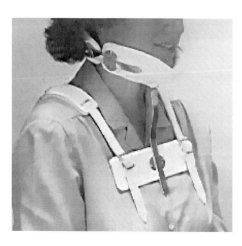

FIGURE 6. SOMI CTO.   **FIGURE 7.** Two-poster orthosis.

Four-poster (Fig. 8)

Design: similar to two-poster but with two anterior and two posterior uprights.
Indications: similar to SOMI.

Daytona (Fig. 9)

Design: consists of an occipital support, mandibular support, and a thoracic extension attached to an adjustable sternal bar. Adjustable sternal bar can relieve chin irritation secondary to proximal brace migration.
Indications: similar to SOMI.

Lerman Minerva CTO
(Fig. 10)

Design: a total contact orthosis made of kydex with anterior and posterior bars. Encompasses the occiput, mandible, upper thorax and forehead. It provides immobilization from C1 to T1, with similar intersegmental immobilization of the cervical spine as a halo except at the C1–C2 segment.
Indications: similar to SOMI. Provides a less invasive alternative to the halo orthosis or an alternative for post-halo immobilization.

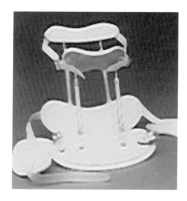

FIGURE 8. Four-poster orthosis.

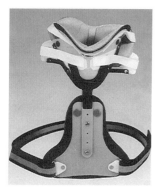

FIGURE 9. Daytona Orthosis.

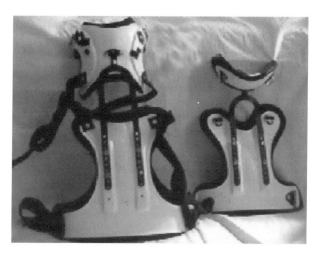

FIGURE 10. Lerman Minerva CTO.

8. Describe the components of a halo vest orthosis.

The halo vest orthosis (Fig. 11) stabilizes the cervical spine by fixing the skull in reference to the chest through an external mechanical apparatus. A rigid metal ring is fixed about the periphery of the skull. A snug fitting fleece-lined plastic vest immobilizes the chest. Adjustable rods and bars hold the ring and vest with respect to each other. This orthosis provides the most effective restriction of cervical motion, especially for the upper cervical region. Traction may be applied to the cervical spine by use of turnbuckles and the superstructure between the halo and the vest.

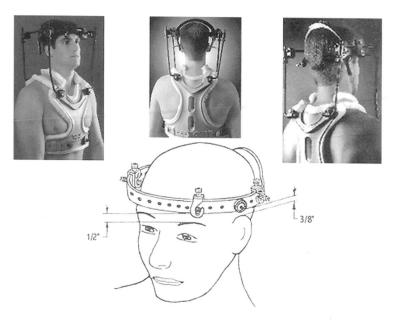

FIGURE 11. Halo orthosis.

9. When should a halo orthosis be prescribed?

Indications for use of a halo skeletal fixator include (1) treatment of select cervical fractures (especially C1 and C2 fractures); (2) postoperative immobilization (e.g., to supplement and protect nonrigid spinal fixation such as C1–C2 wiring; and (3) maintenance of cervical spinal alignment when spinal stability is compromised by tumor or infection and surgical stabilization has not yet been performed or is contraindicated.

10. How is the halo skeletal fixator applied?

The patient is placed supine with the head position controlled by the physician in charge (Fig. 12). The correct ring size (permits 1–2 cm of circumferential clearance around the skull) and vest size are determined. Pin sites are identified. The skin is cleaned with betadine, and pin sites are injected with 1% lidocaine. Anterior pins are placed 1 cm above the orbital rim, below the equator of the skull, and above the lateral two thirds of the orbit. This pattern avoids the temporalis muscle laterally and the supraorbital and supratrochlear nerves and frontal sinus medially. Posterior pins are placed opposite the anterior pins at the 4 o'clock and 8 o'clock positions. The pins are tightened to 8 in/lb (0.9 Nm) in adults. The vest is applied, and the upright posts are used to connect the ring to the vest. Cervical radiographs are obtained to check spinal alignment. The pins are retightened once at 24–48 hours after initial application. The pin sites are cleaned daily with hydrogen peroxide.

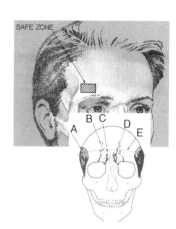

FIGURE 12. Halo pin placement. **A,** Temporalis muscle. **B,** Supraorbital nerve. **C,** Supratrochlear nerve. **D,** Frontal sinus. **E,** Equator. (From Garfin SR, Bottle MJ, Waters RL, Nickel VL: Complications in the use of the halo fixation device. J Bone Joint Surg 68A:320–325, 1986, with permission.)

11. What problems are associated with the use of halo orthosis?

Complications associated with use of a halo orthosis include pin-loosening, pin-site infection, discomfort secondary to pins, scars after pin removal, nerve injury, dysphagia, pin-site bleeding, dural puncture, and pressure sores secondary to vest irritation.

Although the halo is the most restrictive of the various cervicothoracic orthoses, significant motion may occur due in part to difficulty in fitting the brace securely to the chest. Both supine and upright radiographs should be assessed to ensure that cervical alignment and restriction of cervical motion are maintained with changes in posture. A phenomenon termed *snaking* may occur, in which there is movement between individual cervical vertebra without significant motion between the head and the spine. Use of the halo orthosis is not well tolerated in senior citizens or patients with severe rheumatoid arthritis and coexistent hip and knee arthritis. Such patients experience difficulties with ambulation, balance, feeding, and self-care. In such patients rigid spinal fixation to avoid halo use may be the preferred treatment option when possible.

12. What special techniques are required to apply a halo vest orthosis in pediatric patients?

General anesthesia is frequently required. Various ring and vest sizes are required. A CT scan of the skull is obtained to guide pin placement in very small children. It helps to assess skull thickness and to avoid suture lines and bone "fragments" associated with congenital malformations. There is a risk of perforation of the inner table of skull during pin placement in pediatric patients. In patients younger than 2 years of age, use of multiple pin (10–12 pins) inserted with a maximum torque of 2 in-lb is recommended. In children 2–7 years of age, 6–8 pins are used, and the pins are tightened with 4–5 in-lb of torque. For children 7 years of age or older, the adult guidelines for halo placement are used.

13. How are TLSOs classified?

TLSOs are prescribed for disorders involving the thoracic and lumbar region. These braces may be prefabricated (e.g., CASH brace, Jewett brace), custom–molded to the body contours of the individual patient (custom TLSO), or hybrid (prefabricated module customized to a specific patient). Orthoses may be further differentiated on the basis of their intended function:

1. Static support and immobilization (e.g., treatment of stable thoracic and lumbar fractures, postoperative bracing after spine fusion)

2. Deformity correction (spinal deformities such as idiopathic scoliosis, Scheuermann's kyphosis)

3. Postural support (e.g., to relieve axial pain)

14. What motions do thoracolumbosacral orthoses (TLSO) attempt to control?

The thoracic spine is the most stable and least mobile portion of the spinal column. The thorax provides inherent stability with its connecting ribs and sternum. The orientation of the thoracic facet joints is such that rotation is the major motion requiring restriction. This motion is difficult to control and requires a custom-molded orthosis if maiximal motion control is required. The lumbar spine is more mobile with 80–90% of motion occuring at the L4–L5 and L5–S1 segments. Experimental studies have shown that a TLSO can effectively restrict motion between T8 and L4. If motion control is required above T8, a cervical extension should be added to the TLSO. Experimental studies have also shown that a TLSO paradoxically increases motion at the L4–L5 and L5–S1 levels. As a result, a thigh cuff must be added to the TLSO if motion control is desired at L4–L5 and L5–S1.

15. What are the most commonly used types of thoracolumbosacral orthoses (TLSO) and when are they prescribed?

Jewett (Fig. 13)

Design: consists of a three-point fixation system with anterior pads located over the sternum and pubic symphysis and a posterior pad located over the thoracolumbar region. This orthosis restricts flexion but permits free extension. It is reported to be uncomfortable due to force concentration over a small area as a result of its three-point design.

Indication: for pain relief associated with minor stable thoracic and upper lumbar fractures (e.g., fractures secondary to osteoporosis).

CASH (Fig. 14)

Design: the cruciform anterior spinal hyperextension (CASH) orthosis is shaped like a cross with bars and pads anteriorly that are opposed by a posterior thoracolumbar strap.

Indication: as for Jewett

Knight-Taylor (Fig. 15)

Design: pelvic and thoracic bands are connected by a pair of posterior and lateral metal uprights. An interscapular band stabilizes the uprights and serves as an attachment for axillary straps. Over the shoulder straps attempt to limit lateral bending and flexion-extension. A cervical extension may be added. Poor rotational control is provided by this orthosis.

Indications: minor stable fractures and stable soft tissue injuries.

Custom-molded TLSO (Fig. 16)

Design: plastic jacket provides total body contact except over bony prominences. Available in one or two piece construction with anterior, posterior or side-opening styles.

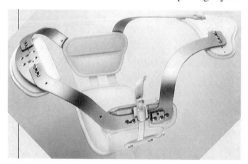

FIGURE 13. Jewett orthosis.

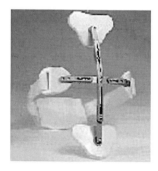

FIGURE 14. CASH orthosis.

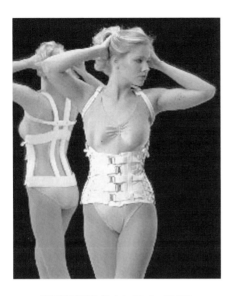

FIGURE 15. Knight-Taylor TLSO.

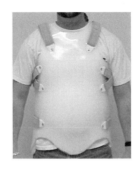

FIGURE 16. Custom-molded TLSO.

Custom-molded TLSO with cervical extension (Fig. 17)

Custom-molded TLSO with thigh cuff (Fig. 18)

Indications: immobilization of the spine between T8 and L4. Provides adequate rotational control for treatment of stable spine fractures in this region.
Design: custom-molded TLSO with attached chin and occiput support
Indications: immobilization of the spine between T2 and T7. Provides adequate rotational control for treating stable spine fractures in this region.
Design: custom-molded TLSO with attached thigh cuff. Thigh cuff may be fixed or may be attached via hinges with a drop lock.
Indications: immobilization of the spine between L4 and S1.

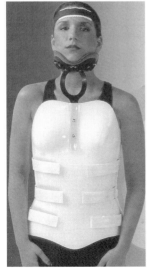

FIGURE 17. Custom-molded TLSO with cervical extension.

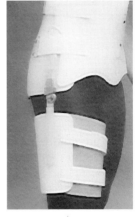

FIGURE 18. Custom-molded TLSO with thigh cuff.

Hyperextension cast (Fig. 19)

Design: custom-molded cast is placed with the patient positioned on a table or frame which extends the injured spine segment.

Indications: treatment of select thoracolumbar fractures (burst fractures without neurologic deficit, Chance fractures involving only bone, certain compression fractures). A good option in unreliable patients who are likely to be noncompliant with bracing.

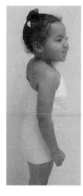 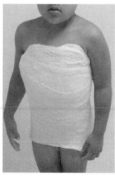 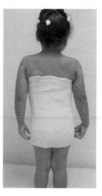

FIGURE 19. Hyperextension cast.

16. When an orthosis is indicated for immobilization of a stable thoracic or lumbar fracture, what is the most important factor in deciding what type of orthosis to prescribe?

In general, the level of injury is the most important factor to consider in orthotic selection for a thoracic or lumbar fracture. A basic principle is that for an orthosis to limit motion in one region of the spine, the orthosis must extend proximal and distal to the level of injury and immobilize the adjacent spinal segments. A TLSO is generally recommended if rigid immobilization is required from the T8–L4 level. If the fracture involves L5, a thigh cuff should be added. If control is required proximal to T8 level, a cervical extension should be added. A halo or Minerva orthosis can effectively immobilize from the T1 level cephalad.

17. When should you consider using an orthosis after a spinal fusion procedure?

At present, spinal fusion procedures are most commonly performed in conjunction with the placement of spinal fixation devices. If the patient is reliable and possesses good bone quality and multiple fixation points are used, postoperative bracing is not mandatory after a spinal instrumentation and fusion procedure. Reasons to consider use of a spinal orthosis following a spinal fusion procedure include:

1. To provide a splinting effect to relieve pain. Use of an orthosis can increase intra-abdominal pressure which has the potential to provide a splinting effect that may help relieve pain during the initial recovery period.

2. To protect spinal implants from excessive forces. Young children tend to become active too soon and may damage spinal fixation. The implants used in children are not as strong as those used in adults. Adults with osteopenia also may require bracing to protect the implant-bone interface. Long fusions from the thoracic spine to the pelvis are another reason to consider an orthosis in patients with less than optimal bone quality.

3. To provide immobilization after a lumbar fusion performed without use of spinal implants.

18. What orthoses are available for treating lumbar and lumbosacral disorders?

The various types of LSOs include corsets, rigid orthoses, orthoses that incorporate the thigh, and sacroiliac orthoses.

Elastic binder (Fig. 20)

Design: broad elastic straps are fastened with Velcro closure.

Sports support (Fig. 21)

Corset (Fig. 22)

Chairback LSO (Fig. 23)

Custom-molded LSO
(Fig. 24)

Sacroiliac orthosis
(Fig. 25)

Indications: for postural support with minimal discomfort. Good choice for a patient with a pendulous abdomen.

Design: Consists of a heavy duty elastic binder with a posterior neoprene pocket. The pocket holds a thermoplastic panel that is heated and contoured to the patient's lumbosacral region.

Indications: for patients whose shape or activity level precludes use of a more restrictive orthosis.

Design: canvas garment with side-pull tightening straps and paraspinal steel stays.

Indications: mechanical low back pain.

Design: composed of a posterior frame of kydex with a fabric abdominal panel. Adjustable laces provide side closure and front straps provide front tightening.

Indications: low back pain exacerbated by lumbar extension.

Design: custom-made from patient mold.

Indications: chronic low back pain of musculoskeletal origin, postsurgical immobilization.

Design: belts that wrap around the pelvis between the trochanters and the iliac crests.

Indications: during pregnancy when laxity of the sacroiliac or anterior pelvic joints may cause pain or for other conditions affecting the sacroiliac joints.

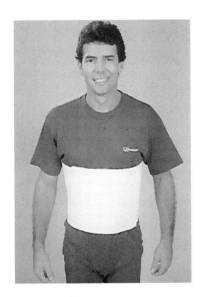

FIGURE 20. Elastic binder.

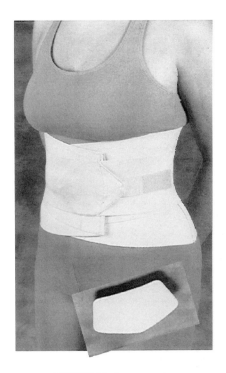

FIGURE 21. Sports support.

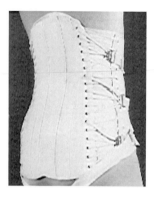

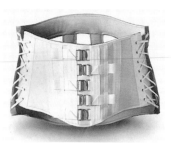

FIGURE 22. Corset.

FIGURE 23. Chairback LSO.

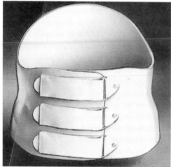

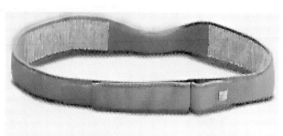

FIGURE 24. Custom-molded LSO.

FIGURE 25. Sacroiliac orthosis.

19. What are the orthosis options for treatment of adolescent idiopathic scoliosis?

Orthoses are recommended for adolescent idiopathic scoliosis patients who have cures of 25–40 ° and who are likely to have significant growth remaining. Patients with curves less than 25° are usually observed for progression, whereas those with curves approaching 50 ° are generally considered for surgical treatment. There is a lower likelihood of successful orthotic treatment in male patients with scoliosis. Options for orthotic treatment include:

Milwaukee Brace. (Fig. 26) Basic components include a custom molded pelvic girdle, one anterior and two posterior uprights extending from the pelvic girdle to a plastic neck ring, corrective pads, straps, and accessories. This brace can be used for all curve types and is the most effective orthosis for curves with an apex above T8. The cosmetic appearance of this brace is a concern to patients and limits compliance.

TLSO (Fig. 27). The TLSO encompasses the pelvis and thorax. Curve correction is obtained through placement of corrective pads within the orthosis. This orthosis is effective for treatment of thoracic curves with an apex located below T8 as well as thoracolumbar and lumbar scoliosis. The best known orthosis in this category is the Boston brace.

Charleston brace (Fig. 28). The Charleston brace is designed to be worn only at night while the patient is lying down. This design permits fabrication of a brace that overcorrects the curve and create a mirror image of the curve. For example, a left lumbar curve is treated by designing a brace that creates a right lumbar curve. The relative success of this brace depends on the flexibility of the spine. It is most effective for single curves in the lumbar or thoracolumbar region. It provides a treatment option for patients who are noncompliant with day-time brace use.

SpineCor brace (Fig. 29). This novel design utilizes fabric pelvic and thoracic harnesses connected by elastic straps. The elastic straps are tightened to provide lateral and rotational corrective forces.

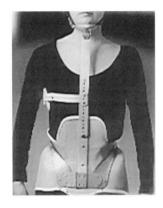

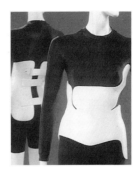

FIGURE 26. Milwaukee brace.

FIGURE 27. TLSO (Boston).

FIGURE 28. Charleston brace.

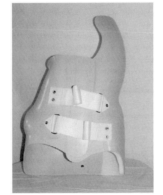

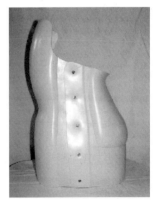

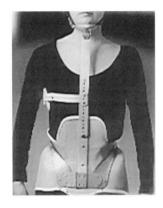

FIGURE 29. Spine Cor brace.

20. What are the orthosis options for treatment of an adolescent with Scheuermann's kyphosis?

The CTLSO (Milwaukee brace) is the primary means of orthotic management of sagittal plane (kyphotic) deformities of the spine in adolescents. Underarm braces may be considered for treatment of low thoracic kyphotic deformities (apex below T9) or thoracolumbar-lumbar Scheuermann's disease.

21. What are the orthosis options for treatment of an adolescent with low back pain and spondylolysis?

Adolescent athletes may sustain injuries to the lumbar region that result in spondylolysis or stress fracture in the pars interarticularis. Various types of braces have been advised for treatment of this condition. Improvement in symptoms following bracing has been reported whether or not healing of the stress fracture occurs. Orthotic options for an adolescent with spondylolysis include a corset, Boston overlap LSO, or a custom TLSO.

BIBLIOGRAPHY

1. Bunch WH (ed): Atlas of Orthotics. American Academy of Orthopaedic Surgeons. St. Louis, Mosby, 1995.
2. Fidler MN, Plasmans MT: The effect of four types of support on the segmental mobility of the lumbosacral spine. J Bone Joint Surg 65A: 943–947, 1983.
3. Garfin SR, Botte MJ, Nickel VL, Waters RL: Complications in the use of the halo fixation device. J Bone Joint Surg 68A:320–325, 1986.
4. Johnson RM, Hart DL, Simmons EF, et al: Cervical orthoses: a study comparing their effectiveness in restricting cervical motion in normal subjects. J. Bone Joint Surg. 59A:332–329, 1977.
5. Rowe DE, Bernstein SM, Riddick MF, et al: A meta-analysis of the efficacy of non-operative treatments for idiopathic scoliosis. J Bone Joint Surg 79A:664–674, 1997
6. Vaccaro AR, Lavernia CJ, Botte M, et al: Spinal orthoses in the management of spine trauma. In Levine AM, Eismont FJ, Garfin SR, Zigler JE (eds): Spine Trauma. Philadelphia, W.B. Saunders, 1998, pp 171–195.

17. PHARMACOLOGIC MANAGEMENT OF CHRONIC PAIN IN SPINAL DISORDERS

Jerome Schofferman, M.D.

1. Define pain.

Pain is an unpleasant sensory or emotional experience associated with actual or potential tissue damage or described in terms of such damage. The key points are that pain is unpleasant and always has both sensory (structural) and emotional (physiological) components. In acute pain, the sensory usually dominates, but there may be anxiety and fear. In chronic pain, there may be depression in addition to the sensory component.

2. Define acute pain.

Acute pain has a recent onset, is usually treatable by specific means, and may be associated with over-activity of the sympathetic nervous system. It is expected to follow a familiar natural history, and resolve naturally or after appropriate treatment.

3. Define chronic pain.

Chronic pain is not just acute pain that does not resolve—it is pain that persists well beyond its expected duration and often associated with significant psychological changes. The psychological changes are usually due to the unremitting pain, not the cause of the chronicity. Specific treatment has been tried and failed. Sympathetic overactivity has been replaced by the vegetative symptoms of sleep disturbance, low energy, changes in appetite and weight, and decreased libido. Often patients have depressed mood.

4. What are some of the types of patients with chronic pain?

There is a spectrum of patients with chronic pain. Some patients have significant nociceptive or neuropathic stimuli, their psychological changes are consistent with the degree of impairment, they function at a level consistent with their disorder, they do the best they can despite their problem, they keep their appointments and follow instructions, and medications appear to work. These people may be called patients with chronic pain. At the other end of the spectrum are true chronic pain patients. They have pain out of proportion to any stimulus, they have psychological and behavioral changes that interfere with their lives, they function at a level far lower than expected for the problem, they miss appointments or fail to follow directions, and they respond poorly to medications and other treatments.

5. What are the types of chronic spine pain?

Chronic pain can be subdivided into nociceptive and neuropathic pains. **Nociceptive pain** is due to a structural disorder that stimulates small nerve endings (nociceptors), for example one or more painful degenerated discs. In addition, when there is direct nerve root compression by a disc herniation or foraminal stenosis, for example, this is a type of nociceptive pain since the nerve root itself contains nociceptive fibers. It may be useful to call nerve root compression pain neurogenic pain.

Neuropathic pain is due to nerve damage or injury. A damaged nerve is the source of the pain even though it is no longer being stimulated. In addition, because the nerve is sensitized, pain increases even further with only minimal stimulation. Examples include a "battered root," arachnoiditis, and complex regional pain syndrome (formerly reflex sympathetic dystrophy).

6. Why is this distinction important?

The distinction is clinically important because some medications are more effective for one type than the other.

7. What are the best drugs for nociceptive pain?

The best drugs for mild-to-moderate nociceptive pain are the nonsteroidal anti-inflammatory drugs (NSAIDs) and the weak opioids. The best drugs for moderate-to-severe nociceptive pain are the strong opioids.

8. What are the best drugs for neuropathic pain?

The drugs of choice for neuropathic pain are the tricyclic antidepressants (TCAs) and anticonvulsants. Some patients respond to opioids, but higher doses may be needed. Some patients may have both nociceptive and neuropathic pain, a mixed pain syndrome.

9. What psychological factors are important in the management of chronic pain?

In one highly regarded functional restoration program, 59% of patients with chronic back pain had *active* psychopathology: major depression in 45%, substance abuse disorder in 19%, and anxiety disorder in 17%.

10. Why is pain management necessary in spinal disorders?

Despite excellent conservative or operative care, some patients do not improve. If a surgeon operates on a patient, but the patient does not get better, it remains that surgeon's responsibility to care for the patient or refer the patient for pain management. It is neither responsible nor ethical to abandon the patient. Other patients with spine pain are not candidates for surgery. They, too, must be treated, and pain management is most likely to help.

11. What are the components of pain management?

Modern pain management may have noninterventional components such as rehabilitation, medications, and psychotherapy. Interventional components may include spinal cord stimulation, intrathecal medication infusions, and facet joint neurotomy.

12. What classes of drugs are most useful for chronic pain?

The opioid analgesics, TCAs, and anticonvulsants, are the classes of medications most useful for chronic pain, although other medications may be helpful for selected patients.

13. What are the classes of analgesics?

Analgesics can be divided into those that act in the periphery and those that act in the central nervous system. Each may have a role in the treatment of chronic spine pain.

14. What are the peripherally acting analgesics?

The peripherally acting analgesics are acetaminophen, aspirin, and NSAIDs. They are useful for mild-to-moderate pain and also act synergistically with centrally-acting analgesics. In addition to their anti-inflammatory effects NSAIDs may produce analgesia by other mechanisms. Empiric support for this includes the facts that analgesia can begin in less than an hour, long before any anti-inflammatory activity could occur, and NSAIDs may relieve pain even when there is no inflammation.

15. What is a good way to select from among the many NSAIDs?

One way to select an NSAID is the speed of onset and duration of analgesia. If it is to be used "as needed" for pain, a drug with a rapid onset is preferred, but the duration of analgesia is shorter. If an NSAID is to be used chronically, a drug with a longer durations of analgesia is preferred, but it may take longer for benefits to occur. It may be necessary to try several NSAIDs because of the variability in patients' responses.

16. What are the most important centrally acting analgesics?

The most important centrally acting analgesics are the opioids. Opioids produce analgesia primarily by binding with opiate receptors in the central nervous system. They work best for nociceptive pain but can be effective for neuropathic pain.

17. Are opioids used for chronic pain by doctors?

Recent surveys have shown that many physicians use opioids for chronic low back pain, osteoarthritis, and other painful musculoskeletal disorders.

18. What concerns prevent doctors from prescribing opioids?

- Fear of producing addiction and dependence
- Fear of causing organ toxicity
- Fear of disciplinary action by medical licensing boards
- Tolerance
- Efficacy

19. Define addiction.

Addiction is a disease that is both psychological and biologic. It is defined as the compulsive use of a psychoactive substance resulting in biological, psychological, or social harm. It is characterized by loss of control.

20. Define dependence.

Chronic opioid use usually causes dependence, a physiologic state induced by chronic use of a psychoactive substance (e.g., alcohol or opioids) and characterized by an abstinence syndrome upon abrupt discontinuation. Dependence is rarely a clinical problem.

21. Define tolerance.

Tolerance is the progressive lack of efficacy of an analgesic. It takes more of the analgesic to provide the same response. However, in some cases of apparent drug tolerance, the medication is not working as well because the disease has progressed or the activity level has increased, either of which produces relative lack of efficacy, but not true tolerance.

22. Is tolerance a limiting factor in long-term use?

No. The experience with the use of long-term opioid analgesics in cancer patients who survive for years has been that tolerance is not a clinical problem. In spine pain, when opioid needs escalate, it is usually because function has increased or there has been progression of the structural disorder, not tolerance.

23. Do opioids produce addiction?

The prevalence of addiction in patients treated with opioids for pain is low. Although opioids may activate an underlying addictive disease, they do not cause it.

24. Are opioids effective for chronic pain?

For years, physicians believed that these drugs were ineffective for long-term treatment and the risks were too great, but their opinions were not based on medical evidence. The evidence published over the past decade is quite convincing that long-term opioid therapy can be safe and effective for many well-selected patients with low back pain and osteoarthritis. Most studies were longitudinal cohort studies, but a few have been randomized and placebo controlled. No recent studies show lack of efficacy. Efficacy has been well maintained in the long-term studies, although none has followed patients for more than a year.

25. Do opioids cause organ toxicity?

Opioids are not toxic to the liver, kidneys, brain, or other organs. Respiratory depression is very rare with oral opioids except in persons with significant pulmonary disease, sleep-apnea syndrome, or other serious medical conditions. There has been no evidence of serious organ toxicity, nor of a high incidence of addictive behavior or abuse.

26. Which opioid is best for chronic pain?

No single opioid has proven superior to others. About 15% of patients are not able to tolerate long-term opioids due to side effects. Of the patients who can tolerate long-term opioids, about 75% experience meaningful pain relief, and most, but not all patients, also experience an increase in function. About 10% of patients who were disabled due to low back pain are able to return to work.

27. Are side effects common with opioids?

Side effects are common but usually can be managed with adjunctive medications.

28. Should physicians who prescribe opioids fear disciplinary action?

No. It is appropriate medical practice to prescribe long-term opioids for chronic pain, and physicians who prescribe opioids for appropriate clinical indications are acting well within the scope of good medical practice.

29. What are some of the side effects of opioids?

Most patients taking opioids have side effects, but the types and intensity vary greatly. The most worrisome are somnolence and changes in mental status. Of interest, chronic severe pain may result in an alteration of cognitive abilities, and when opioids relieve pain effectively, cognitive abilities actually improve. Sedation is common, particularly at initiation of treatment or when doses are raised, but usually improves over time despite continued treatment. If the opioid is effective but sedation is excessive, methylphenidate (Ritalin) can be of value.

Nausea is common, especially when the opioid is first begun. It usually responds to expectant treatment with prochlorperazine (Compazine) or transdermal scopolamine. Constipation occurs in most patients, and prophylaxis is important using dioctyl sodium sulfate (DSS) plus Senokot, 2–4 tablets at night. Other side effects include itching sweating, dry mouth, and dizziness. Occasionally there may be sexual dysfunction due to opioid induced lowered testosterone, which is treated by the use of a testosterone patch.

30. List guidelines that help with safe and effective use of opioids.
- Careful evaluation of the patient
- Written treatment plan that states the goal of therapy
- Informed consent (verbal or written)
- Periodic review to assess and document efficacy, side effects, and problems
- Consultation when necessary
- Maintenance of good medical records

31. What spine problems may respond to long-term opioids?

Opioids should not be used to treat nonspecific pain. There must be a well-defined stimulus that cannot be definitively treated, and the pain level should be consistent with the structural disorder. Aggressive conservative care must have failed, there should be no significant psychological illness or history or addiction or drug abuse, and opioids should be prescribed and refilled in person, not by telephone.

32. What are some of the warning signs that opiods are being abused?

Despite the best screening, some patients abuse or misuse opioid analgesics. If abuse or misuse is suspected, the patient should be referred for consultation to a specialist in addiction medicine. Certain actions have been identified as being highly suggestive of addictive behavior. They include selling prescription drugs, forging prescriptions, repeatedly borrowing drugs from friends or family, concurrent use of large amounts of alcohol, use of any illicit street drugs, the "loss" of prescriptions or pills, seeking prescriptions from other doctors including emergency room personnel, and frequent missed appointments. Other signs that may raise the suspicion of drug abuse include frequent complaints that the dose is too low, requests for specific drugs, unsanctioned dose escalations, or use of the drug to treat other symptoms. However, some of these behaviors may be due to inadequate pain control, sometimes called "pseudoaddiction."

33. What are the ways to use opioids?

There are two ways to prescribe analgesics—pain-contingent and time-contingent dosing. Pain-contingent means taking the analgesic when pain occurs. Time-contingent means taking the analgesic on a regular schedule based on the analgesic half-life of the drug. There is usually better analgesia and less side effects with time-contingent dosing, which avoids large swings in blood or brain levels. It takes more analgesic to reduce severe pain than to maintain mild-to-moderate pain. Time-contingent dosing is almost always preferable for chronic pain, with rescue doses for breakthrough pain.

34. For long-term use, are short-acting opioids indicated?

The short acting opioids such as codeine, hydrocodone (Vicodin and others), or oxycodone (Percocet, Roxicodone) are not usually used for long-term therapy because wide swings in the blood levels lead to poor pain control and more side effects. Rare patients who do better with a short-acting opioid should be prescribed in a time-contingent manner. It is best to use a continuous release or long-acting opioid for long-term opioid analgesic therapy, although short-acting opioids should be available for breakthrough pain.

35. Which opioids are available for long-term use?

There are currently five opioids suitable for long-term use—morphine, oxycodone, methadone, fentanyl, and levorphanol. No single drugs is best for every patient. In fact, some patients respond preferentially to one or two opioids, but not to others, which may make it necessary to try several different ones.

Opioid Analgesics (Narcotics) Most Useful for Chronic Pain

CHEMICAL NAME	BRAND NAMES	DURATION OF ANALGESIA	COMMENTS
Morphine	MS-Contin	8–12 hrs	Multiple dose sizes;
	Oramorph	8 hrs	convenient
Oxycodone	Oxycontin	8–12 hrs	Multiple dose sizes; convenient; expensive
Methadone	Dolophine	8–12 hrs	Very inexpensive
Entamyl	Duramorph	48–72 hrs	Transdermal
Levorphanol	Levo-dromoran	6–8 hrs	Only 2-mg dose size; inconvenient

Continuous-release morphine is reasonably easy to use and highly effective. The opioid is released continuously from the tablet and slowly absorbed from the gut with little accumulation in body tissues. There is effective analgesia for 8–12 hours, and the dosing interval is adjusted accordingly. The continuous-release opioids are available in many dose sizes which makes dose titration convenient. The dose can be titrated upwards once or twice weekly until there is good pain control or significant side effects.

Methadone is a long-acting opioid. It is inexpensive, somewhat more difficult to use, but provides excellent analgesia. This lipophilic drug is well absorbed from the gut and is then distributed in body fat, taking about 5–7 days to reach a steady state. Therefore, the dose should only be adjusted once per week. Once a steady state is reached, there can be 8–12 hours of pain relief.

36. What other opioids are available?

Transdermal fentanyl (Duramorph) is also effective, but there is less dosing flexibility, and some people have difficulty keeping the patches in plate. Levorphanol (Levo-Dromaron) is a long-acting opioid that is also quite effective, but several times in the last few years, the manufacturer was not able to produce sufficient quantities. Therefore it cannot be recommended at this time.

37. Is meperedine (Demerol) ever useful for long-term treatment?

Meperidine should not be used on a long-term basis because it is poorly absorbed, provides unreliable analgesia, and is associated with an unacceptably high level of toxic neurologic side effects.

38. Is there a best dose of an opioid?

The dose and dosing interval is based on the degree and duration of pain relief and side effects until there is good control of baseline pain and minimal side effects. There is no best or correct dose.

39. When are antidepressants used for spine problems?

Antidepressants have many uses in the management of chronic spine problems including the treatment of neuropathic pain, low back pain, sleep disturbance, and depression. TCAs work better than other types of antidepressants for pain. They are most effective for neuropathic pain but also may provide meaningful relief of low back pain.

40. Are antidepressants useful in patients with pain who are not depressed?

Antidepressants are effective in patients with no evidence of depression, the analgesic effect occurs at far lower doses than the antidepressants effect, and the view that antidepresants improve pain through the treatment of a "masked" depression is no longer held.

41. What are some of the antidepressants used in the patient with chronic pain?

Antidepressant Considerations for Patients with Chronic Pain

GENERIC	BRAND NAME	VALUE FOR PAIN	VALUE FOR DEPRESSION	VALUE FOR SLEEP
Nortriptyline	Pamelor	High	Medium	Medium
Amitriptyline	Elavil	High	Medium	High
Desipramine	Norpramin	High	Medium	Low
Trazodone	Desyrel	Low	Low	High
Fluoxetine	Prozac	Low	High	Poor
Sertraline	Zoloft	Low	High	Poor
Paroxetine	Paxil	Low	High	Low
Citalopram	Celexa	Low	High	Low
Doxepin	Sinequan	Low	Medium	High
Bupropion	Wellbutrin	Low	Medium	Poor
Venlafaxine	Effexor	Low	High	High

42. How do we choose the best antidepressant?

The choice of antidepressant depends on the target symptoms—pain, depression, or sleep disturbance. The TCAs nortriptyline (Pamelor), desipramine (Norpramin), and amitriptyline (Elavil) are the antidepressants most effective for pain. Fluoxetine (Prozac), sertraline (Zoloft), paroxetine (Paxil), and citalopram (Celexa) may be the most useful selective serotonin reuptake inhibitors (SSRIs) for depression. Citalopram has very few drug interactions and may be preferred for patients on multiple other medications.

43. What are the usual doses of the tricyclic antidepressants?

The initial dose of nortroptyline, desipramine, or amitriptyline is 10 mg at night, which is then increased every 5 days or so in 10-mg increments to 50 mg. After 50 mg, the dose may be increased in 25 mg increments to a target of 75–100 mg. Fluoxetine is started at 20 mg each morning, sertraline at 50 mg, paroxetine at 20 mg and citalopram at 20 mg. Higher doses are best left to other specialists.

44. What are some of the side effects of the tricyclic antidepressants?

Because the TCAs are sedating, they are usually given at night to help sleep. In some patients there may be excess daytime sedation. Other side effects include dry mouth, urinary retention, constipation, weight gain, blurry vision, and orthostatic hypotension. Usually side effects are mild and decrease with continued use. The SSRIs may cause irritability and sexual dysfunction.

45. What other drugs may be useful for neuropathic pain?

Anticonvulsants can be effective for neuropathic pain, but they rarely, if ever, help low back pain.

46. Which anticonvulsant is most useful?

Gabapentin (Neurontin) is currently used most often, although its use for pain is off-label. It may be useful for neuropathic extremity pain due to iatrogenic nerve injury, arachnoiditis, or prolonged neural compression, and peripheral neuropathy. Gabapentin is started at 300 mg at night, and then increased to 300 mg every 8 hours over the next few days. It is then gradually titrated upwards over several weeks until there is good pain relief or significant side effects. Pain relief may occur at 900 mg per day, but often 1800–3600 mg/day is necessary. Side effects include dizziness, somnolence, ataxia, and headaches, but these are usually seen at the higher dose levels.

47. Are other anticonvulsants also useful?

Clonazepam (Klonopin), a benzodiazepine, may also be useful of neuropathic pain, and is very effective in reducing myoclonic jerks, a potential side effect of opioids. It is started at 0.5 mg at night and increased in 0.5 increments as necessary to a maximum dose of 2 to 4 mg per day in three divided doses. Carbamazine (Tegretol) and sodium valproate (Depakote) may also be helpful for neuropathic pain, but these drugs are more difficult to use, have the potential for many side effects, and are probably best left to pain management specialists.

48. What is the role of muscle relaxants in chronic low back pain?

Their role is very limited. Muscle spasm, strain, or sprain may be primary problems in acute low back pain, may also occur secondary to an underlying disc or joint problem in chronic low back pain, but muscles are rarely a significant cause of chronic pain. Muscle relaxants may have a temporary role in acute low back pain or flares of chronic low back pain, but their use for chronic pain should be limited. They can be sedating and may cause dependence. Little evidence supports that these drugs specifically relax tight muscles. Most of their effect appear to be central rather than peripheral.

49. Which muscle relaxants might be helpful for short-term use?

Cyclobenzaprine (Flexeril) is chemically similar to amitriptyline and may be useful for patients who have a sleep disturbance and decline antidepressants. The dose is 10 mg at night. Baclofen can be effective for the relief of painful spasms, although its effect is in the central nervous system rather than on the muscles. It is started at 10 mg at night and then gradually titrated up to 10 mg every 6 hours. Other muscle relaxants include orphenadrine (Norflex), carisoprodol (Soma), methocarbamol (Robaxin), metaxalone (Skelaxin), and tizanidine (Zanaflex). There is no good evidence to choose one over another. Diazepam (Valium) is too sedating to use regularly, but lorazepam (Ativan) is occasionally effective for "spasms."

50. Are sedatives or hypnotics ever indicated in chronic low back pain?

The role of sedative-hypnotics in chronic spine pain is limited. Chronic sleep disturbance, frequently present in chronic pain, responds better to trazodone or tricyclic antidepressants. However, for occasional sleep problems, especially during flares of chronic pain, a sedative-hypnotic might be useful. Zolpidem (Ambien), 10 mg at bedtime, may be the safest drug, because it is less likely to produce dependence, rebound insomnia, or daytime sedation. Benzodiazepines such as clonazepam or temazepam (Restoril) may also be prescribed for occasional use.

However, the use of sedative-hypnotics for long periods of time is fraught with problems. Long-acting drugs such as diazepam or flurazepam (Dalmane) may accumulate with chronic use and produce cognitive impairment and depression. There may be rebound insomnia when the drugs are discontinued.

51. What is the role of antihistamines in pain?

Antihistamines can help control opioid-induced nausea, vomiting, and itching, but contrary to popular belief, they do not enhance opioid analgesia. Hydroxyzine (Vistaril) and promethazine (Phenergan) are effective for nausea and both hydroxyzine and cetirizine (Zytec) work well for itching. Diphenhydramine (Bendaryl) can also be used, but is more sedating. Antihistamines should not be used as hypnotics as there are far better drugs.

52. How about the topical analgesics?

Capsaicin is a topical analgesic cream that depletes substance P in small nociceptors, and thereby may provide pain relief in patients with peripheral neuropathy, arthritis of small joints, and occasionally complex regional pain syndrome.

Lidoderm, 5% patch, is another useful topical treatment. The patch is applied over small areas of neuropathic pain. Anecdotally, some patients with highly focal nociceptive pain also respond. The patches are worn for 12 hours and then taken off for 12 hours, but the analgesia is sustained.

BIBLIOGRAPHY

1. Atkinson JH, Slater MA, Williams RA, et al: A placebo-controlled randomized clinical trial of nortriptyline for chronic low back pain. Pain 76:287-296, 1998.
2. Hale ME, Fleisschmann R, Salzman R, et al: Efficacy and safety of controlled-release versus immediate-release oxycondone: Randomized, double-blind evaluation in patients with chronic back pain. Clin J Pain 15:179-183, 1999.
3. Jamison RN, Raymond SA, Slawsby EA, et al: Opioid therapy for chronic noncancer back pain. A randomized prospective study. Spine 23:2591-2600, 1998.
4. Joranson De, Ryan KM, Gilson AM, Dahl JL: Trends in medical use and abuse of opioid analgesics. JAMA 283:1710–1714, 2000.
5. Kalso E, McQuay HJ: Opioid sensitivity of chronic noncancer pain. Progress in Pain Research and Management, vol. 14, Seattle, IASP Press, 1999.
6. Max M: Antidepressants as analgesics. In Fields HL, Liebeskind JC (eds): Pharmacological Approaches to the Treatment of Chronic Pain: New Concepts and Critical Issues. Seattle, IASP Press, 1994.
7. McQuay HJ, Tramer M, Nye BA, et al: A systematic review of antidepressants in neuropathic pain. Pain 68:217-227, 1996.
8. Medical Board of California: Action Report: Treatment of Intractable Pain: A Guideline. Sacramento, CA, Medical Board of California, 1996.
9. Portenoy RK: In Fields HL, Liebeskind JC (eds): Pharmacological Approaches to the Treatment of Chronic Pain. Seattle, IASP press, 1994.
10. Rosenberg JM, Harrell C, Ristic H, et al: The effects of gabapentin on neuropathic pain. Clin J Pain 13: 251-255, 1997.
11. Roth SH, Fleischmann RM, Burch FX, et al: Around-the-clock, controlled-release oxycodone therapy for osteoarthritis-related pain. Arch Intern Med 160:853-860, 2000.
12. Schofferman J: Long-term opioid analgesic therapy for severe refractory lumbar spine pain. Clin J Pain 15:136–140, 1999.
13. Schofferman J: Medication considerations in low back pain. In Cole A, Herring S (eds): The Low Back Pain Handbook: A Practical Guide for the Primary Care Physician. Philadelphia, Hanley & Belfus, 1997.
14. Sindrup SH, Jensen TS: Efficacy of pharmacological treatments of neuropathic pain: An update and effect related to mechanism of action. Pain 83:389–400, 1999.
15. Turk DC, Brode MC, Okifuji A: Physicians's attitudes and practices regarding the long-term prescribing of opioids for non-cancer pain. Pain 59:201–208, 1994.

18. COMPLEMENTARY AND ALTERNATIVE MEDICINE TREATMENTS FOR BACK PAIN

Mark A. Thomas, M.D., and Ruijin Yao, M.D., Ph.D.

1. List common treatment approaches to back pain that are considered to be part of complementary and alternative medicine (CAM).

- Manipulation
- Swedish massage
- Acupuncture
- Herbal therapy
- Aromatherapy
- Shiatsu
- Reflexology
- Acupressure
- T'ai chi
- Mind-body treatments
- Magnetic therapy
- Homeopathy
- Prolotherapy
- Nutritional therapy

2. Define chiropractic medicine and chiropractic manipulation.

Chiropractic medicine is a holistic approach to patient care that focuses on the normal relationships among the spinal column, nervous system, and soft tissues. Imbalance or misalignment of the spinal column is considered to be responsible for impaired or abnormal nerve function, resulting in subsequent disease and pain.

Chiropractic manipulation is a realignment or balancing of the spine or extremities to restore normal relationships and health. This goal is achieved by movement of body parts to increase range of motion and to relax muscles.

3. Define somatic dysfunction.

Somatic dysfunction is defined as impaired or altered function of related components of the somatic (body framework) system: skeletal, arthrodial, and myofascial structures and related vascular, lymphatic, and neural elements. Physical findings associated with somatic dysfunction are summarized by the acronym TART:

T = **T**enderness
A = **A**symmetry of bony structures
R = **R**ange-of-motion alterations
T = **T**issue texture changes

4. When is manipulation or manual medicine indicated for treatment of low back pain (LBP)?

Manipulation is useful for patients with acute LBP (< 4 weeks of symptoms) and a related somatic dysfunction who have no progressive neurologic deficit. No supporting data help to define when or how to use manual medicine for the treatment of chronic LBP.

5. What are the goals of manual medicine in the treatment of LBP?

- Restore maximal, painless movement of the musculoskeletal system
- Restore spinal postural balance
- Decrease pain
- Improve global health

6. How does manual medicine achieve a postive effect in the treatment of LBP?

Manipulation is thought to work by:
- Restoring normal and symmetric disc or facet alignment
- Restoring spinal range of motion and optimal muscle function

- Reducing afferent-nociceptor signal transmission to the spinal cord through a gate effect
- Stimulating endorphin release, which increases the pain threshold or reduces pain severity
- Providing a strong placebo effect

7. What are the main manual medicine techniques used to treat LBP?
1. **Thrusting manipulation**
2. **Nonthrusting techniques:** articular mobilization, muscle energy manipulation, strain-counterstrain mobilization, craniosacral therapy, myofascial release, and soft tissue release.

8. What is thrusting manipulation?
Thrusting manipulation is also known as high-velocity, low-amplitude (HVLA) manipulation or mobilization with impulse. Most effective in the lumbar region, it improves the patient's pain-free range of spinal motion. Because patients may experience increased pain immediately after treatment, other pain modalities, such as heat, ice, analgesic medications, and active stretching and strengthening, must be used along with HVLA.

9. How is muscle energy manipulation performed? When is it useful?
Muscle energy manipulation requires that the patient perform a voluntary contraction of muscle in a specific direction, at increasing levels of intensity, against a counterforce applied by the practitioner. For a specific segmental dysfunction, the patient is passively moved to the pathologic barrier to motion and then asked to move away from the barrier with gentle muscle contractions of a 3–5 second duration. After 1–2 seconds of relaxation, the practitioner moves the affected joint directly through the previous pathologic barrier toward the normal physiologic barrier. This technique is commonly applied to segmental dysfunction affecting the lumbar spine segments as well as dysfunction of the pelvis and sacrum.

10. What does muscle energy manipulation accomplish in the treatment of LBP?
Muscle energy techniques lengthen shortened or contracted paraspinal muscles, relax muscle spasm, and strengthen weak muscle groups. Theoretically, muscle energy therapy also reduces local myoedema, relieves passive congestion, and mobilizes spinal articulations with restricted segmental mobility.

11. What is strain-counterstrain? How is it applied in the treatment of back pain?
Strain-counterstrain is a passive, indirect adjustment technique in which a spinal segment is placed into its position of greatest comfort or "ease" to decrease pain and restore normal segmental motion. After identifying a tender point, the patient is moved into a position of pain relief and maintained in this position for 90–120 seconds. This treatment is time-consuming and passive. Therefore, it must be combined with an active exercise program to achieve a lasting, meaningful outcome.

12. Describe myofascial release.
Myofascial release is a manual therapy that applies tension to tight or painful soft tissues through a combination of manual traction and torsion. The goal of myofascial release is to decrease tightness and restore normal tissue mobility. Direct and indirect release techniques are used. In the direct technique the resistance to tissue motion (the pathologic barrier) is engaged with a constant force from the practitioner's hand until release occurs. In the indirect technique the practitioner moves the tissue along the path of least resistance until free motion is obtained. Because of its passive nature, however, myofascial release needs to be performed in the context of active treatment such as exercise. Myofascial release is commonly used to treat myofascial LBP.

13. What can manual medicine offer the patient with back pain?
Evidence indicates that manual medicine treatment may result in early, albeit temporary relief of LBP. This relief may help the patient to begin an active treatment program with more lasting effect. When patients are appropriately selected (again, the somatic dysfunction must be identified), good outcomes can be obtained. The use of manual medicine techniques remains

controversial, especially for persons with known disc herniation. No evidence demonstrates their long-term efficacy in LBP treatment. It is recommended that treatment be discontinued if the patient experiences no measurable benefit after 6–8 visits over a 2-week period.

14. What physiologic effects of massage are useful in the treatment of back pain?
- Tissue relaxation
- Increased local or regional blood flow
- Disruption or loosening of adhesions
- Reduction of edema by stimulating venous and lymphatic drainage
- Activation of a gate mechanism in the second dorsal lamina with related pain reduction
- Stimulation of sensory fibers to produce a state of reduced adrenocortical stress reactivity
- Centrally mediated effects (reflexology).

15. What are the different types of massage therapy?
There are many different massage schools. The most useful and frequently used schools for treatment of LBP include Swedish massage, acupressure (ischemic compression), shiatsu, reflexology, and structural integration (Rolfing).

16. Describe the five basic stroke types in Swedish massage.
1. **Effleurage** (stroking massage). The practitioner's hands glide over skin with varying degrees of pressure. When performed slowly and rhythmically, it effectively induces relaxation. When gliding is more rapid, effleurage is stimulating.
2. **Petrissage** (kneading) involves compressing the skin and muscle between the thumb and forefinger while pulling the tissue away from underlying muscle or bone. This technique is applied to deeper levels than effleurage.
3. **Friction massage** is applied through circular, longitudinal, or transverse motions, using the fingers, thumb, or heel of the palm to apply sufficient soft tissue pressure to free adhesions. It is applied to scar tissue, ligament, or taut bands in muscle.
4. **Tapotement** (pounding) involves alternating movement of the hands on the back. It is an aggressive, rhythmic technique that includes hacking, cupping, and pummeling. The physiologic effects of tapotement are uncertain.
5. **Vibration** uses the hand or fingertips to deliver a rapidly oscillating motion to soft tissue.

17. Describe shiatsu massage.
Shiatsu is a type of massage that synthesizes Western principles of anatomy and physiology with the Oriental principle of energy flow *(chi)*. Pressure is manually applied over acupuncture meridians to smooth and balance energy flow.

18. What are the major contraindications to massage?
- Malignancy
- Cellulitis
- Lymphangitis
- Recent trauma or bleeding
- Deep venous thrombosis
- Recent scuba diving with rapid ascent (nitrogen bubble release)

19. Is massage an effective therapy for patients with LBP?
Massage therapy is frequently used to treat LBP. Although anecdotal reports consistently cite the benefits of massage in this patient population, little scientific literature documents its efficacy. There is a need for further research in the application of massage in the treatment of LBP.

20. What is acupressure? When is it useful in treating LBP?
Acupressure is the application of thumb or finger pressure to traditional acupuncture points. When applied to a myofascial trigger point, it is called ischemic compression. Acupressure

techniques are reported to achieve a theraputic effect by producing ischemia, muscle relaxation, and reactive hyperemia. When trigger points are identified in back musculature, acupressure techniques may produce rapid muscle relaxation and pain relief. One advantage of acupressure is the ease of application . The patient can use a tennis ball, cane, or other object to provide appropriate pressure independently. Alternatively, a family member or friend can be trained to provide acupressure treatment.

21. How does reflexology work?

Reflexology is based on the tenet that a homuncular map of the body is present on the earlobe, palm, and sole of the foot. Circular deep friction or longitudinal pressure is applied to the specific area on the homunculus that corresponds to an identified area of somatic dysfunction. The goal of this type of treatment is to stimulate and restore a balance of energy in the abnormal tissue.

22. What is mind-body therapy?

The theory of mind-body techniques is based on a belief that the mind and body are inseparable. Most mind-body interventions are movement techniques that seek to enhance awareness of posture and movement. Mind-body therapies include relaxation techniques, cognitive-behavioral interventions, biofeedback, hypnosis, and meditation.

23. Provide a brief description of the types of mind-body therapy that have been used to treat patients with LBP.

1. **Cognitive-behavioral programs** are a component of many established pain treatment centers. These programs focus on educating patients and teaching coping skills in a highly structured group setting under the guidance of a clinical psychologist. They frequently incorporate hypnosis, meditation, and biofeedback techniques.

2. The **Alexander technique** is a method of modifying chronic patterns of back and neck muscle tension through an instructor's verbal direction and awareness exercises. Patients are encouraged to experience a state of proper alignment and functional movement.

3. The **Feldenkrais method** uses multiple repetitions of a particular movement to establish new "engrams." It emphasizes consideration of whole-body effects from even simple motions. The method relies on the capacity to learn new movement patterns and bypass the "thinking mind."

4. **Pilates-based methods** condition the entire musculoskeletal system and assist the patient in recovering from an injury that produces a weak link in the kinetic chain. It emphasizes eccentric muscle contractions with little or no resistance and then reintroduces more aggressive strengthening and function by providing gradually incremental tasks.

5. **T'ai chi** consists of a series of linked, slow, and constant movements. Its origin dates back to 17th century China. Special postures and graceful motion are assumed to achieve a balanced energy flow *(chi)* throughout the body . T'ai chi develops strength, flexibility, and conscious muscle relaxation.

6. **Yoga** is a lifestyle that provides direction in philosophy, ethics, social responsibility, and nutrition. The patient with back pain most commonly practices yoga to improve strength, flexibility, and relaxation. The aims of therapeutic yoga are to increase range of motion and flexibility in the spine and to decrease tightness in the lower extremities.

7. **Therapeutic touch** or energy therapy is based on modulating and balancing the flow of *chi*. The therapist's hands move over the patient's body (physical touch or noncontact "touch"), redirecting and rebalancing the "energy field" of the patient with back pain. The goal of energy therapy is to reduce pain and stress-related symptoms.

24. Define acupuncture.

Acupuncture is the use of fine needles inserted through the skin at various points on the body to treat different illnesses. It is based on the idea that the underlying force in the body is energy *(chi)* and that changes in health represent changes in the balance of *chi* in the body. Through inhibition or facilitation of energy flow, spinal balance and health are restored.

25. How has acupuncture been used for treatment of low back pain?

Use of acupuncture has been reported in the treatment of acute LBP, chronic LBP, myofascial pain syndrome, muscle strain and ligament sprain, and vertebral fractures. Most studies do not substantiate the efficacy of acupuncture or acupuncture-like transcutaneous electrical nerve stimulation for treatment of LBP. A large randomized, controlled trial is needed for further evaluation of these therapies in the treatment of different spinal pathologies. Patient expectations may influence clinical outcome independently of treatment effects. This placebo effect may contribute to the popularity of acupuncture for treatment for back pain.

26. Which is the more effective therapy for back pain—massage or acupuncture?

Few studies compare massage and acupuncture. One randomized trial that compared traditional Chinese medical acupuncture and therapeutic massage concluded that therapeutic massage was effective for persistent LBP and had long-lasting benefits, whereas acupuncture was relatively ineffective.

27. Describe aromatherapy.

Aromatherapy is based on the concept that exposure to specific odors, in the form of essential oils, can have a therapeutic effect through physiologic and emotional changes. Its efficacy is controversial. Oils are extracted from jasmine flowers, almonds, and lavender. Aromatherapy for LBP is commonly provided by the addition of essential oils to therapeutic massage

28. Describe herbal therapy.

Herbal medicine is most often associated with ayurveda, traditional Chinese medicine, or Western herbalism. It is a form of botanical medicine that uses plant extracts to treat various diseases. Patients should be aware that herbal therapies are not without potential for adverse interactions with other medications. In addition, herbal remedies are not regulated by the Food and Drug administration(FDA).

Two herbs commonly used to treat low back pain are arnica and St. John's wort. Arnica, which is derived from a flowering plant, is used for musculoskeletal injuries such as acute lumbar strain. St. John's wort (*Hypericum performatum*) is indicated for the treatment of depression, fibromyalgia, arthritic pain, and neuropathic pain. It is commonly prescribed to treat chronic low back pain. St. John's wort should not be used with psychotropic medications, including other antidepressants.

Other forms of LBP treated by herbs include the following:

1. **Backache:** *Conium maculatum* (hemlock)
2. **Nonspecific muscular pain:** *Aconitum napellus* (monkshood), *Allium sativum* (garlic), *Armoracia rusticana* (horseradish), *Atropa belladonna* (belladonna), *Dryopteris filixmax* (male fern), *Mentha arvensis* var. *piperascens* (Japaneese mint), *Mentha piperita* (peppermint), *Mucuna pruriens* (cowhag), *Picea excelsa* (spruce), *Pinus sylvestris* (scotch pine), *Rhododendron ferrugineum* (rust-red rhododendron), *Tamus communis* (black byrony).
3. **Pain and spasm:** *Petasites hybridus* (petasites)
4. **Topical pain relief:** *Allium cepa* (onion), *Artemisia absinthium* (wormwood), *Baptisia tinctoria* (wild indigo), *Calendula officinalis* (marigold), *Cydonia oblongata* (quince), *Echinacea* species (purple coneflower), *Phragmites communis* (reed herb), *Populus* species (poplar bark), *Rauwolfia serpentina* (rauwolfia), *Ribes nigrum* (black currant), *Sempervivum tectorum* (house leek), *Symphytum officinale* (comfrey), *Thymus serpyllum* (wild thyme)

29. What is magnet therapy?

Magnet therapy attempts to balance the patient's energy field in order to decrease pain. It has become a popular treatment for various musculoskeletal conditions, including low back pain. Magnets are available in small pads and discs for local or circumscribed application and as mattress pads and seat cushions for total body coverage. The strength of the therapeutic magnetic field ranges from 300–5000 gauss.

30. How does magnet therapy work?

In theory, the application of a magnetic field increases blood flow by acting on calcium channels located in vascular muscle. Increased circulation improves tissue oxygenation with subsequent elimination of inflammatory byproducts that elicit pain. Magnets also may influence the metabolism and energy flow in both positive and negative ways. The positive magnetic pole is thought to decrease the metabolic rate (negative effect), whereas the negative pole normalizes the body's metabolic and energy function (beneficial effect). In addition, a membrane-stabilizing effect on nociceptive fibers may occur, rendering these fibers less excitable and reducing the firing frequency of unmyelinated C fibers.

31. What are the contraindications for magnetic therapy?

Magnetic therapy is contraindicated in the presence of implanted electrical devices (pacemakers, defibrillators, neurostimulators), active bleeding, or pregnancy.

32. How effective is magnetic therapy?

Little scientific evidence supports the use of magnetic therapy to treat symptoms of LBP. A pilot study in the U.S. showed that permanent magnet application had no effect on a small group of 20 patients with chronic low back pain. In contrast, placebo-controlled studies in Austria and Japan concluded that magnetic therapy is effective in treating LBP symptoms. The application of magnetic therapy remains controversial. Nevertheless, it is commonly used for low back pain symptoms because of its low cost and minimal side effects.

33 How does homeopathic therapy work?

Homeopathy is based on the theory that disease results from an imbalance in the innate human homeostasis. Homeopathic therapy uses minute or diluted doses of natural substances (homeopathic remedies) that would produce illness in larger or more concentrated doses. These remedies restore health by stimulating the body to restore homeostasis through normal healing and immune mechanisms.

34. Describe prolotherapy and its use in LBP.

Prolotherapy treats back pain that is related to motion and due to weakened or incompetent ligaments and tendons. The injury-repair sequence is initiated by scraping the tissue or adjacent periosteum with a needle and then injecting a dextrose solution to induces fibroblast proliferation and scarring/repair of tissue. Prolotherapy can increase tendon size and strength up to 35–40%. The success rate (less pain, less tenderness) in patients with chronic LBP who have not responded to conventional treatment is reported to be 75% or greater

BIBLIOGRAPHY

1. Atchison JW, Taub NS, Cotter AC, Tellis A: Complementary and alternative medicine treatments for low back pain. In Lox DM (ed): Physical Medicine and Rehabilitation: Low Back pain. Hanley & Belfus, 1999, pp 561–586.
2. Bronfort G: Spinal manipulation: Current state of research and its indications. Neurol Clin 17:91–111, 1999.
3. Collacott EA, Zimmerman JT, White DW, Rindone JP: Bipolar permanent magnets for the treatment of chronic low back pain: A pilot study. JAMA 283:1322–1325, 2000.
4. Ernst E: Massage therapy for low back pain: A systematic review. J Pain Symptom Manage 17:65–69, 1999.
5. Gadsby JG, Flower MW: Transcutaneous electrical nerve stimulation and acupuncture- transcutaneous electrical nerve stimulation for chronic low back pain. Cochrane Database Syst Rev 2: CD000210, 2000.
6. Hurley D: Massage is better than acupuncture (and in the short term better than self care) in reducing pain and disability in patients with chronic lower back pain. Aust J Physiother 47(4):299, 2001.
7. Kalauokalani D, Cherkin DC, Sherman KJ, et al: Lessons from a trial of acupuncture and massage for low back pain: patient expectations and treatment effects. Spine 26:1418–1424, 2001.
8. Lee TL: Acupuncture and chronic pain management. Ann Acad Med Singapore 29:17–21, 2000.
9. Pellegrino MJ: Complementary medicine. In Pellegrino MJ (ed): Inside Fibromyalgia. Columbus, OH, Anadem, 2001, pp 117–128.
10. Rurlan AD, Brosseau L, Welch V, Wong J: Massage for low back pain. Cochrane Database Syst Rev (4) CD001929, 2000.

19. DISABILITY EVALUATION

Stephen L. Demeter, M.D., M.P.H.

1. What are the definitions of impairment, disability, and handicap?

An **impairment** is the inability to complete successfully a specific task based on insufficient intellectual, creative, adaptive, social, or physical skills. A **disability,** on the other hand, is a medical impairment that prevents remunerative employment, desired social or recreational activities, or other personal activities. According to the American Medical Association's guidelines, "An impaired individual is **handicapped** if there are obstacles to accomplishing life's basic activities that can be overcome only by compensating in some way for the effects of the impairment. Such compensation or accommodation often entails the use of assisted devices."

An example serves well. A person who has had an amputation of the fifth digit on the right hand has a medical impairment. Loss of function results from the anatomic deficit. If the person is a physician, this medical impairment may translate into no disability. On the other hand, if the person is a concert pianist, the same medical impairment may create total disability. Thus, disability is task-specific, whereas impairment merely reflects an alteration from normal body functions.

2. What is an impairment evaluation?

An impairment evaluation is a medical evaluation. Its purpose is to define, describe, and measure the differences in a particular person compared with either the average person (e.g., an IQ of 86 compared with the normal expected average of 100) or prior capabilities (e.g., a preinjury IQ measured at 134 compared with the current level of 100). Such differences may take the form of anatomic deviations (e.g., amputations), physical abnormalities (e.g., decreased motion of a joint, decreased strength surrounding that joint, or abnormal neurologic input), physiologic abnormalities (e.g., diminished ability to breathe or electrical conduction disturbances in the heart), or psychological (e.g., diminished ability to think and reason or to remember).

3. Who performs an impairment evaluation?

Impairment evaluation should be performed only by professionals with a background in medical practice. Doctors of medicine and osteopathy are the logical choices. However, other professionals also possess such training and background and often perform impairment evaluations. Examples include doctors of chiropractic, dentists, optometrists, psychologists, and physical therapists.

4. How does an impairment evaluation differ from a normal history and physical examination?

The goal of an impairment evaluation is to define deviations from normalcy. Having or arriving at a specific diagnosis/diagnoses is often useful and helpful. However, a specific diagnosis is not the end result in an impairment evaluation as it is in the standard history and physical examination. Both evaluations require appropriate educational background, skill, thoroughness, and dedication. The results of the standard history and physical belong to the patient. The results of an impairment evaluation often do not; they usually are given to attorneys, insurance companies, or governmental agencies (e.g., workers' compensation boards or the Social Security Department). This point often raises an interesting legal concept. Physicians are not allowed to disclose medical information to anyone but the patient. To whom does such confidentiality apply in an impairment evaluation? Usually it exists between the physician and the referring agency or party as opposed to the person evaluated.

Another basic distinction is that the impairment evaluation report centers on the questions that were asked by the referring party. For example, if the physician is asked to evaluate a person for a specific injury, such as arm amputation or dysfunction, the entire process centers on the arm. The end result is a report that describes the injury, differences in the function level of the arm from a normal person's, and a prognosis for future recovery. This information is then used by other parties to determine appropriate compensation. Other diagnoses discovered during the evaluation may be irrelevant.

5. How does a disability evaluation differ from an impairment evaluation?

A disability evaluation is a comprehensive evaluation based on various factors. One of these factors is medical impairment. Other factors may include a person's age, educational background, educational capabilities, and other social factors. Such elements are used by the system to which the worker has applied for relief. For example, a person whose right arm has been amputated may be capable of entering the work force in some other capacity. If the person is young enough, smart enough, and sufficiently motivated, he or she may be capable of performing remunerative activities in some other job market. The referring agency uses such factors when determining whether a person is totally or partially disabled and which benefits are applicable.

6. What is workers' compensation?

According to Elisburg, "Workers' compensation is a disability program to provide medical economic support to workers who have been injured or made ill from an incident arising out of and in the course of employment. It is a complex $70 billion a year program in the United States that involves nearly sixty different systems." This program originated as a social experiment by Bismarck in Germany in the 1880s. It is a "no-fault" compensation system designed to replace the traditional tort system, under which a worker had to sue his employer or get benefits. Unfortunately, the deck was stacked against the employee for various reasons. To rectify this problem, many states developed workers' compensation systems. The last state to do so was Mississippi in 1949. The federal government has similar systems. These systems often are industry-specific and have variable rules regarding impairment, disability, and compensation.

7. What is Social Security Disability (SSD)?

According to the Social Security Administration, SSD is defined as "the inability to engage in any substantial gainful activity by reason of any medically determinable physical or mental impairment(s) which can be expected to result in death or which has lasted or can be expected to last for a continuous period of not less than 12 months." In addition, for a person under the age of 18, disability can exist "if he or she has a medically determinable impairment(s) that is of comparable severity" to impairment in an adult. To comply with these definitions, a person may have a single medical impairment or multiple impairments that, when combined, are of such severity that the person can no longer perform his or her previous occupation or sustain any remunerative activity after age, education, and prior work experience are considered.

Two groups of people are eligible for SSD. Under Title II, Social Security Disability Insurance (SSDI) provides cash benefits for disabled workers and their dependents who have contributed to the Social Security Trust Fund through taxes. Title XVI (Supplemental Security Income [SSI]) provides a minimal income level for the needy, aged, blind, and disabled. People qualify for SSI because of financial need. Under SSI, financial need is said to exist when a person's income and resources are equal to or below an amount specified by law.

8. What is the cost of disability?

This question is difficult to answer. For example, if a worker is injured on the job, what defines the cost of disability? Is it the cost of time off work? Is it the medical expenses (e.g., physician's fees, operative costs, prescription costs, physical therapy, rehabilitation costs)? Is it the cost of paying the worker while he or she is out of work? Is it offset by the fact that the worker's spouse had to return to work? Is it the money to fund the social programs and human resource departments needed to fill out the forms and provide the benefits? Ultimately, of course, all of these factors must be considered.

The aggregate cost of disability in the United States in 1980 was $177 billion or approximately 6.5% of the gross domestic product. Medical expenditures in 1987 totaled $336 billion. Approximately 51% of disability costs are for medical care and other goods and services provided to the disabled. Approximately 39% of the overall cost comes from lost earnings and approximately 10% from the labor market losses of household members or persons with disabilities.

9. Who wrote the "rules" for impairment evaluation?

Disability is a big business in the United States and other countries. Various institutions pay the costs, such as state governments (workers' compensation), the federal government (e.g., veterans or longshoremen), insurance companies, or self-insured employers. Many systems that pay for disability have their own rules and regulations, including rules about the performance and rating of the impairment evaluation. The most commonly used system is a formal set of rules developed by the American Medical Association, which is constantly updated. Another major source of guidelines is the Social Security System. The rules and regulations found in these sources are vastly different. For example, the Social Security Administration recognizes only total impairment. The AMA *Guides* fractionates impairment from 1% to 100%. Highly specific rules are applied to these impairments in each set of guidelines. The impairment evaluator must be thoroughly familiar with the system that he or she is required to use.

10. Define the concept "whole person impairment."

In the AMA *Guides,* whole person impairment reflects the amount of impairment in a given individual. A person who is totally impaired has 100% whole person impairment. A person whose right arm was amputated at the shoulder has a 60% impairment of the whole person. A person with coronary disease may have whole person impairment ranging from 0% to 100%. It depends on the degree of deviation from normal.

11. What is maximum medical improvement (MMI)?

This concept, which is used in impairment evaluation, states that a person has achieved MMI if no more substantial improvement is anticipated with time and/or further treatment. Treatment may include medications, surgery, physical therapy, or other types of rehabilitation. Most impairment systems demand that the person achieve MMI before a final impairment rating can be given. This rating is then used as a basis for the final disability settlement.

12. What is apportionment?

A few states use a concept called apportionment. For example, if a male worker applies for disability benefits because of a toxic gas inhalation, some states take into consideration the fact that he was a two pack a day smoker for the past 20 years. The fact that he was a smoker may have contributed to loss of lung function. The physician evaluating the worker for impairment can quantitate only the current amount of loss of lung function. This loss may have occurred because of the toxic inhalation, the smoking, or a combination of both. When a state or system uses apportionment, it requires the physician to estimate the amount of impairment created by a specific injury or factor as opposed to all other factors that contribute to the total impairment value. Some states ignore this concept and recognize that for any impairment that may have been caused by occupational injury, the occupational injury must be considered the sole cause. California, on the other hand, requires apportionment; the physician in the above case is required to state, for example, that 60% of the impairment was caused by toxic inhalation and 40% by cigarette smoking. Clearly, apportionment requires a great deal of skill and educational background.

13. How does one perform an impairment evaluation?

One starts with the questions that are asked by the referring party. For example, if the examinee's right arm has been amputated, one centers on the amputation. One does not do a complete history and physical examination if it is not requested, called for, or appropriate. On the other hand, the body part that was injured and/or specified in the referral is evaluated thoroughly. This evaluation may take the form of a history, physical examination, specialized physical examination techniques, radiographs and other types of body imaging studies, physiologic testing, and other types of examinations. The evaluation must answer specific questions not only in respect to specific body parts but also in respect to the evaluating system. For example, some evaluating systems require certain tests to be performed and ignore the results from other types of testing. The impairment evaluator must understand thoroughly the system so that the appropriate diagnostic examinations can be performed?

14. What is a functional capacity assessment?

This concept, derived from ergonomists and physical therapists, has been extended to involve other body systems and other types of tests. A functional capacity assessment basically refers to how much a person is capable of doing. In other words, we can measure a person's flexibility in a given joint, the neurologic input to the muscle surrounding that joint, and the strength of the muscles. Then we can determine the physical capability of that joint. This capability may be measured in terms of how much weight can be lifted, how many times it can be lifted, or for how long the person can perform the same activity. These results, called functional capacity assessment, are linked to the specifications of a job. For example, if a man is capable of lifting, on a sustained basis, only 20 pounds (although on a rare basis he is capable of lifting as much as 50 pounds) and the job entails lifting, on an infrequent basis, 60–80 pounds, we might determine that the man is not fit or qualified for the job.

15. What is the American with Disabilities Act?

In 1990 Congress passed the Americans with Disabilities Act (ADA). This law protects people with disabilities from discrimination and mandates accommodations for disabled employees, customers, clients, patients, and others. It prohibits discrimination in public or private employment, governmental services, public accommodations, public transportation, and telecommunication. The ADA defines a person with a disability in three ways: "(1) any person who has a physical or mental impairment that substantially limits one or more of the individual's major life activities, (2) any person who has a 'record of' a substantially limiting impairment, and (3) any person who is 'regarded as' having a substantially-limiting impairment, regardless of whether the person is in fact disabled."

According to the ADA, before an offer for a job, an employer may not inquire about an applicant's impairment or medical history. In addition, inquiries about past injuries and/or workers' compensation claims are expressly prohibited. An employer, however, may conditionally offer a position based on completion of a medical examination or medical inquiry—but only if such examinations or inquiries are made of all applicants for the same job category and the results are kept confidential. A postoffer medical evaluation may be more comprehensive. A job offer may be withdrawn only if the findings of the medical examination show that a person is unable to perform the essential functions of a job, even with a reasonable accommodation, or if the person poses a direct threat to his or her own health or safety or to the health and safety of others, even with reasonable accommodation. Obviously, it is important to have the list of the essential functions of a job for comparison.

16. How do I fill out back-to-work forms?

Functional capacity assessment(s) often comes into play. Some of the basic principles from the ADA are also applicable. One starts with a description of the job—primarily its essential functions, although peripheral functions that, on occasion, may arise also may be included. For assembly-line workers, the job description may include where they have to stand, how many times they have to bend over, whether they have to pick up a part, how heavy the part is, how often they do this activity, and various other ergonomic issues. Ideally, one then matches the person's capability with the requirements of the job. For example, if we can measure how long examinees can stand, how often they can bend, how much bending they care capable of doing, and what strength they have, we should be able to say whether they are capable of returning to their job or whether they need to be assigned to modified and/or restricted duties.

In most circumstances, we do not achieve this perfect state of knowledge and blending of worker with job. When faced with this decision, we have two choices: we can either refer the person for appropriate testing, or we can make an "educated guess," based on experience, knowledge, and background. The more educated the examiner and the better his or her understanding of the job requirements, the more valid his or her determination will be.

17. How do I fill out the forms from the Social Security Department?

Social Security forms frequently cross a physician's desk. They are often multipaged evaluation questions and can be daunting. They are intended to provide background information to the impairment and disability evaluator in the Social Security System. An independent impairment examination also may be performed on such patients. Your report is used to provide background information so that a more accurate and appropriate evaluation can be made. As the patient's treating physician, often you have insights and background that otherwise would not be available to the medical or disability evaluator. You are *not* performing an impairment evaluation when you fill out such forms; that is someone else's job.

18. During his work, a man slips on ice while delivering packages. He has sudden onset of pain and discomfort in his lower back. The pain radiates down the right leg. In addition, numbness and tinging also radiate down the right leg after rest and pain relievers. He is given physical therapy, with some relief. Unfortunately, 2 years later, he has a similar injury. An MRI discloses a herniated disc at the L4–L5 interspace. He has surgery because of persistent and disabling symptoms. He has a successful outcome and has now returned to the work force. He is basically asymptomatic except for mild discomfort in the lower back with prolonged sitting and standing. Does the man have an impairment? If so, how much?

Certainly the man has an impairment because of anatomic deviation from normalcy. Using the AMA *Guides,* he has 10% impairment of the whole person because of the herniated disc and neurologic abnormalities, despite the fact that he has had a successful operation and is relatively asymptomatic.

19. The same man returns to work and slips and falls again. His symptoms are severe. He has pain with minimal activity. He can no longer do sports activities, which he enjoyed in the past. Sexual intercourse is uncomfortable. Does he have an impairment? If so, how much?

The man continues to have impairment caused by the first and second injuries and exacerbated by the third. However, no further impairment is awarded. The 10% impairment that he received originally (although he was essentially asymptomatic) was given because of the known risk for further problems as time passes. Thus, there is no increase in the impairment rating.

BIBLIOGRAPHY

1. American Medical Association: Guides to the Evaluation of Permanent Impairment, 4th ed. Chicago, American Medical Association, 1993.
2. Barth PS: Economic costs of disability. In Demeter SL, Anderson GBJ, Smith GM (eds): Disability Evaluation. St. Louis, Mosby, 1996, pp 13–19.
3. Bell C: Overview of the Americans with Disabilities Act and the Family and Medical Leave Act. In Demeter SL, Andersson GBJ, Smith GM (eds): Disability Evaluation. St. Louis, Mosby, 1996, pp 582–591.
4. Demeter SL: Appendix A. In Demeter SL, Andersson GBJ, Smith GM (eds): Disability Evaluation. St. Louis, Mosby, 1996, pp 606–607.
5. Demeter SL: Contrasting the standard medical examination and the disability examination. In Demeter SL, Andersson GBJ, Smith GM (eds): Disability Evaluation. St Louis, Mosby, 1996, pp 68–72.
6. Demeter SL, Smith GM, Andersson GBJ: Approach to disability evaluation. In Demeter SL, Andersson GBJ, Smith GM (eds): Disability Evaluation. St. Louis, Mosby, 1996, pp 2–4.

 7. Elisburg D: Workers' compensation. In Demeter SL, Andersson GBJ, Smith GM (eds): Disability Evaluation. St. Louis, Mosby, 1996, pp 36–44.
 8. Greenwood JG, History of disability as a legal construct evaluation. In Demeter SL, Andersson GBJ, Smith GM (eds): Disability Evaluation. St Louis, Mosby, 1996, pp 5–12.
 9. Mather JH: Social Security disability systems. In Demeter SL, Andersson GBJ, Smith GM (eds): Disability Evaluation. St. Louis, Mosby, 1996, pp 45–51.
10. Matheson LN: Functional capacity evaluation. In Demeter SL, Andersson GBJ, Smith GM (eds): Disability Evaluation. St. Louis, Mosby, 1996, pp 168–188.
11. Smith GM, Demeter SL, Washington RJ: The disability-oriented medical evaluation and report. In Demeter SL, Andersson GBJ, Smith GM (eds): Disability Evaluation. St. Louis, Mosby, 1996, pp 68–72.
12. Social Security Administration, U.S. Department of Health and Human Services: Disability Evaluation under Social Security. Social Security Administration Publication No. 64-039/ICN 468600, Washington, DC, 1994.

V. Surgical Management of the Spine: General Considerations

20. INDICATIONS FOR SURGICAL INTERVENTION IN SPINAL DISORDERS

Vincent J. Devlin, M.D., and Paul Enker, M.D., FRCS, FAAOS

1. Why is the indication for a spine procedure of such critical importance?

Poor patient selection guarantees a poor surgical result despite how expertly a surgical procedure is performed.

2. What factors determine success after a spinal procedure?

The critical factors that determine success after spinal surgery are the surgical indication (I), surgical technique (T), patient psychosocial factors (PS), and biologic unknowns (BU). It is critical to perform surgery for the appropriate indication with technical proficiency. However, patient psychosocial factors (workmens' compensation, litigation, depression) or biologic unknowns (the multitude of factors that affect healing of a spinal fusion or neural recovery after decompression) can negatively influence the outcome of appropriate and well-executed surgery in powerful ways. Furthermore, these factors are often beyond the control of the surgeon. The relationship among these factors has been summarized in a formula by Enker:

$$\text{Surgical success} = \frac{I \times T}{PS^4 \times BU}$$

3. What are the three major indications for spinal procedures?
- Decompression
- Stabilization
- Realignment

4. Name common indications for spinal decompression procedures.

Spinal decompression is indicated for symptomatic spinal cord or nerve root impingement. Common indications for decompression procedures include disc herniation, spinal stenosis, and cord and/or nerve root impingement secondary to tumor or infection.

5. Name common indications for spinal stabilization procedures.

Spinal stabilization is performed when the structural integrity of the spinal column is compromised to prevent initial or additional neurologic deficit, spinal deformity, or intractable pain. Common indications to perform a spinal stabilization procedure include fractures, tumors, spondylolisthesis, and spinal instability after laminectomy.

6. Name common indications for spinal realignment procedures.

Spinal realignment procedures are performed to correct spinal deformities. Spinal deformities may result from single-level spinal pathology (e.g., spondylolisthesis, fracture, tumor) or from pathology involving multiple spinal levels (kyphosis, scoliosis).

7. How are indications for spinal surgery prioritized?

Indications for spinal surgery are prioritized based on the physician's responsibility to prevent irreversible harm to the patient as a result of spinal pathology and the window of time within which surgical intervention is effective. Although there is no universally accepted classification, surgical indications can be separated into three broad categories :

1. **Emergent indications.** Patients in this category are likely to experience a negative outcome if surgery is not performed emergently. Examples include patients with cauda equina syndrome (most commonly due to a massive lumbar disc herniation) and patients with progressive loss of motor function (e.g., secondary to fracture or spinal tumor).

2. **Urgent indications.** Patients in this category have a serious spinal condition and require surgical intervention to prevent development of a significant permanent neurologic deficit or spinal deformity. Absence of a severe initial neurologic deficit or progressive neurologic deficit permits the opportunity for additional spinal imaging studies, preoperative medical optimization and development of a comprehensive surgical plan that enables the procedure to be performed under ideal conditions on an urgent basis. Examples include patients with unstable spinal fractures as well as certain spinal tumors and infections.

3. **Elective indications.** Patients in this category have the opportunity to explore nonsurgical treatment alternatives and carefully evaluate the risk-benefit ratio of surgical vs. nonsurgical treatment. Examples include patients with degenerative spinal problems (e.g., stenosis, disc herniation, discogenic pain syndromes) and spinal deformities (scoliosis, kyphosis).

8. Is severe back pain an indication for spinal surgery?

Only in limited specific circumstances. Back pain is a symptom, not a diagnosis. The lifetime prevalence of back pain exceeds 70%. Surgery is not indicated for nonspecific low back pain. However, back pain may be a prominent symptom in patients with neural impingement, spinal instability, or certain spinal deformities. In such situations, appropriate spinal decompression, stabilization, and realignment may improve back pain symptoms related to serious underlying spinal pathology. In select degenerative disorders spinal fusion is a reasonable option following adequate nonsurgical treatment if a definite nocioceptive focus is identified in a patient without negative psychosocial factors. Caution is crucial when the indication for surgery is pain because this complaint is often subjective and personal and surgical results are uniformily poor when issues of secondary gain exist.

9. When is surgery indicated for a lumbar disc herniation?

Cauda equina syndrome is the only emergent indication for surgical treatment of a lumbar disc herniation. If a patient is developing a progressive motor deficit it is reasonable to intervene promptly. Indications for elective lumbar disc excision include :

- Functionally incapacitating leg pain in a specific nerve root distribution
- Nerve root tensions signs with or without neurologic signs
- Failure of nonoperative treatment for at least 4–8 weeks

It is critical to confirm that MRI findings correlate with the patient's symptoms before to considering surgical treatment.

10. When is surgical treatment indicated for lumbar spinal stenosis?

Patients with spinal stenosis generally present with varying combinations of low back and buttock pain, neurogenic claudication, and lower extremity radicular symptoms. Severe progressive neurologic deficits are not typically present, although they can occur. Surgery is considered for patients who have failed nonsurgical management, patients with persistent functional incapacity, and patients with neurologic deficits and persistent leg pain. The patient's general medical condition should not pose a contraindication to surgery. The patient should be educated about realistic expectations and goal after surgical treatment. Surgical goals include improved function, decreased pain, and improved or halted progression of neurologic deficits.

11. What are the indications for surgical treatment of cervical radiculopathy due to cervical disc herniation?

- Persistent or recurrent arm pain unresponsive to nonoperative treatment
- Progressive functional neurologic deficit
- Static neurologic deficit associated with significant radicular pain

The patient must have positive imaging studies that correlate with clinical findings.

12. What are the indications for surgical treatment of cervical stenosis?

Patients with cervical radiculopathy secondary to foraminal stenosis with nerve root compression should be distinguished from patients with cervical myelopathy or patients with a combination of radiculopathy and myelopathy. Surgical indications for cervical radiculopathy are identical to those for a cervical disc herniation. Surgical treatment of cervical myelopathy is recommended for patients with progressive neurologic deficit or progressive impairment of function (especially ambulation) in the absence of sustained remisssion of symptoms.

13. When is surgical intervention indicated for spinal infection?

- Open biopsy to obtain tissue for culture when closed biopsy has failed or is considered dangerous
- Failure of medical management with persistent pain and elevated erythrocyte sedimentation rate and/or C-reactive protein levels
- Drainage of an abscess
- Decompression for spinal cord and/or nerve root compression with associated neurologic deficit
- Correction of progressive or unacceptable spinal deformity
- Correction of progressive or unacceptable spinal instability

14. When is surgical intervention indicated for primary spinal tumors?

- Open biopsy to obtain tissue for definitive diagnosis
- Failure of medical therapy (e.g., chemotherapy, radiation)
- For treatment of tumors known to be resistant to medical therapy
- Decompression for spinal cord and/or nerve root compression with associated neurologic deficit
- Correction of progressive or unacceptable spinal deformity
- Correction of progressive or unacceptable spinal instability

15. What are the indications for surgical intervention for metastatic spinal tumors?

- Open biopsy to obtain tissue for definitive diagnosis
- Treatment for tumors resistant to radiotherapy and/or chemotherapy
- Decompression for spinal cord and/or nerve root compression with associated neurologic deficit
- Correction of progressive or unacceptable spinal deformity
- Correction of progressive or unacceptable spinal instability
- Intractable pain and/or neurologic deterioration during radiation therapy despite steroids
- Impending pathologic fracture/instability

16. When is surgical treatment indicated for spinal fractures?

Surgical treatment is indicated for unstable spine fractures. Clinical stability has been defined as the ability of the spine under physiologic loads to limit the patterns of displacement so as not to damage or irritate the spinal cord or nerve roots and, in addition, to prevent incapacitating deformity or pain due to structural changes.[4,5] Specific classifications for fractures involving all levels of the spine are used to guide treatment.

17. What factors are considered in deciding whether surgical treatment is indicated for adolescent idiopathic scoliosis?

Indications for surgical treatment are based on curve magnitude, clinical deformity, risk of curve progression, skeletal maturity, and curve pattern. Curves greater than 50° should undergo surgical treatment because of the risk for continued curve progression in adulthood. Curves in the 40–50° range are analyzed on an individual basis. Curves greater than 40 degrees with documented progression are indicated for surgery. Curves greater than 40 degrees in skeletally immature patients (e.g., premenarchal female) should be treated surgically because of the natural history of continued curve progression with growth. Clinical deformity plays a role in decision-making for select lumbar curves (35–40°). Some curves cause marked waist-line asymmetry and may be considered for surgery on this basis. Sagittal plane alignment is also an important consideration. In a small subgroup of patients with severe thoracic hypokyphosis or actual thoracic lordosis, surgical treatment should be considered even if the coronal plane curve is less than 40°.

18. What are some common indications for surgical treatment of adult scoliosis?

Unlike adolescent patients with scoliosis, adult patients commonly present for evaluation of back pain symptoms. Indications for surgical treatment of adult patients with scoliosis include pain, progressive deformity, cardiopulmonary symptoms, neurologic dysfunction, and cosmesis.

19. When is revision surgery indicated after an initial spinal procedure that has failed?

Surgery is indicated only if surgically correctable pathology is present and the patient's symptoms can be explained on the basis of this pathology. Often there is a poor correlation between imaging studies and a patient's symptoms. For example, not all patients with radiographic evidence of pseudarthrosis are symptomatic. Severity of pain or disability, in and of itself, is not an indication for additional spinal surgery. Commonly encountered problems for which revision spinal surgery may provide benefit in the appropriate patient include:
- Recurrent or persistent disc herniation
- Recurrent or persistent spinal stenosis
- Postlaminectomy instability
- Lumbar disc space infection following lumbar discectomy
- Symptomatic pseudarthrosis
- Flatback syndrome

20. Describe some of the common indications for posterior spinal instrumentation and fusion procedures.

Posterior spinal decompression and stabilization. Symptomatic spinal stenosis is typically decompressed from a posterior approach. Concomitant posterior fusion and spinal instrumentation can restore posterior spinal column integrity and prevent future spinal deformities. A wide range of pathology (e.g., fractures, tumors, spondylolisthesis) requiring decompression and fusion can also be treated from a posterior approach

Posterior correction of spinal deformities. A wide spectrum of spinal deformities can be treated with posterior spinal fusion combined with posterior spinal instrumentation

Restoration of the posterior spinal tension band. Maintenance of normal spinal alignment through application of dorsal tension forces against an intact anterior spinal column is termed the *tension band principle*. When spinal pathology compromises the structural integrity of the posterior spinal column, posterior spinal arthrodesis and posterior spinal instrumenation is required to restore biomechanics of the spinal column

21. Describe the common indications for anterior spinal instrumentation and fusion procedures.

Anterior spinal decompression and stabilization. Spinal infections and tumors most commonly involve the intervertebral disc and/or vertebral body. Debridement, decompression, arthrodesis and stabilization are most directly achieved from an anterior approach.

Anterior correction of spinal deformity. Anterior fusion combined with use of anterior spinal instrumentation is an effective method for treatment of select cases of scoliosis and other spinal deformities.

To enhance arthrodesis. The anterior spinal column provides a highly vascularized fusion bed which promotes successful arthrodesis. The addition of an anterior fusion increases the rate of successful arthrodesis when a posterior spinal instrumentation and fusion is performed for challenging cases.

Anterior release or destabiliztion to enhance posterior spinal deformity correction. Improved correction of rigid spinal deformities using posterior spinal instrumentation can be achieved by resection of disc or bone from the anterior spinal column.

To restore anterior spinal column lead sharing. Normally 80% of axial load is transmitted through the anterior spinal column and 20% through the posterior spinal column. Restoration of anterior spinal load sharing is required to restore stability to mechanically compromised spinal segments.

22. What are common indications for performing combined anterior and posterior spinal fusion and instrumentation?

- Spinal pathology that compromise anterior spinal column load sharing as well as the posterior spinal tension band (e.g., isthmic spondylolisthesis, vertebral destruction of major proportions due to tumor, infection, trauma)
- To enhance arthrodesis (e.g., pseudarthrosis repair, treatment of postlaminectomy instability)
- Treatment of severe spinal deformities (e.g., adult scoliosis, rigid spinal deformities)
- To prevent crankshaft (congenital scoliosis, neuromuscular scoliosis, early-onset idiopathic scoliosis)

An anterior column fusion can be performed either through a posterior approach or through a separate anterior surgical approach depending on clinical circumstances.

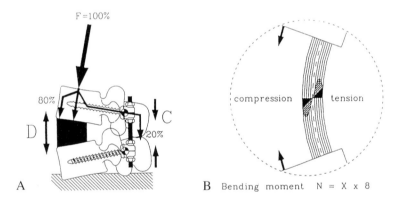

FIGURE 1. Anterior column load sharing and the posterior tension band principle. The normal biomechanics of the lumbar spine is such that 80% of axial load passes through the anterior spinal column and 20% of load passes through the posterior spinal column (**A**). The posterior spinal column is controlled by the erector muscles of the trunk, which apply dorsal compression forces against an intact anterior spinal column (tension band principle). The efficacy of the tension band principle directly depends on the intactness of the anterior spinal column (**B**) (From Harms J: Screw-threaded rod system in spinal fusion surgery. Spine State Art Rev 6:541–575, 1992, with permission.)

BIBLIOGRAPHY

1. Bridwell KH, DeWald RL. The Textbook of Spinal Surgery, 2nd ed. Philadelphia, Lippincott-Raven, 1997.
2. Enker P: Formula for a successful surgical outcome. Presented at the Fourth Annual International Spine Workshop, Cleveland Spine and Arthritis Center at Lutheran Hospital, Cleveland, OH February, 1992.
3. Fardon DF, Garfin SR, et al (eds): Orthopaedic Knowledge Update – Spine 2. Rosemont, IL, American Academy of Orthopaedic Surgeons, 2002.
4. Garfin SR, Vaccaro AR (eds): Orthopaedic Knowledge Update – Spine. Rosemont, IL, American Academy of Orthopaedic Surgeons, 1997.
5. White AA, Panjabi MM: Clinical Biomechanics of the Spine, 2nd ed. Philadelphia, J.B. Lippincott, 1990.

21. WHEN NOT TO OPERATE FOR SPINAL DISORDERS

Vincent Devlin, M.D., and Paul Enker, M.D., FRCS, FAAOS

1. In what situations is it unrealistic to perform surgery for a patient with a spinal disorder?

Decisions can only be made on a case-by-case basis after a complete physical exam, imaging work-up, and medical risk assessment have been completed. Some situations in which spinal surgery would not be advised include:

- When the general medical condition of the patient contraindicates an appropriate surgical procedure
- In the presence of global spinal pathology not amenable to focal surgical treatment (e.g., diffuse degenerative disc changes involving the cervical, thoracic, and lumbar spine may be beyond surgical remedy)
- When severe osteopenia prevents secure internal fixation
- Loss of soft tissue coverage over the posterior aspect of the spine
- Severe infection that cannot be eradicated
- Lack of correlation between imaging studies and the patient's symptoms
- Patients with unrealistic expectations and goals with respect to surgical outcome
- Patients with profound psychological disorders

2. How is surgical decision-making for degenerative spinal disorders different from decision-making for spinal disorders secondary to trauma, tumor, or infection?

Spinal disorders secondary to tumor, trauma, and infection frequently require surgical intervention on an emergent or urgent basis. These disorders are structural problems in which surgical decision-making involves determination of the need for spinal decompression and the optimal surgical procedure to restore spinal biomechanics. Degenerative spinal problems usually require surgery on an elective basis. The patient has the opportunity to maximize available nonsurgical treatment options before considering surgery. Decision-making for degenerative disorders not only involves restoration of spinal biomechanics but also encompasses a multitude of psychologic and socioeconomic issues. It is important that patients undergoing elective spine surgery for degenerative disorders be educated about realistic expectations and goals regarding pain and physical function in relation to surgery.

3. What surgeon factors negatively influence the decision to proceed with a spinal operation?

Spinal surgery has a high risk of serious complications, including problems such as permanent neurologic deficit. This type of surgery should be performed by surgeons with the prerequisite training and experience. There is little role in modern spinal surgery for the surgeon who performs only occasional spine surgery. The current trend is for spinal surgery to be performed by orthopedic surgeons or neurosurgeons who devote the majority of their practice to the diagnosis and treatment of spinal disorders in facilities with adequate equipment and support staff.

4. What patient factors can be modified before a spinal fusion procedure to improve surgical outcome?

- Nutritional status (poor nutritional status increases the risk of infection and wound-healing problems)
- Smoking (nicotine decreases fusion success and increases risk of postoperative pulmonary complications)

- Use of nonsteroidal anti-inflammatory medication (decreases fusion rate and inhibits platelet function)
- Assessment and treatment of osteoporosis (decreases fusion rate and compromises spinal fixation)

5. What patient psychosocial factors may negatively influence the decision to proceed with a spinal operation?

Alcoholism, drug dependence, severe depression or other psychologic disturbance (e.g., borderline personality), ongoing litigation, and social disarray.

6. What physical findings suggest a poor prognosis if lumbar surgery is performed?

A brief screening for nonorganic signs as described by Waddell is valuable. These signs include:

- Tenderness (superficial and/or nonanatomic)
- Simulation (low back pain with axial loading of the skull or rotation of shoulders and pelvis)
- Distraction (marked improvement of pain on straight leg raising with distraction)
- Regional disturbance (nonanatomic findings on sensory and motor examination)
- Overreaction (disproportionate pain behaviors during examination)

The presence of three of more of these signs suggests a poor prognosis after lumbar spine surgery.

7. Why is the presence of degenerative disc changes, disc herniation, or spinal stenosis on MRI an insufficient basis for determining the need for surgical intervention?

MRI of the spine is a highly sensitive but not highly specific. Many findings reported on spinal imaging studies are common in ayymptomatic individuals. Decisions about the need for surgical intervention must rely on correlation of symptomatology and imaging studies. In certain situations, pain provocation procedures are a crucial part of surgical decision-making.

8. A 50-year-old male executive presents to the office of a surgeon after a lumbar MRI scan ordered by his primary care physician. The patient has experienced symptoms of intermittent mechanical low back pain without radiculopathy over the past 3 months. According to the radiologist's report, the patient has severe degenerative disc disease. The patient is extremely worried and is interested in having the disease corrected with an operation. Is surgical treatment indicated?

No. Degeneration of the lumbar intervertebral disc is part of the normal aging process and is not properly termed a disease. In a study of lumbar MRI scans in asymptomatic subjects, degenerative disc changes were seen in 34% of patients between 20 and 39 years, 59% of patients between 40 and 50 years and in 93% of patients between 60 and 80 years of age.[2] This patient should be evaluated with standing radiographs of the lumbar spine and undergo a detailed history and physical examination. If evaluation reveals no serious underlying problem, the patient can be reassured and nonsurgical treatment can be initiated.

9. A 15-year-old football player is evaluated on a preseason exam and reports a history of intermittent low back pain. Presently he is not experiencing low back pain symptoms. Radiographs show an L5 spondylolysis. Is surgical treatment indicated?

No. The patient is asymptomatic, and prophylactic surgery is not indicated. Children and adolescents with spondylolysis and low-grade spondylolisthesis usually respond to nonoperative treatment measures and often can avoid surgery.

10. A 40-year-old man is referred for consultation after a lumbar MRI showed a large extruded disc fragment at L5–S1 level. The patient noted the onset of severe back and radicular pain 1 month ago. Since that time, the patient reports greater than 50% reduction in back and leg pain. The patient reported initial mild weakness of ankle plantarflexion, which

has improved. The patient has no difficulty with gait and has no symptoms to suggest cauda equina syndrome. The patient is presently working at an office job. Should surgery be recommended at this time?

No. This patient is likely to experience a good outcome with nonsurgical treatment. Prognostic factors that suggest a positive outcome with nonoperative care include:

- A large disc extrusion or sequestration
- Progressive return of neurologic function within the first 12 weeks
- Relief or > 50% reduction in leg pain within the first 6 weeks of onset
- Absence of spinal stenosis
- Absence of pain with crossed straight leg raising
- Positive response to corticosteroid injection
- Limited psychosocial issues

11. When is revision lumbar spinal surgery contraindicated?

Revision spinal surgery is contraindicated in the absence of surgically correctable pathology. Severity of pain or disability, in and of itself, is not an indication for additional surgery. Patients with problems such as recurrent herniated discs, spinal instability, or spinal stenosis are potential candidates for additional surgery. Patients with scar tissue (arachnoiditis, perineural fibrosis), systemic medical disease, and psychosocial instability have symptoms that are nonmechanical in nature and should be treated with strategies other than surgery.

12. When is surgery for spinal tumors unlikely to provide significant patient benefit?

Each patient must be evaluated on an individual basis. However, situations in which the risk of surgery for metastatic spine tumors may outweigh patient benefit include:

- Widespread metastatic disease with involvement of all spinal regions(cervical, thoracic and lumbar spine)
- Life expectancy less than three months
- Poor immunologic status (e.g., bone marrow suppression secondary to chemotherapy or radiotherapy)
- Poor nutritional status (increased risk of infection and poor wound healing)
- Poor pulmonary function (if anterior surgical approach indicated)
- Recurrent spinal cord compression due to renal or lung carcinoma
- Immunosuppressed patients with marked deformity and paralysis

13. When can pyogenic spinal infections be treated without surgery?

The majority of spinal infections can be managed effectively with appropriate antibiotic therapy and brace treatment. Biopsy and blood cultures are mandatory to select appropriate antibiotic therapy. Parenteral antibiotics should be administered for a minimum period of 6 weeks. Effectiveness of antibiotic therapy can be assessed with serial erythrocyte sedimentation rates and C-reactive protein levels. The indications for surgical intervention are limited and well-defined.

14. What types of spinal fractures can be treated without surgery?

Cervical spine

- Most atlas (C1) fractures
- Type 1 and type 3 odontoid (C2) fractures
- Most hangman's fractures (C2) except type 3 injuries
- Subaxial cervical compression fractures without posterior ligamentous injury
- Isolated undisplaced fractures of the posterior elements

Thoracic and lumbar spine

- Most compression fractures
- Burst fractures with < 25° kyphosis and < 50% canal compromise in neurologically intact patients

BIBLIOGRAPHY

1. Asdourian PL: Metastatic Disease of the Spine. In Bridwell KH, DeWald RL (eds): The Textbook of Spinal Surgery. 2nd ed. Philadelphia, Lippincott-Raven, 1997, pp 2007–2050.
2. Boden SD, Davis DO, Dina T, et al: Abnormal magnetic resonance scans of the lumbar spine in symptomatic subjects. J Bone Joint Surg 72A:403–408, 1990.
3. Federowicz SG, Wiesel SW. An alogorithm for the multiply operated low back patient and treatment of operative complications. Semin Spine Surg 3:175–183, 1991.
4. Maguire JK: Nonsurgical management of acute injuries to the spine. In Fardon DF, Garfin SR (eds): Orthopaedic Knowledge Update – Spine 2. Rosemont, IL, American Academy of Orthopaedic Surgeons, 2002, pp 167–176.
5. Saal JA: Natural history and nonoperative treatment of lumbar disc herniation. Spine 21: 2S–9S, 1996.
6. Slucky AV, Eismont FJ. Spinal infections. In Bridwell KH, DeWald RL (eds): The Textbook of Spinal Surgery, 2nd ed. Philadelphia, Lippincott-Raven, 1997, pp 2141–2183.
7. Waddell G, McCulloch JA, Kummel EG, Venner RTM: Non-organic physical signs in low back pain. Spine 5: 117–125, 1980.

22. PREOPERATIVE ASSESSMENT AND PLANNING FOR PATIENTS UNDERGOING SPINE SURGERY

Vincent J. Devlin, M.D., and William O. Shaffer, M.D.

1. Name five factors that influence morbidity and mortality after spinal surgery.
- Type of procedure
- Whether elective or emergency
- Chronologic age of the patient
- General health of the patient
- Facility where surgery is performed (e.g., experience of surgeons, anesthesiologists, intensivists; availability of state-of-the-art imaging and spinal monitoring)

2. What types of elective spinal procedures are associated with the lowest risk of complications and perioperative morbidity?
When performed in patients without significant medical comorbidities, the following elective spinal procedures have the lowest risk profiles:
- Lumbar microdiscectomy
- Lumbar laminectomy
- Anterior cervical discectomy and fusion
- Single level lumbar spinal fusion (anterior or posterior)
- Fusions for adolescent idiopathic scoliosis

3. What types of spinal procedures are associated with a high risk of complications and perioperative morbidity?
- Revision spinal deformity procedures
- Same-day multilevel anterior-posterior spinal procedures
- Emergent spinal procedures for tumor, infection and trauma
- Fusions for spinal deformities in patient with neuromuscular scoliosis

4. What types of patients are at increased risk of complications after spinal surgery?
- Pediatric patients with spinal deformities secondary to neuromuscular disease
- Patients > 60 years of age requiring extensive fusion procedures, especially anterior fusions or anterior/posterior fusions
- Patients with major preoperative neurologic deficits
- Patients requiring surgery for tumor or infection
- Patients with a history of chronic steroid use
- Patients with multiple medical comorbidities

5. Once a patient has decided to pursue elective spine surgery, what three general issues require attention before the day of surgery?
1. Appropriate interdisciplinary medical evaluation to confirm that the patient is a reasonable medical candidate for anesthesia and proposed surgery
2. Coordination of equipment and personnel required for the surgical procedure
3. Patient education regarding diagnosis, treatment, and eventual recovery, including discharge planning

Exact details vary with patient factors (pediatric vs. adult patients, associated medical comorbidities), procedure type (decompression vs. fusion), magnitude of surgery (number of levels fused, anterior vs. posterior vs. combined procedures), and surgical setting (outpatient vs. inpatient).

6. List the components of a typical preoperative evaluation for a patient who is to undergo spinal surgery.

- Complete medical history and physical exam
- Appropriate radiographs and spinal imaging studies
- Appropriate preoperative testing based on age and medical history, such as chest radiograph, EKG, complete blood count with differential, chemistry panel, bleeding profile (prothrombin time, partial thromboplastin time, bleeding time), urine analysis, type and cross match (if blood transfusion required). A pregnancy test should be obtained for females > 12 years of age.
- Evaluation by an internist (for patients over 50 years of age or patients with significant medical problems)

7. List key points to assess during the preoperative medical evaluation of a patient undergoing major spinal reconstructive surgery.

Cardiovascular: cardiac risk factors, presence of carotid disease, history of transient ischemic attacks, presence of peripheral vascular disease and/or vascular claudication, history of thromboembolic disease.

Pulmonary: specific problems noted with neuromuscular disorders, severe thoracic scoliosis, chronic obstructive pulmonary disease (COPD), emphysema, and smoking.

Neurologic: document preoperative neurologic deficits; assess ability to cooperate with wake-up test if needed.

Hematologic: history of abnormal bruising or bleeding. Instruct patient to discontinue aspirin and nonsteroidal anti-inflammatory medication at least 2 weeks before surgery; assess issues regarding blood donation and blood transfusion.

Endocrine: assess risk factors for osteoporosis; optimize control of blood glucose in diabetic patients.

Nutritional status: assess nutritional status because deficits result in impaired wound healing and increased risk of infection.

Patient habits: history of smoking, alcohol use, analgesic use, drug abuse.

Psychological factors: assess barriers to recovery.

8. What is the leading cause of death after noncardiac surgery?

Cardiac events in the perioperative period are the leading cause of death after noncardiac surgery.

9. What test is useful to assess patients at risk of a cardiac event before spinal surgery?

A dobutamine stress echocardiography is recommended before elective spine surgery for:

- Patients of any age with a history of previous coronary artery disease, congestive heart failure, myocardial infarction, or smoking
- All patients 65 years of age or older

10. How is cardiac risk stratified before surgery?

Guidelines for cardiac risk stratification developed by the American College of Cardiology and American Heart Association include assessment of:

1. **Clinical risk factors**
   - Major: unstable coronary syndromes, decompensated congestive heart failure (CHF), significant arrthymia, severe valvular disease
   - Intermediate: mild angina pectoris, prior myocardial infarction, compensated CHF, diabetes mellitus, renal insufficiency
   - Minor: advanced age, abnormal EKG, rhythm other than sinus, low functional capacity, history of stroke, uncontrolled hypertension
2. **Procedural risk factors**
   - High risk: major emergency surgery, vascular surgery, any procedure that is prolonged with large fluid shifts, blood loss, or both

- Intermediate risk: general orthopaedic procedures, carotid endarterectomies, peritoneal and thoracic procedures
- Low risk

3. **Patient's functional status:** rated as excellent, moderate, or poor.

Application of an algorithm based on these guidelines leads to a decision to proceed with surgery, to cancel surgery pending coronary artery intervention, or to delay surgery for additional noninvasive cardiac testing.

11. What are the risk factors for perioperative stroke?

Major risk factors include advanced age, history of transient ischemic attacks, hypertension, cardiac abnormalities, diabetes, and prior stroke. Patients with a history of transient ischemic attacks should be referred for a duplex ultrasonography before undergoing an elective spine procedure. Carotid bruits in the absence of symptoms do not necessarily warrant additional work-up.

12. List disorders associated with cardiac dysfunction as well as spinal deformity.

Muscular dystrophy (e.g., Duchenne's, Becker's), Marfan's syndrome, Charcot-Marie Tooth disease, Friedreich's ataxia, and congenital myotonia are associated with a variety of cardiac disorders. There is an association between congenital scoliosis and congenital heart disease.

13. When is a pulmonary consultation advisable before spinal surgery?

- Thoracic spinal deformities
- Neuromuscular spinal deformities
- Patients with known pulmonary problems (asthma, COPD, emphysema) or smoking history
- Infantile or juvenile scoliosis

14. What results on preoperative arterial blood gas testing suggest the presence of significant pulmonary disease?

A baseline arterial carbon dioxide pressure ($PaCO_2$) of greater than 50 or chronic hypoxemia should raise concern about the possibility of pulmonary hypertension or cor pulmonale. Such patients have an increased risk of postoperative respiratory failure.

15. Which patients are likely to require ventilatory support after spinal surgery?

Patients are usually extubated immediately after surgery, and the criteria for extubation are not different for patients after spinal procedures. Exceptions include:

- Patients with significant preoperative impairment of pulmonary function
- Patients undergoing same-day multilevel anterior and posterior fusion procedures involving extensive blood loss and fluid shifts
- Patients undergoing extensive anterior or circumferential cervical surgery due to risk of postoperative neck edema with resultant airway obstruction

16. Why are smokers at increased risk of complications following spinal procedures compared to non-smokers?

Smoking increases the risk of cardiopulmonary problems after surgery (e.g., atelectasis, pneumonia). Cessation of smoking 2 months before surgery reduces the risk of pulmonary complications fourfold. Smoking also decreases the rate of successful spinal fusion.

17. List key points relating to neurologic assessment before spinal procedures.

- Document the presence of any preoperative neurologic deficits.
- Determine the patients's ability to cooperate with a wake-up test (if needed).
- Consider a neurology consultation if a history of seizure disorder is present.
- Obtain neurosurgery consultation if spinal deformity correction is planned in a patient with a CNS shunt.

18. Why is nutritional assessment important? How is a patient's nutritional status quantified?

Malnutrition increases the chance of postoperative infection and wound healing complications. Serum albumin < 3.5 mg/dl, total lymphocyte count < 1500–2000 cells/mm, transferrin < 200 mg/dl, and prealbumin < 20mg/dl are considered to represent clinical malnutrition.

19. What are the options for blood transfusion if significant blood loss is anticipated during a spinal procedure?

Autologous blood (use of the patient's own blood). This is the safest blood available and carries the lowest risk. Most commonly, blood is collected before the date of surgery and stored until the day of surgery. Candidates for this option typically have a hematocrit of at least 34%, weigh at least 100 pounds, are 12–75 years old, and do not have significant medical comorbidities. The patient's own blood may be salvaged during surgery through use of a cell saver. This method of blood conservation decreases the need for transfusion.

Directed donor blood. The patient may specify family members or selected individuals to donate blood before surgery. In general, a safety margin is not provided to the patient by selecting his or her blood donors. Approximately 70% of directed donors are first-time donors, whereas approximately 70% community donors are repeat donors. It has been shown that repeat donors are safer than first-time donors. In addition, when directed donor blood comes from blood relatives, it needs to be irradiated before transfusion to prevent the rare occurrence of graft vs. host disease in the recipient.

Allogenic blood (from the community blood pool). Allogenic blood transfusion is not without risk. The approximate risk of disease transmission and related complications has been estimated as follows:

HIV-1(AIDS)	1: 1,900,000
HTLV-1/11	1: 641,000
Hepatitis C virus (non-A non-B)	1: 600,000
Hepatitis B virus	1: 180,000
Red blood cell bacterial contamination	0.3–2/1000
Allergic reaction	1:100
Hemolytic transfusion reaction	1:6,000
Fatal hemolytic transfusion reaction	1:100,000

20. What can be done before surgery to stimulate increased red blood cell mass in the patient with decreased hemoglobin secondary to blood donation or chronic anemia?

Iron supplementation combined with Epogen or Procrit can be used to increase red blood cell mass before surgery in select patients. An autologous blood donation program also ensures increased marrow production of blood. Hematology consultation is valuable for complex cases.

21. Does the presence of diabetes increase the risk of complications associated with spine surgery?

Yes. The presence of diabetes increases the risk of impaired wound healing and wound infection in patients undergoing spine surgery. In addition, insulin-dependent diabetic patients who undergo decompression for radiculopathy have less favorable outcomes, especially if peripheral neuropathy is present. Optimization of blood glucose levels preoperatively can result in improved wound healing and decreased infection rates.

22. What laboratory tests can be used as a screen for alcoholism in the preoperative period?

Increased red-cell mean corpuscular volume (MCV) and increases in the hepatic enzyme gamma glutamyltranferase have been described as confirmatory markers for alcoholism.

23. What problems may occur in alcoholic patients who undergo spine surgery?

- Alcohol withdrawal symptoms (autonomic dysfunction, seizures, hallucinations)
- Altered metabolism of medications including anesthetic agents

- Abnormal hemostasis due to decrease in vitamin K-dependent clotting factors and platelet abnormalities
- Metabolic abnormalities: hypoglycemia, ketoacidosis, malnutrition, nutrient deficiencies (thiamine, folate and magnesium).

24. What problems are encountered after spinal procedures in patients who abuse opioids or benzodiazapines?

Postoperative problems include difficulty with pain control due to drug tolerance as well as patient anxiety.

25. List basic equipment/facility requirements for undertaking complex spinal surgical procedures.

- Spinal implants and ancillary instrumentation
- Power equipment (e.g., Midas Rex drill)
- Imaging capability (radiographs, fluoroscopy)
- Radiolucent spine table
- Spinal monitoring
- Surgical microscope
- Anesthesiologist familiar with hypotensive anesthetic techniques and wake-up test
- Blood recovery system (cell saver)
- Bone bank access
- Appropriate intensive care unit, medical and surgical intensive care facilities and specialists

26. What is the best way to ensure that a patient has been adequately educated about diagnosis, treatment, and recovery before an elective spinal procedure?

Arrange a conference with the patient and his or her significant others before surgery. Important points to cover during this meeting include:

- Review patient's specific spinal problem and treatment alternatives.
- Review pertinent diagnostic studies.
- Explain specific surgical procedures using spine models (incisions, bone graft, implants, FDA status of spinal devices).
- Discuss realistic expectations and goals of surgical treatment (pain relief, deformity correction, neurologic improvement, likely outcome of procedure).
- Discuss possible surgical complications and obtain informed consent.
- Confirm arrangements for blood donation, cessation of aspirin and anti-inflammatory medication, cessation of smoking, spinal monitoring, review of wake-up test (if needed), orthosis (if needed), and hospital tour and familiarization.
- Order any additional imaging studies required for preoperative planning.
- Review final recommendations and evaluations by consultants (anesthesiologist, internist, intensivist).
- Outline events on the day of surgery for the patient and family: check-in procedures and waiting area, duration of surgery, and patient's postoperative location and status (ICU vs. step down vs. standard floor vs. outpatient; discuss need for postoperative ventilatory support).
- Review anticipated hospital course/discharge arrangements: length of stay, discharge planning concerns, work-related issues, psychologic support during recovery period, and chemical dependency issues related to use of narcotic medication.

27. What common complications should be explained to the patient before performing a procedure for decompression of the spinal cord and /or nerve roots?

- Neurologic injury
- Dural tear
- Spinal instability
- Persistent or increased back and/or extremity pain

- Blood loss
- Wound infection
- Complications related to the surgical approach
- Potential need for subsequent spinal surgery including stabilization
- Medical complications—urinary tract infection, myocardial infarction, deep vein thrombosis
- Anesthetic complication
- Arachnoiditis (scarring of nerves)
- Death

28. What common complications should be explained to the patient before surgical procedures that involve spinal instrumentation and fusion?

- Implant/bone graft failure, misplacement, dislodgement
- Neurologic injury, including paralysis and loss of bowel and bladder control
- Pseudarthrosis (failure of fusion)
- Bone graft donor site pain
- Infection
- Blood loss
- Diseases transmitted by blood transfusion or allograft bone
- Dural tear
- Persistent or increased back and/or extremity pain
- Need for subsequent spinal surgery
- Medical complications: urinary tract infection, myocardial infarction, pneumonia, deep vein thrombosis, pulmonary embolism, stroke
- Allergic reaction (to drugs, metallic devices)
- Surgical approach-related complications (e.g., hernia, retrograde ejaculation in men, vascular injury, visceral injury)
- Visual difficulty or blindness
- Pressure sores on chest, facial areas, pelvis, and lower extremities
- Anesthetic complication
- Death

BIBLIOGRAPHY

1. Baldus C, Blanke K: Preoperative nursing care. In Bridwell KH, DeWald RL (eds): The textbook of spinal surgery, ed. 2, Philadelphia, 1997, Lippincott-Raven, pp 3–10.
2. Boachie-Adjei O: Implications of malnutrition in the surgical patient. . In Bridwell KH, DeWald RL (eds): The textbook of spinal surgery, ed. 2, Philadelphia, 1997, Lippincott-Raven, pp 101–112.
3. Brown CW, Orme TJ, Richardson JD: The rate of pseudarthrosis in patients who are smokers and patients who are non-smokers. A comparison study. Spine 11:942–943, 1986.
4. Devlin VJ, Williams DA: Decision making and perioperative care of the patient. In Margulies JY, Aebi M, Farcy JP (eds). Revision Spine Surgery. Mosby, St. Louis, 1999, pp 297–319.
5. Eagle KA, Berger PB, Calkins H, et al: ACC/AHA guidelines update for perioperative cardiovascular evaluation for noncardiac surgery-executive summary. J Am Coll Cardiol 39:542–553, 2002.
6. Faciszewski T, Jensen R, Rokey R, Berg R: Cardiac risk stratification of patients with symptomatic spinal stenosis. Clin Orthop Rel Res 384:110–115, 2001.
7. Reeg SE: A review of comorbidities and spinal surgery. Clin Orthop Rel Res 384:101–109, 2001.
8. Rubin FH: Preoperative and perioperative issues in the orthopaedic surgical patient. Oper Techn Orthop, 12:60–63, 2002.
9. Smith GF: Perioperative care of the spine patient. In White AH (ed): Spine Care—Operative Treatment. St. Louis, Mosby, 1995, pp 964–983.

23. SPINAL ARTHRODESIS AND BONE-GRAFTING TECHNIQUES

Eric W. Edmonds, M.D., and Munish C. Gupta, M.D.

1. Define spinal arthrodesis.

Spinal arthrodesis is defined as the elimination of motion across an intervertebral segment as a result of bony union (fusion). During surgery adjacent bone surfaces are decorticated, bone graft is applied, and spinal instrumentation or subsequent external immobilization is used to decrease motion at the surgical site and facilitate fusion.

2. What are the three main categories of spinal arthrodesis procedures?

Anterior fusion, posterior fusion and combined anterior and posterior fusion (also called 360° fusion, circumferential fusion, or global fusion).

3. What is the role of spinal instrumentation in spinal arthrodesis procedures?

Spinal instrumentation may be used to correct a spinal deformity or to stabilize a spinal segment whose structural integrity has been compromised by spinal pathology such as a fracture, tumor, or infection. Spinal instrumentation may be used to limit intersegmental motion and to create a favorable mechanical environment that increases the likelihood of successful fusion. The primary goal in any procedure using spinal instrumentation is to achieve a successful fusion. Spinal implants will ultimately fail unless osseous union is achieved.

4. Name common indications for performing a spinal arthrodesis and provide at least one clinical example for each indication.

- Trauma: burst fractures, fracture-dislocations, flexion-distraction injuries
- Tumor: pathologic spine fracture secondary to metastatic or primary tumor
- Infection: spinal instability due to disc space infection or vertebral osteomyelitis
- Rheumatologic disorders: C1–C2 instability due to rheumatoid arthritis
- Spinal deformities: scoliosis, kyphosis, congenital deformities
- Degenerative spinal disorders: degenerative spondylolisthesis with spinal stenosis

5. What factors influence successful healing of a spinal fusion?

1. Type of bone graft used (autograft, allograft, synthetic biomaterials)
2. Local factors
   - Quality of the soft tissue bed into which bone graft is placed
   - Method of preparation of the graft recipient site
   - Mechanical stability of the spine segment(s) to be fused
   - Graft location(anterior vs. posterior spinal column)
3. Systemic host factors
   - Metabolic bone disease(ex. osteoporosis)
   - Nutrition
   - Perioperative medication
   - Smoking

6. How does tobacco use interfere with spinal fusion?

Cigarette smoking has been shown to interfere with bone metabolism and inhibit bone formation. The rate of nonunion in smokers who have undergone spine fusion is higher than in nonsmokers.

7. What common medications can interfere with healing of a spinal fusion?

Certain medications impair fusion if used in the perioperative period because they inhibit or delay bone formation. Examples include nonsteroidal antiinflammatory drugs (e.g., ibuprofen, toradol) and chemotheraputic agents (e.g., methotrexate).

8. What are the common sources for bone graft used in spinal arthrodesis procedures?

Graft options for spinal fusion include autograft, allograft, and synthetics. Sources for autograft bone include the patient's fibula, ribs, and ilium. Autograft may be procured as a structural or nonstructural graft. The ratio of cancellous to cortical bone varies depending on the bone graft site and technique of graft procurement. Allograft bone is human cadaveric bone that can be stored as either a fresh-frozen or freeze-dried preparation. It is available in a variety of shapes and composition similar to autograft bone. Synthetics available for use in fusion procedures include ceramics, demineralized bone matrix (DBM) and bone morphogenetic proteins (BMP).

9. Discuss fundamental differences between cortical and cancellous bone graft in spinal applications.

Cortical bone can be used to provide immediate structural stability. Cortical bone is incorporated by creeping substitution, which occurs slowly over years. Cancellous bone provides a porous matrix essential for osteogenesis in areas not requiring immediate structural support. Cancellous bone is incorporated much more rapidly than cortical bone because of direct bone apposition onto the scaffold provided by bony trabeculae.

10. Compare and contrast the healing potential of the anterior spinal column and posterior spinal column with respect to spinal fusion.

Biomechanical factors are different in the anterior and posterior spinal columns. An estimated 80% of the body's load passes through the anterior spinal column, and 20% passes through the posterior spinal column. Thus, bone graft placed in the anterior column is subjected to compressive loading that promotes fusion. In the anterior spinal column, the wide bony surface area combined with the excellent vascularity of the fusion bed creates a superior biologic milieu for fusion. In contrast, bone graft placed in the posterior column is subjected to tensile forces, which provide a less favorable healing environment. In the posterior spinal column, fusion is more dependent on biologic factors such as the presence of osteogenic cells, osteoinductive factors, and the quality of the soft tissue bed into which the graft material is placed. Thus, the posterior spinal column is a more challenging environment in which to achieve a spinal fusion.

11. What anatomic structures provide potential sites for posterior spinal arthrodesis?

In the cervical region, posterior spinal fusions are achieved by applying bone graft to the lamina , facet joints, and spinous process. In the thoracic and lumbar regions, the lamina, facet joints, spinous processes and transverse processes are available sites for arthrodesis.

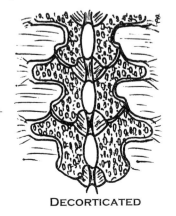
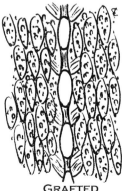

FIGURE 1. Posterior spinal arthrodesis.

DECORTICATED   GRAFTED

12. What type of bone graft is recommended for posterior spinal fusion procedures?

Autogenous cancellous iliac crest bone graft is generally recommended for use in posterior spinal fusion procedures. This type of graft has the highest rate of successful arthrodesis in posterior fusions. Allograft bone alone does not achieve a sufficiently high fusion rate to warrant its use in adult patients for posterior fusions. However, in pediatric patients success has been reported using allograft bone for posterior fusion procedures for scoliosis. Success in this setting is likely due to the greater potential for osseous union inherent in pediatric patients and the creation of local bone graft by meticulous decortication of the posterior bony structures. In general, if autogenous iliac graft is in short supply in a particular patient undergoing posterior fusion, some form of autogenous bone (e.g., rib) or a mixture of local bone graft and a graft extender (morselized allograft, DBM) is recommended to increase the likelihood of successful posterior fusion.

13. What type of bone graft is recommended for anterior spinal fusion procedures?

Both autograft and allograft bone graft have been reported to provide reasonable fusion rates in the anterior spinal column. The higher rate of fusion obtained with autograft must be weighed against the morbidity of harvesting large sections of autogenous bone graft from the pelvis. Use of anterior and/or posterior spinal instrumentation can improve fusion rates when structural allograft bone grafts are used.

14. Explain the difference between nonstructural and structural bone grafts.

Bone grafts placed in the anterior spinal column may be classified as nonstructural or structural grafts. Nonstructural grafts (also termed "morselized" grafts) typically consist of particles of cancellous bone (e.g., from the iliac crest) placed into a defect in the anterior spinal column (e.g., after discectomy). This type of graft is intended to promote arthrodesis between adjacent vertebral bodies. The graft itself does not restore structural stability to the anterior spinal column. Use of adjunctive spinal instrumentation is generally required to facilitate bony union. Structural grafts contain a cortical bone surface that can provide mechanical support during the process of fusion consolidation. Anterior bone graft constructs may be classified according to location as strut grafts, interbody grafts, or transvertebral grafts.

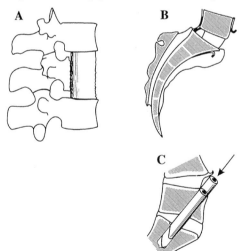

FIGURE 2. Anterior graft constructs may be described as strut grafts (**A**), interbody grafts (**B**) or transvertebral grafts (**C**). (From Devlin VJ, Pitt DD: The evolution of surgery of the anterior spinal column. Spine State Art Rev 12: 493–528, 1998, with permission.)

15. What graft options are available for interbody fusion in the cervical, thoracic, and lumbar spinal regions?

In the **cervical region,** the most frequently used interbody graft material is iliac bone graft. Both autograft and allograft bone graft are commonly used. The most common interbody graft configuration is the tricortical horseshoe-shaped graft described by Smith and Robinson. Fusion cage technology has also been applied to cervical interbody fusion in recent years.

In the **thoracic region,** graft options include rib graft, autogenous iliac graft, structural and nonstructural allograft and fusion cages combined with autograft and/or allograft.

In the **lumbar spine,** both nonstructural and structural grafts are used depending on a variety of factors. Structural graft options for interbody fusion include autograft (iliac crest), allograft (femur, ilium, tibia), and a variety of interbody fusion cage devices that are generally used in combination with nonstructural bone graft.

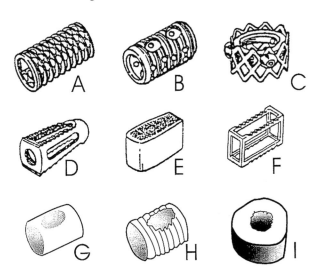

FIGURE 3. Options for lumbar interbody fusion. **A,** Ray cylindrical threaded fusion cage. **B,** BAK cylindrical threaded fusion cage. **C,** Surgical titanium mesh. **D,** Tapered (lordotic) fusion cage. **E,** Iliac crest autograft or allograft bone. **F,** Carbon fiber fusion cage. **G,** Nonthreaded femoral cortical bone dowel. **H,** Threaded femoral cortical bone dowel. **I,** Femoral ring allograft. (From Devlin VJ, Pitt DD: The evolution of surgery of the anterior spinal column. Spine State Art Rev 12: 493–528, 1998, with permission.)

16. What are fusion cages?

Fusion cages are devices intended to provide structural support to the anterior spinal column after removal of an intervertebral disc or vertebral body. These devices are generally used in conjunction with bone graft. The cage is intended to restore immediate mechanical stability to the anterior spinal column and provide a favorable environment for the process of bone graft healing. Cages are available in a variety of shapes and materails (titanium, carbon fiber, cortical bone). Cages can be implanted from either an anterior or posterior surgical approach and typically are used in conjunction with anterior and/or posterior spinal instrumentation.

17. What graft options are available after corpectomy in the cervical, thoracic, and lumbar spinal regions?

In the **cervical region,** one- or two- level corpecotmies are most commonly reconstructed using tricortical iliac autograft combined with spinal instrumentation. For reconstruction of two or more vertebral levels, a fibular graft (either autograft or allograft) or a fusion cage is most commonly used in combination with spinal instrumentation.

In the **thoracic and lumbar regions,** a wide variety of structural graft options are available including autograft, allograft, fusion cages, and bone cement (PMMA). Adjunctive spinal instrumentation is used in combination with these strut grafts (see table).

Anterior Column Reconstruction Options After Corpectomy

GRAFT OPTIONS	ADVANTAGES	DISADVANTAGES
Autograft—iliac crest	Combination of cancellous bone (promotes osseous union) and cortical bone (provides structural support)	Low initial strength Curved geometry Donor site morbidity
Autograft—fibula	Straight geometry High initial strength	Cortical bone Slow osseous incorporation Donor site morbidity
Autograft—rib	Can be harvested during surgical exposure	Low initial strength precludes use as a structural graft
Allograft—structural (e.g., femur, tibia)	High initial strength No donor site morbidity Versatile Can be filled with autograft	Slow osseous incorporation Low risk of disease transmission
Vascular graft—rib	Relative ease of harvest Rapid healing even in compromised fusion bed	Low initial strength requires use of adjunctive mode of structural support
Vascular graft—fibula	High initial strength Straight geometry Rapid healing even in compromised fusion bed	Technical procedure time-consuming Donor site morbidity
Bone cement (PMMA)	No donor morbidity Adequate resistance to compressive loading	Biologically inert Finite lifespan Late loosening and failure
Titanium mesh fusion cage	High strength No donor site morbidity Can be trimmed to fill any bonydefect Serrations provide resistance to shear forces	Subsidence in osteopenic bone may be problematic Osseous integration uncertain Long-term follow-up unknown

From Devlin VJ, Pitt DD: The evolution of surgery of the anterior spinal column. Spine State Art Rev 12: 493–528, 1998, with permission.

18. What is the most common indication for placement of a transvertebral graft?

A transvertebral graft is most commonly used in the surgical treatment of high-grade lumbar spondylolisthesis when a reduction or resection procedure is undesireable. Typically a fibular autograft or allograft is placed from either a posterior or anterior approach to bridge L5 and the sacrum. The graft is typically combined with posterolateral spinal fusion and instrumentation.

19. When does a surgeon use the anterior iliac crest or the posterior iliac crest for harvesting bone grafts?

Factors to consider in selecting the graft site include the volume of bone graft required and the patient's position during surgery. The posterior iliac crest can supply a greater volume of bone than the anterior iliac crest. Patient position during surgery is also a factor. When the patient is in the prone position, the posterior third of the ilium is more easily accessible, whereas in the supine position the anterior third of the ilium is easier to access.

20. List complications associated with harvesting autograft from the ilium.

- Infection
- Donor site pain
- Superior gluteal artery injury
- Damage to the sciatic nerve
- Meralgia paresthetica, or lateral femoral cutaneous nerve injury

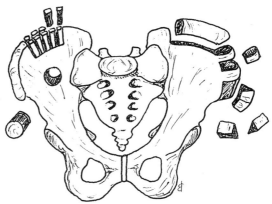

FIGURE 4. Types of anterior and posterior iliac grafts.

- Pelvic fracture
- Sacroiliac joint violation
- Lumbar hernia
- Cluneal nerve transection

21. When harvesting a fibula for autogenous grafting, what three technical considerations can help prevent surgical complications?

1. Localization of the fibular head and peroneal nerve to prevent neural injury
2. Avoidance of graft harvest from the distal fourth of the fibula to preserve ankle stability
3. Reflection of peroneal muscles to prevent transection

22. Either osteotomes or power saws may be used to harvest a cortical graft. In what situation is each technique preferred?

Osteotomes are used when corticocancellous and cancellous bone is harvested. Power saws (oscillating saws or pneumatic drills) are best used to obtain structural bone grafts (e.g., tricortical strut grafts). Use of a power saws avoids creating microfractures, which can weaken a structural bone graft.

23. Define pseudarthrosis after a spinal fusion procedure.

Pseudarthrosis is defined as the failure of an attempted fusion to heal within 1 year after surgery.

24. What are the major risk factors for pseudarthrosis following a spinal fusion procedure?

- Biologic factors: tobacco use, medication (steroids, nonsteroidal anti-inflammatories), deep wound infection
- Mechanical factors: inadequate spinal fixation
- Inadequate surgical technique: inadequate preparation of the fusion site
- Graft-related factors: inadequate volume of bone graft, allograft use in posterior fusions

25. How is a failed spine fusion diagnosed?

Clinical symptoms such as localized pain over the fusion site should prompt suspicion of a pseudarthrosis. Confirmatory tests include structural imaging tests (plain radiographs, polytomography, computed tomography, technetium bone scan), functional imaging tests (flexion-extension radiographs) and surgical exploration of the fusion mass. Radiographic findings that suggest pseudarthosis include broken or loose spinal implants, progressive spinal deformity after surgery, and discontinuity in the fusion mass on radiography. Surgical exploration is the most reliable method of determining whether a fusion has successfully healed.

26. Does the presence of a pseudarthrosis after an attempted spinal fusion always cause symptoms?

No. Although many patients who develop a pseudarthosis report pain symptoms, this is not always the case. Fusion success does not always correlate with patient outcome.

BIBLIOGRAPHY

1. Cleveland M, Bosworth DM, Thompson FR: Pseudoarthrosis in the lumbosacral spine. J Bone Joint Surg 30A:302, 1948.
2. Cobb JR: Technique, after-treatment, and results of spine fusion for scoliosis. Am Acad Orthop Surg 9:65, 1952.
3. Fischgrund JS, Mackay M, Herkowitz HN, et al: Degenerative lumbar spondylolisthesis with spinal stenosis: A prospective, randomized study comparing decompressive laminectomy and arthrodesis with and without spinal instrumentation. Spine 22:2807–2812, 1997.
4. Hibbs RA: An operation for progressive spinal deformities. N Y Med J 93:1013, 1911.
5. McDonnell MF, Glassman SD, Dimar JR II, et al: Perioperative complications of anterior procedures on the spine. J Bone Joint Surg 78A:839–847, 1996.
6. Sandhu HS, Grewal HS, Parvataneni H: Bone grafting for spinal fusion. *Orthop Clin North Am* 30:685–698, 1999.

24. PROCEDURES FOR DECOMPRESSION OF THE SPINAL CORD AND NERVE ROOTS

Munish C. Gupta, MD

1. What steps can spinal surgeons follow to maximize the likelihood of a successful outcome after spinal decompression procedures?

- Rely on high-quality imaging studies (computed tomography [CT], magnetic resonance imaging [MRI], CT-myelography) for preoperative planning.
- Operate only when the clinical history and physical examination correlate with spinal imaging studies.
- Use prophylactic intravenous antibiotics.
- Minimize exposure-related damage to spinal structures (muscles, ligaments, facet joints, bone, nerve tissue).
- Operate with adequate light and exposure, and use loupe magnification or a microscope.
- Confirm that the proper surgical level(s) have been exposed by taking an intraoperative radiograph
- Assess spinal stability before wound closure. Perform a spinal fusion if spinal instability has been created as a result of the procedure or if spinal instability was present before surgery

2. Distinguish among laminotomy, laminectomy, and laminoplasty.

All three procedures are performed through a posterior approach and are intended to provide posterior decompression of neural structures. A **laminotomy** consists of partial lamina or facet joint removal to expose and decompress the nerve root and/or dural sac. A **laminectomy** consists of removal of the spinous process and the entire lamina to achieve decompression. A **laminoplasty** provides decompression of the neural elements by enlarging the spinal canal with a surgical technique (Fig. 1) that avoids removal of the posterior spinal elements. Various laminoplasty techniques permit preservation and reconstruction of the posterior bone and ligamentous structures of the spinal column without the need for fusion (see Fig. 4.)

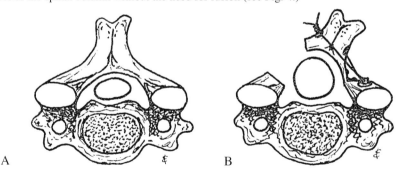

FIGURE 1. Cervical laminoplasty: **A,** Preoperative. **B,** Postoperative.

3. Distinguish among anterior discectomy, corpectomy, and vertebrectomy.

An **anterior discectomy** procedure is indicated for removal of a pathologic intervertebral disc or to relieve anterior neural compression localized to the level of the disc space. The space formerly occupied by the disc is usually filled with bone graft or fusion cages (Fig. 2). A **corpectomy** (*corpus,* another word for vertebral body) entails removal of the vertebral body combined with removal of the superior and inferior adjoining discs (Fig. 3). The resultant anterior spinal column defect is reconstructed with an anterior bone graft or fusion cage and usually stabilized with anterior and/or posterior spinal instrumentation. A corpectomy is indicated to relieve anterior neural compression that extends behind a vertebral body or to remove a vertebral body whose structural integrity is compromised (e.g., tumor, infection, fracture).

A **vertebrectomy** is a more radical procedure consisting of removal of the posterior spinal elements (spinous process, lamina, pedicles) in addition to removal of the vertebral body. This procedure creates severe spinal instability and is usually performed in conjunction with an anterior and posterior spinal instrumentation and fusion.

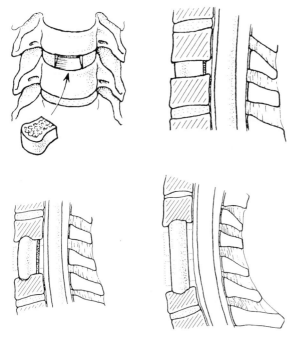

FIGURE 2. Anterior cervical decompression: discectomy. (From Miller, EJ, Aebi M: Anterior fusion of the cervical spine. Spine State Art Rev 6:459–474, 1992, with permission.)

FIGURE 3. Anterior cervical decompression: corpectomy. (From Miller, EJ, Aebi M: Anterior fusion of the cervical spine. Spine State Art Rev 6:459–474, 1992, with permission.).

4. Describe treatment for spinal cord compression with myelopathy due to cranial settling and instability at the occipital cervical junction in patients with rheumatoid arthritis.

A posterior laminectomy of C1 and occipitocervical fusion is performed. The rheumatoid pannus usually decreases in size after stability is provided by posterior fusion. In rare cases, an anterior transoral resection of the odontoid process is performed.

5. What is a transoral decompression ? Describe two indications for this procedure.

Transoral decompression is performed through the mouth. Surgical dissection through the posterior pharynx permits exposure of the odontoid process, C1 arch, and the base of the skull. Anterior surgical access to the occipitocervical junction is required for treatment of tumors (e.g., chordoma in the region of the clivus) and for resection of the odontoid process in rheumatoid arthritis patients with irreducible C1–C2 subluxations.

6. What are the options for surgical decompression of a C5–C6 disc herniation?

An anterior approach is most commonly used to remove a cervical disk herniation, especially when it is large and located centrally. A discectomy is performed by removing the majority of the disk and leaving the lateral annulus on either side intact. The posterior annulus and posterior longitudinal ligament are removed, and any loose disc fragments are removed from the epidural space. After the disk is removed, a bone graft is placed in the disk space. Typically, an anterior cervical plate is applied as well. Another surgical option is to perform a posterior laminoforaminotomy. This approach is suitable for removal of disc fragments located posterolaterally but does not provide sufficient exposure for safe removal of central disc herniations.

7. What are the indications for a cervical laminotomy?

A cervical laminotomy is performed for a posterolateral disk herniation or foraminal stenosis. The lamina and facets are partially removed to provide posterior exposure of the nerve root and adjacent disc. Direct decompression of the nerve root is termed a **foraminotomy**.

8. When is the posterior surgical approach considered for decompression of cervical spinal stenosis?

Posterior surgical approaches for cervical spinal stenosis are most commonly recommended when three or more levels require decompression. An important prerequisite to successful decompression from a posterior approach is the presence of a neutral to lordotic sagittal alignment, which permits dorsal migration of the spinal cord away from anterior compressive pathology.

9. When is the anterior surgical approach considered for decompression of cervical spinal stenosis?

Anterior surgical approaches for treatment of cervical spinal stenosis are widely used for treatment of cervical spinal stenosis in patients with three or fewer levels of involvement. Successful decompression can be achieved regardless of whether the patients has lordotic, neutral, or kyphotic sagittal plane alignment. Multilevel discectomy and interbody fusion are appropriate when neural compression is localized to the level of the disc space. Anterior corpectomy and strut grafting are appropriate when cord compression extends beyond the disc level or when a significant kyphotic deformity is present.

10. When is a combined anterior and posterior approach considered for treatment of cervical spinal stenosis?

- Multilevel cervical stenosis requiring three or more levels of anterior decompression
- Multilevel cervical stenosis requiring two or more levels of corpectomy
- Multilevel cervical stenosis associated with cervical kyphotic deformity
- Rigid posttraumatic or postlaminectomy kyphotic deformities

11. Compare the advantages and disadvantages of cervical laminectomy, cervical laminoplasty, and cervical laminectomy with fusion for treatment of multilevel cervical spinal stenosis.

Cervical laminectomy has been widely used for decompression of cervical stenosis with satisfactory results in a high percentage of patients. Its advantage is its simplicity. Disadvantages include the tendency to produce segmental instability, postoperative kyphotic deformity and late neurologic deterioration in certain patients.

Cervical laminoplasty has been popularized to address some of the problems associated with cervical laminectomy. Retention of the posterior spinal elements decreases the likelihood of postoperative spinal instability and extensive postoperative epidural scar formation. Because the procedure is performed without fusion, cervical motion is preserved. However, postoperative neck pain may be problematic after laminaplasty procedures.

Cervical laminectomy combined with lateral mass fusion and plate fixation continues to play a role in the treatment of multilevel cervical spinal stenosis. It is effective means of decompressing the spinal canal in patients with neutral or lordotic cervical alignment. Fusion prevents the development of postoperative kyphosis and can improve neck pain symptoms. Disadvantages include loss of cervical motion and the complexity of the procedure.

12. What nerve root injury is most common after cervical laminectomy or laminoplasty?

C5 nerve root dysfunction is the most common nerve root problem after cervical laminectomy or laminoplasty. Nerve root dysfunction may be noted immediately after surgery, or it may develop 1–5 days after surgery. The exact cause of C5 dysfunction is not entirely clear, but it has been attributed to the following factors: (1) the C5 root is the shortest cervical root; (2) C5 is usually located at the midpoint of the decompression—the segment that undergoes the greatest dorsal shift after decompression; and (3) C5 root deficits are easily detectable on clinical exam because the C5 root provides sole innervation to the deltoid muscle.

13. Give three examples of clinical situations in which a cervical corpectomy is indicated.

A corpectomy is indicated for anterior spinal cord compression due to (1) tumor, extending into the spinal canal; (2) fracture with retropulsion of bony fragments into the spinal canal, and (3) ossification of the posterior longitudinal ligament in a patient with kyphotic deformity.

14. What factors are involved in determining the appropriate surgical approach for treatment of a thoracic disc herniation?

Factors to consider in determining the appropriate surgical approach (anterior vs posterior) include:

- Location of the disc herniation relative to the spinal cord (central, centrolateral, lateral)
- Level of the disc herniation (upper thoracic, midthoracic, thoracolumbar junction)
- Nature of the herniated disc material (calcified vs. noncalcified)
- Surgeon's familiarity with different surgical approaches

15. Is laminectomy a reasonable approach for treatment of a thoracic disc herniation?

No! Midline laminectomy approaches should be avoided because of their poor historical results. This approach is associated with a high rate of complications, including paraplegia. Laminectomy provides poor access to the centrolateral aspect of the disc space, and retraction of the spinal cord is not advised because of the risk of paraplegia.

16. What anterior surgical approaches are used for treatment of a thoracic disc herniation?

Open thoracotomy approach: best for disc herniations between T4 and T12.

Thoracoscopic approach: easiest for midthoracic disc herniation but requires specialized equipment and training.

Transsternal or medial clavisectomy approach: anterior access to T2–T4 is difficult with the first two approaches and may require one of these more complex approaches. Both are associated with significant exposure-related morbidity.

17. What posterior surgical approaches are used for treatment of a thoracic disc herniation?

Costotransversectomy approach: the transverse process–rib articulation is disrupted, and the portion of the rib overlying the disc is removed. This approach provides posterolateral access to the vertebral body and the disc.

Lateral extracavitary approach: this approach is similar to but more extensive than the costotransversectomy approach. Portions of the transverse process, rib head, pedicle, and facet are resected to provide more extensive access to the disc space.

Transpedicular approach: this midline approach involves removal of the facet joint and medial portion of the pedicle to achieve access to the portion of the disc space lateral to the spinal cord without the need to retract this structure.

18. Describe the three basic steps involved in performing a thoracic or lumbar corpectomy after the exposure has been performed, including ligation of the segmental vessels.

1. The discs above and below the target vertebral body are removed. This procedure facilitates removal of the vertebral body by providing reference landmarks for the depth and position of the spinal canal.

2. The vertebral body is then removed. The anterior two-thirds of the vertebral body is rapidly removed with a rongeur, osteotome, or burr. The remaining posterior wall of the vertebral body is thinned with a burr. This procedure facilitates the more delicate removal of the posterior vertebral cortex with a curette or Kerrison rongeur to expose the spinal canal, posterior longitudinal ligament, and dural sac.

3. The space created after corpectomy is filled with a structural bone graft or a cage to restore anterior column support. Anterior and/or posterior spinal implants are used to provide additional stability.

19. Give three indications for performing a corpectomy in the thoracic and/or lumbar spine.

1. Burst fracture with retropulsion of bone into the spinal canal causing anterior cord compression.

2. Tumor extending from the posterior part of the vertebral body into the spinal canal.

3. Infection when the vertebral body has collapsed with retropulsed material in the canal, resulting in anterior spinal cord compression.

20. In treatment of spinal infections, when is an anterior surgical approach indicated?

An anterior approach is used most commonly in the treatment of spinal infections because the disc space becomes infected and the purulent material enters the anterior epidural space, resulting in anterior neural compression. An anterior approach is also indicated for drainage of a paravertebral abscess, which typically forms along the anterior or anterolateral aspect of the spinal column.

21. In treatment of spinal infections, when is a posterior surgical approach indicated?

A posterior approach is used when an epidural abscess develops posterior to the dural sac in the absence of anterior disc space infection. In this case, a laminectomy or bilateral laminotomies is performed.

22. Describe three techniques for decompression of a thoracolumbar burst fracture with a retropulsed fragment that causes neurologic injury.

1. Indirect decompression achieved by use of posterior spinal instrumentation, fusion, and "ligamentotaxis"

2. Direct posterolateral decompression via a laminectomy or transpedicular approach, combined with use of posterior spinal instrumentation and fusion

3. Direct anterior deompression with corpectomy and reconstruction, combined with anterior and/or posterior spinal instrumentation

23. What structures typically compress the spinal cord and nerve roots in patients with congenital scoliosis or kyphosis?

Spinal cord compression in congenital scoliosis and kyphosis is frequently caused by the posterior part of a hemivertebra . When scoliosis is present, a pedicle at the apex of the curvature may compress the spinal cord and nerve roots.

24. Describe two ways that decompression can be performed to treat such problems.

1. Perform a first-stage transthoracic or transabdominal anterior approach and then a vertebrectomy, including removal of the pedicle. Subsequent posterior decompression and spinal stabilization also are required.

2. Remove the pedicle, transverse process, rib, and portion of the body compressing the spinal cord via a posterolateral approach. Posterior spinal stabilization is performed as part of the procedure.

25. What determines the approach for decompression of a lumbar disc herniation?

The primary factor guiding selection of the operative approach is the location of the disc fragment. Disc herniations located in the central or posterolateral region of the spinal canal are easily removed through a laminotomy approach. Disc herniations located in the foraminal and extraforaminal zone are most directly decompressed through a paraspinal approach.

26. Describe a lumbar laminotomy procedure for removal of a disc herniation.

A laminotomy is performed on the side of the disc herniation. An intraoperative radiograph is taken to confirm the proper level of exposure. Sufficient bone and ligamentum flavum are removed to permit visualiztion of the lateral edge of the nerve root. Retraction of the nerve root and removal of the disc fragment are performed under magnification (loupes or microscope).

27. Describe a paraspinal approach for removal of a foraminal lumbar disc herniation.

The muscles attached to the midline bony structures are left intact. An incision is made in the fascia lateral to the midline. Blunt dissection is carried down to the transverse processes. The transverse processes are identified, and the intertransverse membrane is exposed. A radiograph is obtained to confirm that the correct spinal level has been exposed. The intertransverse membrane is then cut, the nerve root is retracted medially and the disc herniation is removed.

28. What are the surgical options for decompression of lumbar spinal stenosis?

Single or multilevel laminotomy. This technique can be used for single-level or multilevel stenosis when the neural compression is localized to the level of the disc space. This technique has the advantage of preserving the stability provided by midline bony and ligamentous structures. It is somewhat more difficult than a laminectomy when performed for multilevel stenosis (Fig. 4).

Single-level or multilevel laminectomy. This technique may be used for any type of spinal stenosis problem and is required for treatment of congenital lumbar spinal stenosis. The disadvantage of this technique is its tendency to destabilize the spinal column (see Fig. 4).

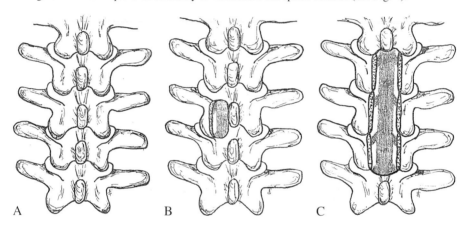

FIGURE 4. Lumbar decompression. **A,** Preoperative. **B,** Laminotomy. **C,** laminectomy.

29. When should the surgeon perform a spinal arthrodesis after decompression for lumbar spinal stenosis?

- Intraoperative destabilization (removal of more than 50% of both facets or complete removal of a single facet joint)
- Patients with significant lumbar scoliosis
- Patients with spondylolisthesis or lateral listhesis

BIBLIOGRAPHY

1. Boos M, Min K: Vertebrectomy and spinal cord decompression. In Weinstein SL (ed): Pediatric Spine Surgery, 2nd ed. Philadelphia, Lippincott Williams & Wilkins, 2001, pp 255–268
2. Gupta MC, Benson DR: Thoracolumbar fractures and fracture-dislocations. In Moehring HD, Greenspan A (eds): Fractures: Diagnosis and Treatment, New York, McGraw-Hill, 2000, pp 59–68.
3. McLone DG: Chiari malformation. Images Pediatr Neurosurg 32:164,
4. O'Hara R, Silvaggio V, Donaldson III WF, Kraus DR: Surgery for rheumatoid arthritis of the cervical spine. In Bridwell K, DeWald R (eds): The Textbook of Spinal Surgery, 2nd ed. Philadelphia, Lippincott-Raven, 1997, pp 1439–1456.
5. Spencer DL, Bernstein AJ: Lumbar intervertebral disc surgery. In Bridwell K, DeWald R (eds): The Textbook of Spinal Surgery, 2nd ed. Philadelphia, Lippincott-Raven, 1997, pp 1547–1560.
6. Truumees E, Herkowitz HN: Lumbar spinal stenosis: Treatment options. AAOS Instructional Course Lectures, vol. 50, 2001, pp 153–161.

25. SURGICAL APPROACHES TO THE CERVICAL SPINE

Kern Singh, M.D., and Alexander R. Vaccaro, M.D.

1. What are the various surgical approaches to the anterior and posterior cervical spine?
1. **Anterior**
   Transoral
   Extra/lateral/ retropharyngeal
   Anterolateral (Smith-Robinson)
2. **Posterior:** midline

2. What are the major palpable posterior anatomic landmarks and their corresponding cervical levels?
- Posterior scalp: occiput
- First palpable spinous process: C2 spinous process
- Most prominent spinous process at cervicothoracic junction: vertebral prominens (C7)

3. Describe the posterior exposure of the upper cervical spine.
The patient is placed into a reverse Trendelenburg position with a midline incision made from the external occipital protuberance to the spinous process of C2. The C2 vertebra (axis) has a large lamina and bifid spinous process that provides attachments for the rectus major and inferior oblique muscles. The bony topography between the lamina and the lateral mass of the axis is indistinct. Surgical dissection on the occiput and the ring of the atlas should be done in a careful manner. It is advisable to use gentle muscle retraction and bovie (monopolar and bipolar) cauterization rather than any forceful subperiosteal stripping.

4. What is the significance of the ligamentum nuchae?
The ligamentum nuchae (Fig. 1) represents the midline fascial confluence. Dissection should be carried through this ligament to decrease blood loss and to maintain a stout tissue layer for closure.

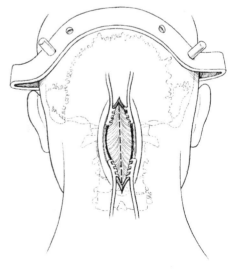

FIGURE 1. Ligamentum nuchae. (From Winter R, Lonstein J, Denis F, Smith M: Posterior Upper Cervical Procedures: Atlas of Spinal Surgery. Philadelphia, W.B. Saunders, 1995, p 21, with permission.)

5. What structure is at risk with lateral dissection of the atlas?

The vertebral artery lies lateral to the ring of the atlas (Fig. 2); therefore, the dissection should not be carried more than 1.5 cm lateral to the posterior midline and 8–10 mm laterally along the superior C1 border to avoid injury to the vertebral artery. Once the greater occipital nerve is encountered and the fragile venae commitantes of the paravertebral venous plexus are exposed, further lateral dissection endangers the vertebral artery. If bleeding is encountered from damage to the cavernous sinus between C1 and C2, packing and hemostatic agents are usually adequate to control bleeding. Monopolar bovie is ineffective in stopping bleeding involving the cavernous sinus because of the absence of an intimal lining. If vertebral artery injury occurs, direct repair or ligation is necessary for control of hemorrhage.

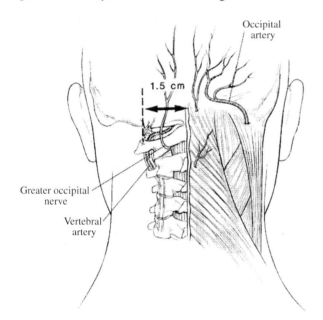

FIGURE 2. Vertebral artery. (From Winter R, Lonstein J, Denis F, Smith M: Posterior Upper Cervical Procedures: Atlas of Spinal Surgery. Philadelphia, W.B. Saunders, 1995, p 23, with permission.)

6. Describe the course of the vertebral artery in the cervical spine.

The vertebral artery arises from the subclavian artery. It enters the transverse foramen at C6 in 95% of people and courses upward through the foramina above. At C1, the vertebral artery exits from the foramen, courses medially on the superior groove of the posterior ring of the atlas, and enters the foramen magnum to unite with the opposite vertebral artery to form the basilar artery.

7. Where is the vertebral artery injured most frequently in upper cervical spine exposures?

The vertebral artery is injured most frequently just lateral to the C1–C2 facet articulation and at the superior lateral aspect of the arch of C1.

8. Why is the patient placed in a reverse Trendelenburg position?

The reverse Trendelenburg position allows venous drainage toward the heart with less bleeding during the procedure.

9. Describe the posterior exposure of the lower cervical spine.

The midline posterior exposure is the most common approach used in the cervical spine. As mentioned previously, dissection should be carried through the ligamentum nuchae to minimize blood loss. Once the tips of the spinous processes are identified at the appropriate levels through radiographic confirmation, subperiosteal dissection of the posterior elements is then carried out.

10. What functional consequences may arise from lateral dissection of the paraspinal muscles?

Lateral dissection carries the potential risk of denervation of the paraspinal musculature. Inadequate approximation of the posterior cervical musculature may lead to a fish gill appearance of the posterior paraspinal muscles and possible loss of the normal cervical lordosis.

11. Why is it important to expose only the levels to be fused, especially in children?

A process termed *creeping fusion extension* is common in children and occurs when unwanted spinal levels are exposed during the fusion procedure.

12. During the transoral approach to the odontoid, what is the key palpable landmark in determining exposure location?

The anterior tubercle of the atlas. The vertebral artery lies a minimum of 2 cm from this anatomic landmark within the foramen transversarium.

13. Describe the transoral exposure to the upper cervical spine.

Transoral retractors are inserted to expose the posterior oropharynx (Fg. 3). A soft rubber catheter is placed through the nostril and looped about the uvula to facilitate its cephalad retraction. The area of the incision is infiltrated with 1:200,000 epinephrine. A midline 3-cm vertical incision centered on the anterior tubercle of the atlas is made through the pharyngeal mucosa and muscle. The anterior longitudinal ligament and tubercle of the atlas are exposed subperiosteally, and the longus colli muscles are mobilized laterally. A high-speed burr may be used to remove the anterior arch of the atlas to expose the odontoid process (Fig. 4).

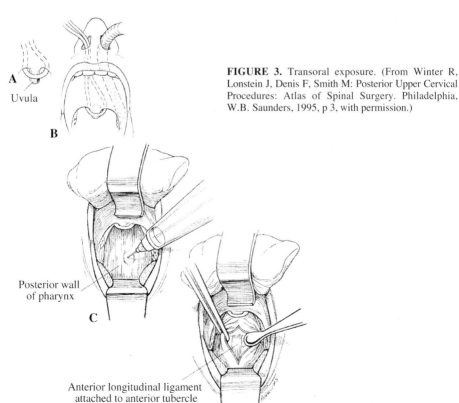

A

Uvula

B

FIGURE 3. Transoral exposure. (From Winter R, Lonstein J, Denis F, Smith M: Posterior Upper Cervical Procedures: Atlas of Spinal Surgery. Philadelphia, W.B. Saunders, 1995, p 3, with permission.)

Posterior wall of pharynx

C

Anterior longitudinal ligament attached to anterior tubercle of C1

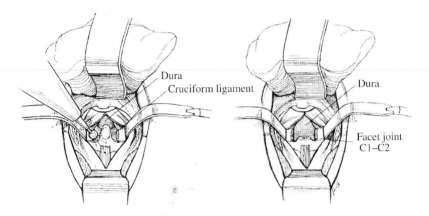

FIGURE 4. Removal of C1 arch. (From Winter R, Longstein J, Denis F, Smith M: Posterior Upper Cervical Procedures: Atlas of Spinal Surgery. Philadelphia, W.B. Saunders, 1995, p 5, with permission.)

14. What preoperative patient care factors must be addressed before undergoing a transoral decompression?

All oropharyngeal or dental infections must be treated before elective surgery because wound infections rates are high with this approach. The oral cavity is cleansed with chlorohexidine before surgery, and after surgery perioperative antibiotics are given for 48–72 hours (often a cephalosporin and metronidazole).

15. Describe the incision and superficial dissection for the retropharyngeal approach to the upper cervical spine.

A skin incision is made along the anterior aspect of the sternocleidomastoid muscle and is curved toward the mastoid process. The platysma and the superficial layer of the deep cervical fascia are divided in the line of the incision to expose the anterior border of the sternocleidomastoid. The sternocleidomastoid muscle is retracted anteriorly, and the carotid sheath laterally (Figs. 5 and 6).

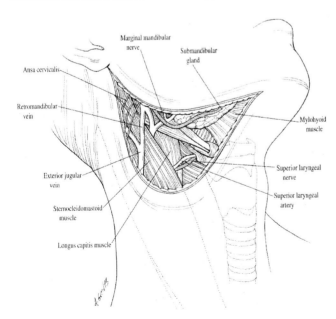

FIGURE 5. Anterior retropharyngeal approach. (From Winter R, Lonstein J, Denis F, Smith M: Posterior Upper Cervical Procedures: Atlas of Spinal Surgery. Philadelphia, W.B. Saunders, 1995, p 10, with permission.)

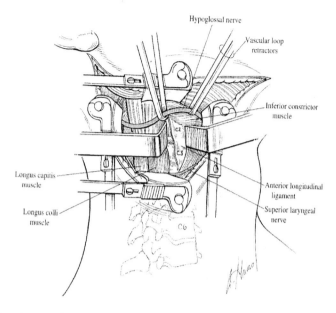

Hypoglossal nerve

Vascular loop retractors

Inferior constrictor muscle

Longus capitis muscle

Longus colli muscle

Anterior longitudinal ligament

Superior laryngeal nerve

FIGURE 6. Anterior retropharyngeal approach– deep dissection. (From Winter R, Lonstein J, Denis F, Smith M: Posterior Upper Cervical Procedures: Atlas of Spinal Surgery. Philadelphia, W.B. Saunders, 1995, p 11, with permission.)

16. What two vessels are ligated once the sternocleidomastoid is retracted?
The superior thyroid artery and the lingual vessels.

17. What is the importance of the facial artery as an anatomic landmark?
The facial artery helps to identify the location of the hypoglossal nerve, which lies adjacent to the digastric muscle.

18. Stripping of what muscle helps to identify the anterior aspect of the upper cervical spine and basiocciput?
The longus colli.

19. Describe the functional consequence of excessive retraction on the superior laryngeal nerve.
Excessive retraction may cause hoarseness and an inability to sing high notes.

20. What nerve may be potentially injured in this approach, resulting in a painful neuroma?
The marginal branch of the facial nerve.

21. Name the palpable anatomic landmarks used to identify the level of exposure of the lower cervical spine.
The angle of the mandible (C2–C3), the hyoid bone (C3), and the cricoid cartilage (C6–C7).

22. Describe the anterior lateral or Smith-Robinson approach to the lower or subaxial cervical spine.
A transverse incision is made over the interspace of interest in Langer's lines to improve the cosmetic appearance of the surgical scar. The incision is carried slightly laterally beyond the anterior border of the sternocleidomastoid muscle and almost to the midline of the neck. The subcutaneous tissue is divided in line with the skin incision. The platysma may be divided along the line of the incision, or its fibers may be bluntly dissected and its medial-lateral divisions retracted (Fig. 7). The anterior border of the sternocleidomastoid is identified, and the fascia anterior to this

muscle is incised. The sternocleidomastoid is retracted laterally and the strap muscles are retracted medially to permit incision of the pretracheal fascia medial to the carotid sheath. The sternocleidomastoid and carotid sheath are retracted laterally, and the strap muscles and visceral structures (trachea, larynx, esophagus, thyroid) are retracted medially. The anterior aspect of the spine, including the paired longus colli muscles, are now visualized.

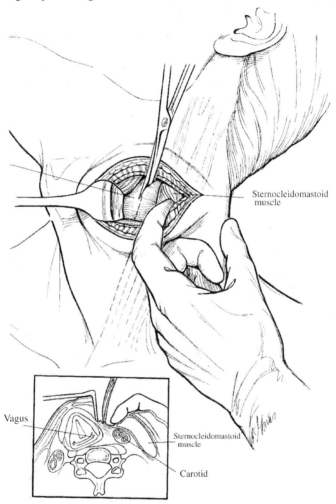

FIGURE 7. Exposure of the lower anterior cervical spine. (From Winter R, Lonstein J, Denis F, Smith M: Posterior Upper Cervical Procedures: Atlas of Spinal Surgery. Philadelphia, W.B. Saunders, 1995, p 53, with permission.)

23. What is the function of the platysma muscle and its corresponding innervation?

The platysma is an embryologic remnant serving no functional importance. It receives its innervation from the seventh cranial nerve.

24. Once the platysma and the superficial cervical fascia are divided, what neurovascular structure is at risk for injury?

The carotid sheath contains three neurovascular structures: internal jugular vein, carotid artery, and vagus nerve.

25. What structures are at risk when dissecting through the pretracheal fascia of the neck?

The superior and inferior thyroid arteries may be injured during dissection through the pretracheal fascial layer. Dissection is normally done in a longitudinal manner, using digital dissection.

26. What fascial layer is encountered after dissection through the pretracheal fascia?

After dissection through the pretracheal fascia, the prevertebral fascia or retropharyngeal space is encountered. The prevertebral fascia is split longitudinally, exposing the anterior longitudinal ligament. The longus colli muscle is elevated bilaterally and retracted laterally until the anterior surface of the vertebral body is exposed.

27. What structures are at risk when the dissection is carried too far laterally on the vertebral body in the subaxial spine?

Dissection carried too far laterally may risk injury to the vertebral artery traversing through the foramen transversarium or damage the sympathetic plexus.

28. What are the advantages and disadvantages of approaching the cervical spine anteriorly from the right or left side?

Smith and Robinson advocated using the left-sided approach to decrease the risk of damaging the recurrent laryngeal nerve. On the right side, the nerve loops beneath the right subclavian artery and then travels in a relatively horizontal course in the neck, increasing its chances of damage to exposure in this region. Most right-handed surgeons find the right-sided approach more accessible because the mandible is not an obstruction. A right-sided exposure also avoids damage to the thoracic duct, and the cervical esophagus is less retracted because of its normal anterior position on the left side of the neck.

29. Name the potential causes of dysphagia after anterior cervical surgery.

Dysphagia may be secondary to postoperative edema, hemorrhage, denervation (recurrent laryngeal nerve), or infection. If persistent dysphagia is present, a barium swallow or endoscopy should be considered.

30. Damage to the sympathetic chain may result in what clinical condition?

Horner's syndrome, which is manifested by a lack of sympathetic response resulting in anhydrosis, ptosis, miosis, and enopthalmus. The cervical sympathetic chain lies on the anterior surface of the longus colli muscles posterior to the carotid sheath. Subperiosteal dissection is important to prevent damage to these nerves. Horner's syndrome is usually temporary; permanent sequelae occur in less than 1% of cases.

31. Describe the rare but serious complication of esophageal perforation.

Patients usually manifest symptoms in the postoperative period related to development of an abscess, tracheoesophageal fistula, or mediastinitis. The usual treatment consists of intravenous antibiotics, nasogastric feeding, drainage, debridement, and repair.

BIBLIOGRAPHY

1. An H: Surgical Approaches to the spine. In An H, Cotler J (eds): Spinal Instrumentation, 2nd ed. Philadelphia, Lippincott Williams & Wilkins, 1999, pp 31–58.
2. An H: Surgical Exposures and fusion techniques of the spine. In An H (ed): Principles and Techniques of Spine Surgery. Baltimore, Williams & Wilkins, 1998, pp 31–62.
3. Cappucino A, McAfee P, Glastein C: Anterior retropharyngeal approaches to the upper cervical spine. In Bridwell K, DeWald R (eds): The Textbook of Spinal Surgery, 2nd ed. Philadelphia, Lippincott Williams & Wilkins, 1996, pp 227–236.
4. Winter R, Lonstein J, Denis F, Smith M: Atlas of Spinal Surgery. Philadelphia, W.B. Saunders, 1995, pp 1–104.

26. ANTERIOR SURGICAL APPROACHES TO THE THORACIC AND LUMBAR SPINE

Mohammad E. Majd, M.D., Douglas H. Musser, D.O., Frank P. Castro, M.D., and Richard T. Holt, M.D.

1. What are the indications for an anterior surgical approach to the thoracic and lumbar spine?
- Anterior spinal decompression and stabilization (e.g., tumor, infection, fracture)
- Anterior correction of spinal defomity (e.g., scoliosis)
- To enhance arthrodesis (e.g., for treatment of posterior pseudarthrosis)
- Anterior release or destabilization to enhance posterior spinal deformity correction (e.g., for treatment of severe, rigid spinal deformities)
- To improve biomechanics of posterior implant constructs (e.g., to restore anterior column load sharing when anterior spinal column integrity has been compromised)
- To enhance restoration of sagittal alignment
- To eliminate asymmetric growth potential (e.g., congenital scoliosis)

2. List situations in which an anterior thoracic or lumbar surgical approach may not be advised.
- Patients who have undergone prior anterior surgery to the same spinal region. In this situation dissection is difficult because of adhesions with increased risk for visceral or vascular injury.
- Patients with poor pulmonary function may have an unacceptable risk of complications after an anterior thoracic approach.
- Patients with extensive calcification of the aorta are not ideal candidates for anterior lumbar approaches. Extensive mobilization of the great vessels is required and is associated with an increased risk of vascular complications.

3. What surgical approaches may be used to expose the upper thoracic spine (T1–T4)?
Access to the T1 vertebral body is generally possible through a standard anterior cervical approach medial to the sternocleidomastoid muscle. Anterior exposure between T1 and T3 is difficult; options for exposure include a modified sternoclavicular approach, a third-rib thoracotomy or a median sternotomy. Each approach has advantages and disadvantages, depending on patient anatomy, type of spinal pathology, number of levels requiring exposure, and type of surgery required.

4. What standard surgical approach is used to expose the anterior aspect of the spine between T2 and T12?
The anterior aspect of the thoracic spine between T2 and T12 is approached by a thoracotomy.

5. What is the preferred method of positioning the patient for an approach to the thoracic spine?
The lateral decubitus position with an axillary roll under the down-side axilla (Fig. 1). Many surgeons prefer approaching the thoracic spine from the left side because it is easier to work with the aorta than the vena cava. However, the type of spinal pathology may dictate the side of approach. For example, in the anterior treatment of scoliosis, the surgical approach should be on the convex side of the curve.

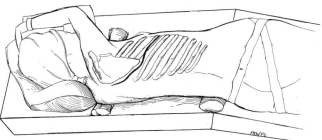

FIGURE 1. Positioning of the patient for an anterior approach to the thoracic spine. (From Majd ME, et al: Anterior approach to the spine. In Margulies JY, et al (eds): Revision Spine Surgery. St. Louis, Mosby, p 139, with permission.)

6. What factors determine the level of rib excision when the thoracic spine is exposed through a thoracotomy approach?

If the procedure requires exposure of a long segment of the thoracic spine (e.g., for treatment of scoliosis or kyphosis), a rib at the proximal end of the region requiring fusion is removed. For example, removal of the fifth rib allows exposure from T5 to T12.

If the patient requires treatment of a single vertebral body lesion, the rib two levels proximal to the involved vertebral body is removed. Alternatively, the rib directly horizontal to the target vertebral level at the mid-axillary line on the anteroposterior (AP) thoracic spine x-ray is removed.

If the surgeon requires only a limited exposure (e.g., to excise a thoracic disc herniation), the rib that leads to the disc should be removed (e.g., the eighth rib is removed for a T7–T8 disc herniation).

7. What are some tips for counting ribs after the chest cavity has been entered during a thoracotomy?

The first cephalad palpable rib is the second rib. The first rib is generally located within the space occupied by the second rib and cannot be easily palpated. The distance between the second and third rib is wider than the distance between the other ribs. Application of a marker on a rib with subsequent radiographic verification is important to identify the level of exposure.

8. In the course of an anterior exposure of the thoracic spine, the parietal pleura is divided longitudinally over the length of the spine. What landmarks may be used for identification of critical anatomic structures?

The vertebral bodies are located in the depressions, and the discs are located over the prominences (Fig. 2). The segmental vessels are identified as they cross the vertebral bodies (depressions). This has been referred to as the "hills-and-valleys" concept (i.e., discs are the hills and vertebral bodies are the valleys).

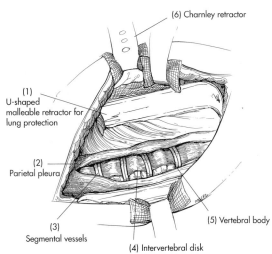

(6) Charnley retractor

(1) U-shaped malleable retractor for lung protection

(2) Parietal pleura

(3) Segmental vessels

(4) Intervertebral disk

(5) Vertebral body

FIGURE 2. Intraoperative view of the anterior exposure of the thoracic spine. (From Majd ME, et al: Anterior approach to the spine. In Margulies JY, et al (eds): Revision Spine Surgery. St. Louis, Mosby, p 142, with permission.)

9. After the initial surgical exposure, what study should be obtained by the surgeon before proceeding with an anterior discectomy or corpectomy?

A radiograph or fluoroscopic view should be obtained to confirm that the correct spinal level has been exposed. Even if one knows anatomy very well, mistakes can be made. This strategy is very important because wrong-level surgery is not an uncommon claim in malpractice lawsuits against spine surgeons.

10. Are there any risks associated with ligation of the segmental artery and vein as they cross the vertebral bodies?

Ligation of the segmental vessels is required to obtain comprehensive exposure of the vertebral body. Unilateral vessel ligation is safe. However, ligation too close to the neural foramina may damage the segmental feeder vessels to the spinal cord. Temporary and reversible occlusion of segmental vessels may be used when the risk of paraplegia is high (congenital kyphoscoliosis, severe kyphosis, patients who have undergone prior anterior spinal surgery with vessel ligation). If there is no change in spinal potential monitoring after temporary vessel occlusion, permanent ligation may be carried out. In contrast, bilateral ligation, as required for aneurysm surgery, has been associated with paraplegia.

11. After thoracotomy, placement of a chest tube is necessary. What are the proper placement criteria?

The chest tube should be placed at the anterior mid-axillary line at least two interspaces from the incision. Placement of the chest tube too posteriorly has potential for kinking and can cause subsequent blockage of drainage in the supine position. In addition, posterior placement is uncomfortable and painful when the patient lie supine.

12. During a thoracic spinal exposure via thoracotomy, a creamy discharge is noted in the operative field. What anatomic structure has been violated?

The thoracic duct. Thoracic duct injuries are uncommon. Most injuries heal without intervention. Repair or ligation of the area of leakage can be attempted. Leaving the chest tube in place for several additional days can be considered. This strategy may help to avoid a chylothorax by allowing the thoracic duct to heal. If a chylothorax should develop postoperatively, nonoperative treatment via chest tube drainage, a low fat diet, and hyperalimentation are recommended as initial treatments.

13. What is the standard surgical approach for exposure of the anterior aspect of the spine between T10 and L2 (thoracolumbar junction)?

Exposure in this region is achieved through a transdiaphragmatic thoracolumbar approach, also termed a *thoracophrenolumbotomy* (Fig. 3). The patient is positioned as for a thoracotomy. The incision typically begins over the tenth rib and extends distally to the costochondral junction,

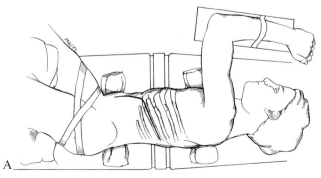

FIGURE 3. A, Positioning of the patient for an anterior approach to the thoracolumbar junction. (*continued*)

A

FIGURE 3. (*continued*) **B,** Intraoperative view of exposure of the thoracolumbar region. Note how the diaphragm requires detachment from its insertion along the lateral chest wall. (From Majd ME, et al: Anterior approach to the spine. In Margulies JY, et al (eds): Revision Spine Surgery. St. Louis, Mosby, pp 146, 147, with permission.)

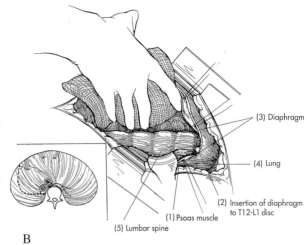

(3) Diaphragm

(4) Lung

(2) Insertion of diaphragm to T12-L1 disc

(1) Psoas muscle

(5) Lumbar spine

B

which is transected. The incision extends distally into the abdominal region as required. Dissection through the layers of the abdominal wall is carried out, and the periotoneum is mobilized from the undersurface of the diaphragm. The diaphragm is then transected from its peripheral insertion. The peritoneal sac and its contents are mobilized off the anterolateral aspect of the lumbar spine. This strategy provides the surgeon with wide continuous exposure of the spine across the two major body cavities (thoracic cavity and abdominal cavity).

14. A patient with an L1 lesion underwent an uneventful left-sided thoracoabdominal approach and corpectomy of L1. After surgery the patient complained of weakness of left hip flexion and difficulty in climbing stairs. What is the most probable cause of this problem?

In this case, the most probable cause is retraction and mobiliztion of the psoas muscle with trauma to the muscle during surgery. The patient's symptoms should gradually improve without further treatment. The psoas major muscle attaches on both sides to the last thoracic and all five lumbar vertebral bodies. The psoas major is innervated by the anterior rami of the upper lumbar nerves. Its principal actions are flexion and medial rotation of hip joint. In addition, the muscle flexes the lumbar spine both anteriorly and laterally. In the sitting position, the psoas muscle is relaxed and permits kyphosis of the lumbar spine. In the standing position, the psoas muscle is taut and thus induces physiologic lumbar lordosis.

15. What are the surgical approach options for exposure of the lumbar spine and lumbosacral junction?

The most commonly used surgical approaches to the lumbar spine and lumbosacral junction are the retroperitoneal flank approach and the medial incision retroperitoneal approach. Less commonly used approaches include the transperitoneal approach and the laparoscopic approach.

16. Describe a medial incision retroperitoneal approach to the lumbar spine.

In a medial incision retroperitoneal approach (Fig. 4), the patient is positioned supine. A left paramedian or midline incision is typically used. A transverse incision is also an option. The rectus sheath is incised, and the muscle is retracted to expose the transversalis fascia. The fascia is incised to enter the retroperitoneal space. Alternatively, if exposure only of L5–S1 is required, the retroperitoneal space can be entered below the arcuate line, thus avoiding the need for incising any fascia. The periotoneal sac is swept off the abdominal wall and anterior aspect of the spine to complete initial exposure.

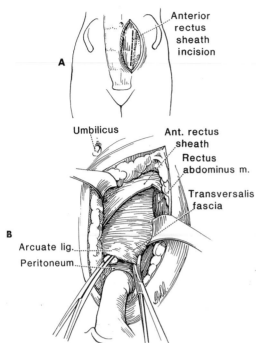

Anterior rectus sheath incision

A

Umbilicus

Ant. rectus sheath

Rectus abdominus m.

Transversalis fascia

B

Arcuate lig.

Peritoneum

FIGURE 4. Anterior exposure of the lumbar spine through a paramedian retro-peritoneal approach. **A,** A longitudinal incision is made through the fascia over-lying the rectus muscle to expose the mus-cle belly. **B,** The arcuate ligament marks the point of entry into the retroperitoneal space. Using a sponge stick caudad to the ligament in a gentle sweeping motion, the surgeon pushes down and toward the mid-line to free the peritoneal sac from the fas-cia and displace it toward the midline, thereby exposing the spine. (From Majd ME, et al: Anterior approach to the spine. In Margulies JY, et al (eds): Revision Spine Surgery. St. Louis, Mosby, p 151, with permission.)

17. What are the advantages and disadvantages of a medial incision retroperitoneal approach?
Advantages
- Provides excellent exposure from L2 through S1.
- This muscle-sparing approach is less painful than a muscle-incising approach.
- The direct anterior exposure facilitates graft placement and anterior decompression.
Disadvantages
- It cannot easily provide exposure above L2.
- The anterior peritoneum is thin and easily perforated in this area.
- Use of this approach is best limited to cases with moderate spinal deformity (scoliosis < 40° or kyphosis < 25°)

18. Describe a retroperitoneal flank approach.
   In the retroperitoneal flank approach (Fig. 5), the patient is typically positioned in the lateral decubitus position with the left side upward. After an oblique skin incision, the layers of the ab-dominal wall are transected (external olique, internal oblique and transversus abdominis). The transversalis fascia is incised, and the peritoneum is mobilized medially to permit exposure of the psoas muscle, which overlies the anterolateral aspect of the spine.

19. What are the advantages and disadvantages of the retroperitoneal flank approach?
Advantages
- Allows exposure of the entire lumbar spine and lumbosacral junction.
- The extensile nature of this approach allows exposure above L2.
- Useful for cases of severe spinal deformity (scoliosis > 40° or kyphosis > 25°).
Disadvantages
- This muscle-incising approach is more painful than a muscle-splitting approach.
- Muscle hernias can occur.
- Exposure of the L5–S1 disc can be more difficult than with the medial incision approach.

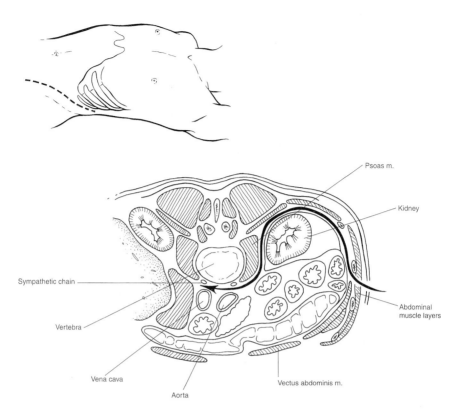

FIGURE 5. The retroperitoneal flank approach to the lumbar spine may be performed with the patient in the lateral position or the supine position. Dissection passes anterior to the psoas muscle to expose the spine. (From An HS: Surgical exposure and fusion techniques of the spine. In An HS (ed): Principles and Practice of Spine Surgery. Baltimore, Williams & Wilkins, 1985, p 56, with permission.)

20. What are the disadvantages of a transperitoneal approach?

Extensive mobilization of the abdominal organs and packing of the intestinal contents out of the operative field increases operative time and complications. Manipulation of the abdominal contents increases the risk of postoperative ileus and intestinal adhesions. There is also a higher risk of retrograde ejaculation in male patients compared with the retroperitoneal approach.

21. What are some of the potential complications of an anterior approach to the lower lumbar and lumbosacral spine?

- Surgical sympathectomy
- Vascular injury
- Ureteral injury
- Deep vein thrombosis
- Incisional hernia
- Retrograde ejaculation

22. During the retroperitoneal exposure of the lumbosacral spine, approximately what percentage of cases is complicated by vascular injuries?

The overall rate of vascular injury during anterior lumbar spine surgery has been reported as 15%. Vascular injuries occur twice as often with the paramedian approach compared with the flank approach. These intraoperative injuries are usually recognized during surgery and repaired with simple suture techniques. The postoperative morbidity rate is low, and the major complication rate of deep venous thrombosis or arterial embolization is low (2%).

23. What is the most important factor in avoiding vascular injury during anterior lumbar spine surgery?

Knowledge of the relationship of vascular structures to the anterior lumbosacral spine is the key to avoiding vascular complications during anterior exposure of the spine (Fig. 6).

First, the surgeon should plan exactly how many anterior disc spaces require exposure. If exposure of only the L5–S1 disc is required, the necessary dissection is limited. However, if exposure of the L4–L5 level or multiple anterior disc levels is required, extensive vascular mobilization is needed, and the exposure will be complex.

Next, the surgeon should assess the level of the bifurcation of the aorta and vena cava. Most commonly the great vessels bifurcate at the L4–L5 disc space or at the upper part of the L5 vertebral body. However, the location of the bifurcation may vary from L4 to S1.

For exposure of the L5–S1 disc, it is necessary to ligate the middle sacral artery and vein, which lie directly over the L5–S1 disc. Exposure of the L5–S1 disc is usually achieved by working in the bifurcation of the aorta and vena cava.

For exposure of the L4–L5 disc it is generally necessary to mobilize branches originating from the distal aorta and vena cava as well as from the external iliac artery and vein. These branches tether the great vessels to the anterior aspect of the spine and limit safe left-to-right retraction of the vascular structures overlying the L4–L5 disc space. It is especially critical to identify and securely ligate the iliolumbar vein and various ascending lumbar veins. Failure to control the vessels before attempting to retract the great vessels off the L4–L5 disc can result in uncontrolled hemorrhage and even death. The segmental vessels overlying the L4 vertebral body and proximal vertebral levels may also require ligation, depending on how many levels require exposure.

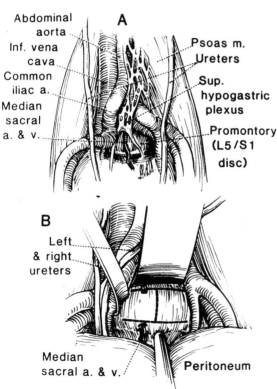

Abdominal aorta
Inf. vena cava
Common iliac a.
Median sacral a. & v.
A
Psoas m.
Ureters
Sup. hypogastric plexus
Promontory (L5/S1 disc)

B
Left & right ureters
Median sacral a. & v.
Peritoneum

FIGURE 6. Anterior anatomy at the lumbosacral junction. **A,** Anatomic structures related to the anterior L4–S1 region—ureter, sympathetic plexus, aorta, vena cava and bifurcation of these vessels. **B,** Exposure of the L5–S1 disc following ligation of the middle sacral vessels. Note that both the left and right ureters are retracted toward the right side. (From Majd ME, et al: Anterior approach to the spine. In Margulies JY, et al (eds): Revision Spine Surgery. St. Louis, Mosby, p 152, with permission.)

24. A 46-year-old man underwent implantation of two BAK fusion cages in the L5–S1 disc space through an anterior surgical approach. Four months after the initial surgery he complained of increased back pain. Radiographs revealed a halo around the cages and anterior migration of the devices. The surgeon decided to revise the cages through an anterior retroperitoneal approach. During the procedure scar tissue made exposure difficult, and the surgeon was concerned that an injury to the ureter had occurred. What is the best way to evaluate for this problem? What treatment is indicated if a ureteral injury exists?

Intravenous injection of 5 cc of methylene blue can appear within 5–10 minutes in the surgical field and confirm the ureteral injury. Urologic consultation and repair or stenting of the ureter are required. Placement of a ureteral stent before surgery helps to identify the ureter during revision anterior surgical procedures and may help to prevent this complication.

25. A 40-year-old man underwent a L5–S1 anterior lumbar interbody fusion with implantation of a anterior fusion cage. He complains of erectile dysfunction after the procedure. What should the surgeon advise the patient?

The patient should be advised that prognosis for recovery is good because erection is not controlled by any of the neural structures that course over the anterior aspect of the L5–S1 disc. The patient's difficulty is not related to the anterior approach; other underlying causes should be evaluated.

Erection is predominantly a parasympathetic function through control of the vasculature of the penis. The parasympathetic fibers responsible for erection originate from the L1–L4 nerve roots and arrive at their target area via the pelvic splanchnic nerves. Somatic function from the S1–S4 levels is carried through the pudendal nerve.

Anterior spine surgery at the L5–S1 level has the potential to disrupt the superior hypogastric plexus. This sympathetic plexus crosses the anterior aspect of the L5–S1 disc and distal aorta. The superior hypogastric plexus controls bladder neck closure during ejaculation. Failure of closure of the bladder neck during ejaculation causes ejaculate to travel in a retrograde direction into the bladder and can result in sterility.

26. During an endoscopic approach to the lumbosacral junction, the bovie is used to coagulate the middle sacral artery and vein. This technique, as opposed to bipolar electrocoagulation or a suture ligation of the middle sacral artery and vessel, increases the risk for what complication?

Retrograde ejaculation. This complication has been reported more commonly with the endoscopic approach to the lumbosacral junction than with an open surgical approach. This finding has been attributed to use of a bovie with subsequent damage to the sympathetic plexus. The reported incidence in the literature is between 2% and 17%. Male patients undergoing an anterior L5–S1 exposure should always be forewarned of this possible complication. Many surgeons do not offer an anterior exposure to men in their reproductive years for fear of this complication and its medical/legal ramifications.

27. After the left-sided retroperitoneal approach to the lumbar spine, the patient wakes up complaining of coolness in the right lower extremity compared with the left. Palpation of pulses demonstrates good dorsalis pedis and posterior tibia pulses bilaterally, and the right leg does appear to be cooler than the left leg. How are these clinical findings explained?

The sympathetic chain lies on the lateral border of the vertebral bodies and is often disrupted during an anterior surgical exposure. A sympathectomy effect occurs and allows increased blood flow to the left leg compared with the right. This process explains the temperature increase and occasional swelling noted in the lower extremity on the side of the surgical exposure. Patients should be forewarned of this possible result of an anterior spine procedure and told that it will not impair the ultimate outcome surgery.

28. After a left-sided retroperitoneal exposure of the lumbosacral junction, the patient awakens in the recovery room complaining of increased pain in the left lower extremity. The left leg is noted to be cooler than the right leg. What test should be ordered immediately?

An arteriogram should be ordered on an emergent basis. This clinical scenario cannot be explained on the basis of a sympathectomy effect by which the ipsilateral leg on the side of the exposure becomes warmer. When the distal extremity on the side of the exposure becomes cooler, it is usually due to dislodgement of an arteriosclerotic plaque. Thus, assessment of the vasculature with an arteriogram is the study of choice to determine whether the plaque has lodged in the trifurcation in the popliteal fossa. Immediate consultation with an experienced vascular surgeon is appropriate.

29. The technique for implantation of an artificial disc requires the surgeon to place the implant as far posteriorly as possible along the vertebral endplates. During the procedure for one type of artificial disc, sequential dilators are placed in the L5–S1 interspace until a loud pop is heard or felt. This noise represents the disruption of the posterior longitudinal ligament. Aside from fainting, what should the surgeon do if a large return of blood is noted in the wound after this popping noise?

In the case of rapid bleeding after distraction and disruption of the posterior longitudinal ligament, the presumptive diagnosis is disruption of the epidural venous plexus. The most appropriate technique at this point is to place gel foam soaked with thrombin into the posterior aspect of the interspace and then remove the distraction from the interspace. After several minutes the bleeding will stop, and the procedure may continue.

BIBLIOGRAPHY

1. Baker JK, Reardon PR, Reardon MJ, et al: Vascular injury in anterior lumbar surgery. Spine 18:2227–2230, 1993.
2. Devlin VJ, Pitt DD: The evolution of surgery of the anterior spinal column. Spine State Art Rev 12: 493–528, 1998.
3. DeWald RL: Anterior exposures of the thoracolumbar spine. In Bridwell KH, DeWald RL (eds): The Textbook of Spinal Surgery, 2nd ed. Philadelphia, Lippincott-Raven, 1997, pp 253–260.
4. Majd ME, Harkess JW, Holt RT, et al: Anterior approach to the spine. In Margulies JY, Aebi M, Farcy JP (eds): Revision Spine Surgery. Mosby, 1999, pp 138–155.
5. Watkins RG: Surgical Approaches to the Spine, New York, Springer-Verlag, 1983.
6. Winter RB, Lonstein JE, Denis F, et al: Paraplegia resulting from vessel ligation. Spine 21(10):1232–1234, 1996.
7. Winter RB, Lonstein JW, Denis F, Smith MD. Atlas of Spine Surgery. Philadelphia, W.B. Saunders, 1995.

27. POSTERIOR SURGICAL APPROACHES TO THE THORACIC AND LUMBAR SPINE

Vincent J. Devlin, M.D.

1. Describe the options for patient positioning for posterior surgical approaches to the thoracic and lumbar spinal regions

Typically patients are positioned prone on an operative frame for posterior approaches to the thoracic and lumbar spine. Exceptions include use of a lateral decubitus position during simultaneous anterior and posterior surgical procedures and use of a partial decubitus position for costotransversectomy approaches.

2. What are the basic types of positioning frames for posterior spinal procedures?

Four-post frame: Two proximal pads are placed beneath the pectoral region and two distal pads are placed in the region of the anterior superior iliac spines. The hip joints and lower extremities are positioned parallel with the trunk.

Wilson frame: Longitudinal curved pads are attached to a frame and can be raised or lowered to alter lumbar lordosis.

Knee-chest frame: The patient's hips and knees are positioned at 90° and the patients's abdominal and lower extremity mass is supported by the patient's knees.

3. Discuss major considerations for selecting the appropriate positioning frame for a specific spinal procedure.

A four-post frame is preferred for multilevel fusion procedures. This type of frame permits extension of the hips and thighs, which preserves or enhances lumbar lordosis. Use of a frame that decreases lumbar lordosis (Wilson frame, knee-chest frame) is preferred for lumbar discectomy procedures. Decreasing lumbar lordosis facilitates access to the lumbar spinal canal as the distance between the spinous processes and lamina is increased. Care is necessary when selecting a frame for spinal stenosis decompressions. Spinal stenosis patients are symptomatic in extension. Positioning such patients on a frame that decreases lumbar lordosis and flexes the spine may result in failure to fully appreciate the extent of neural decompression required to relieve symptoms.

4. Outline the steps involved in a midline posterior exposure of the thoracic and lumbar spine.

- Incise the skin and subcutaneous tissues with a scalpel.
- Place Weitlander and cerebellar retractors to tamponade superficial bleeding by exerting tension on surrounding tissues.
- Electrocautery dissection is carried out down to the level of the spinous processes.
- Cobb elevators and electrocautery are used to elevate the paraspinous muscles from the lamina at the level(s) requiring exposure. This provides sufficient exposure for discectomy and laminectomy procedures.
- If a fusion is planned, Cobb elevators and electrocautery are used to elevate the paraspinous muscles laterally to the tips of the transverse processes on each side. Subsequently the facet joints are excised and prepared for fusion. Care is taken to preserve the soft tissue structures (interspinous ligaments, supraspinous ligaments and facet capsules) at the transition between fused and nonfused levels.
- Hemostasis is maintained by coagulating bleeding points with electrocautery and packing with surgical sponges.

5. Where are blood vessels encountered during posterior spinal exposures?

The arterial blood supply of the posterior thoracic and lumbar spine is consistent at each spinal level (Fig. 1). Arteries are encountered at the lateral border of the pars interarticularis, the upper medial border of the transverse process, and in the intertransverse region. Sacral arteries exit from the dorsal sacral foramen. The superior gluteal artery enters the gluteal musculature and may be encountered during iliac crest bone grafting.

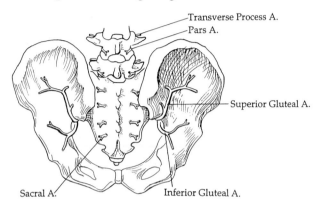

FIGURE 1. Blood vessels encountered during posterior midline approach. (From Wiesel SW, et al (eds): The Lumbar Spine, 2nd ed. Philadelphia, W.B. Saunders, 1996, with permission.)

6. What methods are used to guide the surgeon in exposing the correct anatomic levels during a posterior approach to the thoracic or lumbar spine?

A combination of methods is used to guide exposure of correct anatomic levels:
- Preoperative radiographs are reviewed to determine bony landmarks and presence of anatomic variants that may affect numbering of spinal levels (i.e., altered number of rib-bearing thoracic vertebra, lumbarized or sacralized vertebra).
- Intraoperative bony landmarks are referenced: C7 (vertebra prominens), T8 (inferomedial angle of the scapula), T12 (most distal palpable rib), L4–L5 (superior lateral edge of ilium).
- An intraoperative radiograph with a metallic marker at the level of exposure is obtained. A permanent copy should be made to document the correct level of exposure for every procedure.

7. How is the location of the thoracic pedicle identified from the posterior midline approach?

The general location of a thoracic pedicle can be determined by crossing a horizontal line at the midportion of the transverse process and a vertical line at the junction between the lamina and transverse process. The exact location of the pedicle at each thoracic level varies slightly and has been determined by Lenke.[2] A power burr is used to remove the outer bony cortex and expose the entry site to the pedicle.

8. How is the location of the lumbar pedicle identified from the posteror midline approach?

The lumbar pedicle is located at the intersection of two lines. The vertical line passes along the lateral aspect of the superior articular process and passes lateral to the pars interarticularis. The horizontal line passes through the middle of the transverse process, where it joins the superior articular process.

9. What is a costotransversectomy approach?

A costotransversectomy approach is a posterolateral approach to the thoracic spine (Fig. 2). It provides unilateral access to the posterior spinal elements, lateral aspect of the vertebral body, and anterior aspect of the spinal canal without the need to enter the thoracic cavity. Exposure includes resection of the posteromedial portion of the rib and transverse process. This approach was initially developed for drainage of tuberculous abscesses. It remains useful for biopsies and disc excision in patients who cannot tolerate a formal thoracotomy. It does not provide sufficient exposure to permit placement of an anterior strut graft.

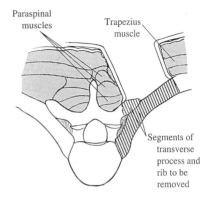

FIGURE 2. Costotransversectomy approach. (From Winter RB, Lonstein JE, Dennis F, Smith MD (eds): Atlas of Spine Surgery. Philadelphia, W.B. Saunders, 1995, with permission.)

10. What is a lateral extracavitary approach?

A lateral extracavitary approach is a posterolateral extrapleural approach to the thoracic spine and thoracolumbar junction (Fig. 3). It provides greater exposure of the anterior spinal column and anterior aspect of the spinal canal than is achieved with a costotransversectomy. This approach requires removal of portions of the rib, costotransverse joint, facet, and pedicle. The exposure achieved is sufficient to permit corpectomy and placement of an anterior strut graft.

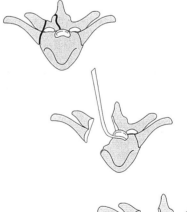

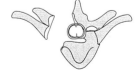

FIGURE 3. Lateral extracavitary approach. (From Amundson GM, Garfin SR: Posterior spinal instrumentation for thoracolumbar tumor and trauma reconstruction. Semin Spine Surg 9:262, 1997, with permission.)

11. What is a transpedicular approach?

After the spine is exposed by a posterior midline approach, the pedicle can be used as a pathway to access anterior spinal column pathology. A pedicle tunnel is created with specialized curets. Subsequently bone and disc material can be removed through the pedicle channel. This approach can be used for a variety of procedures, including biopsy, discectomy, corpectomy, and osteotomy throughout the thoracic and lumbar spinal regions. Spinal instrumentation can be placed concurrently to provide spinal stabilization and deformity correction.

12. Describe the paraspinal approach to the lumbar spine.

The paraspinal (Wiltse) approach is a posterolateral approach to the lumbar region (Fig. 4). It utilizes the plane between the multifidus and longissimus muscles. It permits direct access to disc herniations and spinal stenosis located in the extraforaminal zone without the need to resect the pars interarticularis or facet complex. It is also a useful approach for lumbar intertransverse fusion and instrumentation procedures.

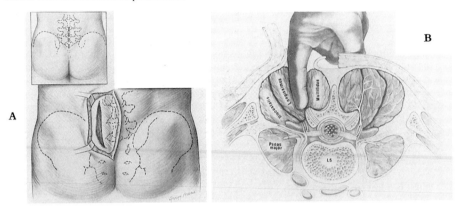

FIGURE 4. Lumbar paraspinal approach. (From Zindrick MR, Selby D: Lumbar spine fusion: Different types and indications. In Wiesel SW, Weinstein JN, Herkowitz H, et al (eds): The Lumbar Spine, 2nd ed, vol. 1. Philadelphia, W.B. Saunders, 1996, p 609, with permission.)

13. What is a PLIF approach?

Posterior lumbar interbody fusion (PLIF) refers to placement of intracolumnar implant(s) into a lumbar disc space from a posterior approach (Fig. 5). The disc space must be prepared to receive the interbody device. Steps involved in this process include laminectomy, discectomy, restoration of disc space height, and decortication of the vertebral endplates. One interbody device is generally placed on each side of the disc space, and posterior pedicle instrumentation is used to stabilize the spinal segment.

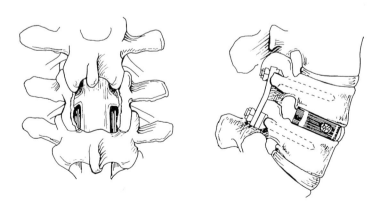

FIGURE 5. Posterior lumbar interbody fusion (PLIF). (From Zindrick MR, Wiltse LL, Rauschning W: Disc herniations lateral to the intervertebral foramen. In White AH, Rothman RH, Ray CD (eds): Lumbar Spine Surgery: Techniques and Complications. St. Louis, Mosby, 1987, p 204, with permission.)

14. What is a TLIF approach?

Transforaminal lumbar interbody fusion (TLIF) refers to placement of intracolumnar implant(s) into a lumbar disc space through a unilateral posterior approach (Fig. 6). Unilateral removal of the pars interarticularis and facet complex provides posterolateral access to the disc space. This technique minimizes the need for significant retraction of neural elements and preserves the contralateral facet complex. The working space is sufficient to permit placement of two interbody fusion devices through a unilateral approach. Posterior pedicle instrumentation is used to stabilize the spine segment.

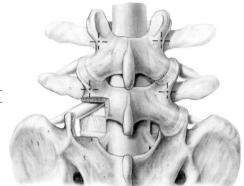

FIGURE 6. Transforaminal lumbar interbody fusion (TLIF). (Courtesy of DePuy AcroMed, Raynham, MA.)

BIBLIOGRAPHY

1. Lenke LG: Posterior and posterolateral approaches to the spine. In Bridwell KH, DeWald RL (eds): The Textbook of Spinal Surgery. Philadelphia, Lippincott-Raven, 1997, pp 193–216.
2. Lenke LG, Rinella A, Kim Y: Freehand thoracic pedicle screw placement. Semin Spine Surg 14:48–57, 2002.
3. Steffee AD, Sitkowski DJ: Posterior lumbar interbody fusion and plates. Clin Orthop 227:99–102, 1988.
4. Wiltse LL, Bateman JG, Hutchinson RH, Nelson WE: The paraspinal sacrospinalis-splitting approach to the lumbar spine. J Bone Joint Surg 50A:919–926,1968.
5. Winter RB, Lonstein JE, Denis F, Smith MD: Atlas of Spine Surgery. Philadelphia, W.B. Saunders, 1995.

28. CERVICAL SPINE INSTRUMENTATION

Kern Singh, M.D., and Alexander R. Vaccaro, M.D.

1. What are the goals of cervical spinal implants?

(1) To immobilize an unstable segment; (2) to promote bony union, fusion, and soft tissue healing; (3) to correct spinal deformity; and (4) to decrease the need for extended external immobilization.

2. Define spinal instability.

Spinal instability is defined as segmental hypermobility under physiologic loading, which may lead to neurologic dysfunction or excessive spinal segment displacement if not treated or stabilized.

3. How are the various types of cervical spinal implants classified?

1. **Anterior**
   Occiptocervical
   Odontoid
   Upper cervical (C1–C2)
   Subaxial (C3–C7)

2. **Posterior**
   Occiptocervical
   Upper cervical (C1–C2)
   Subaxial (C3–C7)

4. What are the indications for instrumentation of the occipitocervical junction from a posterior approach?

- Trauma
- Ligamentous instability
- Select odontoid fractures
- Rheumatoid arthritis (basilar invagination)
- Infection
- Neoplasm
- Intractable pain
- Select skeletal dysplasias
- Arnold Chiari malformation
- Select metabolic bone diseases

5. What types of fixation are available for surgical stabilization of the occipitocervical junction?

1. **Anterior options** (Fig. 1A): C2 to clivus plating
2. **Posterior options** (Fig. 1B)
   Wires / Cables
   Plates, wires / screws
   Rod-plate, wires/ screws
   Rods, wires/screws

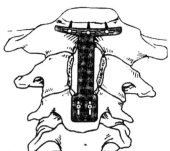

FIGURE 1. Occipitocervical fixation options. **A,** Anterior option. *(continued)*

A

B

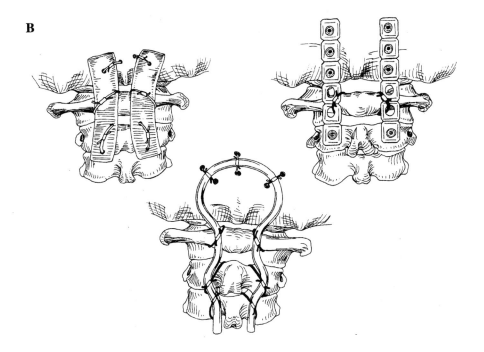

FIGURE 1. *(continued)* Occiptocervical fixation options. **B,** Posterior options.

6. Describe the principles involved in posterior occipitocervical segmental fixation.

The original occipitocervical plate was de-signed by Roy-Camille. The plates were pre-molded with a 105° angulation designed to restore the nor-mal sagittal plane curvature of the occipitocervical junction. A midline approach is used. Great care is afforded not to disturb the venous cavernous sinus between the C1 and C2 facet joint articulation and the vertebral artery approximately 1.5 cm from the posterior midline of C1 (8–10 mm along the superior margin of C1). The plate is secured to the subaxial spine traditionally with lateral mass screws, at C2 with an isthmus or pedicle screw, and at the occiput with unicortical or bicortical screws. The most dense bone of the skull is in the midline at the inion. Drilling of bicortical screws may risk injury to the meninges or venous sinus penetration during drilling (Fig. 2).

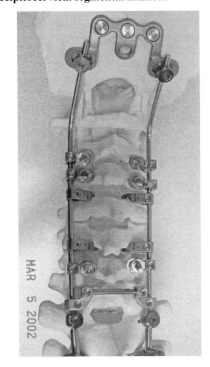

FIGURE 2 *(right).* Saw bone model demonstrating occipto-cervical plate-rod system.

7. What are the indications for spinal implant placement in the upper cervical spine?

Atlantoaxial instability due to traumatic causes (unstable odontoid fractures, transverse ligament disruption, odontoid nonunion, unstable os odontoideum) or nontraumatic disorders (rheumatoid arthritis, congenital and metabolic disorders).

8. What types of implants are used to stabilize the atlantoaxial (C1–C2) joint?
   1. **Anterior:** transarticular screws (Fig. 3A)
   2. **Posterior**

   Tapes (Fig. 3B)   Wires/cables (Figs. 4 and 5)   Screw-rod constructs
   Rod clamps (Fig. 3C)   Transarticular screws (Fig. 6)

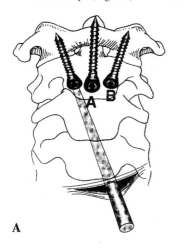

A

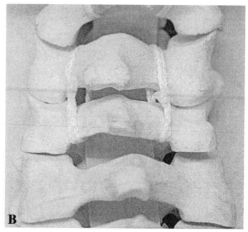

B

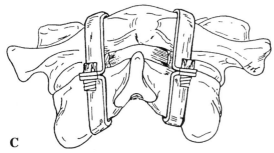

C

FIGURE 3. C1–C2 fixation techniques. **A**, Anterior atlantoaxial screw fixation. **B**, Tape (secure strand). **C**, Rod/clamp.

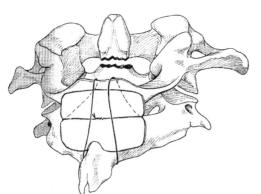

FIGURE 4 *(right)*. Gallie wiring technique. (From Winter R, Lonstein J, Denis F, Smith M: Anterior upper cervical procedures. In Atlas of Spine Surgery. Philadelphia, W.B. Saunders, 1995, p 29, with permission.)

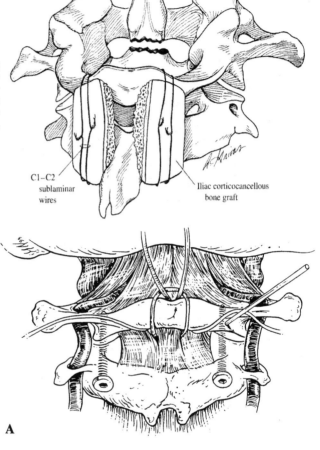

FIGURE 5 *(left)*. Brooks wiring technique. (From Winter R, Lonstein J, Denis F, Smith M: Anterior upper cervical procedures. In Atlas of Spine Surgery. Philadelphia, W.B. Saunders, 1995, p 28, with permission.)

C1–C2 sublaminar wires

Iliac corticocancellous bone graft

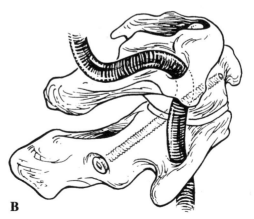

FIGURE 6 *(left)*. C1–C2 transarticular screw fixation. **A**, Anteroposterior view. **B**, Lateral view.

A

B

9. Describe the Gallie and Brooks wiring procedures.

The **Gallie technique** begins with passage of a sublaminar wire (double-looped) from caudal to cranial under the posterior arch of C1. After wire passage, a piece of cortical cancellous graft is harvested and shaped to conform to the posterior processes of C1 and C2. The two free ends of the wire are passed through the leading wire loop and then over the graft and around or through the spinous process of the axis. The free ends of the wire are then twisted in the midline, thereby securing the graft position between C1 and C2 (see Fig. 4)

The **Brooks procedure** involves the passage of dual or doubled sublaminar wires (cables/tape) from caudal to cranial under the arch of C2 and then C1. After the passage of the wire, two separate triangular or rectangular corticocancellous grafts are harvested and placed over the posterior elements of C1 and C2. The ends of the wires on each side are then tightened together, thereby securing the position of the grafts (see Fig. 5).

10. What are the advantages and disadvantages of the Gallie and Brooks procedures?

The main disadvantage of both procedures involves the passage of sublaminar wires. Although the Gallie procedure is adequate in resisting flexion moments, the Brooks procedure is more biomechanically sound in resisting extension and axial rotation. Neither procedure compares biomechanically to the stability afforded by transarticular screw fixation.

11. Describe the procedure of C1–C2 transarticular facet screw fixation.

After exposing the posterior C1–C2 facet complex and inferior margin of the inferior articular process of C2, the isthmus of C2 is palpated bilaterally. This guides placement of the percutaneous transarticular screws, which traverse the inferior articular process of C2, the isthmus of C2, the superior endplate of C2, and the lateral mass of C1 (see Fig. 6).

12. What are the advantages of transarticular screw fixation vs. posterior wiring procedures?

Improved stability in all modes of motion testing. Posterior wiring constructs shift the axis of rotation posteriorly so that C1 now rotates around the wired graft complex. This construct cannot offer significant resistance to posterior shear forces. However, transarticular C1–C2 screws are nearly 10 times stiffer in rotation than posterior wiring, thereby decreasing the potential of pseudarthrosis (0.6%).

13. What complications may be associated with transarticular screw placement?

Spinal cord and vertebral artery injury are the two most common complications. Unilateral hypoglossal nerve paralysis has been reported secondary to a long screw projecting anterior to the occipital condyle.

14. Describe the fixation of choice for select odontoid fractures treated anteriorly.

One or two screws may be used to stabilize a type 2 odontoid fracture. The critical transverse outer diameter for the placement of two 3.5-mm cortical screws is 9 mm. Cadaveric biomechanical studies have demonstrated that one central screw that engages the cortical tip of the dens is just as effective as two screws. Two screws better counter the rotational forces created by the alar ligaments. Single-screw options include the use of a single 4.5-mm cannulated Herbert screw or a single 4- to 4.5-mm standard lag screw (Fig. 7).

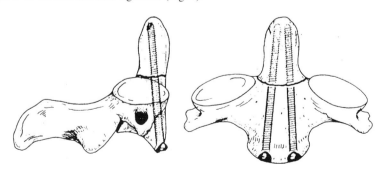

FIGURE 7. Odontoid screw fixation. **Left,** Lateral view. **Right,** Anteroposterior view.

15. Describe the anatomic characteristics of body habitus or fracture pattern that may increase the difficulty of odontoid screw placement.

Short neck, thoracic kyphosis, barrel chest deformity, and a fracture pattern that requires a flexed position to obtain and maintain fracture reduction.

16. What are the major contraindications to the use of odontoid screw fixation?

Odontoid fractures associated with comminution of one or both atlantoaxial joints, a sagittal plane fracture that courses posterior superiorly to anterior inferiorly, a pathologic fracture with compromised bone quality, and significant osteoporosis.

17. What are the mostly commonly used implants in the lower subaxial cervical spine?

1. **Anterior:** plates and screws
2. **Posterior**

| Tapes | Lateral mass plates/ rods and screws |
| Wires/ cables | Pedicle screws and rods or plates |

18. What are the indications for anterior cervical plating?

To decrease the incidence of graft subsidence and dislodgement, to minimize kyphotic collapse of the fused interspace, to improve fusion success, and to minimize the need for external immobilization.

19. Describe the features of the first anterior cervical plates.

The original Caspar (Aesculap Instrument Company, San Francisco, CA) and Orozco (Synthes Spine, Paoli, PA) systems were nonconstrained, load-sharing plates that required bicortical screw purchase. Because of the nonconstrained nature of the screw–plate interface, excessive motion at the screw–plate junction occasionally led to screw loosening or pull-out. This problem required engaging the posterior vertebral cortex to minimize screw loosening.

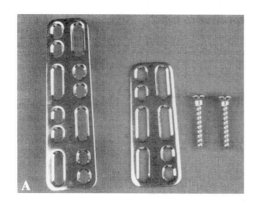

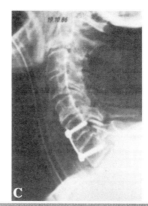

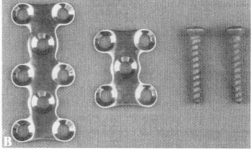

FIGURE 8. First-generation anterior cervical plates. **A**, Caspar plates. **B**, Orozco (H-type) plates. **C**, Note the posterior vertebral body cortex perforation on this lateral radiograph.

20. What are some of the newer anterior cervical plating systems available to the spine surgeon?

Because of the technical difficulty associated with bicortical screw purchase, constrained systems that firmly lock the screws to the plate were developed. One plate system uses an expandable cross-split head that locks into the plate after insertion of a small central bolt (Synthes Spine, Paoli, PA). Securing the screws to the plates allows a more direct transfer of the applied forces from the spine to the plate and improved construct stiffness without the need for bicortical purchase. Other systems use screw head coverage mechanisms (ring locks, blocking heads) to secure the screw to the plate.

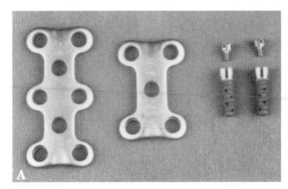
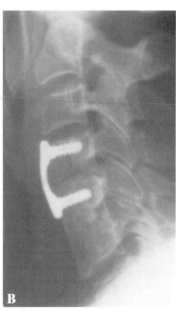

FIGURE 9. Anterior cervical locking plate (Synthes Spine, Paoli, PA). **A,** The screw head is locked to the plate by insertion of a conical bolt, thereby ensuring angular stability between the plate and the screws. **B,** Anterior cervical locking plate application after interbody fusion. Note that penetration of the posterior vertebral body cortex is not required to achieve a stable implant construct.

21. Describe the different biomechanical missions of available anterior cervical plate systems.

Plates may have a constrained (screw heads lock to plate) or nonconstrained screw–plate interface. Vertebral screws may be unicortical or bicortical. Plates may be considered to have a dynamization function if the screw is able to migrate in an angular manner in a round screw hole or migrate superiorly or inferiorly in a slotted screw hole nest.

22. What factors are directly related to screw pull-out force with anterior cervical plating?

Bone mineral density as determined by dual-energy x-ray absorptiometry (DEXA) and insertional torque.

23. What is the current consensus regarding cervical plating and pseudarthrosis rates?

Clinically, the fusion rate of one-level cervical interbody fusions is not significantly improved with anterior cervical plate fixation. Pseudarthrosis, delayed union, and graft collapse are decreased in multilevel fusions with anterior cervical plating. Multiple-level corpectomies (three or more) followed by stand-alone anterior cervical plating are prone to failure due to plate host bone repetitive loading stresses over the long plate lever arm. This results in screw-host bone failure, usually at the inferior plate margin, and loss of fixation. In these clinical situations, prior to failure, the surgeon should consider either rigid posterior cervical segmental fixation or postoperative immobilization in a halo vest.

24. What are some of the common complications related to anterior cervical spine surgery?

Hoarseness and dysphagia due to soft tissue dissection and esophagus and trachea retraction. Anterior cervical plate failure has been reported by several authors, particulary when long, multisegmental plate constructs have been used. Plate and screw migration may result in anterior soft tissue irritation and possible erosion involving the esophagus. Extensive soft tissue scar often covers anterior cervical implants and may afford some soft tissue protection if implant prominence is less than or equal to 5 mm.

25. What is a buttress plate?

A buttress or junctional plate is an alternative to long segment anterior cervical plates, which are subject to large cantilever forces, particularly at the caudal plate-screw-bone junction. The buttress plate spans only the caudal or cephalad graft-host junction, thereby theoretically preventing graft extrusion. The plate is most commonly used at the caudal end of the graft where the cantilever forces are the greatest. A surgeon should strongly consider supplemental posterior segmental fixation in the setting of a long anterior strut graft fusion and junctional plate stabilization.

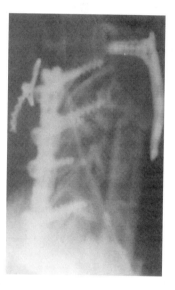

FIGURE 10. The buttress plate prevents anterior fibula graft dislodgment in combination with posterior cervical lateral mass stabilization.

26. What are the indications for posterior subaxial cervical instrumentation?

Fusion and stabilization for fracture, posterior stabilization after an anterior nonunion, an adjunctive stabilization procedure after a long segment anterior fusion, or fusion and stabilization after a posterior decompression for cervical myelopathy.

27. Describe the Bohlman triple wiring technique.

After exposure of the posterior cervical elements to the lateral margins of the lateral masses, a 2- or 3-mm right-angle burr is used to create a hole on each side of the base of the spinous process at the spinolaminar line. The burr hole is placed in the superior third of the superior vertebral spinous process and in the inferior third of the inferior vertebral spinous process. A 16- or 18-gauge wire, cable, or tape is then placed through one spinous process hole and circled around its respective spinous process. This procedure is followed by wire passage through the other spinous process with circling of its spinous process. The wire ends are then twisted to themselves. Separate wires are then passed through each set of burr holes at each level. These wires are used to secure a corticocancellous bone graft to the decorticated posterior elements on each side of the spinous processes.

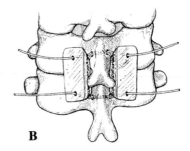

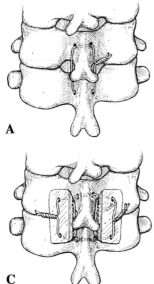

FIGURE 11. **A, B,** and **C,** Steps in the Bohlman triple-wire technique. (From An H, Cotler J (eds): Spinal instrumentation, 2nd ed. Philadelphia, Lippincott Williams & Wilkins, 1999, p 204, with permission.)

28. What are the most common complications associated with posterior cervical wiring techniques and their causes?

Loss of wire fixation due to wire failure or bony pull-out is the most common complication. Factors that determine fixation success or failure include bone quality, patient age, and method of postoperative immobilization.

29. What are the advantages of lateral mass and pedicle screw fixation vs. posterior wiring?

Cervical lateral mass and pedicle screw fixation afford a significant increase in rotational and extension stability compared with posterior wiring techniques. Spinal implant fixation to the lateral mass and pedicles obviates the need for intact laminae or spinous processes. The major contraindication to this technique is the presence of osteoporotic bone.

30. Describe the techniques for placement of lateral mass screws.

The three most commonly used techniques for lateral mass screw placement, as described by Roy-Camille, Magerl, and An, are summarized in the table below and illustrated in Figure 12 (on following page).

TECHNIQUE	ROY-CAMILLE	MAGERL	AN
Starting position (lateral mass)	Center	1 mm medial and 1–2 mm cephald to the center	1 mm medial to the center
Cephalad tilt	0	30	15
Lateral tilt	10	25	30

31. At what levels are lateral mass screws considered to be dangerous?

At C2, there is significant risk of injury to the vertebral artery with a laterally directed mass screw. At C7, the lateral mass is small, and a lateral mass screw risks causing C8 nerve root irritation.

32. What is the role of pedicle screws in the cervical spine?

Pedicle screws are useful and relatively safe at the C2 and C7 levels, especially in the absence of vertebral artery passage in the foramen transversarium of C7 (Fig. 13). Pedicle screw placement at the C3–C6 levels is currently under study as a potential means of rigid posterior subaxial stabilization.

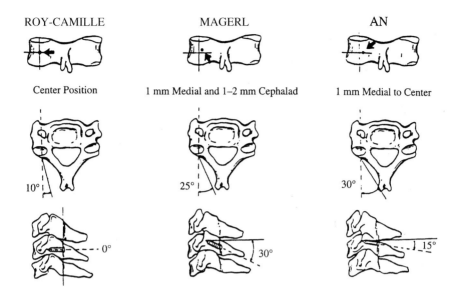

ROY-CAMILLE   MAGERL   AN

Center Position   1 mm Medial and 1–2 mm Cephalad   1 mm Medial to Center

10°   25°   30°

0°   30°   15°

FIGURE 12. Techniques for lateral mass screw placement.

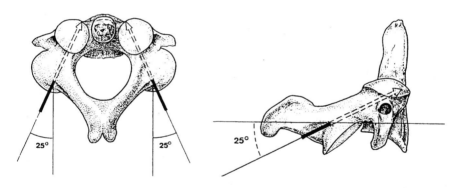

25°   25°   25°

FIGURE 13. Guidelines for C2 pedicle screw placement.

33. Summarize the role of cervical spinal implants.

Cervical spinal implants are intended to supplement a well performed fusion technique. If the performance of a fusion is suboptimal, regardless of the implant used, clinical failure is a high possibility.

BIBLIOGRAPHY

1. Abdu W, Bohlman H: Techniques of subaxial posterior cervical spine fusions: An overview. Orthopedics 287–295, 1992.
2. Connolly J, Esses S, Kostuik J: Anterior cervical fusion: Outcome of patients fused with and without anterior cervical plates. J Spinal Dis 9:202–206, 1996.
3. Montane I, Eismont F, Green B: Traumatic occipitoatlantal dislocation. Spine 16:112–116, 1991.
4. Sutterlin C, McAfee P, Warden K, et al: A biomechanical evaluation of cervical spine stabilization in a bovine model: static and cyclical loading. Spine 13:795–802, 1988.
5. Vaccaro A, Singh K: Instrumentation for cervical spinal trauma. In An H, Cotler J (eds): Spinal Instrumentation, 2nd ed. Philadelphia, Lippincott Williams & Wilkins, 1999, pp 31–58.
6. Winter R, Lonstein J, Denis F, Smith M: Atlas of Spinal Surgery. Philadelphia, W.B. Saunders, 1995, pp 1–104.

29. THORACIC AND LUMBAR SPINAL INSTRUMENTATION

D. Greg Anderson, M.D., Adam C. Crowl, M.D., and Vincent J. Devlin, M.D.

GENERAL CONSIDERATIONS

1. Summarize the functions of spinal instrumentation in thoracic and lumbar fusion procedures.

1. **Enhance fusion.** Spinal implants function to immobilize spinal segments during the fusion process and increase the rate of successful arthrodesis.

2. **Restore spinal stability.** When pathologic processes (e.g., tumor, infection, fracture) compromise spinal stability, spinal implants can restore stability.

3. **Correct spinal deformities.** Spinal instrumentation can provide correction of spinal deformities (e.g., scoliosis, kyphosis, spondylolisthesis).

4. **Permit extensive decompression of the neural elements.** Complex spinal stenosis problems requiring extensive decompression create spinal instability. Spinal instrumentation and fusion prevent development of post-surgical spinal deformities leading to recurrent spinal stenosis.

2. Why is surgical stabilization of the spine considered a two-stage process?

In the short term, stabilization of the spine is provided by spinal implants. However, long-term stabilization of the spine occurs only if fusion is successful. If the fusion does not heal, spinal implants eventually fail. The surgeon influences this process through meticulous fusion technique, selection of the appropriate location for fusion (anterior, posterior or combined anterior and posterior fusion), and use of appropriate spinal implants to adequately support the spine during this process.

3. What is meant by the terms *tension band principle* and *load-sharing concept*?

In the normal spine, the posterior spinal musculature maintains normal sagittal spinal alignment through application of dorsal tension forces against the intact anterior spinal column. This is termed the **tension band principle**. The posterior spinal musculature can function as a tension band only if the anterior spinal column is structurally intact. Biomechanical studies have shown that in the normal spine approximately 80% of axial load is carried by the anterior spinal column and the remaining 20% is transmitted through the posterior spinal column. This relationship is termed the **load-sharing concept**. See Figure 1.

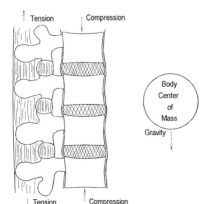

FIGURE 1. Anterior column load-sharing and posterior tension band principle.

4. What is the relevance of the load-sharing concept to the selection of appropriate spinal implants?

Load sharing between an instrumentation construct and the vertebral column is a function of the ratio of the axial stiffness of the spinal instrumentation and the axial stiffness of the vertebral column. If the anterior spinal column is incompetent, the entire axial load must pass through the posterior spinal implant. In the absence of adequate anterior column support, normal physiologic loads exceed the strength of posterior spinal implant systems. In this situation, posterior spinal implants will fail by fatigue, permanent deformation, or implant migration through bone. Thus, it is critical to reconstruct an incompetent anterior spinal column when using posterior spinal implant systems.

POSTERIOR SPINAL INSTRUMENTATION

5. What three posterior spinal instrumentation systems are considered to be the precursors of contemporary posterior spinal instrumentation systems?

Harrington instrumentation, Luque instrumentation, and Cotrel-Dubousset instrumentation.

6. What is Harrington instrumentation?

After its introduction in 1960, Harrington instrumentation continued to be used successfully for over 25 years for treatment of various spinal pathologies. Harrington initially used a single rod with ratchets on one end in combination with a single hook at each end of the rod. Distraction forces were applied to obtain and maintain correction of spinal deformites. Shortcomings of this system included the need for postoperative immobilization to prevent hook dislodgement as well as inability to correct and maintain sagittal plane alignment. Various modifications were introduced to address these problems, including square-ended hooks, use of compression hooks along a convex rod, and use of supplemental wire fixation (Fig. 2).

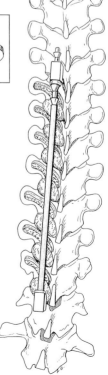

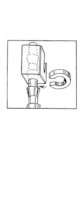

FIGURE 2. Harrington instrumentation. (Adapted from Winter RB, Lonstein JE, Denis F, Smith MD: Atlas of Spine Surgery. Philadelphia, W.B. Saunders, 1995, with permission).

7. What is Luque instrumentation?

In the 1980s Luque introduced a system that provided segmental fixation consisting of wires placed beneath the lamina at multiple spinal levels (Fig 3). Wires were tightened around rods placed along both sides of the lamina. Corrective forces were distributed over multiple levels thereby decreasing the risk of fixation failure. This eliminated the need for postoperative immobilization and provided better control of sagittal plane alignment than Harrington instrumentation.

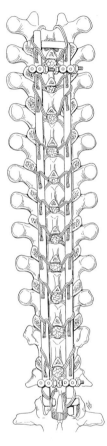

FIGURE 3. Luque instrumentation. (Adapted from Winter RB, Lonstein JE, Denis F, Smith MD: Atlas of Spine Surgery. Philadelphia, W.B. Saunders, 1995, with permission.)

8. What is Cotrel-Dubousset instrumentation?

In 1984 Cotrel and Dubousset introduced their segmental fixation system, which used multiple hooks and screws placed along a knurled rod . The use of multiple fixation points obviated the need for postoperative immobilization and permitted selective application of compression and distraction forces along the same rod by altering hook direction. A rod rotatation maneuver was introduced in an attempt to provide improved three-dimensional correction of scoliosis. Modern posterior segmental spinal instrumentation systems integrate use of hook, wire, and screw fixation (Fig. 4).

9. What is meant by the term *posterior segmental spinal fixation*?

Posterior segmental spinal fixation is a general term used to describe a variety of contemporary posterior spinal instrumentation systems. A complete implant assembly is termed a **spinal construct**. Typically, spinal instrumentation constructs consist of a **longitudinal member** (rod or plate) on each side of the spine connected by **cross-linking devices** to increase construct stability. **Segmental fixation** is defined as the connection of the longitudinal member to multiple vertebra within the construct. Options for achieving segmental fixation include the use of hook,

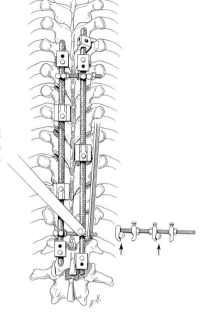

FIGURE 4. Cotrel-Dubousset instrumentation. (Adapted from Winter RB, Lonstein JE, Denis F, Smith MD. Atlas of Spine Surgery. Philadelphia, W.B. Saunders, 1995, with permission.)

wire, and pedicle screw **anchors**. Various corrective forces can be applied to the spine by means of these segmental anchors including compression, distraction, rotation, cantilever bending, and translation. An example of a contemporary posterior segmental spinal fixation system is the Isola system developed by Asher and colleagues (Fig. 5).

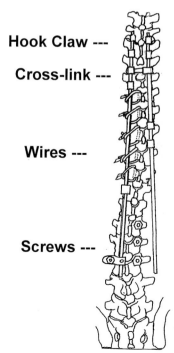

Hook Claw ---

Cross-link ---

Wires ---

Screws ---

FIGURE 5. Contemporary posterior segmental spinal instrumentation.

10. Describe the use of hook anchors in posterior segmental spinal constructs.

Hook anchors may be placed above or below the T1–T10 transverse processes, under the thoracic facet joints, and above or below the thoracic and lumbar lamina. When blades of adjacent hooks face each other, this is termed a **claw configuration**. Compression forces can be applied to adjacent opposing hooks thereby securing the hooks to the posterior elements. A claw may be composed of hooks at a single spinal level (intrasegmental claw) or hooks at adjacent levels (intersegmental claw). Hooks placed in a claw configuration provide more secure fixation than a single hook anchor. For this reason, claw fixation is typically used at the proximal and distal ends of spinal constructs.

11. Describe the use of wire anchors in posterior segmental spinal contructs.

Wire anchors (and more recently cables) can be placed at every level of the spine. Possible attachment points for wire anchors include the base of the spinous process or the sublaminar position. Spinous process wires are placed through a hole in the base of the spinous process and remain outside the spinal canal. Sublaminar wires require careful preparation of the cephalad and caudad interlaminar spaces to minimize the risk of neurologic injury as wires are passed beneath the lamina and dorsal to the neural elements.

12. Describe the use of pedicle screw anchors in posterior spinal contructs.

Pedicle screw anchors can be used throughout the thoracic and lumbar spinal regions. Pedicle screw anchors allow control of all three vertebral columns from a posterior approach and provide the most secure spinal anchor site. In the thoracic region, screw placement is initiated at the base of the transverse process near the region of the superior facet and pars interarticularis. Exact position of the entry site is adjusted, depending on the specific level of the thoracic spine. In the lumbar region, the entry site for screw placement is located at the upslope where the transverse process joins the superior articular process just lateral to the pars interarticularis. Screws are directed into the pedicle and engage the vertebral body. Correct screw placement is subsequently confirmed by palpation, imaging and electrophysiologic monitoring techniques. A variety of options exist for linking a screw to the longitudinal member. The longitudinal member may consist of either a plate or a rod.

ANTERIOR SPINAL INTRUMENTATION

13. What are the two main types of anterior spinal instrumentation?

Anterior spinal implants may be broadly classified as extracolumnar or intracolumnar implants. **Extracolumnar implants** are located on the external aspect of the vertebral body and span one or more adjacent vertebral motion segments. Extracolumnar implants consist of vertebral body screws connected to a longitudinal member consisting of either a plate or a rod. Extracolumnar implants are generally placed on the lateral aspect of the thoracic and lumbar vertebral bodies with screws placed in a coronal plane trajectory. **Intracolumnar implants** consist of implants that reside within the contour of the vertebral bodies that they span. They may consist of bone, metal, or synthetic materials. Intracolumnar implants may or may not possess potential for biologic incorporation within the anterior spinal column.

14. Contrast the utility of anterior plate and rod systems.

Plate systems (Fig. 6A) are useful for short-segment spinal disorders (one or two spinal levels). Tumors, burst fractures, and degenerative spinal disorders requiring anterior fusion over one or two levels are indications for use of an anterior plate system. The use of a plate system is problematic when significant coronal or sagittal plane deformity exists or when multiple anterior vertebral segments require fixation. Technical difficulties arise as restoration of spinal alignment is required prior to plate application in the presence of significant spinal deformity.

Anterior rod systems (Fig. 6B) offer advantages in comparison to plate systems. In short-segment spinal problems, anterior rod systems permit corrective forces to be applied directly to

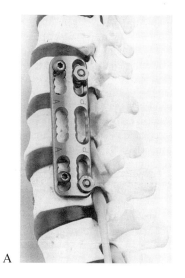
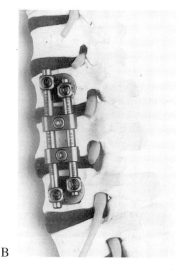

A   B

FIGURE 6. Anterior extracolumnar implants: Plate system (**A**) and Rod system (**B**). (From Devlin VJ, Pitt DD: The evolution of surgery of the anterior spinal column. Spine State Art Rev 12:493–528, 1998, with permission.)

spinal segments, thereby restoring spinal alignment. For example, in the presence of a kyphotic deformity secondary to a burst fracture, initial distraction provides deformity correction and facilitates subsequent placement of an intracolumnar implant. Subsequent compression of the anterior graft or cage restores anterior load sharing and enhances arthrodesis. In long-segment spinal problems (e.g., scoliosis) single or double rod systems can be customized to the specific spinal deformity requiring correction.

15. What are some guidelines for placement of vertebral body screws when using an anterior plate or rod system?

The screws should be parallel to the vertebral endplates. In the axial plane, the screws should be parallel with or angle away from the vertebral canal. The screw tips should purchase the far cortex of the vertebral body but should not protrude more than 5 mm beyond this point (Fig. 7).

FIGURE 7. Correct placement of anterior vertebral body screws. (From Zindrick MR, Selby D: Lumbar spine fusion: Different types and indications. In Wiesel SW, Weinstein JN, Herkowitz H, et al (eds): The Lumbar Spine, 2nd ed. Philadelphia, W.B. Saunders, 1996, p 607, with permission.)

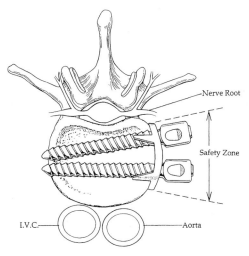

Nerve Root

Safety Zone

I.V.C.   Aorta

16. Describe three possible functions of intracolumnar implants.

Intracolumnar implants may be differentiated based on their intended function:

1. **Promote fusion.** Intracolumnar implants that have potential for biologic incorporation include autograft bone (e.g., ilium, fibula), allograft bone (tibia or femur), and titanium mesh or carbon fiber cages filled with bone graft. Such implants are typically used after discectomy or corpectomy to reconstruct the anterior spinal column through spinal fusion.

2. **Function as a spacer.** Certain intracolumnar implants (e.g., polymethylmethacrylate) are intended to function as an anterior column spacer despite lack of potential for biologic incorporation.

3. **Preserve motion.** An emerging concept is the use of a disc spacer to maintain segmental mobility, stability, and disc space height without fusion. Such intervertebral disc protheses are currently under investigation in the United States.

17. What factors should be considered in choosing among autograft, allograft, and cage devices when an intracolumnar implant is indicated?

Autograft remains the gold standard from the standpoint of fusion success. However, significant donor site morbidity is associated with procurement of a structural autograft. Allografts provide good early strength but have a lower and slower fusion rate compared to autograft. In addition, use of allografts exposes the patient to the infectious risk associated with donor tissue. Cage devices possess excellent strength and provide the advantage of mechanical interdigitation with vertebral receptor sites, thereby decreasing risk of dislodgement (Fig. 8). Cage devices can be filled with cancellous autograft to promote fusion. However, cage devices may subside into the vertebral bodies, resulting in loss of anterior column height. In addition, radiographic assessment of anterior column fusion can be difficult in the presence of cage devices.

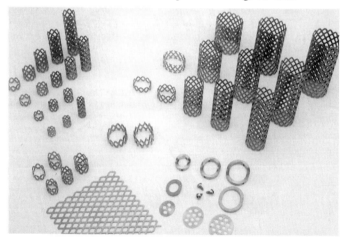

FIGURE 8. Intracolumnar implants—Titanium surgical mesh cages may be easily contoured to reconstruct anterior spinal column deficiencies (courtesy of DePuy AcroMed, Raynham, MA).

18. When is it reasonable to use polymethylmethacrylate (PMMA) as a spacer to reconstruct an anterior spinal column defect?

Currently PMMA is used in two situations:

1. **Anterior spinal reconstruction of metastatic vertebral body lesions in patients with a finite lifespan.** When used for this purpose, PMMA is subject to tensile failure and loosening secondary to development of a fibrous membrane at the cement-bone interface.

2. **Reconstruction of osteoporotic compression fractures.** Vertebroplasty and kyphoplasty procedures involve the injection of PMMA into the vertebral bodies to alleviate pain secondary to acute and subacute fracture.

19. What are the approach options for placement of an intracolumnar implant?

Intracolumnar implants may be placed through anterior, posterior, or lateral surgical approaches. The best approach depends on the location and type of spinal pathology requiring treatment. Recently, minimally invasive approaches have been popularized for placement of intracolumnar implants.

BIBLIOGRAPHY

1. An HS, Cotler JM: Spinal Instrumentation. Baltimore, Williams & Wilkins, 1999.
2. Asher MA, Strippgen WE, Heinig CF, Carson WL. Isola implant system. Semin Spine Surg 4:175–192, 1992.
3. CotrelY, Dubousset J, Guillaumat M. New universal instrumentation in spine surgery. Clin Orthop 227: 10–23, 1988.
4. Devlin VJ, Pitt DD: The evolution of surgery of the anterior spinal column. Spine State Art Rev 12 493–528, 1998.
5. Enker PE, Steffee AD. Interbody fusion and instrumentation. Clin Orthop Rel Res 300:90–101, 1994.
6. Harrington PR: The history and development of Harrington instrumentation. Clin Orthop 227:3–5, 1988.
7. Harms J: Screw-threaded rod system in spinal fusion surgery. Spine State Art Rev 6:541–577, 1992.
8. Kaneda K, Abumi K, Fujiya M: Burst fractures with neurologic deficits of the thoracolumbar-lumbar spine: Results of anterior decompression and stabilization with anaterior instrumentation. Spine 9: 788–795, 1984.
9. Luque ER: The anatomic basis and development of segmental spinal instrumentation. Spine 7:256–259, 1982.
10. Vaccaro AR, Garfin SR: Pedicle-screw fixation in the lumbar spine. J Am Acad Orth Surg 3:262–274, 1995.

30. INSTRUMENTATION AND FUSION OF THE SPINE TO THE SACRUM AND PELVIS

Joseph Y. Margulies, M.D., Ph.D., Vincent J. Devlin, M.D., and William O. Shaffer, M.D.

1. List common indications for a fusion across the lumbosacral motion segment.
- L5–S1 spondylolisthesis
- Degenerative disorders involving the L5–S1 level
- Spinal pathology affecting the lumbosacral junction, such as tumor, infection, or fracture
- Spinal deformities
  Neuromuscular scoliosis associated with pelvic obliquity
  Degenerative lumbar scoliosis
  Adult idiopathic scoliosis with associated degenerative changes at L5–S1
  Extension of a prior scoliosis fusion due to degenerative changes below previously fused levels

2. List complications associated with fusion across the lumbosacral junction.
- Pseudarthrosis
- Loss of lumbar lordosis resulting in flatback syndrome
- Recurrent or worsening spinal deformity
- Implant loosening or failure
- Sacroiliac pain or arthrosis
- Pelvic stress fracture

3. Why is the L5–S1 level considered the most difficult level of the spine to fuse?
Unfavorable biomechanical conditions. The lumbosacral junction is a transition zone between the highly mobile L5–S1 disc and the relatively immobile sacropelvis. Tremendous loads are transferred across the lumbosacral junction (up to 11 times body weight) as axial weight-bearing forces are transmitted from the vertebral column to the pelvis. In addition, the oblique orientation of the L5–S1 disc results in increased shear forces across this level.

Unique anatomy of the sacrum and pelvis. The sacrum is composed of cancellous bone and possesses limited sites for screw fixation. The large diameter S1 pedicle provides less secure screw purchase compared to proximal vertebral levels. Surgeons may utilize additional fixation sites within the sacrum or extend fixation to the ilium in order to increase the strength of anchor sites below the L5 level. Since iliac fixation does not typically include sacroiliac fusion, normal motion of the sacroiliac joint may increase the risk of implant failure or loosening.

4. What is the "80–20 rule" of Harms? How is it relevant to L5–S1 fusion procedures?
Biomechanical studies of the lumbosacral region have demonstrated that approximately 80% of axial load is transmitted through the anterior spinal column and the remaining 20% is transmitted through the posterior column. Spinal fusion and instrumentation procedures that do not restore anterior column load sharing across the lumbosacral junction are destined for failure.

5. Explain why it is more difficult to achieve successful fusion between T10 and the sacrum compared with fusion between L4 and the sacrum.
Long-segment fusion constructs (e.g., T10–S1) have a higher rate of failure than short-segment constructs (e.g., L4–S1) because of the following factors:
- Increased risk of pseudarthrosis. The pseudarthosis rate increases as the number of levels undergoing fusion increases.

- Increased forces placed on distal sacral fixation. Increasing the number of instrumented levels proximal to the sacrum increases the lever arm exerted by the proximal spine on the distal sacral implants. The degree of strain on S1 screws increases as the number of segments immobilized above the sacrum is increased. These unfavorable biomechanical factors increase the risk of distal fixation failure.

6. What types of anterior spinal implants are used when arthrodesis is performed across the lumbosacral junction?

The most common anterior implants utilized when arthrodesis is performed across the lumbosacral junction are intracolumnar implants. These include structural bone graft (autograft or allograft) as well as fusion cages (e.g., titanium mesh, carbon fiber) used in combination with autograft, allograft, or bone morphogenetic protein. Extracolumnar implants are used less commonly than in other spinal regions because of the close proximity of vascular structures and the bony contour of the lumbosacral junction, which make implant placement difficult. Low-profile implants such as large diameter cancellous screws are useful to secure bone grafts between adjacent vertebral bodies.

7. What options are most commonly used for posterior implant fixation in the sacrum and pelvis when arthrodesis is performed across the lumbosacral motion segment?

- S1 pedicle screws: directed medially into the S1 pedicle and body
- S1 alar screws: directed laterally into the sacral ala at the level of S1
- S2 alar screws: directed laterally into the sacral ala at the level of S2
- Iliac fixation: rods or bolts are directed within the cortices of the ilium
- Intrasacral (Jackson) rods: a rod is directed within the sacral ala from proximal to distal

8. Describe the technique of S1 pedicle screw placement.

The dorsal bony cortex at the base of the superior S1 articular process is removed with a rongeur or burr. A pedicle probe is directed perpendicular to the sacrum and directed medially and angled toward the S1 endplate. Careful penetration of the anterior cortex of the sacrum permits bicortical screw purchase and increases screw purchase.

9. Describe the technique of laterally directed screw placement at the level of S1.

The screw entrance point is located just distal to the L5–S1 facet joint in line with the dorsal S1 neural foramen. A starting point is created with a burr or drill in this area. A probe is placed through the sacrum until it contacts the anterior sacral cortex. The desired trajectory is 35° laterally and parallel with the S1 endplate. Length of this pilot hole is determined with a depth gauge. The anterior sacral cortex is then perforated in a controlled fashion to achieve bicortical fixation.

10. What structures are at risk when a screw is placed through the anterior cortex of the sacrum?

Medially directed S1 screws which are directed parallel to the upper S1 endplate or toward the sacral promontory do not endanger any neurovascular structures with the exception of the middle sacral artery and vein. If a screw is inserted in a straightforward direction without medial angulation, the L5 nerve root is at risk of injury where it crosses the anterior sacrum. Screws placed laterally at the S1 level have a greater potential to injure critical structures including the lumbosacral trunk, internal iliac vein and sacroiliac joint.

11. When is it reasonable to perform a fusion across the sacrum with only bilateral S1 screw fixation?

Bilateral S1 screw fixation is effective for short segment instrumentation and fusion across the lumbosacral junction (i.e., L4 or L5 to sacrum). A typical instrumentation construct consists of bilateral lumbar pedicle screws at each proximal level undergoing fusion. Supplemental anterior structural grafts and/or cages are utilized to provide anterior column load sharing as needed.

12. List situations in which S1 screw fixation should be supplemented with additional fixation strategies.

Indications for use of S1 screw fixation combined with additional sacropelvic fixation include:

- Long-segment scoliosis fusions that extend to the sacrum(ex. neuromuscular scoliosis)
- For correction of pelvic obliquity
- Stabilization and/or reduction and fusion of high grade spondylolisthesis
- Lumbar revision surgery (e.g., osteotomy for lumbar flatback syndrome; decompression and fusion for degeneration, pain and stenosis below a long-segment fusion to L5)

13. Describe the technique for placement of iliac fixation.

A rongeur is used to remove bone from the region of the posterior superior iliac spine (PSIS) at the level of S2–S3. As the PSIS is the most prominent part of the posterior pelvis, the ilium in this region must be made level with the sacrum to prevent implant prominence (Fig. 1). A blunt probe is used to develop a channel for insertion of a screw or rod between the cortices of the iliac bone along a trajectory extending from the posterior superior iliac spine and passing above the greater sciatic notch toward the anterior inferior iliac spine. Typically an anchor of at least 80 mm in length can be safely placed in adult patients.

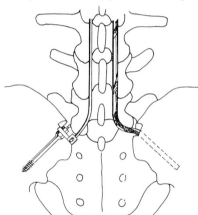

FIGURE 1. Iliac fixation. A rod is inserted on the right side and an iliac screw is inserted on the left side. (From Chewning SJ: Pelvic fixation. Spine State Art Rev 6:359–368, 1992, with permission.)

14. What risks may be associated with iliac fixation?

- Need for extensive surgical exposure which can be associated with increased bleeding and prolonged operative time
- Injury to surrounding neurovascular structures including the superior gluteal artery, sciatic nerve and cluneal nerves
- Potential for damage to the acetabulum or hip joint by misdirected anchor placement
- Implant prominence leading to the need to remove implants after fusion has occurred
- Sacroiliac pain

15. Describe the technique for placement of an intrasacral rod.

A rod is inserted into the lateral sacral mass through the canal of a previously placed S1 pedicle screw. The rod and screw interlock within the sacrum providing secure fixation. The implants are "buttressed" by the posterior ilium. Fixation provided by this technique is superior to fixation provided by S1 screws alone (Fig. 2).

16. What is transsacral fixation?

In cases of high grade isthmic spondylolisthesis (grades 3 and 4) screws and/or bone grafts may be placed across the L5–S1 disc space and obtain purchase in both the L5 and S1 vertebrae.

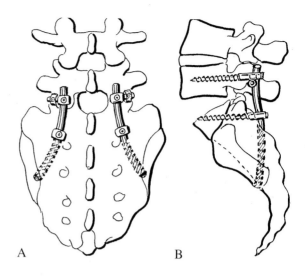

FIGURE 2. Anteroposterior (**A**) and lateral (**B**) views of the lumbosacral junction depicting an intrasacral rod construct. (From Margulies JY, Armour EF, Kohler-Ekstrand C: Revision of fusion from the spine to the sacropelvis: Considerations. In Margulies JY, Aebi M, Farcy JP (eds): Revision Spine Surgery. Mosby, St. Louis, 1999, pp 623–630, with permission.)

A   B

Traditionally a fibular graft is placed from either a posterior approach (from S1 to L5) or anterior approach (from L5 into S1). The addition of screw fixation from the upper sacrum across the L5–S1 disc space and into the L5 vertebral body increases the fusion rate and decreases the risk of graft fracture.

17. What is a sacral bar?

This type of fixation uses rod(s) that spans the sacrum passing from ilium to ilium. Initially sacral bars were used for fixation of sacral fractures. They have been modified to serve as an anchor within the pelvis to form the basis for complex reconstruction procedures involving fusion across the lumbosacral region (Fig. 3).

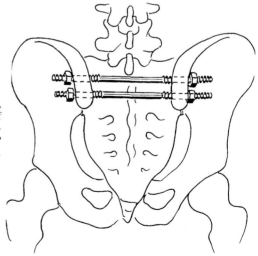

FIGURE 3. Sacral bars. (From Margulies JY, Armour EF, Kohler-Ekstrand C: Revision of fusion from the spine to the sacropelvis: Considerations. In Margulies JY, Aebi M, Farcy JP (eds): Revision Spine Surgery. Mosby, St. Louis, 1999, pp 623–630.)

18. What is a two-bolt iliac construct?

Fixation in the ilium has traditionally been inserted within the column of bone located immediately above the sciatic notch. Iliac fixation may also be inserted into the column of bone located immediately below the upper edge of the ilium. The combination of upper and lower iliac fixation creates a stable foundation permitting reconstruction of complex lumbosacral instabilities (e.g., after tumor resection) and is termed a two-bolt iliac construct (Fig. 4).

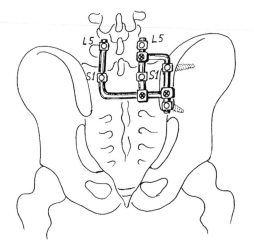

FIGURE 4. A foundation in the pelvis based on two L5 screws, two S1 screws and two unilateral iliac screws (two-bolt iliac construct) connected by longitudinal members. (From Margulies JY, Armour EF, Kohler-Ekstrand C. Revision of fusion from the spine to the sacropelvis: Considerations. In Margulies JY, Aebi M, Farcy JP (eds): Mosby, St. Louis, 1999, pp p623–630, with permission.)

19. What is meant by the lumbosacral pivot point in relation to the biomechanics of lumbosacral fixation?

The stability provided by sacropelvic fixation devices has been conceptualized in relation to a pivot point located at the posterior aspect of the L5–S1 disc (at the intersection of the middle osteoligamentous column and L5–S1 disc) (Fig. 5). S1 screw fixation provides the least resistance to counteract flexion moments around the pivot point compared with other sacropelvic fixation techniques. The addition of a second point of sacral fixation provides improved fixation compared to use of S1 fixation alone. However, iliac fixation provides the most stable method of sacropelvic fixation because it extends fixation for a greater distance anterior to the lumbosacral pivot point than any other technique.

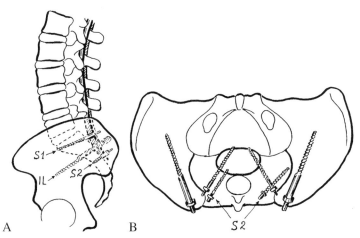

FIGURE 5. A, Lateral view of the lumbopelvic junction with S1 and S2 screws in the sacrum and iliac screws. **B,** Axial view of the pelvis with S1 screws, S2 screws in two variations, and iliac screws. (From Margulies JY, Armour EF, Kohler-Ekstrand C: Revision of fusion from the spine to the sacropelvis: Considerations. In Margulies JY, Aebi M, Farcy JP (eds): Revision Spine Surgery. Mosby, St. Louis, 1999, pp 623–630, with permission.)

20. What type of brace should be prescribed if the surgeon wishes to restrict motion across the lumbosacral junction?

The surgeon should prescribe a TLSO with a thigh cuff. Lumbar orthoses which do not immobilize the thigh increase rather than decrease motion across the L5–S1 level.

21. Summarize the techniques that a surgeon can use to increase the rate of successful fusion across the L5–S1 segment.

- Perform an L5–S1 interbody fusion with a structural spacer (e.g., allograft, autograft, fusion cage) to restore anterior column load sharing and increase likelihood of successful arthrodesis
- Use multiple fixation points within the sacropelvic unit (iliac fixation is the most stable type of fixation)
- Cross-link the longitudinal members in the region of the sacrum
- Use an appropriate orthosis to restrict lumbosacral motion

BIBLIOGRAPHY

1. Boachie-Adjei O, Dendrinos GK, Ogilvie JW, et al: Management of adult spinal deformity with combined anterior-posterior arthrodesis and Luque-Galveston instrumentation. J Spinal Disord 4:131–141, 1991.
2. Chewning SJ: Pelvic fixation. Spine State Art Rev 6:359–368, 1992.
3. Cunningham BW, Lewis SJ, Long J, et al: Biomechanical evaluation of lumbosacral reconstruction techniques for spondylolithesis. Spine 27:2321–2327, 2002.
4. Devlin VJ, Asher MA: Biomechanics and surgical principles of long fusions to the sacrum. Spine State Art Rev 10:515–529, 1996.
5. Jackson R, McManus A: The iliac buttress: a computed tomographic study of sacral anatomy. Spine 18:1318–1328, 1993.
6. Lebwohl NH, Cunningham BW, Dmitriev A, et al. Biomechanical comparison of lumbosacral fixation techniques in a calf spine model. Spine 27:2312–23270, 2002
7. Margulies JY, Floman Y, Farcy JP, Neuwirth MG (eds): Lumbosacral and Spinopelvic Fixation. Lippincott-Raven, Philadelphia, 1996.
8. Margulies JY, Armour EF, Kohler-Ekstrand C: Revision of fusion from the spine to the sacropelvis : Considerations. In Margulies JY, Aebi M, Farcy JP (eds): Revision Spine Surgery. Mosby, St. Louis, 1999, pp 623–630
9. McCord DH, Cunningham BW, Shono Y, et al: Biomechanical analysis of lumbosacral fixation. Spine 17:S235–S243, 1992.

31. INTRAOPERATIVE SPINAL MONITORING

Robin H. Vaughn, Ph.D., and Vincent J. Devlin, M.D.

1. What is intraoperative spinal monitoring?

Intraoperative spinal monitoring refers to the various techniques used to assess functional integrity of the nervous system during surgical procedures that place these structures at risk.

2. What criteria need to be met if intraoperative spinal monitoring is used during spinal surgery?

Three criteria need to be met if monitoring is used during spinal surgery:
1. Neurologic structures are at risk.
2. Those structures can be monitored reliably and efficiently by qualified personnel.
3. The surgeon is willing and able to alter surgical technique based on information provided.

3. List common types of spinal procedures during which monitoring is used.

- Correction of spinal deformities (scoliosis, kyphosis, spondylolisthesis)
- Insertion of spinal fixation devices (e.g., pedicle screw placement)
- Decompression at the level of the spinal cord
- Surgical treatment of spinal cord tumors

4. Which intraoperative personnel perform spinal monitoring? What are their qualifications?

A variety of personnel may provide spinal monitoring services, including:
- Certified neurophysiologic intraoperative monitoring technologist (CNIM): usually a registered electroencephalography (EEG) technologist who has completed a course of study, demonstrated competence in acquiring intraoperative data over a number of cases, and passed a nationally recognized technologist examination. No state license is available.
- Audiologist (CCC-A): certified audiologist with a minimum of a masters degree in audiology and related neurophysiology. Passing a nationally recognized audiology examination is required. There is no requirement to document surgical case experience or intraoperative skills. A license is available in most states.
- Neurophysiologist: noncertified neurophysiologist with a minimum of a masters degree and often a doctorate in neurophysiology or neurosciences. Demonstration of intraoperative monitoring proficiency is not required. No state license is available.
- Neurophysiologist D.ABNM: Neurophysiologist with a minimum of a masters and often a doctorate degree in audiology, neurophysiology, or neurosciences. Requirements include passing a written and oral nationally accredited board examination with a minimum of 300 documented monitored surgical cases. A state license is available only in audiology.
- Physician: usually a neurologist who may work with or without technicians. The physician is not required to pass any nationally recognized or accredited board examinations. A state license is available.

5. What neurologic structures are at risk during spinal procedures?

- Spinal cord and/or nerve roots at the surgical site
- Spinal cord and/or nerve roots remote from the surgical site (e.g., placed at risk of injury from positioning of extremities, head, or neck)
- Optic nerve

6. What mechanisms may be responsible for neurologic injury during spine procedures?

- Direct injury due to surgical trauma (e.g., during spinal canal decompression or placement of spinal implants)

- Traction and/or compression of neural structures during spinal realignment and deformity correction
- Ischemia resulting in decreased perfusion affecting the spinal cord and nerve roots over multiple levels (e.g., ligation of critical segmental vessels supplying the spinal cord, sustained hypotension resulting in ischemic injury to neurologic structures)
- Compressive neuropathy as a result of patient positioning during surgery

7. What is the rate of spinal cord injury associated with reconstructive surgical procedures performed for spinal deformities?

< 1%.

8. What is the rate of nerve root injury reported for complex spinal reconstructive procedures such as adult thoracolumbar scoliosis correction?

10%.

9. What techniques are available for monitoring spinal cord function?

- Stagnara wake-up test
- Somatosensory-evoked potentials (SEPs)
- Motor-evoked potentials (MEPs)
- Ankle clonus test

10. What is the technique of choice for monitoring nerve root function during spinal surgery?

Electromyographic (EMG) monitoring.

11. What is the Stagnara wake-up test?

The Stagnara wake-up test is used to assess the gross integrity of spinal cord motor tract function during spinal surgery. Discussing this test with the patient before surgery increases its success. During the procedure anesthesia is temporarily reduced to a degree where the patient is able to follow simple commands (move both hands and then both feet). Most patients have no recollection of being awakened, and those who recall do not report the experience to be unpleasant. This test does not provide information about spinal cord sensory tract function or individual nerve root function. In addition, it cannot be administered in a continuous fashion during surgery.

12. What are SEPs?

SEPs are a modification of the basic EEG in which a cortical or subcortical response to repetitive stimulation of a peripheral mixed nerve is recorded at sites cephalad and caudad to the operative field. Data including signal amplitude (height) and latency (time of occurrence) are recorded continuously during surgery and compared with baseline data. SEPs provide direct information about status of the spinal cord sensory tracts (located in the dorsal medial columns of the spinal cord). SEPs provide only indirect information about the status of the spinal cord motor tracts (located in the anterolateral columns of the spinal cord).

13. Discuss important limitations of SEPs.

SEPs directly assess spinal cord sensory tracts but provide only indirect information about motor tracts. Damage to the spinal cord motor tracts can occur without a concomitant change in SEPs. SEPs are better for detecting mechanical damage than ischemic damage to motor tracts because these cord regions have different blood supplies. The spinal cord motor tracts are supplied by the anterior spinal artery, whereas the spinal cord sensory tracts are perfused by radicular arteries. In addition, recording of SEPs is not a sensitive technique for monitoring individual nerve root function.

14. What factors other than neurologic injury can have an adverse effect on SEP recordings?

Operating room power equipment, halogenated anesthetic agents, hypothermia, and hypotension.

15. When is the best time to collect baseline SEP data during a spinal procedure?

The best time to collect baseline SEP data is after completion of the surgical exposure because this timing eliminates the variables of anesthetic level and patient core temperature.

16. When should the surgeon be notified about changes in SEPs?

The surgeon should be notified when SEPs show a 50–60% reduction from baseline amplitude or a 10% increase from baseline latency.

17. What protocol should be followed if SEP deterioration occurs during surgery?

The surgeon and anethesiologist should remain calm and communicate with the spinal monitoring personnel as the following steps are taken:

1. Check that the electrodes have not become displaced.
2. Increase the concentration of inspired oxygen.
3. Elevate the mean blood pressure.
4. Stop further inhalation anesthetic agents.
5. Discontinue spinal instrumentation including release of any distraction forces.
6. Irrigate the wound with warm saline.
7. Send an arterial blood gas to assess for an unrecognized metabolic abnormality or unrecognized low hemoglobin.
8. If SEPs fail to return, a wake-up test should be performed.
9. Depending on the patient's response to the wake-up test and the specific spinal problem requiring treatment, spinal instrumentation may require removal.
10. Use of steroids (spinal injury protocol) may be considered.

18. What are MEPs?

MEPs are electrical impulses measured in peripheral nerves and muscles in response to stimulation of the cerebral cortex or the spinal cord. These impulses travel through the corticospinal tracts. Changes in MEPs indicate possible disruption of motor pathways. The motor cortex may be stimulated by electrical or magnetic means. The spinal cord is stimulated by electrical means using percutaneous-percutaneous electrodes, nasopharyngeal electrodes, or transcranial electrodes. MEPs can be recorded either from a peripheral mixed nerve (NMEP) or directly from muscle (MEP-EMG).

19. What is the advantage of using MEPs?

MEPs can provide information about the functional integrity of the spinal cord motor tracts that cannot be obtained using SEPs. In many institutions, MEPs are used in combination with SEPs to provide a direct measure of both spinal cord sensory and motor tract function, thereby increasing the efficacy of spinal monitoring.

20. What is the role of EMG monitoring during spinal procedures?

EMG is used to assess the functional integrity of individual nerve roots. EMG techniques are classified into two categories based on method of elicitation: mechanical and electrical. Mechanically elicited EMGs are used during the dynamic phases of surgery (pedicle screw preparation and insertion, nerve root manipulation). Electrically elicited EMGs should be used during the static phases of surgery (immediately before or after pedicle screw placement).

21. How does a surgeon use EMG to check that screws have been properly placed within the lumbar pedicles?

The surgeon places an EMG probe onto the pedicle screw and electrically stimulates the screw. If the pedicle wall is intact, the passage of electrical current will be restricted and the adjacent nerve root will not be stimulated. If the pedicle wall has been fractured, current passes through the pedicle wall and stimulates the adjacent nerve root. This results in contraction of the associated peripheral muscle, which is recorded as an EMG. Electrical thresholds for EMG activity consistent with safe screw placement have been determined and provide a reference for clinical practice.

22. What is the difference between *burst* and *train* EMG?

Burst EMG activity is indicative of a nerve root being mechanically irritated resulting in a brief burst of muscle activity of a few seconds' duration. Multiple irritations or insults result in the muscle going into spasm, which is termed train. **Train EMG** activity is consistent with nerve root injury and must be dealt with immediately because it often predicts postoperative motor nerve deficit.

23. How is intraoperative spinal monitoring used to prevent neurologic injury secondary to patient positioning?

Paraplegia or quadriplegia may result from hyperextension positioning of the stenotic cervical or lumbar spine. Spinal monitoring of both upper and lower extermity neurologic function can permit prompt recognition and repositioning, thereby preventing permanent neurologic deficit. Monitoring of ulnar nerve SEPs is performed to assess possible brachial plexopathy due to changes in arm positioning. During anterior procedures, monitoring of peroneal nerve and femoral nerve function is performed. Peroneal nerve monitoring can alert staff to the onset of an impending peroneal nerve palsy secondary to pressure of the leg against the operating room table. A permanent injury can be averted by moving the patient's leg or adjusting the padding. Monitoring of femoral nerve function can alert the surgeon to excessive traction on the iliopsoas muscle and the adjacent nerve roots during an anterior procedure and prevent femoral nerve injury.

24. What is the ankle clonus test?

Ankle clonus is the rhythmic contraction of the calf muscles following sudden passive dorsiflexion of the foot. Clonus is produced by elicitation to the stretch reflex. In the normal awake person, clonus cannot be elicited because of central inhibition of this stretch reflex. The clonus test relies on the presence of central inhibition and clonus to confirm that the spinal cord and peripheral neurologic structures are functionally intact. Neurologically intact patients emerging from general anesthesia normally have temporary ankle clonus bilaterally. Absence of transient ankle clonus has been correlated with neurologic compromise.

25. Is any technique available for monitoring optic nerve function during spinal surgery?

No. Ischemic optic neuropathy has been reported in association with spinal procedures performed in the prone position. Increased intraocular perfusion pressure causes decreased ocular perfusion with resultant visual loss. There is no known effective treatment for this complication.

26. A 50-year-old woman is undergoing surgical treatment for adult scoliosis consisting of multilevel anterior discetomies and fusion followed by posterior spinal instrumentation (pedicle screws) and fusion. What intraoperative spinal monitoring techniques are indicated for this type of surgical procedure?

The goal of intraoperative monitoring is to detect the onset of a surgically induced neurologic injury and permit timely intervention to prevent permanent neurologic injury. No single spinal monitoring technique can achieve this goal. A combination monitoring procedures is required. A combination of SEPs and MEPs is required to optimally assess spinal cord function. EMG techniques are required to assess nerve root function. A Stagnara wake-up test can be performed if significant deterioration of SEPs and/or MEPs occurs during surgery. A clonus test may be performed as an additional confirmatory test to document intact spinal cord function.

BIBLIOGRAPHY

1. Bridwell KH, Lenke LG, Baldus C, et al: Major intraoperative neurologic deficits in pediatric and adult spinal deformity patients: Incidence and etiology at one institution. Orthop Trans 21:109–115, 1997.
2. Gugino LD, Aglio LS, Segal ME, et al: Use of transcranial magnetic stimulation for monitoring spinal cord motor paths. Semin Spine Surg 9:315–336, 1997.

 3. Hoppenfeld S, Gross A, Lonner B: The ankle clonus test for assessment of the integrity of the spinal cord during operations for scoliosis. J Bone Joint Surg 79A:208–212, 1997.
 4. Owen JH: Monitoring during surgery for spinal deformities. In Bridwell KH, DeWald RL (eds): The Textbook of Spinal Surgery, 2nd ed. Philadelphia, Lippincott-Raven, 1997, pp 39–60.
 5. Owen JH. The application of intraoperative monitoring during surgery for spinal deformity. Spine 24: 2649–2662, 1999.
 6. Owen JH: Cost efficacy of intraoperative monitoring. Semin Spine Surg 9:348–352, 1997.
 7. Padberg AM, Komanetsky RE, Bridwell KH, et al: Neurogenic motor evoked potentials: A prospective comparison of stimulation methods. J Spinal Disord 11:21–24, 1997.
 8. Sloan TB: Anesthesia during spinal surgery with electrophysiological monitoring. Semin Spine Surg 9: 302–308, 1997.
 9. Vauzelle C, Stagnara P, Jouvinroux P: Functional monitoring of spinal cord activity during spinal surgery. Clin Orthop 93:173–178, 1973.

32. ANESTHESIA AND RELATED INTRAOPERATIVE CONSIDERATIONS IN SPINE SURGERY

Ashit C. Patel, M.D., William O. Shaffer, M.D., and Vincent J. Devlin, M.D.

1. What are the top ten areas of concern in relation to perioperative anesthesia care for spinal surgery patients?
1. Assessment of patient-specific risk factors
2. Assessment of procedure-specific risk factors
3. Airway management
4. Maintenance of normothermia
5. Invasive monitoring requirements
6. Fluid management (crystalloid, colloid, transfusion, autotransfusion)
7. Neurologic monitoring
8. Intraoperative positioning
9. Preparation for intraoperative disasters
10. Postoperative assessment and coordination of postoperative care

2. What patient-specific risk factors are emphasized during the preoperative anesthetic evaluation?

Cardiac. Pediatric patients have a low incidence of coronary diseases unless neuromuscular disease is present. In adult patients, cardiac assessment is crucial and is based on cardiac risk factors and cardiac symptoms.

Pulmonary. Restrictive lung disease may be present in patients with thoracic scoliosis or spinal deformities secondary to neuromuscular disease. Smoking, chronic obstructive pulmonary disease and asthma are additional factors that influence perioperative management.

Hemostasis. A history of abnormal bruising or bleeding should be investigated. Nonsteroidal anti-inflammatory medication and aspirin should be discontinued at least 2 weeks before surgery. A laboratory coagulation profile is advised before surgery.

Neurologic. Important concerns include the presence/absence of neurologic deficit, stability of the cervical spine as it influences intubation technique, and possible need for an intraoperative wake-up test.

3. What patient populations are at increased risk of latex allergy?

Patient populations with an increased risk of latex allergy include patients with myelodysplasia, congenital genitourinary tract abnormalities, spinal cord injuries, cerebral palsy, ventriculoperitoneal shunts, and health care workers. Anaphylaxis may occur intraoperatively, and latex allergy must be included in the differential diagnosis of intraoperative emergenies. A detailed history is the best means of detecting patients at risk. Patients with a history of latex allergy are treated with premedication (diphenhydramine, ranitidine, predinisone). A latex-free environment is provided in the operating room.

4. How do anesthesiologists estimate anesthetic risk and anticipate outcome associated with surgery?

Anesthesiologists perform a preanesthetic assessment and assign an American Society of Anesthesiologist (ASA) physical classification:

CLASS	DESCRIPTION
1	Normal, healthy patient
2	Patient with mild systemic disease
3	Patient with severe systemic disease that limits activity but is not incapacitating
4	Patient with an incapacitating disease that is a constant threat to life
5	Moribund patient who is not expected to survive 24 hours with or without surgery
E	Patient undergoing an emergency procedure

5. What types of spinal procedures are associated with an increased risk of complications and perioperative morbidity?
- Revision spinal deformity procedures
- Same-day multilevel anterior-posterior spinal procedures
- Multilevel anterior spinal fusions
- Fusions for spinal deformities in patients with neuromuscular scoliosis
- Emergent procedures for tumor, infection, and trauma

6. When is fiberoptic intubation the preferred method for intubation?
Patients with an unstable cervical spine (e.g., fracture, rheumatoid arthritis, odontoid hypoplasia) or severe cervical stenosis are best managed with fiberoptic intubation.

7. What types of spinal procedures require placement of a double-lumen endotracheal tube?
Thoracic spine procedures performed with the assistance of thoracosopy require endobronchial intubation and single-lung ventilation to maintain a safe working space within the thoracic cavity. Anterior thoracic spine procedures performed through an open thoracotomy approach for exposure of the spine above the level of T8 also benefit from single-lung ventilation. Single-lung ventilation decreases the difficulty of retracting the lung from the operative field in the upper thoracic region. For open procedures below the T8 level, the lung can more easily be retracted out of the operative field without the need for single-lung ventilation.

8. What complications have been reported in association with hypothermia during surgery?
Complications reported in association with intraoperative hypothermia (core temperature $< 35.5°$ C) include myocardial depression, cardiac arrhythmias, thrombocytopenia, decreased mobilization of calcium, prolongation of drug half-lives, and lactic acidosis.

9. What steps can be taken to prevent hypothermia during spine surgery?
- Use of forced-air warming systems
- Use of fluid warmers
- Use of humidified, warmed (40°C) inspired gases
- Use of warm lavage for wound irrigation
- Warming of the operating room

10. What are the requirements for hemodynamic monitoring during spinal procedures?
The minimum requirements for major spine procedures include two large-bore peripheral intravenous lines and intra-arterial blood pressure monitoring. Central venous pressure monitoring is considered when:
- Expected intraoperative blood loss is expected to exceed 50% of blood volume
- Major fluid shifts are anticipated
- Preoperative asssessment suggests that traditional signs of fluid management will be difficult to assess
- Special intraoperative management is planned (e.g., hypotension, hemodilution)

11. What is the best way to monitor fluid administration during major spinal reconstructive procedures?

Careful fluid calcuations and hourly recording of estimated blood loss are the most effective method to monitor fluid administration. Fluid replacement calculations must account for deficit, maintenance, third-space loss, and blood loss. Initially crystalloid solution is administered. Administration of colloid solution (e.g., 5% albumin or 6% hetastarch) or blood should be considered for surgery exceeding 4 hours or blood loss exceeding 25% of blood volume. There is no universally accepted threshold at which to transfuse blood. Factors to consider include patient age, concomitant disease, and concern about perfusion of the optic nerve. Because deliberate hypotensive anesthesia decreases renal blood flow and glomerular filtration rate, urine output does not accurately reflect the patient's level of hydration. Monitoring of central venous pressure combined with heart rate and direct arterial pressure can provide additional valuable information regarding hemodynamics.

12. What methods can be used to reduce allogeneic blood transfusion during spine surgery?
- Preoperative autologous blood donation
- Preoperative marrow stimulation (erythropoietin)
- Acute normovolemic hemodilution
- Intraoperative salvage (use of cell saver)
- Hypotensive anesthesia technique
- Accepting a lower threshold (hemoglobin = 9, hematocrit = 27) before transfusion

13. What problems are associated with use of a cell saver?
- Improper suctioning technique can lead to hemolysis
- Coagulopathy (loss of fibrinogen and platelets in salvaged blood)
- Potentially toxic materials may be infused to the patient (e.g., thrombin)
- Pulmonary complications due to tissue debris that accompanies washed cells
- Hemoglobinuria
- Inability to remove cancer cells and bacteria

14. How does hypotensive anesthesia help control hemorrhage?

Hypotensive anesthesia involves the deliberate reduction of blood pressure using pharmacologic agents (e.g., sodium nitroprusside) to limit blood loss during spinal surgery. As a result, hemorrhage associated with exposure of the spine and decortication of bone is decreased. Epidural bleeding points can be more easily identified and controlled. The mean blood pressure must be such that tissue perfusion in vital tissue sites away from the field is maintained.

15. List contraindications to the use of hypotensive anesthesia.
- Severe cardiac disease
- Arteriosclerosis
- Visceral or kidney disease
- Significant hypertension
- Pulmonary insufficiency
- Glaucoma
- Incomplete spinal cord injury (due to potential for neurologic deterioration as a result of decreased perfusion of neural structures)

16. What are the options for monitoring neurologic function during spinal procedures?

A variety of methods are used to monitor neurologic function during spinal surgery including:
- Somatosensory-evoked potentials (SEPs)
- Motor-evoked potentials (MEPs)
- Electromyography (EMG)
- Stagnara wake-up test
- Ankle clonus test

17. What are the anesthesia requirements for the different spinal monitoring techniques?

During the course of a spinal procedure, a variety of spinal monitoring techniques may be used to assess different components of the nervous system (e.g., spinal cord sensory tracts, spinal cord motor tracts, nerve roots). Anesthesia techniques and spinal monitoring techniques require coordination at different stages throughout the procedure.

- Stagnara wake-up test requires use of short-acting anesthetic agents (e.g., nitrous oxide, propofol) or agents that can be quickly reversed (e.g., opiods, benzodiazepines).
- SEPs. The most common anesthetic technique used in conjunction with SEPs involves low dose inhalation agents in combination with intravenous infusion of sedative agents and analgesics. Muscle relaxation has no direct deleterious effect on SEPs.
- MEPs. The anesthetic technique must be modified based on the type of MEP used (e.g., stimulation of motor cortex vs. spinal cord, electrical vs. magnetic stimulation).
- EMG. The level of muscle relaxation must be maintained at 2–3 twitches out of a train of four. If the level of relaxation is too great, the sensitivity of EMG to nerve root compromise is reduced.

18. What difficulties have been reported in association with use of the Stagnara intraoperative wake up test?

- Extubation secondary to patient movement
- Dislodgement of intravenous access
- Air embolus
- Dislodgement of spinal implants
- Difficulty using the test in patients with reduced capacity (e.g., mental retardation, deafness, language barrier)
- Contamination of the surgical field

19. List important considerations in positioning patients for a spinal procedure in the prone position.

Most patients readily tolerate spine surgery in the prone position. Important considerations include:

- The head should be kept at or slightly above the level of the heart to maintain brain perfusion. The head-down postion should be avoided because it decreases intraocular perfusion pressure.
- Cushioning should be placed beneath the forehead and chin, to keep the eyes, chin, and face free of pressure.
- The upper extremities should be positioned with the shoulders below 90° of abduction.
- Padding should be placed beneath the elbow to protect the ulnar nerve from compression.
- The abdomen should be free of compression to reduce venous backflow through Batson's plexus into the spinal canal.
- The breast, chest, and iliac areas should be adequately padded to prevent compression injury.
- If the surgical procedure involves lumbar fusion, the hips should be extended to create a lordotic alignment of the lumbar spinal segments.
- Male genitalia should be free of compression.
- Sequential compression stockings should be placed to prevent venous pooling in the lower extremities.
- The Foley catheter should be secured to prevent dislodgement.

20. List important considerations in positioning a patient for a spinal procedure in the lateral decubitus position.

The lateral decubitus position is commonly used for surgical procedures involving the anterior aspect of the thoracic and lumbar spine. Important considerations include:

- Neutral alignment of the head and cervical spine
- Protection of the dependent eye and ear from pressure
- Placement of an axillary roll to relieve pressure on the dependent shoulder and prevent compression of the neurovascular bundle by the humeral head
- Protection of the peroneal nerve in the dependent leg with a pillow
- Placement of a pillow between the legs to prevent pressure from bony prominences
- Sequential compression stockings to prevent venous pooling in the lower extremities

21. What are the major concerns when the kneeling or tuck position is used for spinal procedures?

The extreme degree of hip and knee flexion required to achieve this position is not feasible for many patients, especially those with total joint replacements. This position can significantly compromise perfusion to the lower extremities, resulting in ischemia, thrombosis, compartment syndrome, and neurologic deficits. This position is not commonly used. Its use should be restricted to shorter spinal procedures such as lumbar discectomy.

22. What are the major concerns with use of the sitting position for spinal procedures?

The sitting position is preferred by some surgeons for procedures involving the posterior cervical spine. The major advantage of this position is reduced blood pooling in the surgical field and potentially reduced blood loss because of improved venous drainage. The airway is easily accessible, and optimal ventilation of lungs is facilitated. The disadvantages include systemic hypotension and the creation of a negative pressure gradient that may result in air entrainment and venous air embolus (VAE). Careful management and monitoring are essential to prevent serious complications associated with this operative position. Prior hydration and gradual transfer to the sitting position avoid undue systemic hypotension. Insertion of a central venous pressure catheter is recommended to monitor intravascular pressure, confirm the diagnosis of air embolism, and potentially retrieve air in the event that a large embolus obstructs cardiac outflow. A precordial Doppler placed on the right chest is a sensitive marker for sounds of air embolus.

23. What intraoperative disasters can occur during spinal procedures?

- Excessive bleeding
- Disseminated intravascular coagulation (DIC)
- Malignant hyperthermia
- Deterioration in neurologic status
- Air embolus
- Tension pneumothorax

24. What is DIC?

DIC is the intravascular consumption of coagulation factors and platelets that leads to diffuse and excessive hemorrhage. Normally tissue injury initiates hemostasis and results in the formation of thrombus. In DIC the inciting factors render the local control mechanisms inadequate, and intravascular clot formation is precipitated. The conversion of plasminogen to plasmin triggers the fibrinolytic mechanism, resulting in diffuse hemorrhage. Subsequent renal failure, liver dysfunction, respiratory distress, shock, and thromboembolic phenomenon can lead to multisystem failure and death.

25. How is DIC diagnosed?

If the surgeon encounters diffuse, excessive hemorrhage during surgery, a coagulation panel should be drawn. Platelets levels below 100,000/mm^3, fibrinogen levels below 100 mg/mm^3, and fibrin split products (FSP) levels above 40 gm/ml define DIC. Treatment is immediate transfusion of fresh frozen plasma (contains 10,000 platelets/ml) fibrinogen, and other coagulation factors. Platelet packs should be transfused as well.

26. What factors may contribute to the development of DIC during spine surgery?

- Blood transfusion (transfusion reaction)
- Massive tissue destruction (extensive dissection, combined front back procedures)
- Sepsis
- Hypotension (unplanned and uncontrolled)
- Preexisting medical conditions (cancer, leukemia)

27. Define air embolus.

VAE has been reported in association with spinal surgery in the prone or sitting position. Air may enter the venous system during spine surgery as multiple venous channels remain open above the level of the heart. VAE may occur if the venous pressure at the level of the wound is less than the surrounding atmospheric pressure. Turbulence on the Doppler monitor and sudden decrease in the end-tidal carbon dioxide, followed by compromise of vital signs, suggest VAE. If air continues to enter, hypotension, arrhythmias, hypoxemia, and cardiac arrest may occur. Treatment consists of discontinuing nitrous oxide from the gas mixture and flooding the wound with saline to prevent further air entrainment. If the patient is in the sitting position, the head of the table should be lowered to allow the patient to be placed in the supine position.

28. What is malignant hyperthermia (MH)?

MH is an uncommon inherited disorder of skeletal muscle characterized by a hypermetabolic response of skeletal muscle to anesthetic agents (primarily halogenated agents and depolarizing muscle relaxants). An important pathophysiologic process in this disorder is intracellular hypercalcemia. Intracellular hypercalcemia activates metabolic pathways that, if left untreated, result in depletion of adenosine triphosphate, high temperature, acidosis, and cell death. No simple preoperative diagnostic test is available. Disorders associated with MH include myopathies (e.g., central core disease), Duchenne muscular dystrophy, and osteogenesis imperfecta.

29. How is MH diagnosed and treated?

Hypercarbia may be an early sign. Other signs include tachypnea, tachycardia, muscle rigidity, increased temperature, and decreased oxygen saturation. The following steps should be taken immediately when MH is diagnosed:

1. Discontinue inhalation agents and succinylcholine.
2. Conclude surgery.
3. Hyperventilate with 100% oxygen.
4. Administer dantrolene intravenously at 2.5 mg/kg.
5. Titrate dantrolene and bicarbonate to heart rate, body temperature, and $PaCO_2$.
6. If significant metabolic acidosis is present, administer 2–4 mEq/kg bicarbonate.
7. Change the anesthesia circuit.
8. Treat arrhythmias with procainamide. (Avoid calcium channel blockers because they may induce hyperkalemia in the presence of dantrolene.)
9. Elevation of body temperature should be managed with external ice packs in addition to gastric, wound, and rectal lavage.
10. Administer fluid and diuretics to maintain urine output.
11. Transfer patient to an intensive care setting.

BIBLIOGRAPHY

1. American Society of Anesthesiologists: New classification of physical status. Anesthesiology 24: 111, 1963.
2. Cotter TP, Goelzer SL: Anesthesia in cervical spine surgery. In White AH, Shofferman JA (eds): Spine Care—Operative Treatment. Mosby, St. Louis, 1995, pp 939–949.
3. Faciszewski T, Winter RB, Lonstein JE, et al: The surgical and medical perioperative complications of anterior spinal fusion surgery in the thoracic and lumbar spine in adults. A review of 1223 procedures. Spine 20:1592–1599, 1995.
4. Murray DJ, Forbes RB: Anesthetic considerations. In Weinstein SL (ed): Pediatric Spine Surgery, 2nd ed. Philadelphia, Lippincott Williams & Wilkins, 2001 pp 3–32.
5. Nielsen CH. Preoperative and postoperative anesthetic considerations for the spinal surgery patient. In Bridwell KH, DeWald RL (eds): The Textbook of Spinal Surgery. Philadelphia, Lippincott-Raven, 1997, pp 31–38.
6. Rose SH, Elliott BA, Horlocker TT: Anesthesia, positioning, and postoperative pain management for spine surgery. In The Adult Spine: Principles and Practice, 2nd ed. Philadelphia, Lippincott-Raven, 1997, pp 703–718.
7. Stevens WR, Glazer PA, Kelley SD, et al: Opthalmic complications after spinal surgery. Spine 22:1319–1324, 1997.
8. Tosi LL, Slater JE, Shaer C, et al: Latex allergy in spina bifida patients: Prevalence and surgical implications. J Pediatr Orthop 13:709–712, 1993.

33. POSTOPERATIVE MANAGEMENT AND COMPLICATIONS AFTER SPINE SURGERY

John M. Gorup, M.D., Vincent J. Devlin, M.D., and William O. Shaffer, M.D.

1. What types of complications may present in the early postoperative period after spinal procedures?

The spectrum of spine procedures ranges from outpatient lumbar discectomy to complex anterior and posterior multilevel fusion procedures. Health care providers must be knowledgeable about the following:

- Procedure-specific complications (e.g., problems related to surgical approach or spinal implants)
- General postsurgical complications (may involve the neurologic, pulmonary, cardiovascular, and gastrointestinal systems. Nutritional and pain control issues are additional important considerations.)

2. List potential causes of neurologic deficits diagnosed after spine procedures.

- Direct intraoperative neural trauma (e.g., during decompression procedures, as a result of neural impingement by spinal implants)
- Spinal deformity correction (e.g., L5 root injury during spondylolisthesis reduction)
- Acute vascular etiology (e.g., intraoperative hypotension, disruption of crucial segmental vessels supplying the spinal cord during anterior surgical approaches)
- Subacute vascular etiology (neurologic deterioration has been reported to develop 24–96 hours after spinal deformity surgery and has been attributed to a vascular etiology)
- Patient positioning during surgery (e.g., brachial plexopathy, compressive neuropathy involving the peroneal nerve)
- Postoperative bleeding with resultant epidural hematoma and neural compression

3. What are the components of neurologic assessment after spinal surgery?

Initial neurologic assessment after spine surgery should include assessment of upper and lower extremity neurologic function (motor strength, sensation). Neurologic examination should be performed every 2 hours for the first 24 hours, every 4 hours for the next 48 hours, and then once a shift until discharge. The onset of neurologic deterioration has been documented 96 hours after a surgical procedure in patients who were initially thought to be neurologically stable.

4. Describe the clinical presentation of a postoperative epidural hematoma.

Epidural hemorrhage involving the cervical or thoracic region compresses the spinal cord and typically produces an acute, painful myelopathy. Epidural hematoma involving the lumbosacral region typically presents as cauda equina syndrome. Causes include persistent postoperative hemorrhage, coagulopathy-induced bleeding, and spinal cord malformations. Treatment is emergent spinal decompression.

5. What is cauda equina syndrome?

Cauda equina syndrome is a complex of low back pain, bilateral lower extremity pain and/or weakness, saddle anesthesia, and varying degrees of bowel and/or bladder dysfunction. Treatment is prompt surgical decompression. Neurologic assessment must include evaluation of bowel and bladder function in the postoperative period to permit prompt recognition of this syndrome. Inadequate decompression of lumbar spinal stenosis is a risk factor for development of cauda equina syndrome in the postoperative period.

6. After an uneventful posterior spinal instrumentation procedure for idiopathic scoliosis in a teenage patient, unilateral anterior thigh numbness and discomfort are noted. What is the most common cause of this problem?

Pressure injury to anterior femoral cutaneous nerve secondary to intraoperative positioning. If there is no associated motor deficit and the sensory exam confirms a deficit limited to the distribution of the anterior femoral cutaneous nerve, the diagnosis is confirmed. The prognosis for recovery is good.

7. An adult patient with grade 1 L5–S1 isthmic spondylolisthesis undergoes L5–S1 posterior spinal instrumentation (pedicle fixation), decompression, and fusion. Before surgery the patient experienced only right leg symptoms. After surgery the patient reports relief of right leg pain but has a new left L5 radiculopathy that was not present before surgery. What are the likely causes?

A problem related to the left L5 pedicle screw with resultant neural impingement must be ruled out. Radiographs can be helpful in ruling out gross screw misplacement. However, a CT scan is the best test because it can provide an axial view and depict the exact screw location in relation to the L5 nerve root. Other potential causes for new-onset left leg pain include intraoperative nerve root injury, inadequate L5 nerve root decompression, L5–S1 disc herniation, and postoperative hematoma.

8. What is the incidence of ophthalmic complications after spinal surgery? What are the risk factors?

The incidence of significant visual complications after spine surgery is on the order of 1 case per 100 spine surgeons per year. Risk factors include smoking, hypertension, diabetes, vascular disease, intraoperative hypotension, and blood loss > 5 liters. The cause is multifactorial. Increased intraocular pressure associated with the prone position is considered to be the critical factor. An eye check should be included in the postoperative neurologic assessment. Symptoms or abnormal exam findings should prompt an opthamology consultation.

9. What pulmonary complications may occur after spine procedures?

Atelectasis, pneumonia, pleural effusion, pneumothroax, acute respiratory distress syndrome, pulmonary thromboembolism, and respiratory failure.

10. What factors are associated with an increased risk of pulmonary complications after spine surgery?

Pulmonary complications are frequently noted in patients with nonidiopathic scoliosis, mental retardation, advanced age, and chronic obstructive pulmonary disease. Patients undergoing anterior thoracic spine procedures and combined anterior and posterior spinal procedures associated with large blood loss and fluid shifts have an increased risk of postoperative pulmonary problems. Anterior cervical surgery, especially multilevel corpectomies, is associated with an increased risk of postoperative upper airway obstruction. Overnight intubation should be considered for high-risk patients.

11. Can hemothrorax or pneumothorax occur during or after posterior spinal procedures?

Yes. During posterior surgical procedures, the chest cavity may be entered inadvertently if dissection is carried too deeply between the transverse processes. This complication should be considered when a thoracoplasty is performed to decrease rib prominence as part of a posterior procedure for scoliosis. A tension pneumothorax may result from respirator malfunction or rupture of a pulmonary bleb. Insertion of a central venous pressure (CVP) line in the operating room may result in a pneumothorax that is not diagnosed before beginning the surgical procedure. Prompt diagnosis and chest tube insertion are required.

12. After an anterior thoracic fusion performed through an open thoracotomy approach, a patient has persistent high chest tube outputs after the fourth postoperative day. The fluid has a milky color. What diagnosis should be suspected?

Chylothorax. Injury to the thoracic duct or its tributaries may not be recognized intraoperatively and lead to leakage from the lymphatic system into the thoracic cavity. Treatment consists of continued chest tube drainage and decreasing the patient's fat intake. Hyperalimentation is of benefit during this period. Failure of these measures may require surgical exploration and repair of the lymphatic ductal injury.

13. What is acute respiratory distress syndrome (ARDS)?

ARDS results from diffuse, multilobar capillary transudation of fluid into the pulmonary interstitium, which dissociates the normal relationship of alveolar ventilation with lung perfusion. Persistent perfusion of poorly ventilated lung regions creates a shunt that results in hypoxia. ARDS has many causes, including fluid overload, massive transfusion, sepsis, malnutrition, and cardiac failure. Typically ARDS presents several days after surgery with fever, respiratory distress, reduced arterial oxygen, and diffuse bilateral infiltrates on chest radiographs. Treatment includes ventilator support with positive end-expiratory pressure (PEEP) to promote ventilation of previously trapped alveoli and minimize shunting.

14. When should a chest tube be removed after an uncomplicated anterior thoracic spinal procedure?

A chest tube is generally left in place for 48–72 hours after an anterior thoracic spinal procedure. No universal criteria define when a chest tube should be removed after anterior thoracic spine surgery. Unlike cardiac and pulmonary surgical procedures, anterior spinal procedures disrupt bony anatomy and stimulate a fracture-healing response with formation of serous fluid. This serous fluid can be absorbed by the pleura. Recommended criteria for chest tube removal range from 30–100 ml chest tube output in an 8-hour observation period. In addition, chest tube removal is generally deferred until the patient has been extubated after surgery.

15. Are deep vein thrombosis and pulmonary embolism significant problems after spine procedures?

Yes. The exact rate of these complications is difficult to define and ranges from 0.9% to 14%, depending on the patient population and type of spinal procedure. The application of sequential pneumatic compression stockings to the lower extremities before, during, and after surgery has been shown to reduce the rate of deep vein thrombosis. The use of pharmacologic agents for anticoagulation is not routine because of potential complications of epidural bleeding, cauda equina syndrome, and wound hematoma. Patients at increased risk of deep vein thrombosis (e.g., prolonged immobility, paralysis, prior venous thromboembolism, cancer, obesity, staged adult scoliosis procedures) can be considered for additional preventive measures, including prophylactic placement of a vena cava filter or serial postoperative screening (e.g., duplex ultrasonography). The use of pharmacologic agents can be considered for prophylaxis in specific high-risk cases on an individual basis.

16. You are called to assess a 49-year-old man in the recovery room immediately after an anterior L4–S1 fusion performed via a left retroperitoneal approach. The nurse reports that the left leg is cooler than the right leg. The patient reports severe left leg pain. What test should be ordered?

An emergent arteriogram and a vascular surgery consultation are indicated. The scenario is consistent with a vascular injury. The temperature change should not be attributed to the sympathectomy effect that is routinely noted following anterior lumbar surgery (in which increased temperature is noted on the side of the exposure).

17. A healthy 40-year-old woman underwent a 12-hour revision procedure consisting of anterior T10–sacrum fusion and posterior spinal instrumentation and fusion from T2 to pelvis. Blood loss was 5000 ml, and the patient received 6 units of packed red cells, 2 units of fresh frozen plasma, and 12 liters of crystalloid in the operating room. During the first 2 hours after surgery, this 60-kg patient had a urine output of 30 cc and CVP = 2. What is the problem?

Hypovolemia. Decreased urine output in this otherwise healthy patient is a sign of fluid volume deficit due to third spacing as fluid volume is pulled out of the vascular space into the interstitial space. Complete blood count (CBC), platelet count, electrolyte panel, coagulation profile, and ionized calcium levels should be checked immediately. Tranfusion of packed cells, fresh frozen plasma, platelets, and additional crystalloid should be administered based on these results. Cardiovascular status should be monitored with serial assessment of blood pressure, heart rate, urine output, and CVP measurements.

18. Describe the pathophysiology of the syndrome of inappropriate antidiuretic hormone secretion (SIADH). What are the diagnostic findings and treatment?

SIADH results in the retention of water by the body, causing serum hypoosmolality and urine hyperosmolality. Serum sodium is less than 130 mEq/L, serum osmolality is less than 275 mOsm/L, and urine sodium is greater than 50 mEq/L. Treatment is fluid restriction; if fluid must be given, it should be isotonic. In patients with SIADH, urine output generally returns to normal by the third postoperative day. There is approximately a 7% incidence of SIADH after spinal surgery. This condition must be differentiated from decreased urine output as a result of hypovolemia because the treatment for hypovolemia is fluid replacement. Decreased urine output due to hypovolemia is distinguished from SIADH since both urine and serum hyperosmolality are noted in the presence of hypovolemia.

19. What is the most common gastrointestinal problem after spinal surgery? What are the causes?

Ileus. Common causes include general anesthesia, prolonged use of narcotics, immobility after surgery, and significant manipulation of intestinal contents during anterior surgical procedures. Clinical findings include abdominal distention, abdominal cramping/discomfort, and pain. Diet restriction is the initial treatment. Nasogastric suction is instituted as needed for symptomatic relief.

20. What is Ogilvie's syndrome?

Acute massive dilation of the cecum and ascending and transverse colon in the absence of organic obstruction is termed Ogilvie's syndrome. Patients present with normal small bowel sounds and a colonic ileus. It is a dangerous entity that can result in cecal dilation and rupture. Death has been reported. The incidence appears to be increasing and may be related to use of patient-controlled analgesia (PCA). Diagnosis is made with an upright kidney-ureters-bladder (KUB) radiograph. Treatment consists of decompressing the colon with a rectal tube, colonoscopy, and, in some cases, cecostomy.

21. When should a patient be started on a diet after a spine fusion?

An abdominal assessment should be performed. The patient should have bowel sounds and should not be vomiting. After bowel patency has been confirmed, the patient may be given ice chips. If they are tolerated, the patient may progress to a clear liquid diet. This intake routine should be observed for 24 hours before advancing to a regular diet.

22. Define superior mesenteric artery syndrome.

This syndrome refers to bowel obstruction in the region where the superior mesenteric artery crosses over the third portion of the duodenum. In general, it is seen in thin patients who undergo significant correction of spinal deformity. Patients present with persistent postoperative vomiting. Physical exam reveals hyperactive, high-pitched bowel sounds. Treatment includes complete restriction of oral intake, gastric decompression with a nasogastric tube, adequate intravenous hydration, and initiation of hyperalimentation if symptoms persist. Patients should be encouraged to lie in the prone or left lateral position. If symptoms persist, general surgery intervention is occasionally indicated.

23. What are the most common genitourinary complications after spine surgery?

Urinary retention is frequently seen after spine procedures when a Foley catheter has not been used. It is associated with the use of epidural analgesia and PCA. Urinary tract infection is the most common complication in spinal patients who are treated with a Foley catheter. This complication is readily treated with antibiotic therapy.

24. What is the most common non–life-threatening postoperative complication in a patient over age 60 who undergoes a spinal fusion?

Transient confusion and delerium.

25. A nurse reports that a patient has developed a small amount of wound drainage 5 days after a posterior lumbar decompresssion and fusion for spondylolisthesis. The discharge planner has already made arrangements to transfer the patient to a skilled nursing facility later that day. What should you advise?

The patient's transfer should be cancelled, and the patient should remain hospitalized to permit evaluation by the surgical team. As a general principle, postoperative spine patients with wound drainage should not be discharged from the hospital because they generally require surgical exploration of the wound if drainage persists past the fourth or fifth postsurgical day. The differential diagnosis includes wound infection, seroma, and cerebrospinal fluid (CSF) leak. Expectant management and oral antibiotic treatment have no role.

Wound drainage should be cultured. Routine lab tests, including CBC with differential, erythrocyte sedimentation rate, and C-reactive protein levels should be obtained. Aspiration of the wound may be performed under sterile conditions. Persistent wound drainage or aspiration of purulent fluid mandates operative exploration and debridement. Clinical findings associated with postoperative spine infections may be minimal or nonexistent. Potential clinical findings include general malaise, spinal pain out of proportion to the expected typical postoperative course, and a low-grade fever. If infection is suspected on clinical grounds, surgical exploration should be undertaken.

26. What is the incidence of dural tears associated with spinal decompression procedures? How are dural tears managed?

The incidence of dural tear is approximately 1/20 in primary cases, increasing to 1/6 in revision cases. Dural tears recognized in the operating room are best treated with water-tight closure of the dura and soft tissues at the time of the index procedure. Fibrin glue and, more recently, ready-made glues can be used to augment the repair. When dural tear is suspected in the postoperative period (e.g., clear drainage on the postoperative surgical dressing), the patient can initially be maintained on strict bedrest in the head-down position. If drainage persists, a percutaneous catheter can be inserted proximally to divert CSF into a closed sterile drainage system to permit healing of the dura. If this approach fails to resolve the problem, open surgical repair is required.

27. What is the most common method used for pain management after an extensive spinal fusion procedure?

Intravenous opioid injections are the most widely used method for postoperative pain management after spine surgery. In the alert and cooperative patient, opioids are typically administered by PCA. With frequent dosing from the PCA with 1–2 mg of morphine or its equivalent, only the most difficult cases need further adjustment of the dosing. Meperidine (Demerol) should be avoided because of the potential for accumulation of the toxic metabolite normeperidine, which can lead to agitation, delerium, and seizures. Other options include opioids delivered in the epidural or intrathecal space. However, these techniques require additional surveillance of the patient to reduce the risk of side effects. Intercostal nerve blocks can provide substantial analgesia for thoracic and abdominal wall pain after anterior spinal procedures. Nonsteroidal anti-inflammatories such as ketorolac (Toradol) can reduce opioid requirements but are contraindicated in the postfusion patient because of their adverse effect on bone healing.

28. What complications are associated with early care of the quadriplegic patient?

Respiratory insufficiency, pneumonia, pressure ulceration, gastric bleeding, urinary retention with bladder distention and calculus formation, joint contracture, autonomic dysreflexia, skeletal osteoporosis, and psychological withdrawal.

29. Define reflexive dysenergia.

Reflex dysenergia is a reflex increase in blood pressure due to an obstructed viscus in a quadriplegic patient. A patient with a dangerously high blood pressure who is quadriplegic should be evaluated for an obstructed viscus (e.g., bladder or bowel obstruction).

30. How are steroids dosed after acute spinal cord injury? What is the most common complication of steroids in this setting?

A loading dose of 30 mg/kg of methylprednisolone is given within 8 hours of injury, followed by an infusion of 5.4 mg/kg/hr for 23 hours. If the loading dose is given within 3 hours of injury, the infusion is continued for 47 hours. The most common complication is wound infection (7% of patients).

BIBLIOGRAPHY

1. An HS, Glover JM: Complications and revision surgery in adult spinal deformity. In Bridwell KH, De-Wald RL (eds): The Textbook of Spinal Surgery, 2nd ed. Philadelphia, 1997, Lippincott-Raven, pp 797–820.
2. Devlin VJ, Williams DA: Decision making and perioperative care of the patient. In Margulies JY, Aebi M, Farcy JP (eds): In Revision Spine Surgery. St. Louis, Mosby, 1999, pp 297–319.
3. Fujita T, Kostuik JP, Huckell CB, et al: Complications of spinal fusion in adult patients more than 60 years of age. Orthop Clin North Am 29:669–678, 1998.
4. Postoperative visual loss registry. Available at www.asaclosedclaims.org.
5. Smith GF: Perioperative care of the spine patient. In White AH (ed): Spine Care—Operative Treatment. St. Louis, 1995, Mosby, pp 964–983.
6. Transfeldt EE: Complications of treatment. In Lonstein JF, Winter RB, Bradford DS, Ogilvie JW (eds): Moe's Textbook of Scoliosis and Other Spinal Deformities, 3rd ed. Philadelphia, W.B. Saunders, 1995, pp 451–481.
7. Tredwell SG: Complications of spinal surgery. In Weinstein SL (ed): The Pediatric Spine. New York, Raven Press, 1994, pp 1766–1775.

34. REVISION SPINE SURGERY

Joseph Y. Margulies, M.D., Ph.D., Vincent J. Devlin, M.D.,
and William O. Shaffer, M.D.

GENERAL CONSIDERATIONS

1. Why should the term *failed back surgery syndrome* be abandoned?

Failed back surgery syndrome is an imprecise term used to refer to patients with unsatisfactory outcomes after spine surgery. This term does not identify a diagnosis responsible for persistent symptoms and implies that additional treatment will not provide benefit. A better approach is to perform an appropriate assessment to differentiate problems amenable to additional surgical treatment from those for which further surgery would not likely provide benefit. Additional surgery can be considered for appropriate candidates. Patients unlikely to benefit from additional surgery can be directed toward appropriate nonsurgical management strategies.

2. Poor outcome after an initial spinal procedure is frequently attributed to one of the "three Ws". What are they?

1. **Wrong patient:** inappropriate patient selection for the initial surgical procedure led to a poor outcome. Examples include:
   - The patient indicated for spinal decompression or fusion had pathologic findings that could not be expected to benefit from the operation.
   - The patient's psychosocial circumstances and expectations created a barrier to success (e.g., IV drug abuse, spousal abuse, litigation).

2. **Wrong diagnosis:** inadequate imaging studies or incomplete preoperative assessment led to misdiagnosis and selection of an inappropriate surgical technique not likely to benefit the patient (e.g., decompression at the wrong level or side for a disc herniation based on mislabeled diagnostic studies).

3. **Wrong surgery:** technical problems were associated with the inital procedure or the initial procedure was inadequate to address all aspects of the patient's spinal pathology. Examples include:
   - Incorrect placement of spinal implants resulting in neural impingement
   - Inadequate decompression of spinal stenosis
   - Unstable instrumentation construct with subsequent implant failure or dislodgement
   - Failure to maintain or restore lumbar lordosis resulting in flatback syndrome
   - Failure to stabilize and fuse when a decompression is performed at an unstable spinal segment (unstable spondylolisthesis with coexistent spinal stenosis)

3. What additional factors can lead to a poor outcome after a spinal procedure?

- Unavoidable complication after appropriately performed surgery (e.g., infection, pseudarthrosis)
- Failure to diagnose a significant surgically related complication (e.g., pseudarthrosis, instability, persistent neural compression)
- Neurologic injury
- Complications related to the surgical approach (e.g., vascular injury, recurrent laryngeal nerve injury)
- Medical complications (MI, stroke, pulmonary embolus)
- Recurrence or progression of an underlying disease process (e.g., metastatic disease, infection, myelopathy, rheumatoid arthritis)
- Patient selection. Certain types of patients have a significantly increased risk of complications (e.g., Charcot spinal arthropathy, Parkinson's disease, neuromuscular spinal deformities, neurofibromatosis).

- Inadequate postoperative rehabilitation
- Surgeon inexperience. Surgeons who do not devote the majority of their practice to spine surgery are unlikely to master the sophisticated techniques of modern spine surgery.

4. What important factors should be assessed during the history and intial evaluation of a patient with continuing symptoms after spine surgery?

- Are the present symptoms the same, better, or worse after surgery?
- Are the current symptoms similar to or different from those present before surgery?
- Were the indications for the initial or most recent surgery appropriate?
- Did intraoperative complications occur? (Review the operative report if possible.)
- Was there a period in which the patient had relief of preoperative symptoms (pain-free interval)?
- Were any complications recognized in the postoperative period?
- Are the present symptoms predominantly radicular pain, axial pain, or both?
- Do ongoing legal entanglements exist?

5. What is the significance of a pain-free interval following a spinal decompression procedure?

The presence or absence of a pain-free interval following a spinal decompression procedure (e.g., lumbar laminectomy) can provide a starting point for determining the most likely causes of persistent symptoms:

- When the patient has no immediate relief, the wrong operation or wrong diagnosis should be suspected.
- When the patient has immediate relief but symptoms recur within weeks to months after the operation, new pathology or a complication of the initial operation should be suspected.
- When the patient has good relief initally but symptoms recur months to years later, new pathology or pathology secondary to an ongoing degenerative process should be suspected.

6. What are important points to assess on physical examination in the patient being evaluated for possible revision spine surgery?

A general neurologic assessment and regional spinal assessment should be performed. The presence of nonorganic signs (Waddell signs) should be assessed. Global spinal balance in the sagittal and coronal planes should be assessed. The physical exam is tailored to the particular spinal pathology under evaluation. For cervical spine disorders, shoulder pathology, brachial plexus disorders, and conditions involving the peripheral nerves should not be overlooked. For lumbar spine problems, the hip joints, sacroiliac joints, and prior bone graft sites should be assessed. Examination of peripheral pulses is routinely performed to rule out vascular insufficiency. Consider degenerative neurologic or muscle-based problems, such as amyotrophic lateral sclerosis.

7. What diagnostic imaging tests are useful in the evaluation of patients following prior spinal surgery?

The sequence of imaging studies in the postoperative patient is similar to assessment for primary spine surgery. Imaging studies are indicated to confirm the most likely cause of symptoms based on a comprehensive history and physical examination.

Radiographs. Standing posteroanterior (PA) and lateral spine radiographs are the intial imaging study. Lateral flexion-extension radiographs play a role in the diagnosis of postoperative instability or pseudarthrosis. Assessment of spinal deformities is best accomplished with standing 36-inch PA and lateral radiographs.

MRI, CT, and CT-myelography. The most appropriate study is selected based on the patient's symptoms, the presence or absence of spinal implants, and the specific spinal problem requiring assessment. MRI provides optimal visualization of the neural elements and associated bony and soft tissue structures. However, MRI is subject to degradation by metal artifact that may arise from microscopic debris remaining at the initial surgical site or from spinal implants (especially non-titanium implants). CT remains the optimal test to assess bone detail. Spiral CT is the preferred test for diagnosis of pseudarthrosis. CT myelography is of great utility in evaluation of the previously operated spine, especially in the presence of spinal deformity or extensive metallic spinal implants.

Linear tomography. Remains a valuable study for detection of pseudarthrosis.

Technetium bone scan. Provides valuable information for the diagnosis of pseudarthrosis, infection, and metastatic disease in the patient who has undergone prior spine surgery.

Discography. Can be helpful in localization of a pain generator for low back pain symptoms and can play a role in assessment of degenerative disc changes above or below a prior spinal fusion.

8. What *surgical* options are available for patients who experience persistent symptoms following spine surgery?
- **Decompression** of neural elements (spinal cord, cauda equina, nerve roots)
- **Realignment** of spinal deformities. Options include use of a corrective implant, discectomy or osteotomy.
- **Spinal stabilization.** The load-bearing capacity of the vertebral column is restored in the short term by spinal implants and on a long-term basis by spinal fusion.

Failure of a spinal procedure to improve a neurologic deficit, to correct a spinal deformity, to achieve a solid fusion, or to relieve associated pain is reason to assess the feasibility of revision spinal surgery.

9. What are the basic principles to follow when performing revision spinal surgery?
- Adequate preoperative assessment
- Optimization of the patient for spine surgery (smoking cessation, nutritional status)
- Perform definitive surgical procedures (combined anterior and posterior procedures often required)
- Adequate neural decompression
- Restoration or maintenance of sagittal alignment
- Adequate internal fixation
- Restoration of anterior spinal column load-sharing
- Use of autologous bone graft somewhere within the instrumentation construct
- Appropriate postoperative immobilization
- Postoperative rehabilitation

10. What nonsurgical treatment options are available for patients who fail to improve after spinal surgery and do not have a surgically correctable spinal problem?
- Intensive rehabilitation
- Spinal cord stimulation
- Dorsal column stimulation
- Oral narcotics
- Intrathecal narcotics (implantable drug pump)

REVISION SURGERY AFTER PRIOR SPINAL DECOMPRESSION

11. When a patient undergoes a spinal decompression procedure and reports no improvement in symptoms immediately after surgery, what are the most likely causes to consider?

Operation at the incorrect level, inadequate decompression, incorrect preoperative diagnosis or psychosocial issues predisposing to failure.

12. When a patient undergoes a spinal decompression procedure and reports temporary relief of symptoms followed by early recurrence of symptoms (within days to weeks), what are the most likely causes to consider?

Postoperative hematoma, infection (discitis, osteomyelitis, epidural abscess), meningeal cyst, and facet or pars fracture.

13. When a patient undergoes a spinal decompression procedure and reports temporary relief of symptoms followed by recurrence of symptoms within weeks to months after the index procedure, what are the most likely causes to consider?

Recurrent disc herniation, perineural scarring, infection, and unrealistic patient expectations regarding surgical outcome.

14. When a patient undergoes a spinal decompression procedure and reports temporary relief of symptoms followed by recurrence of symptoms more than 6 months after the index procedure, what are the most likely causes to consider?

Recurrent spinal stenosis and spinal instability. Recurrent spinal stenosis commonly presents as lateral stenosis secondary to disc space collapse after a discectomy. Risk factors for instability after lumbar decompression procedures include recurrent disc surgery at the L4–L5 level, multilevel decompression in patients with osteoporosis, and multilevel decompression in patients with scoliosis, especially if the deformity is flexible based on preoperative bending radiographs.

Classification of Problems After Spinal Decompression Procedures

1. Lack of improvement immediately after surgery with persistent or unchanged radicular symptoms

A. *Wrong preoperative diagnosis*

Tumor	Psychosocial causes
Infection	Discogenic pain syndrome
Metabolic disease	Decompression performed too late

B. *Technical error*

Surgery performed at wrong level(s)	Failure to treat both spinal stenosis and disc
Inadequate decompression performed	protrusion when necessary
Missed disc fragment	Conjoined nerve root

2. Temporary relief with recurrence of pain

A. *Early recurrence of symptoms (within 6 weeks)*
Hematoma
Infection
Meningeal cyst

B. *Midterm failure (6 weeks to 6 months)*

Recurrent disc herniation	Arachnoiditis
Stress fracture of pars interarticularis	Unrealistic patient expectations regarding surgical
Battered root syndrome	outcome

C. *Long-term failure (greater than 6 months)*
Recurrent stenosis
Adjacent level stenosis
Segmental spinal instability

15. What is the incidence of recurrent lumbar disc herniation following lumbar microdiscotomy?

The incidence of recurrent lumbar disc herniation is 5–10%.

16. What is the incidence of postoperative wound infection after a lumbar microdiscectomy?

1%.

REVISION SURGERY AFTER PRIOR SPINAL FUSION

17. What two factors obtained from the patient's history can be used to arrive at a differential diagnosis for persistent symptoms after spinal fusion surgery?

The differential diagnosis for persistent symptoms following spinal fusion surgery has been categorized according to:

- Time of appearance of symptoms in relation to the most recent fusion procedure
- Predominance of leg vs. back symptoms

Classification of Problems after Spinal Fusion Procedures

TIME OF APPEARANCE	BACK PAIN PREDOMINANT	LEG PAIN PREDOMINANT
Early (weeks)	Infection	Neural impingement by fixation devices
	Wrong level fused	Foraminal stenosis due to change in
	Insufficient levels fused	spinal alignment (e.g., after spinal
	Psychosocial distress	osteotomy)
Midterm (months)	Pseudarthrosis	Neural compression due to pseudarthrosis
	Adjacent level degeneration	Adjacent level degeneration
	Sagittal imbalance	Graft donor site pain
	Graft donor site pain	
	Inadequate reconditioning	
	Fixation loose, displaced or broken	
Long-term (years)	Pseudarthrosis	Adjacent level stenosis
	Adjacent level instability	Adjacent level disc herniation
	Acquired spondylolysis	
	Compression fracture adjacent	
	to fusion	
	Adjacent level degeneration	
	Abutment syndrome	

18. Define pseudarthrosis.

Pseudarthrosis is defined as failure to obtain a solid bony union 1 year after an attempted spinal fusion. The diagnosis of pseudarthrosis is suggested by the presence of continued axial pain and the absence of bridging trabecular bone on plain radiographs. Other findings which suggest the presence of pseudarthrosis include: abnormal motion on flexion-extension radiographs, loss of spinal deformity correction and spinal implant loosening or failure.

19. What factors influence the rate of pseudarthrosis following a spinal fusion procedure?
- The number of levels fused
- Fusion technique (anterior, posterior, circumferential)
- Use of internal fixation
- Use of autograft bone
- Underlying pathologic condition for which the fusion was performed
- Patient-related factors—age, smoking, osteoporosis, medications (e.g., NSAIDs)
- Use of external immobilization
- Radiographic criteria used to define fusion

20. What is the most reliable method for diagnosis of a pseudarthrosis?

Radiographs, linear tomography, SPECT bone scans, and CT scans have been used to diagnose pseudarthrosis. No test is completely reliable. CT scans with two-dimensional and possibly three-dimensional reconstructions are the preferred radiographic imaging test for diagnosis of pseudarthrosis. However, the most reliable method for diagnosis of pseudarthosis remains surgical exploration of the fusion mass.

21. What is the most reliable technique for achieving a successful fusion in a patient who developed a pseudarthrosis after a posterior L4–L5 fusion procedure?

The technique most likely to result in successful fusion is a combination of an L4–L5 interbody fusion and posterior fusion with pedicle fixation.

22. What is a transition syndrome?

Spinal fusion causes increased stress on adjacent spinal motion segments that can lead to adjacent level spinal instability, spinal stenosis, and/or disc herniation. This clinical scenario has been termed a transition syndrome. Treatment generally involves decompression and extension of the spinal fusion and spinal instrumentation.

23. What is the incidence of postoperative wound infection after a posterior lumbar fusion without spinal instrumentation? After a posterior lumbar fusion with use of spinal intrumentation? After anterior lumbar fusion?
- Posterior fusion without instrumentation: 3–5%
- Posterior fusion with spinal instrumentation: 3–8%
- Anterior spinal fusion: 0.6%

REVISION SURGERY FOR SPINAL DEFORMITY

24. What common problems may require revision surgery after an initial surgical procedure for spinal deformity?
- Pseudarthrosis
- Back pain secondary to implant prominence or implant failure
- Adjacent level disc degeneration or instability
- Coronal plane imbalance
- Sagittal plane imbalance (flatback syndrome)
- Junctional kyphotic deformity
- Residual rib prominence
- Infection
- Crankshaft phenomenon

25. What is the crankshaft phenomenon?

Crankshaft phenomenon refers to continued anterior spinal growth after a posterior spinal fusion in a skeletally immature patient, resulting in increased spinal deformity. Risk factors include skeletal immaturity (Risser stage 0, premenstrual), surgery before the peak growth period, and large residual curves after initial surgery. Prevention is by anterior spinal fusion in addition to posterior spinal fusion in patients at risk of developing crankshaft phenomenon.

26. What procedure is advised to treat a severe rib prominence that persists after posterior spinal fusion and instrumentation for scoliosis?

An unsightly rib prominence can be treated with a thoracoplasty. This procedure involves resection of the medial portions of the ribs over the prominence.

27. Describe the surgical treatment for flatback syndrome.

Flatback syndrome refers to symptomatic loss of sagittal plane balance primarily through straightening of the normal lumbar lordosis. Symptoms include pain and inability to stand upright with the head centered over the sacrum without bending the knees. Patients typically report a sense of leaning forward, thoracic pain, neck pain, and leg fatigue. Surgical treatment options include osteotomies (Smith-Peterson type or pedicle subtraction type), combined anterior and posterior procedures, or vertebral column resection procedures.

BIBLIOGRAPHY

1. Albert TJ, Pinto M, Denis F: Management of symptomatic lumbar pseudarthrosis with anteroposterior fusion: A functional and radiographic outcome study. Spine 25:129–129, 2000.
2. Dubousset J, Herring A, Shufflebarger H: Crankshaft phenomenon in spinal surgery. J Pediatr Orthop 9:541–550, 1989.
3. Hsu SD, Fontaine F, Kelley B, et al: Nutritional depletion in staged spinal reconstructive surgery. Spine 23:1401–1405, 1998.
4. Kostuik JP: The surgical treatment of failures of laminectomy. Spine State Art Rev 11:509–538, 1997.
5. Kostuik JP: Failures after spinal fusion. Spine State Art Rev 11:589–650, 1997.
6. LaGrone M, Bradford DS, Moe JH et al: Treatment of symptomatic flatback after spinal fusion. J Bone Joint Surg 70A:569–580, 1988.
7. Lauerman WC, Bradford DS, Transfeldt EE, et al: Management of pseudarthrosis after arthrodesis of the spine for idiopathic scoliosis. J Bone Joint Surg 73A: 222–236, 1991.
8. Margulies JY, Aebi M, Farcy JP (eds): Revision Spine Surgery. St. Louis, Mosby, 1999.

VI. Degenerative Disorders of the Adult Spine

35. CERVICAL DEGENERATIVE DISORDERS

Paul A. Anderson, M.D.

1. Define cervical spondylosis. What causes it?

Cervical spondylosis is a nonspecific term that refers to any lesion of the cervical spine of a degenerative nature. Cervical spondylosis results from an imbalance between formation and degradation of proteoglycans and collagen in the disc. With aging, a negative imbalance with subsequent loss of disc material results in degenerative changes. Factors such as heredity, trauma, metabolic disorders, certain occupational exposures, and other environmental effects (e.g., smoking) can influence the severity of degeneration.

2. Describe the clinical conditions associated with cervical spondylosis.

Patients with symptomatic cervical spondylosis may present with neck pain (axial pain), cervical radiculopathy, or cervical myelopathy. Most patients with spondylosis have little or no pain. In patients who present with neck pain symptoms, it is unclear whether the spondolytic changes are responsible for pain.

3. Describe the degenerative changes seen on radiographs in patients with cervical spondylosis.

Degenerative changes noted on radiographs include narrowing of the intervertebral disc, sclerosis of the vertebral endplates, and osteophyte formation. As a result, the segmental range of motion is decreased. Similar changes may occur in the facet joints. Rarely, facet degeneration is advanced compared with degeneration of the intervertebral disc. Degenerative changes are observed most frequently at the C5–C6 and C6–C7.

4. Describe the relationship between facet degeneration and disc degeneration.

In the majority of cases, disc degeneration is thought to precede or occur simultaneously with facet degeneration. However, in some cases isolated facet degeneration may be present. Facet-mediated pain is especially prevalent in patients with hyperextension injuries such as rear-end accidents. Extension moments create high-contact forces in the facet joints, which can lead to chronic facet pain even in the absence of radiographic findings.

5. What is the incidence of cervical spondylosis noted on radiographs in *asymptomatic* patients?

Percent of Population with Radiographic Changes by Age Group[1]

20–30	31–40	41–50	51–60	61–70
5%	25%	35%	80%	95%

6. What is the incidence of cervical spondylosis (i.e., cervical disc herniation, degenerative disc changes, cervical stenosis) noted on MRI in *asymptomatic* patients (2)?

	AGE	
	< 40 YR	> 40 YR
Cervical disc herniation	10%	5%
Degenerative disc changes	25%	60%
Cervical stenosis	4%	20%

7. List common causes of chronic neck pain.

Common causes of neck pain include (1) degenerative disc and/or facet disease, (2) neurologic compression syndromes secondary to herniated discs or cervical stenosis, (3) cervical instability, (4) posttraumatic soft tissue or facet injury after whiplash, and (5) inflammatory arthritis, such as rheumatoid arthritis or ankylosing spondylitis.

8. Do patients with chronic neck pain improve with the passage of time?

A natural history study by Gore showed that at 10 years 79% of patients had less pain.[3] Overall, 43% were pain-free, 25% had mild pain, 25% had moderate pain, and 7% had severe pain. The level of pain did not correlate with degenerative changes or other radiographic parameters. However, the pain level was correlated with the severity of the initial pain and whether onset was due to an injury. Chronic disabling symptoms were seen in 18% of patients.

9. Define cervical spinal instability.

Instability is present when the spine is unable to withstand physiologic loads, resulting in significant risk for neurologic injury, progressive deformity, and long-term pain and disability. Instability is not common in patients with cervical spondylosis except in those with stiffness in the middle and lower segments who develop compensatory hypermobility at C3–C4 or C4–C5. This condition can result in degenerative spondylolisthesis and lead to symptomatic cervical myelopathy. Cervical spinal instability may be diagnosed according to the radiographic criteria of White (> 11° angulation, > 3.5-mm translation of adjacent subaxial cervical spine segments).

10. Is surgery indicated for chronic neck pain?

Indications for surgical treatment of patients with axial neck pain are uncommon. Surgery may be indicated for conditions such as instability, posttraumatic facet injuries, and C1–C2 osteoarthritis. Patients with discogenic-mediated neck pain secondary to degenerative disc disease can occasionally be treated surgically. Whitecloud has shown that 60–70% of patients improve following anterior discectomy and fusion. Before surgery patients are evaluated by provocative cervical discography to confirm the source of pain.[5] Poorer results are seen in litigation cases and cases involving more than two cervical levels.

11. List the signs and symptoms commonly present in patients with symptomatic disc herniation.

Signs and symptoms may include neck pain, radicular arm pain, weakness in specific myotome, diminished sensation in specific dermatome, and altered reflexes.

12. Which nonoperative treatment options are effective for cervical disc herniations?

Few studies evaluating the effectiveness of nonoperative treatment are available. A commonly accepted treatment is to decrease the associated inflammatory response with the use of nonsteroidal anti-inflammatory drugs, oral corticosteroids, or epidural and selective nerve root steroid injections. Rest by use of an orthosis such as a soft collar and reduction of activities may be useful. Traction, physical therapy, and manipulation are frequently attempted but are often poorly tolerated in patients with acute cervical disc herniations.

13. List the surgical indications for patients with herniated cervical discs.

Indications for surgery for patients with symptomatic cervical disc herniation include intractable radicular pain and neurologic changes, especially if they are progressive and interfere with quality of life. The neuroimaging study should correlate with clinical symptoms.

14. Is anterior discectomy and fusion the only treatment option for patients with a cervical herniated nucleus pulposus?

No. Alternative surgical techniques include anterior discectomy without fusion, posterior foramenotomy with discectomy, anterior foramenotomy without discectomy, or artificial disc replacement (Fig. 1). In properly selected cases outcomes for all the above techniques are similar to those with anterior discectomy and fusion.

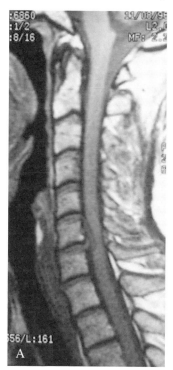

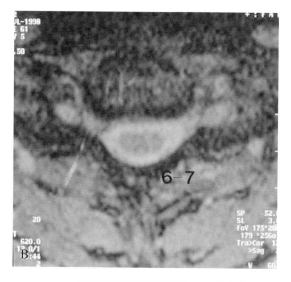

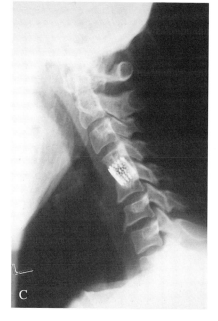

FIGURE 1. **A,** Lateral MRI showing large herniated disc at C6–C7. The patient presented with a C7 radiculopathy. **B,** Axial MRI at C6–C7 showing right posterolateral herniated disc. **C,** Treatment of a C4–C5 disc herniation with anterior discectomy and fusion cage. (*continued*)

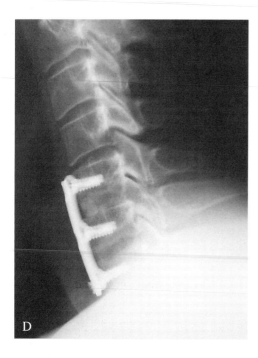

FIGURE 1. (*continued*) **D,** Treatment of C4–C5 and C5–C6 disc herniations with two-level anterior discectomy, interbody grafting and plate fixation.

15. Discuss the indications and results of posterior foramenotomy and discectomy for a herniated cervical disc.

Patients who have acute radiculopathy without longstanding chronic neck pain and posterolateral or intraforamenal soft tissue disc herniation are excellent candidates for posterior foramenotomies. The disc space height should be well preserved, and there should be no associated spinal instability. The advantages of this technique are avoidance of fusion and early return to function. The disadvantages are difficulty in removing pathology ventral to the nerve root, especially an osteophyte, and the potential for instability if more than 50% of the facet is removed. Satisfactory outcomes are seen in 85–90% of properly selected cases.

16. What are the advantages of using an anterior cervical plate after anterior discectomy and fusion?

Anterior cervical plate stabilization prevents graft collapse, maintains alignment (prevents local kyphosis), decreases postoperative brace requirements, and usually allows earlier return to activities such as work or driving.[6] Fusion success and clinical outcome have not been shown to improve with the use of the anterior cervical plate

17. What is the rate of succcessful fusion after an anterior cervical discectomy and fusion procedure?

Pseudarthrosis rates strongly correlate to number of levels arthrodesed.[7]

Pseudarthrosis

One Level Fusion	0–5%
Two Level Fusion	10–20%
Three Level Fusion	30–60%

18. Have allograft or interbody cage devices replaced autograft in the treatment of patients requiring cervical fusion?

Interbody spacer devices and allografts have been developed and used to avoid the morbidity of autogenous bone grafting. Zdeblick and Ducker reported significantly higher rates of nonunion in allograft versus autograft in two level cases, but no difference in one level cases.[8] Newer machined allografts have not been critically examined at this time to determine efficacy. The efficacy of interbody cage devices is currently under investigation.

19. What are the indications for discectomy and interbody fusion versus corpectomy in patients requiring treatment of two-level cervical disc pathology?

Patients with two-level disease may be treated by discectomy and interbody fusion at both sites or by discectomies and removal of the intervening vertebral body, followed by strut grafting. Radiographic results in retrospective series are conflicting. Biomechanical studies strongly favor two-level discectomy over corpectomy. The author's current recommendation is to perform corpectomy only when it is required to complete a neural decompression and when it enhances safety during removal of disc and bone pathology from a narrow spinal canal.

20. Why does degeneration occur at spinal segments adjacent to a prior cervical fusion?

The causes of adjacent segment degeneration are (1) progression of the underlying degenerative disease process, which would occur regardless of whether spinal surgery was performed, and (2) increased load and stress transfer, resulting in accelerated degeneration of the motion segment adjacent to a cervical fusion. No clear evidence determines which process is the more important.

21. What is the potential for development of degenerative changes adjacent to fused cervical spine segments?

Long-term studies after anterior cervical discectomy and fusion indicate that progressive radiographic degenerative changes occur in up to 50% of cases. The incidence of degenerative changes after anterior cervical fusion has been reported to exceed the rate predicted if fusion was not performed. Hilibrand documented new symptomatic radiculopathy or myelopathy at adjacent segments in 20% of patients within 10 years after anterior cervical decompression and fusion. Lifetime analysis indicates that 25% of patients have recurrence of neurologic symptoms by 20 years after an intial surgical procedure.

22. Are the results of fusion cages better than autograft in the treatment of patients requiring cervical interbody fusion?

Single-level intervertebral BAK cages have been shown to have higher fusion success rates and improved clinical outcome compared with autograft in a multicenter randomized study.[9] Two-level cages had slightly poorer outcomes than autograft. Comparison of cages with plates is currently under way.

23. What are the physical findings in patients with cervical spondylotic myelopathy?

Cervical spondolytic myelopathy is often slowly progressive. It is associated with nonspecific symptoms such as generalized fatigue, weakness, clumsiness of hands, loss of balance, gait disturbance, and bladder or bowel impairment. Pain may be lacking or minimal. Physical findings include reduced neck motion, especially in extension; atrophy and weakness of muscles; muscle fasciculation; poor hand coordination; increased muscle tone; ataxia of gait; and the Romberg sign. Reflexes in the upper extremity are variable but are usually increased in the legs. Pathologic reflexes such as Hoffman's, and Babinski's signs and clonus are usually present. Abnormal pinprick and vibratory sensation indicates severe involvement.

24. Discuss the natural history of cervical myelopathy.

The natural history of patients with established cervical myelopathy is poor.[10] Most often there is a slow stepwise worsening with periods of neurologic plateau preceding another episode of deterioration. Rarely, patients present with acute deterioration or even quadriplegia.

25. Is cervical degenerative disc disease the only cause of cervical myelopathy?

No. Other common causes of cervical myelopathy include (1) ossification of the posterior longitudinal ligament (OPPL); (2) large central disc herniations; (3) spinal instability, especially at C3–C4 or C4–C5; and (4) rheumatoid arthritis with associated instability involving the craniocervical, atlantoaxial, or subaxial spinal regions.

26. List common complications associated with anterior cervical discectomy and fusion

Soft tissue injury

• Airway obstruction	< 1%	**Neurologic injury**	1–3%
• Esophagus	< 1%	**Vertebral artery injury**	0–1%
• Recurrent laryngeal nerve	1–2%	**Graft-related complications**	
• Horner's syndrome	< 1%	• Collapse 10–25%	
• Dysphagia		• Dislodgement 5–10%	
Acute (< 3 weeks)	35%	• Nonunion 5–30%	
Chronic	8–18%	**Hardware-related problems** 1–5%	
• Superior laryngeal nerve	1–2%		
• Thoracic duct	< 1%		

27. Describe the typical radiographic and imaging findings associated with cervical spondylotic myelopathy.

A variety of spinal pathology can result in cord compression with subsequent myelopathy. Spinal pathology may occur at a single level or, more commonly, involve multiple spinal levels. Most patients with myelopathy have a congenitally small spinal canal with a mid-sagittal diameter measuring less than 10 mm. Common radiograph findings include anterior and posterior osteophytes, retrolisthesis (expecially at C5–C6 and C6–C7), anterolisthesis (most common at C3–C4 and C4–C5) and acute soft tissue disc herniation. Magnetic resonance imaging (MRI) demonstrates focal cord compression. Cord compression occurs anteriorly in 80% of cases. Posterior compression may result from ligamentum flavum hypertrophy. Plastic deformation of the cord with decreased anteroposterior diameter and increased medial-lateral diameter may be noted. In 20–40 % of cases, an increased signal in the cord is present on MRI and represents myelomalacia.

28. What are the indications for surgery for patients with cervical myelopathy?

Most patients with cervical myelopathy should be treated surgically, unless surgery is contraindicated by age or medical conditions. Increasing numbers of patients with cord compression on MRI but without neurologic symptoms or evidence of myelopathy are being evaluated. In the absence of objective findings or symptoms of myelopathy, such patients are best treated nonoperatively. However, they should be monitored with periodic examinations for the development of cervical myelopathy.

29. List the surgical options for patients with cervical myelopathy.

- Anterior discectomy or corpectomy and fusion combined with anterior spinal instrumentation
- Laminectomy
- Laminoplasty
- Laminectomy and posterior fusion combined with posterior spinal instrumentation
- Anterior decompression and fusion combined with posterior fusion and posterior spinal instrumentation

The anatomic location and cause of neural compression, surgeon preference, and patient's desire are the important factors that determine the surgical approach.

30. Why is laminectomy associated with poorer outcomes compared with anterior cervical decompression for the treatment of cervical myelopathy?

Outcomes after laminectomy deteriorate over time secondary to development of spinal instability and cervical kyphosis.

31. Discuss the indications for and results of cervical laminoplasty.

Laminoplasty increases the mid-sagittal diameter and cross-sectional area of the spinal canal. This procedure directly decompresses the cord dorsally. It also allows posterior displacement of the cord, which indirectly decompresses its ventral surface (Fig. 2). Accepted indications for laminoplasty are a straight or lordotic cervical spine, a stable spine, and multilevel cord compression. It is the preferred technique when only dorsal cord compression is present. Long-term improvement is seen in 60–75 % of patients.[12]

32. List the long-term morbidities associated with laminoplasty.

The limitations and morbidity of laminoplasty include loss of range of motion, chronic neck pain (up to 30% of patients), and recurrent stenosis. Acutely, 3–5% of patients develop a C5 motor neuropraxia, often within 24–48 hours postoperatively. This complication resolves in two-thirds of cases.

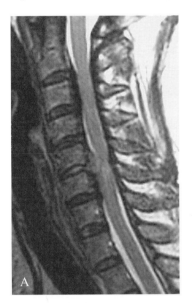

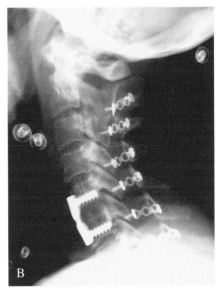

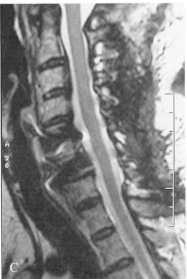

FIGURE 2. A, 60-year-old Japanese woman with severe myelopathy due to C5–C6 herniated disc and multilevel cervical stenosis. Stenosis from C2–C3 through C6–C7 is due to ossification of posterior longitudinal ligament. **B,** Postoperative lateral radiograph following C5–C6 anterior discectomy and fusion with plate fixation combined with laminoplasty from C2 to C7. **C,** Postoperative MRI demonstrating excellent decompression of the spinal canal after anterior and posterior procedures.

33. What are the indications for anterior cervical decompression and fusion for the treatment of cervical myelopathy?

Anterior decompression and fusion are the most accepted treatment for cervical spondylitic myelopathy in patients with ventral cord compression. Reported results indicate that 60–70% of patients experience improvement in neurologic function following surgery. Most surgeons perform anterior decompression for up to three levels of compression, although successful results have been reported with anterior decompression for 4 or 5 levels. Complications related to reconstruction increase significantly as more levels are treated.

34. What pitfalls are associated with the use of anterior cervical plates for multilevel myelopathy cases?

Long reconstructions stabilized by plates are at high risk of failure due to (1) screw pullout at the inferior segment and (2) subsidence of the strut graft into the vertebral body or dislodgement into the retropharynx. Biomechanical studies have shown that excessive forces occur at the caudal vertebral body screws. In multiple level constructs, subsidence from 1 to 3 mm at each level results in increased screw contact forces caudally. Loss of fixation can result in graft dislodgement with subsequent esophageal injury or dysphagia. Additionally, graft resorption commonly occurs at the proximal and distal extent of the graft, where it contacts the vertebral body. If the construct is splinted by a plate, nonunion may result. For these reasons, anterior decompression and fusion combined with posterior spinal instrumentation (typically a screw-rod system) are recommended for use in multilevel cervical reconstructive procedures—specifically, all three-level constructs and certain two-level constructs (e.g., patients with osteopenia). (See Figure 3.)

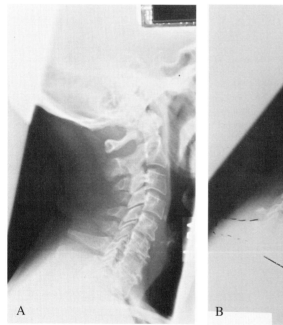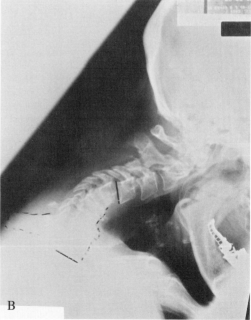

FIGURE 3. A, Preoperative lateral radiograph of a 70-year-old woman with cervical stenosis. **B,** Postoperative radiograph after cervical laminectomy demonstrating development of a post-laminectomy kyphotic deformity. (*continued*)

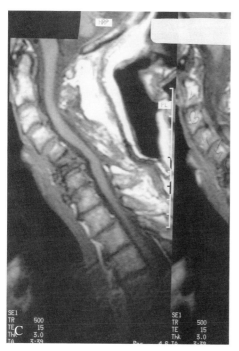
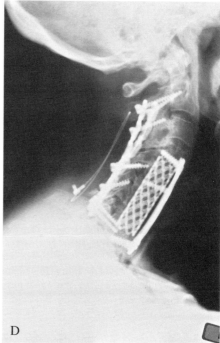

FIGURE 3. (*continued*) **C,** MRI demonstrates persistent cervical stenosis despite posterior decompression. **D,** Anterior and posterior spinal reconstructive surgery is required. Anterior decompression and reconstruction were performed using a cage and plate. Posterior reconstruction was performed using a plate-screw system.

BIBLIOGRAPHY

1. Gore DR : Roentgenographic findings in the cervical spine in asymptomatic persons: a ten-year follow-up. Spine 26:2463–2466, 2001.
2. Boden SD, McCowin PR, Davis DO; et al: Abnormal magnetic-resonance scans of the cervical spine in asymptomatic subjects. A prospective investigation. J Bone Joint Surg 72A:1178–1184, 1990.
3. Gore DR, Sepic SB, Gardner GM, et al: Neck pain: a long-term follow-up of 205 patients. Spine 12:1–5, 1987.
4. Whitecloud TS, Seago RA: Cervical discogenic syndrome: Results of operative intervention in patients with positive discography. Spine 12:313–316, 1987.
5. Wirth FP, Dowd GC, Sanders H, et al: Cervical discectomy. A prospective analysis of three operative techniques. Surg Neurol 53:340–346, 2000.
6. Troyanovich SJ, Stroink AR, Kattner KA, et al: Does anterior plating maintain cervical lordosis versus conventional fusion techniques? A retrospective analysis of patients receiving single-level fusions. J Spin Disord Tech 15:69–74, 2002.
7. Bohlman HH, Emery SE, Goodfellow DB, et al: Robinson anterior cervical discectomy and arthrodesis for cervical radiculopathy. Long-term follow-up of one hundred and twenty-two patients. J Bone Joint Surg 75A:1298–1307, 1993.
8. Zdeblick TA, Ducker TB: The use of freeze-dried allograft bone for anterior cervical fusions. Spine 16: 726–729, 1991.
9. Hilibrand AS, Carlson GD, Palumbo MA, et al: Radiculopathy and myelopathy at segments adjacent to the site of a previous anterior cervical arthrodesis. J Bone Joint Surg 81A:519–528, 1999.
10. Hacker RJ, Cauthen JC, Gilbert TJ, et al: A prospective randomized multicenter clinical evaluation of an anterior cervical fusion cage. Spine 25:2646–2654, 2000.
11. Emery SE: Cervical spondylotic myelopathy: diagnosis and treatment. J Am Acad Orthop Surg 9(6): 376–388, 2001.
12. Seichi A, Takeshita K, Ohishi I et al: Long-term results of double-door laminoplasty for cervical stenotic myelopathy. Spine 26:479–487, 2001.

36. THORACIC DISC HERNIATION

Jeffrey E. Deckey, M.D.

1. What is the incidence of thoracic disc herniation?

The incidence of symptomatic thoracic disc herniation has been reported as 1 per million patients. However, magnetic resonance imaging (MRI) and computed tomography (CT) myelogram studies have shown an incidence ranging between 11% and 37% in asymptomatic patients. Peak incidence occurs in the fifth decade.

2. Describe the clinical presentation of a symptomatic thoracic disc herniation.

The clinical presentation can include axial pain, radicular pain, or myelopathy. Axial thoracic pain may be mechanical but is sometimes confused with cardiac, pulmonary, or abdominal pathology. Radicular complaints consist of pain radiating around the chest wall along the path of an intercostal nerve. Myelolpathy may develop as a result of spinal cord compression. Careful examination for upper motor neuron signs can lead to the diagnosis of myelopathy. Examples include a Romberg sign, Babinski reflex, clonus, ataxic gait, loss of rectal tone, and decreased perianal sensation.

3. At what spinal level do thoracic disc herniations most commonly occur?

Thoracic disc herniation can occur at any level in the thoracic spine. Disc herniation is most common in the lower third of the thoracic spine with the highest percentage reported at the T11–T12 level.

4. Which imaging modalities are useful in the diagnosis of a thoracic disc herniation?

Routine plain radiographs should be performed to rule out osseous abnormalities such as tumors, deformities, or fractures. In addition, plain radiographs are essential as an intra-operative reference to determine if the surgeon is operating at the correct level. MRI is the best imaging modality for assessment of the vertebra, intervertebral discs, and neural elements. CT myelography is helpful for assessment of the degree of spinal cord compression and determining whether there exists calcification of the disc or posterior longitudinal ligament.

5. How is a thoracic disc herniation treated?

Treatment of a thoracic disc herniation depends on the patient's symptoms, physical exam, and radiologic findings.

6. What treatment is recommended for an asymptomatic thoracic disc herniation without spinal cord compression?

Asymptomatic disc herniations without evidence of spinal cord compression require no treatment.

7. What treatment is recommended for a symptomatic thoracic disc herniation without spinal cord compression?

Symptomatic disc herniations without evidence of spinal cord compression should initially be treated nonoperatively. Clinical presentations often vary. The patient's symptoms are often vague. Symptoms may include axial back pain in the thoracic region or radicular pain involving the chest wall with associated numbness. Acute disc herniations resulting in axial pain should be treated with activity modification, nonsteroidal anti-inflammatory drugs, and physical therapy. In patients with radicular complaints, oral corticosteroids or epidural steroid injections can be considered. This approach may provide sufficient pain relief to permit initiation of physical therapy. Nonoperative treatment should be considered for at least 4 to 6 weeks. If symptoms are unrelenting despite nonoperative treatment, surgery may be considered as an option.

8. What treatment is recommended for a symptomatic thoracic disc herniation causing spinal cord compression?

Spinal cord compression may result in myelopathy. Clinical findings may include an ataxic gait and a Romberg sign (the patient loses balance when asked to stand upright with feet together, hands straight out, and eyes closed). Other findings may include lower extremity hyperreflexia, clonus, and the presence of a Babinski reflex. In addition the patient may present with a thoracic sensory level. Patients may also complain of loss of bowel or bladder function. Spinal cord compression with myelopathy or progressive neurologic deficit should be considered for immediate surgical intervention. The use of systemic steroids is controversial because previous studies have focused on cervical spinal cord injury rather than thoracic cord injury.

9. What are the surgical approach options for treatment of a symptomatic thoracic disc herniation?
- Transthoracic anterior approach via a thoracotomy
- Transsternal approach or approach via resection of the medial aspect of the clavicle (for upper thoracic lesions)
- Laminectomy with pediculofacetectomy
- Costotransversectomy
- Lateral extracavitary approach
- Video-assisted thoracoscopic discectomy

10. Which approach should be used for treating a thoracic disc herniation?

Various factors should be considered when selecting a surgical approach for a thoracic disc herniation:
- Level of the herniation
- Location of the herniation in relation to the spinal cord (lateral, paracentral, or central)
- Patient's underlying medical condition
- Number of levels requiring treatment
- Surgeon's familiarity with various approaches

If the patient is medically stable, the disc herniation can be treated via an anterior approach, which includes a transsternal or medial claviculectomy in the upper thoracic spine (T1–T4). In the middle and distal thoracic spine, an anterior transthoracic or thoracoscopic approach can be used (Figs. 1 and 2). If an anterior approach cannot be safely performed for medical reasons, either a costotransversectomy or pediculofacetectomy can be considered. These latter approaches permit reasonable exposure for lateral or paracentral disc herniations but are suboptimal for central disc herniations.

11. How can the surgeon determine the correct surgical level intraoperatively?

Intraoperative determination of the correct surgical level is crucial. Often MRI scout films number the spine counting from C1 downward. Intraoperatively, however, it is often easier to count vertebrae upward from the sacrum or to use the ribs as a reference. Preoperatively, the scout film on the MRI should be performed counting from the lumbar spine upward. In addition, anteroposterior and

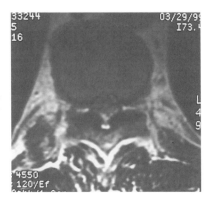

FIGURE 1. Axial MRI image of a T8–T9 central thoracic disc herniation with spinal cord compression in a 55-year-old man.

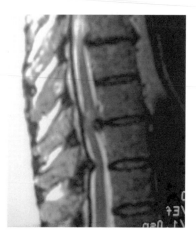

FIGURE 2. Sagittal MRI image of a T8–T9 central thoracic disc herniation with spinal cord compression.

lateral radiographs of the thoracic and lumbar spine should be obtained to determine the number of thoracic and lumbar vertebra present. The ribs should be numbered to correspond with appropriate thoracic levels. In the thoracic spine, the first, eleventh, and twelfth ribs usually articulate only with their corresponding vertebral bodies. Between T2 and T10, the rib heads articulate with the corresponding vertebral body as well as the proximal vertebral body and overlie the intervening disc space.

12. At which level should a thoracotomy be performed for a transthoracic disc resection?

A chest radiograph can be used to determine the slope of the ribs in the thoracic spine. Usually, a thoracotomy is performed one or two levels above the target disc space. This strategy allows a parallel approach to the disc space, thus permitting the use of a microscope if desired. Alternatively, a minithoracotomy can be performed to attempt to decrease approach-related morbidity. The posterior portion of the rib leading to the target disc space is removed (e.g., remove the posterior portion of the ninth rib to access a T8–T9 disc herniation).

13. Is a fusion necessary after thoracic discectomy?

Fusion after thoracic discectomy is controversial. Currently, the addition of a fusion should be considered in cases of multilevel discectomy or underlying Scheuerman's disease with kyphosis and when a significant amount of the vertebral body must be resected to decompress the spinal cord. Instrumentation should be considered when instability is present, when a significant portion of a vertebral body is removed to access the spinal canal, and when kyphosis is likely to develop after decompression.

14. What complications can occur after surgery for thoracic disc herniation?

Complications can include death, deterioration of neurologic function (including complete paralysis), kyphotic deformity, pseudarthosis, instrumentation failure, infection, and various medical complications.

BIBLIOGRAPHY

1. Awwad EE, Martin DS, Smith KR Jr, Baker BK: Asymptomatic versus symptomatic herniated thoracic discs: Their frequency and characteristics as detected by computed tomography after myelography. Neurosurgery 28:180–186, 1991.
2. Currier BL, Eismont FJ, Green BA: Transthoracic disc excision and fusion for herniated thoracic discs. Spine 19:323–328, 1994.
3. Simpson JM, Silveri CP, Simeone FA, et al: Thoracic disc herniation: Re-evaluation of the posterior approach using a modified costotransversectomy. Spine 18:1872–1877, 1993.
4. Vanichkachorn JS, Vaccaro AR: Thoracic disk disease: Diagnosis and treatment. J Am Acad Orthop Surg 8:159–169, 2000.

37. LOW BACK PAIN

Maury Ellenberg, M.D., and Joseph C. Honet, M.D., M.S.

1. Is low back pain (LBP) a common problem?

Yes. Epidemiologic studies show that by the age of 20, 50% of the population has experienced LBP. By age 60 years, the incidence may be as high as 80%, LBP is second only to the common cold when it comes to symptoms prompting a physician visit.

2. What are the most common diagnoses of back pain?

In a number of studies, the most common diagnoses are actually nondiagnoses, such as "nonspecific LBP" or "degenerative disease." More specific diagnoses include compression fracture, spondylolisthesis, malignancy, ankylosing spondylitis, and infection. Approximately 2% are diagnosed with "radiculopathy" or "sciatica."

3. Does back pain have a natural history?

Yes. LBP is usually self-limited. Because the incidence is over 50% and point prevalence in the 10–20% range, it is obvious that most individuals are able to deal with their pain for the period of time until resolution. However, in certain populations, the pain, complaints, and subsequent disability become significant and difficult to resolve. Recurrence over time, which is not predictable, is also part of the natural history.

4. Is there a way to prevent recurrences?

There are ways to try to prevent recurrence, but few have proven effective. It makes sense to learn proper back care, exercises including back, abdominal, and back stabilizer strengthening, and stretches for the back and hamstrings. Patients can be educated to respond to acute episodes with nonsteroidal anti-inflammatory drugs (NSAIDs), ice or heat, and activity maintenance and to expect resolution in 3–7 days.

5. Are there really no abnormalities in people with so-called nonspecific LBP?

There are many abnormalities in the spine of people with LBP. However, there is no conclusive evidence that these abnormalities are responsible for the patient's complaints. Clinical studies have shown a poor correlation between spinal x-ray abnormalities and LBP. Nonetheless, past generations of medical practitioners have told patients that their LBP was due to "arthritis" of the spine. More recently, as computed tomography (CT) scanning and magnetic resonance imaging (MRI) evolved and more abnormalities became visible, surgery has been recommended to remove architecturally observable but nonoffending discs. Even today, degenerative discs are blamed for LBP, lumbar fusion, IDET (heat dissolution of discs), and a variety of other procedures are being performed to fix the problem.

A number of structures can potentially cause LBP. Anatomic studies have determined which structures have free nerve endings that transmit pain sensations, and irritating material has been injected into structures to determine if and where pain is caused. Newer techniques claim to distinguish some of these structures by differential injection, specifically into the facet joint, the sacroiliac joint, or disc (discogram). These remain controversial and are generally only effective in a reliable patient without psychological, legal, or monetary reinforcers.

6. What is the most important tool to assess patients with LBP?

Believe it or not, the history and physical examination remain the mainstays for evaluating LBP, despite the new expensive technology.[1]

7. What factors of the history are most important?

The history is vital and may be more important than physical examination. Determine the on-set and duration of the problem; the reason it occurred; its relation to work, automobile, or other injury; if litigation is involved; and if there is financial remuneration. Define the pain carefully: its location, relationship to position and activity, and time of day it is most prominent. Determine if there are associated symptoms such as pain in an extremity, numbness, or tingling. "Red flags" that may indicate serious pathology include bowel or bladder dysfunction, history of cancer, and generalized disorders such as end stage renal disease, osteoporosis, Paget's disease, AIDS, or drug use. These red flags warrant further testing such as laboratory tests or imaging studies. In acute back pain without red flags, treatment usually only requires a history and physical examination.

Low Back Pain "Red Flags"

Fever	Significant trauma	Failure to improve with treatment
Unexplained weight loss	Osteoporosis	Alcohol or drug abuse
Cancer history	Age > 50 years	

8. Which structures should be examined in a patient with LBP? How is the examination performed?

The physical examination requires demonstration and lots of practice. Keep in mind that few physical exam techniques have been proven to identify the specific structure or disorder that is the cause of pain. The examination should address the low back, pelvis, hips, lower limbs, and gait and should include a neurologic examination for nerve root involvement. Ex-amination points include back motion to look for asymmetric movement, re-creation of pain, and area of mechanically limited motion or guarded motion (so-called spasm). Examine for ten-derness, especially percussion tenderness over bony areas in the back and pelvis; the gait and balance including heel- and toe-walking and squat and return to upright; range of motion (ROM) of the lower extremities; and any muscle tightness, especially the hamstrings and quadriceps. Pay particular attention to hip ROM, which is best examined in the supine position. LBP and hip pain with limited hip range may indicate osteoarthritis or other hip abnormality. A full peripheral neurologic examination should be performed, including testing of reflexes, strength, and sensation.

9. Even though laboratory and imaging studies are not always accurate for diagnosing low back problems, should any tests be performed?

Imaging studies can be used to exclude severe disease. They are indicated only if red flags are present or if there is no improvement after several weeks of treatment. The initial study may be a plain x-ray. Other tests include bone scan, cross-sectional imaging (e.g., CT and MRI), and special tests, such as single photon emission CT (SPECT) scanning and discography. Remember that "abnormal" findings are expected on cross-sectional imaging. If leg pain is present, EMG, which is more specific than imaging, can be performed.

10. Is disability from LBP common?

Patients with disability from LBP present a very different picture from those with acute, acute recurrent, or even chronic LBP who are still functioning. Despite improvements in diagnostic and treatment techniques, disability from LBP has risen astronomically in the last couple of decades (as much as 2500%). We must look beyond pure physical explanation for this rise. Patients with disability from LBP that occurred either spontaneously or, more commonly, from an injury must also be assessed from a psychoemotional, social, and vocational viewpoint.

11. What are signs to look for in identifying the "disability syndrome"?

The most common associations that indicate disability from an injury are *not* physical ones. The best predictors are history of prior injury with time off work, high Minnesota Multiphasic

Personality Inventory (MMPI) scale 3 (hysteria), and high work dissatisfaction scales. History and physical examination features that may help identify this syndrome include past episodes of back pain that led to disability, a long history of tests and surgical procedures, and a very detailed description of the event that generated their problem. Usually the patient reports that someone or something is at fault (e.g., oil on the floor, extra work that the patient was not supposed to do). Pain is often rated as very severe, such as 9 or 10 on a 0–10 scale, with 10 being excruciating pain. The patient may indicate a 10-level pain while sitting comfortably in no apparent distress. Patients may be very demonstrative, grimace, position their bodies in unusual ways, complain of pain with minor movements, and have bizarre gait patterns. Check for Waddell's signs, which indicate that organic abnormality is not the primary factor in the patient's disability. These signs do not prove malingering but merely show that factors other than physical issues are significant contributors.

Signs (Waddell and Others) that LBP is Not Organic

- Simulated axial loading—pressure on the neck leading to LBP
- Simulated rotation—neck extension or rotation with back motion leading to LBP
- General overreaction to physical examination
- Superficial tenderness
- Regional weakness (not following anatomic patterns)
- Widespread nonanatomic distribution of pain
- Regional sensory deficient (not following anatomic patterns)
- Distracted straight-leg raising (e.g., sitting position vs. supine)

12. How do you treat the patient with acute LBP?

The offending structure is not known, and the natural history is to improve regardless of (or despite) treatment. Few treatments have proven to be beneficial, but several things may hasten the healing process. **Reassurance** can be very beneficial. Advise the patient that the process is "benign," will not lead to long-term impairment, and most likely will not need major intervention. **NSAIDs** can give the double benefit of pain relief and decreased inflammation. **Educate** the patient on proper back care and exercises. Other treatments for acute LBP are usually not necessary. Several studies suggest that **manipulation** during the first 3 weeks decreases painful episodes, but this is controversial. Mild exercise may be helpful.

13. Is bed rest helpful?

Bed rest was the mainstay of treatment at one time. However, a number of studies show that patients are better off doing as many normal activities as possible. This seems to shorten the course of disability and allow an earlier return to work. Thus, it is recommended that patients be up and about as much as tolerable and avoid anything that significantly increases pain.

14. What if the pain persists for several weeks after the initial treatment?

If pain persists, it is reasonable to do some minor investigations, staring with lumbosacral spine x-ray. Additional treatment depends on the severity of discomfort and degree to which it interferes with function. More tests and treatment can be performed, but the risk-benefit and cost-benefit ratios should be considered. If the pain remains severe, a regular therapy program can be instituted. Other treatments include trigger point injections with lidocaine (Xylocaine) or lidocaine with steroids; injections are easy to perform.

If pain does not resolve in several months and the individual is not disabled but is distressed, repeat reassurances because patients may fear severe illness. If not already performed, imaging studies are appropriate. Bone scan and MRI should be interpreted cautiously and correlated clinically. Determine the severity of pain perception and how it interferes physically, psychosocially, and psychoemotionally with function. Treatment options include medications such as NSAIDs, tricyclic antidepressants, and acetaminophen; injections including sacroiliac joint, facet joint, and local myofascial trigger points; and alternative medicine techniques such as acupuncture.

15. What about the patient who is disabled by the pain?

Other factors contributing to the pain must be identified. There has been a large movement toward treating "benign" or "nonmalignant" pain problems with opioid medications and various injections, disc dissolution techniques, device insertion (spinal stimulation, morphine pumps), and surgery. However, they are unlikely to treat the entire problem. When etiology is not clearly defined and there are multiple inorganic signs, treat the functional loss and disability. This type of patient is best served by an interdisciplinary team approach (not multidisciplinary) such as a functional restoration program.

16. Who should treat patients with LBP?

A variety of clinicians can initiate treatment, and it is appropriate for a primary care physician to start the process. Unfortunately, by the time patients see a specialist, they may have undergone an MRI and been told the pain is due to disc problems or other misinformation. It is difficult to "unteach" the patient, especially because the general population places such credence on MRI findings. Physiatrists (physical medicine and rehabilitation physicians) are the best next line of treatment. Ideally, a physiatrist would be the best primary physician as well.

17. Should neurosurgeons or orthopedic surgeons be consulted first?

Definitely not! If an internist has a patient with a gastrointestinal or cardiac problem that he cannot solve, does he send the patient to a GI surgeon or thoracic surgeon? No! The patient is referred to a gastroenterologist or cardiologist. After an expert evaluation and treatment, these specialists can make any appropriate surgical referrals. The same should occur with LBP, especially because internists receive less training in rehabilitation than in internal medicine subspecialities. In addition, a surgeon's primary training is in surgery. They will not have the knowledge of the total armamentarium that physiatrists have at their disposal.

18. What is the bottom line for LBP?

- LBP is ubiquitous in the human race and not a disease.
- Degenerative disc disease and some of the anatomic sequelae of facet arthropathy or spurring are usual consequences of aging.
- The natural history of LBP is to improve with or without treatment, but certain treatments can hasten the process and are worthwhile.
- There is little or no correlation between anatomic abnormalities seen on imaging studies and the patient's clinical symptoms or signs.
- It is the physiatrist's job to discover serious problems presenting as LBP by identifying the red flags outlined in the AHCPR guidelines. This guideline is worth requesting (remember that the guideline only applies to acute LBP).
- Treatment comprises reassurance, NSAIDs, and having the patient stay out of bed and be active.
- Disability from LBP is a different disorder than acute LBP, and a host of factors contribute to it. It must be evaluated and treated differently than acute LBP.
- Special injection techniques are sometimes indicated in patients with LBP.

BIBLIOGRAPHY

1. Agency for Health Care Policy and Research: Clinical Practice Guideline 14: Acute Low Back Pain in Adults. Rockville, MD, U.S. Department of Health and Human Services Public Health Service, 1994.
2. Cutler R, Fishbain D, Rosomoff H, et al: Does nonsurgical pain center treatment of chronic pain return patients to work? Spine 19:643–652, 1994.
3. Deyo R, Tsui-Wu Y: Descriptive epidemiology of low back pain and its related medical care in the United States. Spine 12:264–268, 1987.
4. Deyo R, Rainville J, Kent D: What can the history and physical examination tell us about low back pain? JAMA 268:760–765, 1991.
5. Dreyfuss P, Michaelsen M, Pauza K, et al: The value of medical history and physical examination in diagnosing sacroiliac joint pain. Spine 21:2594–2602, 1996.

6. Frymoyer J, Ducker T, Hadler N, et al (eds): The Adult Spine: Principles and Practice, Volume 1. New York, Raven Press, 1991.
7. Haldeman S: Diagnostic tests for the evaluation of back and neck pain. Neurol Clin 14:103–117, 1996.
8. Jensen M, Brant-Zawadzki M, Obuchoswki N, et al: Magnetic resonance imaging of the lumbar spine in people without back pain. N Engl J Med 331:69–73, 1994.
9. Leboeuf-Yde C, Kyvik K: At what age does low back pain become a common problem: A study of 29,424 individuals aged 12–41 years. Spine 23:228–234, 1998.
10. Malmivaara A, Hakkinen U, Aro T, et al: The treatment of acute back pain: Bedrest, exercise, or ordinary activity. N Engl J Med 332:351–355, 1995.
11. Sobel D, Schwartz T: Oh, Your Aching Back: A Sufferer's Guide to the Best Treatment. New Yorker Magazine (Mar):41–45, 1986.
12. Van Tulder M, Assendelft W, Koes B, Bouter LM: Spinal radiographic findings and nonspecific low back pain: A systematic review of observational studies. Spine 22:427–434, 1997.

38. LUMBAR DISC HERNIATION AND DISCOGENIC LUMBAR PAIN SYNDROME

Vincent J. Devlin, M.D.

1. Describe the prevalence and natural history of lumbar disc herniations. How do they differ from the prevalence and natural history of low back pain?

The lifetime prevalence of a lumbar disc herniation is approximately 2%. The natural history of sciatica secondary to lumbar disc herniation is spontaneous improvement in the majority of cases. Among patients with radiculopathy secondary to lumbar disc herniation, approximately 10–25% (0.5% of the population) experience persistent symptoms. These statistics are in sharp contrast to low back pain, which has a lifetime prevalence of 60–80% in the adult population. Although the natural history of acute low back pain is favorable in the majority of patients, the successful management of patients with chronic symptoms remains an enigma.

2. What is the typical history of a patient with a lumbar disc herniation?

Typically there is an attempt to link the onset of back and leg pain with a traumatic event, but frequently patients have experienced intermittent episodes of back and leg pain for months or years. Factors that tend to exacerbate symptoms include physical exertion, repetitive bending, torsion, and heavy lifting. Pain typically begins in the lumbar area and radiates to the sacroiliac and buttock regions. Radicular pain typically extends below the knee in the distrubution of the involved nerve root. Radicular pain may be accompanied by paresthesia and weakness in the distribution of the involved nerve root. Patients with a disc herniation generally report that pain in the leg is worse than low back pain. Pain tends to be exacerbated by sitting, straining, sneezing, and coughing and tends to be relieved with standing or bed rest.

3. Define cauda equina syndrome.

Cauda equina syndrome is defined as a complex of low back pain, sciatica, saddle hypoesthesia, and lower extremity motor weakness in association with bowel or bladder dysfunction. The mode of onset may be slow or rapidly progressive. The most common cause of cauda equina syndrome is a central lumbar disc herniation at the L4–L5 level. Expedient surgical treatment is advised.

4. Outline the physical examination of a patient with a suspected lumbar disc herniation.

The patient should be undressed. Observation may reveal the presence of a limp or a list (sciatic scoliosis). Spinal range of motion is assessed. A complete neurologic examination (sensory, motor, reflex testing) should be performed to identify the involved nerve root. Nerve root tension signs should be evaluated. Hip and knee range of motion should be assessed to rule out pathology involving these joints. Peripheral pulses (dorsalis pedis and posterior tibial) should be assessed to rule out peripheral vascular problems. A rectal exam should be performed in patients suspected of having cauda equina syndrome.

5. What are nerve root tension signs?

Tension signs are maneuvers that tighten the sciatic or femoral nerve and in doing so further compress an inflamed nerve root against a lumbar disc herniation. The supine straight leg raise test (Lasegue's test) and its variants (sitting straight leg raise test, bowstring test, contralateral straight leg raise test) increase tension along the sciatic nerve and are used to assess the L5 and S1 nerve roots. The femoral nerve stretch test (reverse straight leg raise test) increases tension along the femoral nerve and is used to assess the L2, L3, and L4 nerve roots.

6. Compare and contrast sciatica with other common clinical syndromes presenting with low back and/or lower extremity pain symptoms.

Sciatica: Leg pain rather than low back pain is the predominant symptom. Neurologic symptoms and signs are found in a specific nerve root distribution. Nerve root tension signs are present.

Nonmechanical back and/or leg pain: Pain is constant and minimally affected by activity and unrelieved with rest. Pain is usually worse at night or early morning (e.g., spinal tumor, infection).

Mechanical back and/or leg pain: Pain is exacerbated by activity, changes in position or prolonged sitting. Pain is relieved with rest especially in the supine position (e.g., degenerative disc patholgy, spondylolisthesis).

Neurogenic claudication: Low back and buttock pain, radiating leg or calf pain, worse with ambulation, worse with spinal extension, relieved with flexion maneuvers, absent nerve root tension signs (e.g., spinal stenosis).

7. Are routine lumbar radiographs helpful during the initial assessment of patients with a suspected acute lumbar disc herniation?

Routine lumbar radiographs are not typically helpful in the initial evaluation of patients with a suspected acute lumbar disc herniation. Although radiographs may show degenerative changes (disc space narrowing, osteophyte formation), there is a poor correlation between these findings and clinical symptoms because these findings are also present in asymptomatic patients. Guidelines suggested for ordering initial plain radiographs include:

- Patient age over 50 years
- Pain symptoms lasting for greater than 6–8 weeks
- History of trauma, cancer, night pain, rest pain, weight loss, drug or alcohol abuse, steroid use
- Elevated temperature
- Neurologic deficit
- Ankylosing spondylitis

8. What initial treatment is advised for patients with a suspected acute lumbar disc herniation?

Initial treatment options include a short period of bedrest (not to exceed 3 days), oral medications (NSAIDs, aspirin, analgesics), progressive ambulation, and patient education and reassurance. Use of injections such as selective nerve root blocks or epidurals can be considered. As acute pain subsides, physical therapy and aerobic conditioning are advised. If a patient fails to improve with 4–6 weeks of nonsurgical care, further evaluation is indicated. The optimal time for nonsurgical treatment ranges from a minimum of 4 weeks to a maximum of 6 months.

9. When clinical examination suggests the presence of an acute lumbar disc herniation, what is the preferred imaging test to confirm the diagnosis?

Magnetic resonance imaging (MRI) is the preferred imaging test because it provides the greatest amount of information about the lumbar region. It is unparalleled in its ability to visualize pathologic processes involving the disc, thecal sac, epidural space, neural elements, paraspinal soft tissue, and bone marrow. However, caution is indicated when interpreting results of MRI scans due to the high frequency of disc abnormalities in asymptomatic patients. It is critical to correlate imaging findings with clinical examination.

10. At what spinal level are symptomatic lumbar disc herniations most commonly diagnosed?

Most lumbar disc herniations occur at the L4–L5 and L5–S1 levels (90%). The L3–L4 level is the next most common level for a symptomatic lumbar disc herniation.

11. What terms are used to describe lumbar disc pathology noted on MRI?

Terms used to describe lumbar disc pathology noted on MRI include degeneration, annular tear, bulge, protrusion, extrusion, and sequestration (Fig. 1).

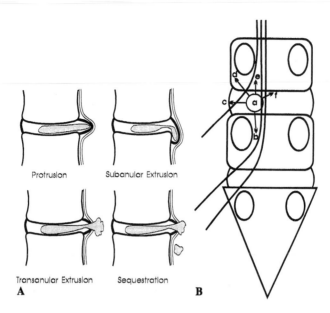

FIGURE 1. The four varieties of disc herniation. (From McCullough JA: Least invasive spine surgery at the L5–S1 level in adults. Spine State Art Rev 11:215–238, 1994, with permission.)

Degeneration: Decreased or absent T2-weighted signal is noted from the intervertebral disc. It is not possible to distinguish symptomatic from asymptomatic degeneration based on MRI.

Disc bulge: Disc material is noted to extend beyond the disc space with a diffuse, circumferential, nonfocal contour. Disc bulges are caused by early disc degeneration and infrequently cause symptoms in the absence of spinal stenosis.

Protrusion: Displaced disc material extends focally and asymmetrically beyond the disc space. The displaced disc material is in continuity with the disc of origin. The diameter of the base of the displaced portion, where it is continuous with the disc material within the disc space of origin, has a greater diameter than the largest diameter of the disc tissue extending beyond the disc space.

Extrusion: Displaced disc material extends focally and asymmetrically beyond the disc space. The displaced disc material has a greater diameter than the disc material maintaining continuity (if any) with the disc of origin.

Sequestration: Refers to a disc fragment that has no continuity with the disc of origin. By definition all sequestered discs are extruded. However, not all extruded discs are sequestered.

12. How is the location of a disc herniation within the spinal canal described?

The location of a disc herniation within the spinal canal is described in terms of a three-floor anatomic house (story 1 = disc space level, story 2 = foraminal level, story 3 = pedicle level) (Fig. 2). The spinal canal is also divided in terms of zones—central, foraminal, and extraforaminal. The central zone is located between the pedicles. The foraminal zone is located between the medial and lateral pedicle borders. The extraforaminal zone is located beyond the lateral pedicle border. This scheme is applicable to lumbar spinal stenosis syndromes as well as lumbar disc problems.

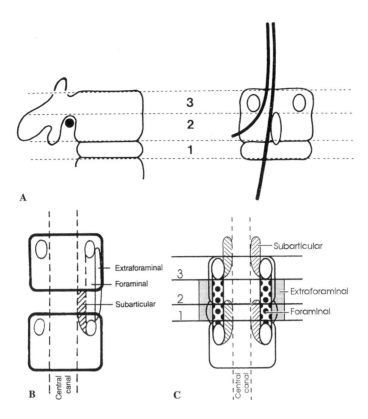

FIGURE 2. Locating the lumbar disc herniation. (From McCullough JA: Microdiscectomy: The gold standard for minimally invasive disc surgery. Spine State Art Rev 11:373–396, 1997, with permission.)

13. How does the location of a disc herniation along the circumference of the anulus of the disc determine the pattern of nerve root compression?

Discs herniations are described by their relationship along the circumference of the anulus fibrosus as central (midline), posterolateral (most common), foraminal, or extraforaminal. The location of the disc herniation determines the pattern of nerve root compression. The nerve roots of the lumbar spine exit the spinal canal beneath the pedicle of the corresponding numbered vertebra and above the caudad intervertebral disc. A posterolateral L4–L5 disc herniation compresses the L5 nerve root (the traversing nerve root of the L4–L5 motion segment). An L4–L5 foraminal or extraforaminal disc herniation compresses the L4 nerve root (the exiting nerve root of the L4–L5 motion segment). A central disc herniation compresses one or more of the caudal nerve roots.

14. What are the indications for surgical treatment for a lumbar disc herniation?

Occasionally an acute massive disc herniation can result in cauda equina syndrome, which is best managed by emergent surgical treatment. However, most patients undergo elective surgical treatment due to failure of radicular pain to improve with nonsurgical treatment. Surgical treatment is directed at improving the patient's leg pain. When the predominant symptom is back pain, symptom relief is unpredictable, and discectomy is not advised. Appropriate criteria for surgical intervention include:

- Functionally incapacitating leg pain extending below the knee within a nerve root distribution
- Nerve root tension signs with or without neurologic deficit
- Failure to improve with four to eight weeks of nonsurgical treatment

- Confirmatory imaging study (preferably MRI) which correlates with the patient's physical findings and pain distribution

15. What surgical procedure is recommended for treatment of a symptomatic lumbar disc herniation?

Open lumbar discectomy using microsurgical technique remains the gold standard for the treatment of a symptomatic lumbar disc herniation (Fig. 3). Important technical points include use of a small incision, limited muscle and bone dissection, and limited removal of displaced or loose disc material. A surgical microscope or headlight and loupe magnification is used to enhance intraoperative visualization. Uncomplicated patients typically go home within 24 hours of surgery and are able to return to work in 1 month. The success rate for relief of leg pain exceeds 90% in appropriately selected patients.

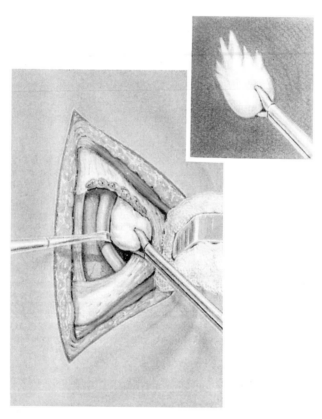

FIGURE 3. Lumbar disc fragment excision. (From McCullough JA: The lateral approach to the lumbar spine. Oper Tech Orthop 1:27, 55, 1991, with permission.)

16. How does the location of a disc herniation influence selection of the appropriate surgical approach?

Disc herniations located within the central spinal canal are treated through an interlaminar surgical approach. Disc herniations located in the extraforaminal zone are treated through an intertransverse surgical approach. The surgical approach for disc herniations located in the foraminal zone is determined by a combination of factors, including the level and size of the disc herniation. (See Fig. 4.)

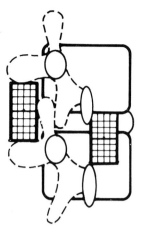

FIGURE 4. The two windows of opportunity into the spinal canal: interlaminar (right) and intertransverse (left). (From McCullough JA: The lateral approach to the lumbar spine. Oper Tech Orthop 1:27, 55, 1991, with permission.)

17. What are the surgical alternatives to microsurgical lumbar discectomy?

A variety of alternative procedures have been proposed. However, no procedure has demonstrated superior surgical outcomes compared with microsurgical lumbar discectomy. Alternative procedures include chymopapain, percutaneous automated discectomy, laser discectomy, and a variety of endoscopic surgical techniques.

18. What complications have been reported in association with microsurgical lumbar discectomy?

Fortunately complications are rare but may include:

- Vascular injury
- Nerve root injury
- Dural tear
- Infection
- Increased back pain
- Recurrent disc herniation
- Cauda equina syndrome
- Medical complications (e.g., thrombophlebitis, urinary tract infection)

19. What is the most common cause of surgical failure after lumbar disc excision?

Poor patient selection is the most common cause of treatment failure following lumbar discectomy. Other factors which may contribute to a poor surgical outcome include prolonged symptoms (> 6–12 months), abnormal pain behavior, workman's compensation situation, litigation, and tobacco use.

20. What is the incidence of recurrent disc herniation after microsurgical lumbar discectomy?

The incidence of recurrent disc herniation following microsurgical lumbar discecetomy is 5–10%. If symptoms are predominantly radicular, repeat lumbar discectomy may be beneficial. If symptoms include a combination of radiculopathy and low back pain, discectomy combined with fusion may be considered in select patients.

21. What is discogenic pain syndrome?

Discogenic pain syndrome has been defined as a continuum of diagnostic categories (internal disc disruption, degenerative disc disease, segmental instability) that reflect various stages of degenerative pathology affecting the intervertebral disc. Patients typically present with various degrees of low back pain and referred lower extremity pain symptoms. Radiographs do not show the presence of structural problems such as scoliosis or spondylolisthesis. MRI studies do not demonstrate disc displacement (e.g., protrusion, extrusion) but instead show degenerative changes such as decreased signal intensity, disc bulging, and annular tears. Treatment is difficult because of the lack of consensus regarding diagnostic criteria and absence of long-term data documenting successful treatment outcomes.

22. Which patients are appropriate candidates for surgical treatment for discogenic pain syndrome?

Lumbar fusion may be considered for treatment of low back pain of discogenic origin in patients who fail to improve after a minimum of six months of appropriate nonsurgical care. However, it is challenging to select surgical candidates who will benefit from lumbar fusion procedures for discogenic back pain. Many spine specialists use discography in an attempt to correlate patient symptomatology and imaging studies. Appropriate surgical criteria include:

- Patients with pain and disability for > 1 year
- Failure of aggressive physical conditioning and conservative treatment for > 6 months
- Single level degeneration on MRI with concordant pain response on discography
- Absence of psychiatric or secondary gain issues

Patients with multilevel disc degeneration (> 2 levels) are considered to be poor candidates for lumbar fusion surgery as procedures typically fail to provide significant benefit for such patients.

23. What surgical options are available for lumbar discogenic pain syndrome?

A wide range of fusion procedures have been advocated. Presently, an interbody fusion procedure is favored by many surgeons because it directly addresses the pain generator. Interbody fusion can be performed through an anterior approach (ALIF, or anterior lumbar interbody fusion) or posterior approach (PLIF, or posterior lumbar interbody fusion). A variety of implants can be used to promote interbody fusion, including autograft, allograft, and fusion cages used with autograft or bone morphogenetic protein. Posterior spinal instrumentation is commonly used in combination with interbody fusion. A posterolateral fusion may be combined with an interbody fusion. Minimally invasive laparoscopic and endoscopic approaches have been popularized in an attempt to decrease exposure-related surgical morbidity. Presently artificial disc replacement is being explored as an alternative to fusion procedures in this population.

BIBLIOGRAPHY

1. McCullough JA: Microdiscectomy: The gold standard for minimally invasive disc surgery. Spine State Art Rev 11:373–396, 1997.
2. McCulloch JA, Young PA: Essentials of Spinal Microsurgery. Philadelphia, Lippincott-Raven, 1998.
3. Weber H: Lumbar disc heniation: A controlled prospective study with ten years of observation Spine 8:131–140, 1983.
4. Zdeblick TA: Discogenic back pain. In Herkowitz HN, Garfin SR, Balderston RA, et al (eds): The Spine. Philadelphia, W.B. Saunders, 1999, pp 749–766.

39. LUMBAR SPINAL STENOSIS

Vincent J. Devlin, M.D.

1. What is lumbar spinal stenosis?

Lumbar spinal stenosis has been defined as any type of narrowing of the spinal canal, nerve root canals, or intervertebral foramen. This narrowing can be caused by soft tissue, bone, or a combination of both. The resultant nerve root compression leads to nerve root ischemia and a clinical syndrome associated with variable degrees of low back, buttock, and leg pain.

2. What are the two main types of spinal stenosis?

The two main types of spinal stenosis are (1) congenital-developmental and (2) acquired spinal stenosis. In the most widely accepted classification, spinal stenosis is subdivided into two congenital-developmental subtypes and six acquired subtypes.

Congenital-developmental stenosis
- Idiopathic
- Achondroplastic

Acquired stenosis
- Degenerative
- Combined congenital and degenerative stenosis
- Spondylolytic or spondylolisthetic
- Iatrogenic (after laminectomy, after fusion after chemonucleolysis)
- Posttraumatic
- Metabolic (e.g., Paget's disease, fluorosis)

3. What is the most common type of spinal stenosis?

The acquired degenerative type.

4. How does degenerative spinal stenosis develop?

Pathologic changes in the lumbar disc and facet joints are responsible for the development of spinal stenosis. With the passage of time, biochemical and mechanical changes in the intervertebral disc decrease its ability to withstand cyclic loading. These changes eventually lead to annular tears, loss of disc height, annular bulging, and osteophyte formation. A degenerative sequence also occurs posteriorly in the facet joint complex. Disc space narrowing increases loading on posterior facet and capsular structures, leading to joint erosion, loss of cartilage, and capsular laxity. Ultimately facet hypertrophy and osteophyte formation occur.

Osteophytes on the inferior articular process encroach medially, resulting in **central spinal canal stenosis.** Ligamentum flavum hypertrophy and annular bulging further contribute to stenosis involving the central spinal canal.

Osteophytes on the superior articular process enlarge anteriorly and medially, resulting in **lateral zone stenosis.** Osteophytes may also form circumferentially at the vertebral margins at the attachment of the anulus in an attempt to autostabilize the motion segment. Portions of these osteophytes, termed uncinate spurs, may protrude from the subjacent vertebral endplate or disc margin into the lateral nerve root canal above and provide an additional source of lateral nerve root entrapment. Loss of disc space height can further decreases the cross-sectional area of the neural foramen, leading to symptomatic lateral zone stenosis.

5. Discuss the epidemiology of spinal stenosis.

Spinal stenosis may present at any age (e.g., congenital type). However, the acquired degenerative type of spinal stenosis typically becomes symptomatic in the sixth and seventh decades of life. The most common levels of involvement in the lumbar region are L3–L4 and L4–L5. Up to 15% of patients with degenerative lumbar spinal stenosis have coexistent cervical spinal stenosis.

6. Describe the typical history reported by a patient with acquired degenerative spinal stenosis.

The typical patient reports the gradual onset of low back, buttock, thigh, and calf pain. Patients may report numbness, burning, or weakness in the lower extremities. The lower extremity symptoms may be unilateral or bilateral, depending on the location of spinal stenosis. Symptoms are exacerbated by activities that promote spinal extension, such as prolonged standing or walking (neurogenic claudication). Maneuvers that permit spinal flexion, such as sitting, lying down, or leaning forward on a shopping cart, tend to relieve symptoms because these positions increase spinal canal diameter. Changes in urinary function or impotence due to lumbar spinal stenosis are rare but occasionally noted.

7. What common conditions should be considered in the differential diagnosis of spinal stenosis?
- Degenerative arthritis involving the hip joints
- Peripheral neuropathy
- Vascular insufficiency
- Metastatic tumor

8. Compare and contrast the presentation of neurogenic claudication and vascular claudication.

Patients with **neurogenic claudication** report tiredness, heaviness, and discomfort in the lower extremities with ambulation. The distance walked until symptoms begin and the maximum distance that the patient can walk without stopping varies from day to day and even during the same walk. Patients report that leaning forward relieves symptoms. Patients may not experience symptoms during activities performed in a flexed posture, such as riding a bicycle or walking uphill. In contrast, activities performed in extension such as walking down hill tend to worsen symptoms. Patients with **vascular claudication** describe cramping or tightness in the calf associated with ambulation. The distance that they are able to walk before symptoms occur is constant. Their symptoms are not affected by posture. They are unable to tolerate walking uphill or cycling.

9. What findings are typically noted on physical examination of the patient with spinal stenosis?

Although most patients with lumbar spinal stenosis have significant subjective complaints, physical examination generally reveals few objective findings. The most frequent physical findings include reproduction of pain with lumbar extension, weakness of the extensor hallucis longus muscle, and sensory deficits over the lower extremities. Neurologic findings not otherwise detectable are sometimes demonstrated by performing a stress test (walking until symptoms occur and repeating the neurologic examination).

10. Summarize the role of radiographs, MRI, CT, and CT-myelography in the assessment of spinal stenosis.

Radiographs. Used to diagnose spinal deformities (scoliosis, spondylolisthesis. lateral listhesis). Flexion-extension radiographs are useful to diagnose spinal instabilities. Radiographs can also exclude pathologic processes such as neoplasm, infection or hip osteoarthiritis.

MRI. The best initial study for the diagnosis of spinal stenosis. In many cases it provides sufficient diagnostic information to eliminate the need for further diagnostic studies.

CT. Its strength is assessment of osseous anatomy in relation to spinal stenosis syndromes. It does not provide optimal soft tissue detail and does not typically visualize the entire lumbar region.

CT-myelography. An excellent test that is generally limited to the presurgical patient because of its invasive nature. It can visualize posturally dependent stenosis of the lumbar spinal canal that is not visible with any other imaging modality.

11. What are the options for nonsurgical management of lumbar spinal stenosis?
- Medication (NSAIDs, analgesics)
- Physical therapy (William's flexion exercises, functional stabilization exercises)
- General fitness and conditioning (cycling, pool exercise)
- Injections (epidurals, selective nerve root blocks)
- Gentle traction
- Transcutaneous electrical nerve stimulation (TENS)
- Lumbar orthoses

12. What are the indications for surgical treatment for patients with spinal stenosis?

Surgical treatment is indicated for patients with severe spinal stenosis accompanied by neurogenic claudication or intractable pain and for patients who fail to improve with appropriate nonsurgical treatment. Surgical treatment for spinal stenosis is elective except in the presence of bowel or bladder dysfunction (cauda equina syndrome).

13. What is the surgical treatment for lumbar spinal stenosis?

Surgical treatment for spinal stenosis consists of spinal decompression to remove structures (lamina, ligamentum flavum, hypertrophied portions of facet joints, uncinate spurs) that are responsible for compression of the dural sac and nerve roots. In certain specific situations a spinal fusion should be performed in addition to a spinal decompression.

14. Explain the basic steps involved in a midline decompresssion procedure for central spinal stenosis between L4 and S1.

A skin incision is made between L3 and S1. The paraspinal muscles are elevated from the lamina between L3 and S1. The L4 and L5 spinous processes are resected. The pars interarticularis is identified at each level to ensure that bone removal does not compromise its integrity. The hypertrophic lamina of L4 and L5 are thinned with a motorized burr to facilitate removal with angled Kerrison rongeurs. Adhesions between the dural sac and surrounding tissue are released with a Penfield elevator. Starting from the L5–S1 interspace, lamina and hypertrophic ligamentum flavum are resected between L4 and S1. The midline decompression should be widened to permit visualization of the lateral border of the dural sac as well as the medial border of the pedicle at each level (Fig. 1).

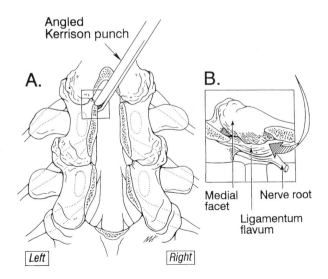

FIGURE 1. Decompression for central spinal stenosis. (From Stambough JL: Technique for lumbar decompression of spinal stenosis. Oper Tech Orthop 7:36–43, with permission.)

15. Explain the basic steps involved in decompression of lateral zone stenosis between L4 and S1.

Clinical evaluation and preoperative imaging studies are reviewed to determine the extent of lateral zone stenosis. Potential sources of neural compression include:

Zone 1 (also called the subarticular zone, entrance zone or lateral recess). Osteophytes from the superior articular process may compress the exiting nerve root in this zone.

Zone 2 (also called the foraminal zone, midzone, pedicle zone or hidden zone). A variety of pathology may cause nerve root impingement, including facet and ligamentum flavum hypertrophy, disc bulges, and uncinate spurs.

Zone 3 (also called the extraforaminal zone, exit zone or far-lateral zone). Nerve root compression may result from disc protrusion, uncinate spurs, facet subluxation, and ligamentous structures.

After the midline decompression is completed, each nerve root in the surgical field must be inspected and decompressed (Fig. 2). Each nerve root is identified along the medial border of its respective pedicle. Medial facet overgrowth and ligamentum flavum hypertrophy are resected with a Kerrison rongeur. The goal is to undercut the facet joint without sacrificing its integrity. The intervertebral disc is palpated or visualized to ensure that it is not causing significant nerve root compression. Resection of disc and/or uncinate spurs is performed as necessary to enlarge the foramen. Adequacy of decompression is checked by assessing the ability to retract the nerve root 1 cm medially and laterally without tension at the entrance zone. In addition, it should be possible to pass a blunt probe dorsal and volar to the nerve root out through the neural foramen (zone 3) without resistance.

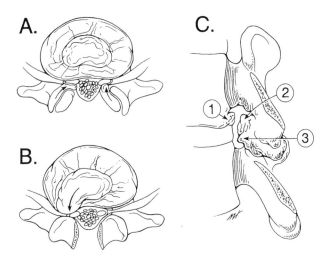

FIGURE 2. Decompression for lateral zone stenosis. **A,** Zone 1—stenosis due to hypertrophy of the superior articular process. **B,** Zone 2—stenosis due to disc bulging and uncinate spurs. **C,** Zone 3—stenosis due to (1) uncinate spur, (2, 3) superior articular process hypertrophy. (From Stambough JL: Technique for lumbar decompression of spinal stenosis. Oper Tech Orthop 7:36–43, with permission.)

16. What complications may occur with lumbar decompression procedures for spinal stenosis?

- Dural tears
- Arachnoiditis
- Infection
- Nerve root injury
- Spinal instability
- Inadequate decompression
- Persistent symptoms
- Recurrent stenosis

17. What are the indications for fusion in lumbar spinal stenosis procedures?

The indications for fusion fall into two broad categories:

1. Preoperative structural problems that predispose to instability after decompression
   - Degenerative spondylolisthesis or lateral listhesis
   - Progressive scoliosis or kyphosis
   - Recurrent spinal stenosis requiring repeat decompression at the same level
2. Intraoperative structural alterations that warrant consideration of a fusion
   - Excess facet joint removal ($> 50\%$)
   - Pars interarticularis fracture or removal
   - Radical disc excision with resultant destabilization of the anterior spinal column

18. What types of fusion are performed for unstable spinal stenosis syndromes?

The most common type of fusion procedure is a posterior fusion combined with posterior pedicle screw fixation. Interbody fusion may be added for patients with severe coronal and sagittal imbalance, rotatory subluxations, marked foraminal stenosis (to provide indirect decompression through restoration of foraminal height), or biologic factors that negatively affect posterior fusion success.

BIBLIOGRAPHY

1. Arnoldi CC, Brodsky AE, Cauchoix J et al: Lumbar spinal stenosis and nerve root entrapment syndromes. Definition and classification. Clin Orthop 115:4–5, 1976.
2. Bridwell KH, DeWald RL (eds): The Textbook of Spinal Surgery, 2nd ed. Philadelphia, Lippincott-Raven, 1997.
3. Devlin VJ: Degenerative lumbar spinal stenosis and decompression. Spine State Art Rev 11:107–128, 1997.
4. Hanley EN JR, Eskay ML: Degenerative lumbar spinal stenosis. Adv Orthop Surg 8:396–403, 1995.
5. Herkowitz HN, Sidhu KSD: Lumbar spine fusion in the treatment of degenerative conditions: Current indications and recommendations. J Am Acad Orthop Surg 3:123–135, 1995.
6. Katz JN, Lipson SJ, et al.: Seven- to ten-year outcome of decompressive surgery for degenerative lumbar spinal stenosis. Spine 21:92–98, 1996.
7. Wiltse LL, Kirkaldy-Willis WH, McIvor GW: The treatment of spinal stenosis. Clin Orthop 115: 83–91, 1976.

VII. Pediatric Spinal Deformities and Related Disorders

40. BACK PAIN IN CHILDREN

Mary Hurley, M.D., and Vincent J. Devlin, M.D.

1. Discuss the epidemiology of back pain in children.

The prevalence of back pain in children is less than in the adult population. Studies report a 10–30% incidence of back pain in children. Only 8% of children seek medical attention for back pain symptoms. Disability or temporary inability to participate in school or sports secondary to back pain occurs in 8% of pediatric patients. Complaints of back pain are rare before age 10 and increase between 12 and 15 years of age. Among pediatric patients who seek evaluation for back pain, the likelihood of diagnosis of a definable cause of symptoms is higher than in adult patients and ranges between 22% and 84% in various studies.

2. What is the differential diagnosis of back pain in children?

1. **Mechanical disorders**
   - Muscle strain
   - Overuse syndrome
   - Fracture
   - Herniated disc
   - Slipped vertebral apophysis
   - Spondylolysis/spondylolisthesis
2. **Developmental disorders**
   - Scheuermann's kyphosis
   - Spondylolysis/spondylolisthesis
3. **Inflammatory disorders**
   - Discitis
   - Vertebral osteomyelitis
   - Tuberculosis
   - Sacroiliac joint infection
   - Rheumatologic disorders
4. **Neoplastic disorders**
   - Benign primary spine tumors
   - Malignant primary spine tumors
   - Metastatic tumors
   - Spinal cord/canal tumors
   - Tumors of muscle origin
5. **Psychogenic Pain**
6. **Referred pain from visceral disorders**
   - Pneumonia
   - Pyelonephritis
   - Retrocecal appendicitis
7. **Idiopathic back pain**

3. What are the most common causes of back pain in skeletally immature patients referred to a tertiary pediatric orthopedic center for evaluation?

Spondylolysis or spondylolisthesis (30%), Scheuermann's disease (30%), spinal tumor or infection (20%), undetermined cause (15%), and referred pain from visceral disorders (5%).

4. Why is the child's age often helpful in narrowing the diagnosis?

No diagnosis is unique to a single age group. However, some generalizations can help in determining the most likely diagnosis:

Less than 10 years old: disc space infection, vertebral osteomyelitis and certain tumors (eosinophilic granuloma, leukemia, astrocytoma, neurobalastoma).

Older than 10 years: disorders involving repetitive loading and trauma, such as spondylolysis, spondylolisthesis, Scheuermann's kyphosis, fractures, lumbar disc herniation, and apophyseal ring injury.

5. What information should be obtained in a history for evaluation of back pain?
- Duration of pain symptoms (acute, greater than 1 month, chronic)
- Location of pain (cervical vs. thoracic vs lumbar)
- Frequency of symptoms (intermittent, constant)
- Aggravating and alleviating factors
- Timing
- History of trauma
- Recreational activites

Red flags that should prompt further work-up include a history of systemic symptoms (fever, weight loss), neurologic complaints (numbness, weakness, bowel or bladder difficulty), and non-mechanical pain (night pain, pain at rest).

6. How should the physical examination be performed?
The physical exam must take place with the child undressed and appropriately gowned. All systems should be examined thoroughly. The child should be observed for posture, stance, and gait. The spine should be assessed for tenderness, alignment, and flexibility. A forward bend test should be performed to assess for symmetry and flexibility. Spinal deformity (kyphosis, scoliosis) should prompt further assessment. Suspicion of underlying disease is prompted by spinal tenderness, decreased spinal range of motion, spasticity, hamstring tightness, and skin abnormalities (hemangioma, midline hairpatch). The neurologic examination should carefully document motor strength, sensation, deep tendon reflexes, and symmetry of abdominal reflexes. The musculoskeletal examination includes assessment of all muscle groups for tenderness or limited range of motion.

7. What laboratory tests are useful for evaluation of back pain in children?
Useful laboratory tests include a complete blood count (CBC) with differential, erythrocyte sedimentation rate (ESR), and C-reactive protein. These tests are recommended for young children with a history of night pain or constitutional symptoms. If a rheumatologic disorder is considered in the differential diagnosis, additional useful tests include a rheumatoid factor, antinuclear antibody (ANA), and HLA-B27.

8. What imaging studies play a role in evaluation of the child with back pain?
- Plain radiographs
- Technetium bone scans
- Computed tomography (CT)
- Magnetic resonance imaging (MRI)

9. When are radiographs indicated for evaluation of the child with back pain?
Anteroposterior (AP) and lateral spinal radiographs are the best first imaging test for a child with back pain. Spinal radiographs are indicated for initial evaluation of children 4 years old or younger, children who report pain symptoms for greater than 1 month, children who report that back pain awakens them from sleep, and children with constitutional symptoms.

10. When is a technetium bone scan indicated for evaluation of a child with back pain?
If a child with back pain has normal spinal radiographs and does not have a neurologic deficit, a technetium bone scan should be obtained. This test is quite sensitive for diagnosing spinal problems such as infections, tumors, and occult fractures. Single-photon emission computed tomography (SPECT) provides increase sensitivity and specificity compared with a planar bone scan and is used when a planar bone scan is negative or equivocal. SPECT is especially helpful in the diagnosis of spondylolysis.

11. When is an MRI scan indicated for evaluation of a child with back pain?

Children presenting with back pain and an abnormal neurologic exam require evaluation with a spinal MRI. MRI is the method of choice for evaluation of the spinal column and neural axis. It is useful for defining abnormalities such as tumor, infection, disc herniation, Arnold Chiari malformation, syrinx, and tethering of the spinal cord. Because it is a noninvasive test, it has largely replaced CT myelography. Disadvantages of MRI include the need for anesthesia when the study is required in very young children and the danger of attributing symptoms to imaging findings that are clinically irrelevant.

12. When is a CT scan indicated for evaluation of a child with back pain?

CT is the method of choice for evaluation of a bone lesion diagnosed on plain radiographs or a technetium bone scan. Spinal CT provides the clearest depiction of bone detail and plays an important role in assessment of fractures, spondylolysis, spondylolisthesis, and tumors.

13. What guidelines aid the practitioner in pursuing an effective and sytematic approach to the child with back pain?

An algorithm has been developed to guide patient assessment based on data obtained from clinical history and physical exam.[1] The algorithm takes into account three factors:

1. Mechanism of injury: clear or unclear
2. Nature of symptoms / physical findings: local vs. systemic vs. neurologic
3. Duration of symptoms: less than 1 month vs. greater than 1 month

The patient may enter into the algorithm at any stage based on findings noted in the history and physical exam. The patient may progress from a lower to a higher level based on the above three factors. The algorithm has four levels:

Level 1

- Mechanism: clear history of specific injury
- Nature of symptoms/findings: symptoms localized to back pain
- Duration of symptoms: less than 1 month
- Studies/ action needed: symptomatic treatment (activity restriction, NSAIDs) and follow-up in 1 month. If symptoms persist, advance to level 2.

Level 2

- Mechanism: history unclear
- Nature of symptoms: back pain without systemic or neurologic signs, minor physical findings (spinal asymmetry, hamstring spasm), progression from level 1
- Duration of symptoms: greater than 1 month
- Studies/ action needed: PA and lateral radiographs of entire spine (LS spine radiographs if spondylolysis/spondylolisthesis suspected). Positive radiographs (Scheuermann's disease, spondylolysis, significant scoliosis) can be referred to a specialist. Patients with negative radiographs can be observed or advanced to level 3, depending on clinical judgment.

Level 3

- Mechanism: history unclear
- Nature of symptoms: back pain with systemic symptoms (fever, weight loss)
- Duration of symptoms: greater than 1 month
- Studies/ action needed: CBC, ESR, C-reactive protein, and bone scan in addition to spinal radiographs. Patients with negative findings on these studies require only symptomatic treatment as most serious disorders have been excluded. Patients with positive studies require specialty referral.

Level 4

- Mechanism: history unclear
- Nature of symptoms: back pain with neurologic deficit or patients advanced from level 3
- Duration of symptoms: generally greater than 1 month but not always
- Studies/ action needed: MRI and/or CT is obtained in addition to level 3 studies (radiographs, CBC, ESR, C-reactive protein, bone scan). Refer patient to surgeon for assessment for surgical treatment.

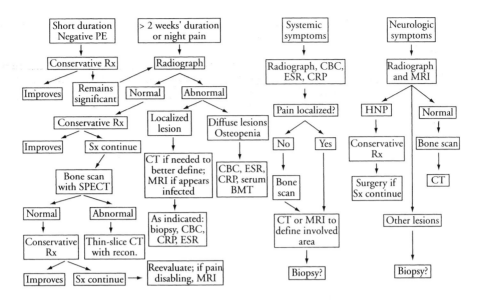

FIGURE 1. Diagnostic algorithm for back pain in children. (From Ecker ML: Back pain. Spine State Art Rev 14:236, 2000, with permission.)

14. How is a muscle strain diagnosed in children?

History and physical exam are usually sufficient to establish the diagnosis of muscle strain. A short history of localized pain, no neurologic findings, and association with physical activity are typical. The pain should resolve within a few weeks. The treatment for muscle strain is activity modification, ice, and NSAIDs. If the pain does not resolve with this treatment, reevaluation is needed.

15. Define spondylolysis.

Spondylosis is a defect in the pars interarticularis. The defect is unilateral in 20% and bilateral in 80% of cases.

16. Who is at risk for spondylolysis?

Children engaged in repetitive activities involving hyperextension of the spine. Commonly associated sporting activities include gymnastics, diving, dancing, wrestling, and football.

17. How is spondylolysis diagnosed?

History and physical examination are important indicators of spondylosis. A history of hyperextension activities should alert the clinician to the possibility of the diagnosis. Patients typically present with back pain radiating into the buttocks. Physical examination reveals tenderness to palpation, hamstring tightness, decreased forward flexion of the lumbar spine and a stiff gait. Lateral radiographs may reveal a pars defect. Oblique views can more clearly delineate the pars interarticularis. Bone scan with SPECT can help define pars defects. CT scan delineates the defect most clearly.

18. How is spondylolysis treated?

Activity modification, bracing, physical therapy, and NSAIDs are the basis of nonoperative therapy. Surgical intervention is rarely needed. Surgical options include repair of the pars defect or a posterolateral fusion.

19. Define spondylolisthesis. How is it diagnosed in children?

Spondylolisthesis is a forward slippage of a vertebra in relation to the adjacent inferior vertebra. The most common type of spondylolisthesis in children is the isthmic type, which occurs when bilateral pars defects allow the upper vertebra to slide forward on the lower vertebra, usually L5 on S1. A standing lateral lumbar radiograph is the best test for making the diagnosis. MRI plays a role when there is a need to assess the intervertebral disc or if a neurologic deficit is present. CT scan plays a role when details about formation of the posterior spinal elements (dysplasia) are indicated.

20. What treatment is recommended for spondylolisthesis?

Low-grade slips (< 30–50%) do not require active treatment if the patient is asymptomatic. Such patients should be followed closely for slip progression through skeletal maturity. Symptomatic low-grade slips should undergo initial nonoperative treatment, including activity modification, physical therapy, NSAIDs, and bracing, before considering surgical treatment (spinal fusion). Higher-grade slips (> 50%) are generally treated with spinal fusion.

21. What is Scheuermann's disease? How does it present in children?

Scheuermann's disease is a disorder of endochondral ossification that alters the development of the vertebral endplate and ring apophysis. It may lead to intraosseous disc herniation, anterior wedging of the vertebral body, and kyphotic deformity. Scheuermann's disease may affect either the thoracic or lumbar region.

In the thoracic region, three consecutive wedged vertebra (> 5°), irregular upper and lower vertebral endplates, apparent loss of disc space height, and increased thoracic kyphosis that does not correct when the patient lies supine are criteria for diagnosis. Patients typically are referred for assessment of the associated kyphotic deformity, which is occasionally associated with pain over the apex of the kyphosis. Scheuermann's kyphosis should be differentiated from postural round back, which is a flexible deformity that reduces when the patient lies supine.

Patients with Scheuermann's disease in the lumbar region present with back pain. Spinal deformity is generally not a significant problem. Patients generally report a history of strenuous physical activity or acute injury. Radiographs show vertebral endplate irregularities, intraosseous disc herniation (Schmorl's nodes), and disc space narrowing.

22. What treatment is recommended for Scheuermann's disaease?

Most patients with Scheuermann's disease involving the thoracic region can be successfully treated with exercise, bracing, and supportive care. Surgical intervention can be considered for persistent pain associated with a kyphotic deformity exceeding 75°. Scheuermann's disease involving the lumbar region is generally treated with activity modification and occasionally with an orthosis.

23. Is idiopathic scoliosis commonly associated with severe pain in children?

No. Idiopathic scoliosis is not a cause of severe back pain in children. Up to one-third of patients with adolescent idiopathic scoliosis report mild, intermittent, and nonspecific back pain. When persistent severe back pain is noted in the presence of a spinal curvature, further work-up is indicated to determine the source of pain. Conditions such as infection, tumor, syringomyelia, or disc herniation may cause secondary scoliosis.

24. What is the difference between discitis and vertebral osteomyelitis?

In the past, a distinction was made between discitis (infection invoving the disc space) and osteomyelitis (infection in the vertebral body). Studies have shown that in children the vascular supply crosses the vertebral endplate from vertebral body to the disc space. As a result, discitis and vertebral osteomyelitis are considered to represent a continuum termed infectious spondylitis. Hematogenous seeding of the vertebral endplate leads to direct spread of infection into the disc space. Subsequently, infection involving the disc space and both adjacent vertebral endplates may progress to osteomyelitis. Vertebral fracture and epidural abscess may occur if the infection is permitted to progress without treatment. *Staphylococcus aureus* is the most frequently isolated bacteria. Tuberculosis is prevalent in developing countries and should be considered in children who have traveled outside of the United States to endemic areas.

25. Describe the presentation, work-up, and treatment for spinal infection in a child.

Children may present with back, abdominal, or leg pain symptoms. The child may limp or refuse to walk. When asked to pick something up from the floor, the child generally avoids bending over and squats in an attempt to keep the spine straight. Some children may appear quite ill with a fever, whereas others are afebrile and report minimal pain.

Radiographs are typically normal during the first month. Bone scans demonstrate increased uptake even in the early stages of infection. MRI is the most sensitive and specific imaging test and demonstrates the extent of the lesion as well as the presence or absence of an epidural abscess. Laboratory studies may be helpful in making the diagnosis. The white blood cell count is elevated in less than 50% of cases. The ESR is elevated in over 90% of patients. C-reactive protein is a more specific indicator of infection and may be useful in diagnosis as well as evaluation of treatment. Blood cultures should be drawn before starting antibiotics, because 50% yield an organism. Disc space cultures are not necessary for diagnosis and yield positive results in only 60% of cases. *S. aureus* is the most commonly isolated organism.

Treatment consists of intravenous antibiotics, casting, or bracing as needed. Surgical treatment is rarely needed. Early in the disease process with minimal tissue destruction, intravenous antibiotics may be sufficient treatment. In the presence of significant bony destruction, kyphotic deformity, or soft tissue abscess, surgical intervention is indicated.

26. How does a lumbar disc herniation present in children?

Lumbar disc herniation is less common in children than adults. In contrast to adults, children commonly have a history of acute injury or chronic repetitive injury. The child may present with back pain and/or radicular leg pain. Physical examination may reveal reduced lumbar range of motion and a positive Lasegue's sign. Neurologic changes and bowel and bladder compromise are rare in adolescents. Initial treatment includes activity reduction, NSAIDs, ice, and physical therapy. Surgery is reserved for prolonged symptoms or neurologic involvement. Whereas 85% of adult patients experience resolution of acute symptoms by 6 weeks, 75% of adolescents do not improve with nonsurgical treatment.

27. What is a slipped vertebral apophysis?

Slipped vertebral apophysis or apophyseal ring fracture is a fracture through the junction of the vertebral body and the cartilagenous ring apophysis. This injury is possible prior to complete fusion of the cartilagenous ring apophysis, which occurs at approximately 18 years of age. Most injuries occur at the L4–L5 or L5–S1 level. This traumatic injury presents most often in males who participate in sports requiring repetitive flexion combined with rotation. Patients present with symptoms similar to a central disc herniation. Surgery is frequently necessary to excise the bone fragment with attached cartilage and disc.

28. What benign spinal tumors are most commonly found in children?

The most common benign tumors involving the spine in children are osteoid osteoma, osteoblastoma, aneurysmal bone cyst, and eosinophilc granuloma (Langerhans cell histiocytosis). Aneurysmal bone cyst, osteoid osteoma, and osteoblastoma typically involve the posterior spinal column. Eosinophilc granuloma typically involves the anterior spinal column and classically manifests as a vertebra plana.

29. What is the most common malignant condition in the pediatric population?

Acute leukemia is the most common malignancy in children. Back pain may be the presenting symptom. This condition should be suspected in a child less than 10 years old with pain at night. Additional findings include anemia, increased white blood cell count, increased ESR, vertebral compression fractures, diffuse osteopenia, and metaphyseal bands.

30. What primary bone tumors are most likely to involve the spine in the pediatric population?

Osteosarcoma and Ewing's sarcoma.

31. What are the most common spinal cord tumors in children?

Astrocytoma and ependymoma.

32. What is the most prevalent malignant condition that produces skeletal metastases in children?

Neuroblastoma. Up to 80% of patients develop spinal metastases.

33. What soft tissue sarcoma is most likely to involve the spine in the pediatric population?

Rhabdomyodarcoma.

34. Do children and adolescents present with nonorganic causes for back pain?

Yes. Children and adolescents may present with back pain for which a specific physical cause cannot be found. Conversion disorders are rare but do occur. Compensation is a consideration in children with an appropriate history, such as a recent motor vehicle accident. "Pain disorder with psychological factors" is the preferred diagnosis when pain is the focus of clinical presentation in the absence of a definite physical cause. Frank discussion with the patient and family may yield an obvious stressor in the family, such as a recent death, divorce, move, or school problems. An integrated approach, including the primary care physician, psychologist or psychiatrist, social worker, and physical therapist, helps to diagnose and treat such patients.

BIBLIOGRAPHY

1. Davids JR, Wenger DR: Back pain in children and adolescents. J Musculoskel Med 19–32, 1994.
2. DeLuca PF, Mason DE, Weiand R, et al: Excision of herniated nucleus pulposus in teenage children and adolescents. J Pediatr Orthop 14:318–322, 1994.
3. Ecker ML: Back pain. Spine State Art Rev. 14:233–248, 2000.
4. Epstein NE: Lumbar surgery for 56 limbus fractures emphasizing noncalcified type 3 lesions. Spine 17: 1489–1496, 1992.
5. Ginsburg GM, Bassett GS: Back pain evaluation in children and adolescents: Evaluation and differential diagnosis. J Am Acad Orthop Surg 5:67–78, 1997.
6. King HA: Back pain in children. Pediatr Clin North Am 31:1083–1095, 1984.
7. Ring D, Johnson CE, Wenger DR: Pyogenic infectious spondylitis in children: The convergence of discitis and vertebral osteomyelitis. J Pediatr Orthop 15:652–660, 1995.

41. PEDIATRIC CERVICAL DISORDERS

Thomas R. Haher, MD

GENERAL CONCEPTS

1. What family of genes regulates development of the vertebral column?

The homeobox or *Hox* genes regulate embryonic differentiation and segmentation of the developing vertebral column.

2. What anatomic features differentiate the immature cervical spine from the adult cervical spine?

Unique anatomic features of the immature cervical spine include hypermobility, hyperlaxity of ligamentous and capsular structures, presence of epiphyses and synchondroses, incomplete ossification, and unique configuration of the vertebral bony elements (e.g., wedge-shaped vertebral bodies).

3. When does the immature cervical spine approach adult size and shape?

The immature cervical spine approaches adult size and shape around age 8 years.

4. How does a child's age affect the pattern of traumatic cervical spine injury?

Before age 8 years, most cervical injuries occur at C3 or above and are associated with a high risk of fatality. After age 8, cervical injury patterns are similar to adults and occur below the C4 level and are less likely to be fatal.

5. How does a child's age affect the position for immobilization during initial evaluation of a suspected traumatic cervical spine injury?

Up to age 8 years, children have a large cranium in relation to their thorax. If children < 8 years of age are immobilized on a routine backboard, the cervical spine will be flexed and fracture deformity may be increased. Use of a double mattress to elevate the thorax or use of a recess for the occiput is recommended.

TORTICOLLIS

6. Define torticollis.

Torticollis is a clinical diagnosis based on head tilt in association with a rotatory deviation of the cranium.

7. What is the most common type of torticollis?

Congenital muscular torticollis is the most common type of torticollis. It presents in the newborn period. Its cause is unknown, but it has been hypothesized to arise from compression of the soft tissues of the neck during delivery, resulting in a compartment syndrome. Radiographs of the cervical spine should be obtained to rule out congenital vertebral anomalies. Clinical exam reveals spasm of the sternocleidomastoid muscle on the *same* side as the tilt causing the typical posture of head tilt toward the tightened muscle and chin rotation to the opposite side. Initial treatment is stretching and is successful in up to 90%. Surgery is considered for persistent deformity after one year of age. Common problems seen in patients with congenital muscular torticollis include congenital hip dysplasia and plagiocephaly (facial asymmetry).

8. What are some other causes of torticollis?

When torticollis presents after the newborn period, the etiology is wide-ranging and may result from pathology involving any structure in the head or neck region:

- Congenital anomalies of the craniocervical junction or upper cervical spine
- Ocular or auditory dysfunction
- Tumors involving the posterior fossa, brainstem or spinal cord
- Osseous tumors (osteoid osteoma, aneurysmal bone cyst)
- Infection
- Inflammatory disorders (juvenile rheumatoid arthritis, disc calcification)
- Fracture
- Rotatory subluxation of the atlantoaxial joints
- Sandifer's syndrome (gastroesophageal reflux and torticollis)

9. What features suggest that torticollis is due to atlantoaxial rotatory subluxation?

Features that suggest that torticollis is due to atlantoaxial rotatory subluxation include prior normal cervical alignment and motion, history of recent upper respiratory infection before developing torticollis (Grisel's syndrome), normal neurologic exam, and spasm in the sternocleidomastoid muscle on the side *opposite* the head tilt. This posture has been termed the "cock robin" deformity. It is distinct from congenital muscular torticollis, in which muscle spasm occurs on the side of the head tilt. Plain radiographs are frequently difficult to interpret but typically show asymmetry of the C1 lateral masses on the AP odontoid view. A dynamic rotational CT scan can be obtained to confirm the diagnosis.

10. How is atlantoaxial rotatory subluxation classified?

Type 1: rotatory displacement without anterior shift of C1
Type 2: rotatory displacement with anterior shift of 5 mm or less
Type 3: rotatory displacement with an anterior shift > 5 mm
Type 4: rotatory displacement with a posterior shift

11. Describe the treatment of atlantoaxial rotatory subluxation.

When the problem is diagnosed early, many children respond well to immobilization with a soft cervical collar and activity restriction. If early follow-up shows persistent subluxation, inpatient treatment with traction via a head halter is indicated. If reduction occurs (confirmed clinically and by CT), immobilzation is continued for at least 6 weeks with a Minerva cast or halo cast. Surgery is indicated for failure of reduction following traction treatment, recurrent subluxation, neurologic involvement and deformities present for more than three months. Posterior C1–C2 arthrodesis is the most commonly performed surgical procedure.

CONGENITAL ANOMALIES

12. What serious problems are associated with congenital anomalies of the cervical region?

Recognition of congenital anomalies involving the cervical region is important because of their association with spinal deformity, spinal instability, and spinal cord and brainstem compression resulting in myelopathy. Other organ system anomalies may be associated with cervical spine anomalies because these systems share common embryonic development.

13. What are some commonly diagnosed cervical spinal anomalies?

Cervical anomalies may be broadly grouped into those located in the upper cervical region (occiput–C2) and those occurring in the subaxial cervical region (C3–C7).

Occiput–C2 region
1. Congenital anomalies associated with neural compression
   - Basilar impression
   - Congenital cervical stenosis
   - Arnold-Chiari malformation
2. Anomalies associated with cervical instability at occiput–C1
   - Occipitalization of C1
   - Down's syndrome

3. Anomalies associated with C1–C2 problems
   - Odontoid anomalies (aplasia, hypoplasia, os odontoideum)
   - Down's syndrome

Subaxial cervical region

1. Anomalies associated with deformity and instability
   - Klippel-Feil anomaly
2. Miscellaneous Disorders
   - Postlaminectomy kyphosis
   - Neurofibromatosis

14. What is basilar impression?

Basilar impression is a downward displacement of the base of the skull in the area of the foramen magnum. It is identified by the protrusion of the tip of the odontoid through the foramen magnum. The most significant clinical problems associated with congenital basilar impression are due to anterior or posterior brainstem compression with or without atlantoaxial instability. It is the most common congenital anomaly of the upper cervical spine.

15. What are the different types of basilar impression?

There are two main types of basilar impression: primary and secondary. The primary type is most common. This congenital anomaly is frequently associated with other vertebral defects, including atlanto-occipital fusion, odontoid abnormalities, Klippel-Feil anomaly, and hypoplasia of the atlas. Secondary basilar impression arises as the result of softening of osseous structures at the base of the skull. Diseases associated with secondary basilar impression include osteomalacia, rickets, Paget's disease, osteogenesis imperfecta, renal osteodystrophy, and rheumatoid arthritis.

16. What clinical problems result from basilar impression?

Patients present with a short neck, painful cervical motion and asymmetry of the skull and face. Additional clinical problems include nuchal pain, vertigo, long tract signs with associated cerebellar ataxia, falling, and lower cranial nerve involvement resulting in dysarthria and dysphagia.

17. How is the diagnosis of basilar impression confirmed radiographically?

The lateral craniocervical radiograph is the initial study obtained. The position of the tip of the dens is assessed in relation to the various skull base lines (McGregor, McRae, Chamberlain). MRI or CT-myelography with sagittal reconstructions is helpful to assess the exact postion of the dens in relation to the foramen magnum and to assess neural compression.

18. What treatment is indicated for symptomatic basilar impression?

Treatment typically involves decompression and stabilization. Options for decompression include anterior transoral odontoid resection or posterior suboccipital craniectomy and C1 laminectomy.

19. What is the Arnold-Chiari malformation?

The Arnold-Chiari malformation is a developmental anomaly in which the brainstem and cerebellum are displaced caudally into the spinal canal. In type 1 Arnold-Chiari malformation the cerebellar tonsils are displaced into the cervical spinal canal. This malformation is associated with other cervical anomalies including basilar impression and Klippel-Feil syndrome. Dense scarring at the level of the foramen magnum may lead to hydromyelia or syringomyelia. Type 2 Arnold-Chiari malformation is a more complex anomaly and is usually associated with myelomeningocele. Cerebellar displacement is accompanied by elongation of the fourth ventricle as well as displacement of the fourth ventricle and cervical nerve roots.

20. How is occipitocervical instability defined radiographically?

Occipitocervical instability is defined as greater than 1mm of translation measured from the basion to the posterior margin of the anterior arch of C1 on lateral flexion-extension views.

21. What is Steel's "rule of thirds"?

Steel noted that the area of the spinal canal at the C1 level in a normal person could be divided into equal thirds with one third occupied by the odontoid process, one third by the spinal cord and one third as empty space (Fig. 1). The empty space serves as a safe zone into which displacement can occur without neurologic impingement. In the presence of atlantoaxial instability, the safe zone may decrease resulting in spinal cord compression.

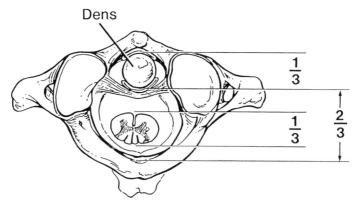

FIGURE 1. Steel's rule. (From Moskovich R: Atlanto-axial instability. Spine State Art Rev 8:533, 1994, with permission.)

22. How is atlantoaxial instability defined radiographically?

Atlantoaxial instability is defined as an increased mobility between the anterior surface of the odontoid and the posterior aspect of the anterior arch of the atlas. This measurement is called the atlantodens interval (ADI) and is measured from lateral flexion-extension radiographs. The upper limit of normal for the ADI in children is 4 mm. An ADI greater than 4 mm is considered pathologic and represents failure of the transverse ligament. An ADI greater than 10 mm suggests failure of the secondary supporting ligaments, including the alar ligaments, with increased risk of neurologic compromise. In patients with chronic atlantoaxial instability the odontoid may be hypermobile resulting in an increased ADI in the absence of clinical symptoms. In this situation, measurement of the space available for the cord (SAC) is more helpful in assessing pathologic instability. The SAC is measured from the posterior margin of the odontoid to the closest posterior sturcture, either the foramen magnum or the posterior ring of C1 (Fig. 2). An SAC < 13 mm indicates insufficient space for the spinal cord and may be associated with neurologic problems.

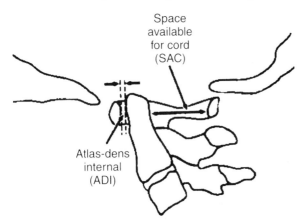

FIGURE 2. Measurements for atlas-dens interval (ADI) and the space available for the cord (SAC) as determined on lateral cervical radiographs. (From Herman MJ, Pizzutillo PD. Cervical spine disorders in children. Orthop Clin North Am 320: 457–475, 1999, with permission.)

23. What are the major causes of nontraumatic atlantoaxial instability?

The major causes can be categorized into three groups:

1. Anomalies of the odontoid process (e.g., os odontoideum)

2. Ligamentous laxity (e.g., Down's syndrome, juvenile rheumatoid arthritis, osteo-chodrodystrophies)

3. Synotosis at adjacent spinal levels (e.g., Klippel-Feil anomaly, occipitalization of the atlas)

24. Define os odontoideum and explain its most likely etiology.

Os odontoideum is an acquired nonunion of the odontoid process. It appears as an ossicle separated from the body of the axis which results from resorption of an occult fracture of the dens. The atlantoaxial joint becomes unstable as the odontoid becomes unable to function as a peg. Associated symptoms range from mild neck pain to myelopathy and sudden death secondary to minor trauma. Surgery is considered in the presence of neurologic deficit, C1–C2 instability > 10 mm on flexion-extension radiographs or persistent neck pain.

25. What patterns of upper cervical instability are seen in patients with Down's syndrome?

Patients with Down's syndrome develop congenital instability of both the atlanto-occipital joints and the atlantoaxial joints. It is important to rule out atlanto-occipital instability prior to performing a fusion of the atlantoaxial joints. In addition, atlanto-occipital instability may develop following a successful atlantoaxial fusion. The underlying problem is generalized ligamentous laxity present in this patient population. Caution is advised when surgical treatment is undertaken in this population because of the high risk of surgical complications.

26. What is the clinical triad described by Klippel-Feil syndrome?

Klippel-Feil syndrome has been classically described as the clinical triad of a short neck, low posterior hairline, and limitation of cervical motion. The spinal anomaly associated with Klippel-Feil syndrome is congenital fusion of the cervical spine. The classic triad is seen in less than 50% of cases. The number of fused segments may vary from two segments to fusion of the entire cervical spine.

27. Why is early recognition of Klippel-Feil syndrome important?

Klippel-Feil anomalies are a marker that should prompt investigation for a wide range of systemic anomalies. Because the embryologic development of cervical spine parallels the development of many other organ systems, a wide range of congenital anomalies may be present, including anomalies involving the genitourinary, cardiovascular, auditory, gastrointestinal, skeletal, and neurologic systems. The most common neurologic abnormality is synkinesis, which causes unconcious mirror movement that mimic movement by the opposite extremity. Associated skeletal system anomalies include Sprengel's deforrmity (failure of descent of the scapula) and cervical ribs.

28. What work-up should be performed for a patient diagnosed with Klippel-Feil syndrome?

Diagnosis of a congenital cervical fusion should prompt assessment of the genitourinary system (renal ultrasound), cardiac system (echocardiogram, cardiology referral), and auditory system (hearing test). Neurologic symptoms should be evaluated with a MRI of the brainstem and cervical spine.

29. Are any patterns of congenital cervical fusion associated with an increased risk of neurologic deficit?

Three fusion patterns are considered to be associated with an increased risk of neurologic problems:

1. C2–C3 fusion with occipitalization of the atlas

2. A long cervical fusion in the presence of an abnormal occipital-cervical junction

3. A single open interspace between two fused spine segments

BIBLIOGRAPHY

1. Copley LA, Dormans JP. Cervical spine disorders in infants and children. J Am Acad Orthop Surg 6:204–214, 1998.
2. Drummond DS. Congenital Anomalies of the Pediatric Cervical Spine. Textbook of Spinal Surgery.2nd Ed, Bridwell KH, DeWald RL(Eds), Lippincott-Raven, Philadelphia, 1997, p951–968.
3. Dubousset J: Torticollis in children caused by congenital anomalies of the atlas. J Bone Joint Surg 68A: 178–188, 1986.
4. Fielding JW, Hawkins RJ: Atlantoaxial rotatory fixation(fixed subluxation of the atlantoaxial joint). J Bone Joint Surg 59A: 37–44, 1977.
5. Hensinger RN, Fielding JW. The cervical spine, in Morrissy RT (ed): Lovell and Winter's Pediatric Orthopaedics, 3rd ed. Philadelphia, JB Lippincott, 1990, p703–740.
6. Hensinger RN, Lang JE, MacEwen GD. Klippel-Feil syndrome: a constellation of associated anomalies. J Bone Joint Surg56A:1246–1253, 1974.
7. Herman MJ, Pizzutillo PD. Cervical spine disorders in children. Ortho Clin of North Am Vol 30 No. 3 457–475, 1999.
8. Herzenberg JE, Hensinger RN, Dedrick DK, Phillips WA. Emergency transport and positioning of young children who have an injury of the cervical spine: the standard backboard may be hazardous. J Bone Joint Surg 71A: 15–22, 1989.
9. Koop SE, Winter RB, Lonstein JE: The surgical treatment of instability of the upper part of the cervical spine in children and adolescents. J Bone joint Surg 66A: 403–411, 1984
10. Moskovich R: Atlanto-axial instability. Spine State Art Rev 8:531–549, 1994.

42. IDIOPATHIC SCOLIOSIS

Vincent J. Devlin, M.D.

1. What is idiopathic scoliosis?

Idiopathic scoliosis is the most common type of scoliosis. At present it is uncertain whether this deformity represents a single disease entity or reflects a similar clinical expression of several different disease states. Idiopathic scoliosis is defined as a spinal deformity characterized by lateral bending and fixed rotation of the spine in the absence of any known cause. The criterion for diagnosis of scoliosis is a coronal plane spinal curvature of 10° or more as measured by the Cobb method. Curves less than 10° are referred to as spinal asymmetry. Idiopathic scoliosis is classified according to age at onset into infantile (0–3 years), juvenile (3–10 years) and adolescent (> 10 years) subtypes. In general, the younger the age at diagnosis, the more likely the deformity is to progress and require treatment.

2. What causes idiopathic scoliosis?

The cause of idiopathic scoliosis is the focus of ongoing research. A significant problem associated with this research is the difficulty in distinguishing whether observed changes are secondary to the spinal deformity or whether they are the cause of the deformity. Areas under investigation include:

- Genetic factors: due to the higher incidence of scoliosis within families compared to the general population
- Central nervous system factors: CNS asymmetry, vestibular dysfunction
- Collagen, muscle, and platelet defects
- Growth and hormonal factors: asymmetric spinal growth patterns, melatonin
- Biomechanical factors

3. List characteristic features of infantile idiopathic scoliosis.

- Common in Europe but rare in the United States (<1% of cases in U.S.)
- Male predominance (vs. adolescent idiopathic scoliosis, which is more common in females).
- Left thoracic curve pattern is most common (vs. adolescent idiopathic scoliosis, in which right-sided thoracic curves are typical).
- Association with plagiocephaly, mental retardation, congenital heart disease, and developmental hip dysplasia.
- Two types have been identified: a resolving type (85%) and a progressive type (15%).

4. How are resolving and progressive infantile curve types distinguished?

Resolving and progressive curve types are distinguished by analyzing the relationship between the apical vertebra of the thoracic curve and its ribs on an anteroposterior (AP) radiograph in order to determine the **rib-vertebral angle difference (RVAD)** and **rib phase.** The rib vertebral angle is determined by a line perpendicular to the endplate of the apical vertebra and a line drawn along the center of the rib (Fig. 1). The rib vertebral angle difference is calculated by subtracting the angle of the convex side from the concave side. A RVAD greater than 20° indicates that curve progression is likely. Rib phase is assessed by determining the amount of overlap between the convex rib head and the apical vertebral body. If the convex rib does not overlap the vertebral body (phase 1), progression is unlikely. As the curve increases, the apical convex rib overlaps the vertebral body (phase 2) and further curve progression is likely.

5. How is infantile idiopathic scoliosis treated?

Resolving type curves are observed with serial physical exams and radiographs. Sleeping in the prone position is recommended. Progressive curves are treated with serial casting followed by a Milwaukee brace. Curves that continue to progress despite orthotic treatment require surgery. Options include anterior and posterior spinal fusion or spinal instrumentation without fusion to delay definitive fusion until the child has achieved additional trunk growth. Posterior fusion alone is not recommended due to the likelihood of the crankshaft phenomenon (persistent anterior spinal growth in the presence of a posterior fusion, leading to recurrent and increasing spinal deformity).

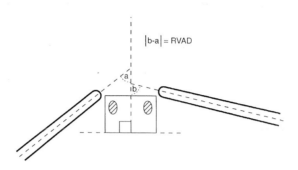

FIGURE 1. The rib-vertebral angle difference (RVAD). (From Ginsberg GM: Scoliosis and kyphosis. In Brown DL, Neumann RD (eds): Orthopedic Secrets. Philadelphia, Hanley & Belfus, 1999, with permission.)

6. What are the characteristic features of juvenile idiopathic scoliosis?

Juvenile idiopathic scoliosis represents a gradual transition from the characteristics of infantile idiopathic scoliosis to those of adolescent idiopathic scoliosis. Its characteristic features include:

- Less common than adolescent idiopathic scoliosis (12–16% of all patients with idiopathic scoliosis).
- Increasing female predominance noted with increasing age (female-to-male ratio is 1:1 between 4–6 years and increases to 8–10:1 between age 6–10 years).
- Curve patterns tend to be right thoracic and double major curve types.
- Approximately 70% of curves progress and require some forms of treatment (bracing or surgery).
- Total spine MRI should be considered in this group (also in infantile idiopathic scoliosis) since spinal deformity may be the only clue to the presence of a coexistent neural axis abnormality potentially requiring treatment.

7. List characteristic features of adolescent idiopathic scoliosis.

- Most common type of scoliosis in children (prevalence is 3% in the general population), but few patients (0.3%) develop curves requiring treatment.
- A female predominance is noted, which increases substantially for larger curves requiring treatment.
- Thoracic curve patterns are generally convex to the right (atypical curve patterns are an indication for MRI).
- Idiopathic scoliosis in adolescence is rarely associated with pain.

8. Describe the initial evaluation for a patient referred for assessment for adolescent idiopathic scoliosis.

1. **Patient history:** includes age of onset of menarche, inquire as to existence of a family history of scoliosis

2. **Physical examination**
- Height and weight
- Observation (look for shoulder, thorax or waist asymmetry).
- Adams forward bend test. The right and left sides of the trunk should be symmetrical. Presence of a thoracic or lumbar prominence suggests scoliosis. Use a scoliometer to quantitate asymmetry.
- Neurologic assessment includes motor strength testing, deep tendon reflexes, abdominal reflexes (abnormalities may indicate intraspinal pathology such as syringomyelia), plantar reflexes, clonus testing.
- Upper and lower extremity assessment includes gait and leg length evaluation.

3. **Radiographic assessment.** A standing posteroanterior (PA) 36-inch cassette radiograph is the initial view obtained. Lateral radiographs are indicated when sagittal plane abnormalities are noted on physical exam, for patients with back pain, when spondylolisthesis is suspected, and for presurgical planning prior to scoliosis correction. Side-bending radiographs are reserved for presurgical planning prior to scoliosis surgery and are not required for initial patient evaluation.

9. What radiographic parameters should be assessed on the PA radiograph?

Identify the end vertebra , apical vertebra, curve location, curve direction, curve magnitude, and Risser sign.

1. **End vertebra.** The top and bottom vertebra that tilt maximally into the concavity of the curve are termed the end vertebra. They are typically the least rotated and least horizontally displaced vertebra within the curve.

2. **Apical vertebra.** The apical vertebra is the central vertebra within a curve. It is typically the least tilted, most rotated, and most horizontally displaced vertebra within a curve.

3. **Curve location.** The curve location is defined by its apex:

Curve	Apex
Cervicothoracic	C7–T1
Thoracic	T2–T11
Thoracolumbar	T12–L1
Lumbar	L2–L4
Lumbosacral	L5–S1

4. **Curve direction.** Curve direction is determined by the side of the convexity. Curves convex toward the right are termed right curves, while curves convex to the left are termed left curves.

5. **Curve magnitude.** The Cobb-Lippman technique is used to determine curve magnitude. Perpendicular lines are drawn with reference to lines along the superior endplate of the upper end vertebra and along the inferior endplate of the lower end vertebra. The angle created by the intersection of the two perpendicular lines is termed the Cobb angle and defines the magnitude of the curve.

6. **Risser sign.** The Risser sign describes the ossification of the iliac epiphysis. The iliac crest is divided into quarters and the stage of ossification is used as a guideline to assess skeletal maturity: grade 0 : absent; grade 1 (0–25%); grade 2 (26–50%); grade 3 (51–75%); grade 4 (76–100%); grade 5 (fusion of epiphysis to the ilium). Risser stage 4 correlates with the end of spinal growth. Risser stage 5 correlates with the end of height increase (Fig. 2).

10. Define structural curve, nonstructural curve, major curve, minor curve, full curve, and fractional curve.

Many patients have a combination of fixed and flexible spinal deformities. Side-bending radiographs are used to assess the flexibility of curves that comprise a spinal deformity. Curves that correct completely when the patient bends toward the convexity of the curve are termed **nonstructural curves.** Curves that do not correct completely are termed **structural curves.** Nonstructural curves permit the shoulders and pelvis to remain level to the ground and permit the head to remain centered in the midline above the pelvis. For this reason, nonstructural curves are also referred to as **compensatory curves**. Over time, compensatory curves may develop structural characteristics. Full curves and fractional curves are distinguished by assessing the angular displacement of the end vertebra of the curve. Curves in which both end vertebrae are tilted from the horizontal are termed **full curves.** Curves that have one end vertebra parallel to the ground are termed **fractional curves.**

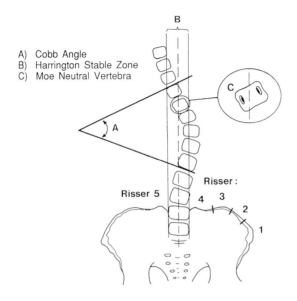

A) Cobb Angle
B) Harrington Stable Zone
C) Moe Neutral Vertebra

FIGURE 2. Measurement for idiopathic scoliosis. Note the Cobb angle **(A)**, Harrington's stable zone **(B)**, Moe's neutral vertebra **(C)**, Risser's staging, and the center sacral line (dashed line). (From Stefko RM, Erickson MA: Pediatric orthopaedics. In Miller MD (ed). Review of Orthopaedics, 3rd ed. Philadelphia, W.B. Saunders, 2000, with permission.)

11. What are the neutral and stable vertebrae?

The neutral vertebrae are the first nonrotated vertebra at the caudal and cranial ends of a curve. Rotation is assessed based on the radiographic appearance of the vertebral pedicle shadow in reference to the lateral margins of the vertebral body (Nash-Moe classification). The stable vertebra is the vertebra bisected by the center sacral line (a vertical line extending cephalad from the S1 spinous process).

12. What is the King-Moe classification?

The King-Moe classification (Fig. 3) of thoracic curve patterns in idiopathic scoliosis distinguishes five curve types as a guide to surgical treatment:

Type 1: S-shaped curve in which both the thoracic and lumbar curves cross the midline and in which the lumbar curve is larger than thoracic curve or less flexible than the thoracic curve.

Type 2 : S-shaped curve in which the thoracic curve is larger or less flexible than the lumbar curve (also called a "false" double major curve).

Type 3: single thoracic curve without a structural lumbar curve.

Type 4: long thoracic curve in which L5 is centered over the sacrum and L4 is tilted into the thoracic curve.

Type 5: double thoracic curve with T1 tilted into the convexity of the upper curve.

The King classification does not address lumbar curves, thoracolumbar curves, double major curves, or triple major curves. It was developed to guide surgical treatment in the era of Harrington instrumentation.

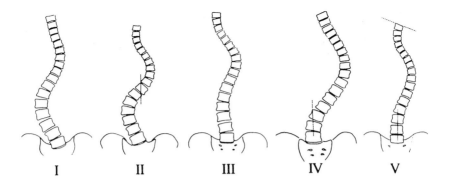

FIGURE 3. Five types of idiopathic scoliosis as defined by King, Moe, Bradford, and Winter.[2] (From Roach JW: Adolescent idiopathic scoliosis. Orthop Clin North Am 30(3), 1999, with permission.)

13. What is the comprehensive classification system for idiopathic scoliosis described by Lenke and colleagues?

As decision-making for scoliosis surgery has become more complex, an alternative classification system has been developed. This classification is based on assessment of both PA and lateral radiographs. Six curve types are identified:

1. Primary thoracic
2. Double thoracic
3. Double major
4. Triple major
5. Primary thoracolumbar or lumbar
6. Primary thoracolumbar or lumbar with a secondary thoracic curve

The six main curve types are subclassified as A, B, or C based on relationship of the center sacral vertical line (CSVL) to the lumbar spine. A thoracic sagittal modifier is assigned to further define curve types based on sagittal plane alignment (Fig 4).

14. What are the treatment options for adolescent idiopathic scoliosis?

The treatment options for adolescent idiopathic scoliosis include observation, orthoses, and operation (the three O's). There is no evidence that exercise programs, electrical stimulation, special diets, chiropractic adjustment, acupuncture, or other nontraditional treatment methods are effective in preventing curve progression or correcting established curves.

15. What is the purpose of observation for adolescent idiopathic scoliosis?

The purpose of observation for adolescent idiopathic scoliosis is to identify and document curve progression and thereby facilitate timely intervention. Curves less than 20° are observed.

16. What are the risk factors for curve progression in skeletally immature patients with idiopathic scoliosis?

- Future growth potential of the patient (assessed by a variety of factors, including Risser stage, Tanner stage, menarche, peak height velocity, triradiate physeal closure)
- Curve magnitude at the time of diagnosis
- Curve pattern (double curves progress more frequently than single curves)
- Female sex (curves in females are more likely to progress than curves in males)

17. What patients with adolescent idiopathic scoliosis are likely to experience progression of untreated curves in adulthood?

Curves measuring less than 30° at maturity are least likely to progress. Curves measuring 30–50° degrees are likely to progress an average of 10–15° over the course of a normal lifetime.

Curves measuring 50–75° at maturity progress steadily at a rate of approximately 1° per year. Lumbar and thoracolumbar curves are more likely to progress than thoracic curves because they lack the inherent stability provided by the rib cage.

			Curve Type	
Type	Proximal Thoracic	Main Thoracic	Thoracolumbar/ Lumbar	Curve Type
1	Non-Structural	Structural (major*)	Non-Structural	Main Thoracic (MT)
2	Structural	Structural (major*)	Non-Structural	Double Thoracic (DT)
3	Non-Structural	Structural (major*)	Structural	Double Major (DM)
4	Structural	Structural (major*)	Structural	Triple Major (TM)
5	Non-Structural	Non-Structural	Structural (major*)	Thoracolumbar/Lumbar (TL/L)
6	Non-Structural	Structural	Structural (major*)	Thoracolumbar/Lumbar-Main Thoracic (TL/L - MT) Lumbar Curve>Thoracic by ≥5°

STRUCTURAL CRITERIA
(Minor Curves)

*Major = Largest Cobb Measurement, always structural
Minor = All other curves with structural criteria applied

Proximal Thoracic: - Side Bending Cobb ≥ 25°
- T2 - T5 Kyphosis ≥+20°

LOCATION OF APEX
(SRS definition)

Main Thoracic: - Side Bending Cobb ≥ 25°
- T10 - L2 Kyphosis ≥20°

CURVE	APEX
THORACIC	T2 - T11-12 DISC
THORACOLUMBAR	T12 - L1
LUMBAR	L1-2 DISC - L4

Thoracolumbar/Lumbar: - Side Bending Cobb ≥ 25°
- T10 - L2 Kyphosis ≥+20°

Modifiers

Lumbar Spine Modifier	CSVL to Lumbar Apex		Thoracic Sagittal Profile T5 - T12		
A	CSVL Between Pedicles		-	(Hypo)	< 10°
B	CSVL Touches Apical Body(ies)		N	(Normal)	10° - 40°
C	CSVL Completely Medial	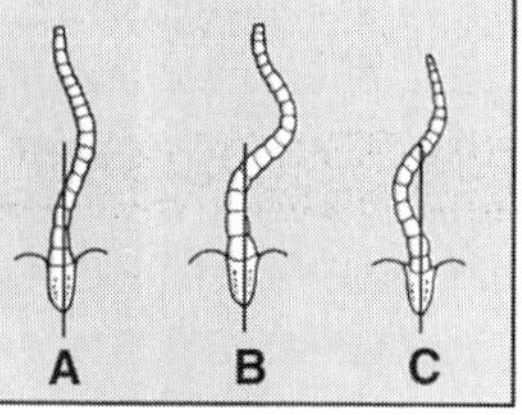 A B C	+	(Hyper)	> 40°

Curve Types (1- 6) + Lumbar Spine Modifier (A, B, or C) + Thoracic Sagittal Modifier (-, N, or +)
Classification (e.g. 1B+):_____

FIGURE 4. Lenke's system of classification for idiopathic scoliosis. (From Hurley ME, Devlin VJ: Idiopathic scoliosis. In Fitzgerald RH, Kaufer H, Malkani AL (eds): Orthopaedics. St. Louis, Mosby, 2000, with permission.)

18. What are the consequences of untreated adolescent idiopathic scoliosis?

Natural history studies of untreated adolescent idiopathic scoliosis in adult patients focus on:

1. **Mortality rate.** The mortality rate of untreated adult patients with adolescent idiopathic scoliosis is comparable to that of the general population. Patients with untreated adolescent idiopathic scoliosis do not typically develop respiratory failure and premature death. Patients with adolescent idiopathic scoliosis must be distinguished from patients with early onset scoliosis (before age 5) who develop severe curves (> 90°). Patients with early onset scoliosis may develop cor pulmonale and right ventricular failure, resulting in premature death.

2. **Pulmonary and cardiac function.** Marked limitation of forced vital capacity does not occur until thoracic curves approach 90° in the absence of marked hypokyphosis. Only in thoracic curve patterns is there a direct correlation between curve magnitude and negative effects on pulmonary function.

3. **Back pain.** The incidence of back pain in adult scoliosis patients is comparable with the

general population. Patients with large lumbar curves report an increased incidence of low back pain, particularly if the apical vertebra develops a significant lateral translation.

4. **Self-image.** Spinal deformity and its negative effect on self image remain a significant issue for many adult scoliosis patients. These issues are frequently the reason adult patients seek treatment for idiopathic scoliosis.

19. When is bracing indicated for adolescent idiopathic scoliosis?

Patients who are Risser stage 0–1 and premenarchal with curves 20–29° are candidates for bracing. In the Risser stage 2–4 patient with a curve of 20–29°, progression of 5° should be documented before bracing is initiated. Patients presenting with curves of 30–40° should be braced immediately if they are skeletally immature. Patients and families should be advised that a spinal orthosis is used to prevent curve progression and generally does not lead to permanent curve improvement. The best predictor of successful brace treatment is the initial correction achieved in the brace. If a curve is corrected by 50% or more upon initiation of bracing, there is a good chance brace treatment will be successful.

20. When is brace treatment contraindicated?

Relative contraindications to brace treatment include:
- Skeletally mature patients
- Curves > 40°
- Thoracic lordosis (bracing potentiates cardiopulmonary compromise)
- Patients unable to cope emotionally with treatment

21. What types of braces are used?

The general types of orthoses used for adolescent idiopathic scoliosis are:
- CTLSO (Milwaukee brace). Used less commonly due to its cosmetic appearance. However, for curves with an apex above T8, it remains the orthosis of choice by many specialists.
- TLSO (e.g., Boston brace). These lower-profile orthoses are better accepted by patients and are indicated for curves with an apex at T8 or below.
- Bending brace (e.g., Charleston brace). This type of brace holds the patient is an acutely bent position in a direction opposite to the curve apex. It is worn only during sleep. It has been advocated as an alternative to full-time bracing regimens.

22. When is surgery indicated for adolescent idiopathic scoliosis?

For the immature adolescent, surgery is indicated for curves > 40° that are progressive despite brace treatment. Select thoracic curves greater than 30° may require surgery if they are progressive and associated with thoracic lordosis (due to concerns about future cardiorespiratory compromise secondary to decreased intrathoracic volume). Select lumbar or thoracolumbar curves greater than 35° associated with significant coronal imbalance and waist line assymmetry may be considered for surgical treatment. In the mature adolescent, surgery is considered for curves greater than 50°. It is not possible to indicate patients for surgery based solely on the coronal Cobb angle. Additional factors to consider in decision-making include sagittal plane alignment, rotational deformity, the natural history of the patient's curve, and the patient's skeletal maturity.

23. What treatment options exist when surgery is indicated?

- Posterior spinal instrumentation and fusion
- Anterior spinal instrumentation and fusion
- Anterior spinal fusion combined with posterior spinal instrumentation and fusion

24. Explain what is involved in a posterior spinal instrumentation and fusion procedure for adolescent idiopathic scoliosis.

The posterior surgical approach is applicable to all idiopathic scoliosis curve types. During the surgical procedure the posterior spinal structures are exposed, the facet joints are excised, and autogenous iliac crest bone graft is packed into the facet joints and over the decorticated posterior spinal elements. Posterior spinal instrumentation is placed and used to correct the spinal deformity. Spinal implants used to achieve fixation to the posterior spinal elements may include hooks, wires (cables) and/or pedicular screws. The typical instrumentation construct consists of two parallel rods attached to the spine at multiple sites (posterior segmental spinal instrumentation). The rods are connected at their cephalad and caudad ends by cross-link devices, thereby creating a rigid rectangular construct (Fig. 5).

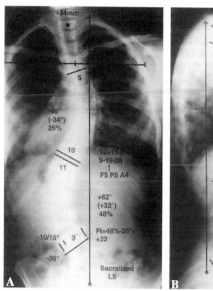
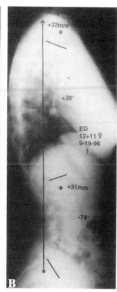
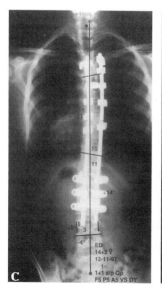
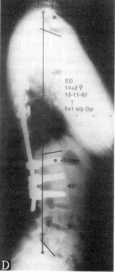

FIGURE 5. Posterior spinal instrumentation and fusion. Preoperative PA (**A**) and lateral (**B**) radiographs of a 13-year old girl with a King-Moe type 1 curve. Postoperative radiographs (**C, D**) show a typical posterior segmental spinal instrumentation construct. (From Asher MA: Anterior surgery for throacolumbar and lumbar idiopathic scoliosis. Spine State Art Rev 12:708–709, 1998, with permission.)

25. Explain what is involved in an anterior spinal instrumentation and fusion procedure for adolescent idiopathic scoliosis.

Anterior spinal instrumentation and fusion procedures (Fig. 6) are most commonly indicated for single thoracic, thoracolumbar, or lumbar curve types. The convex side of the curve is exposed. The thoracic spine is approached via a thoracotomy. The thoracolumbar and lumbar spine is exposed through a thoracophrenolumbotomy, which includes release of the diaphragm attachment to the lateral chest wall. The disc, annulus, and cartilagenous vertebral endplates are excised over the levels undergoing fusion. The disc spaces are packed with morselized bone graft. Structural spacers are placed in the disc spaces in the lumbar region. This structural spacer may be an allograft cortical ring (femur or humerus) or a metallic fusion cage. Vertebral body screws are placed across the vertebral body to engage the opposite vertebral cortex to achieve bicortical fixation. The screws are subsequently linked to rod(s), and corrective forces are applied to the spine. Single- or double-rod systems may be used, depending on a variety of factors such as patient body habitus, curve location, and patient willingness to wear a postoperative orthosis. Minimally invasive approaches utilizing thoracoscopic instrumentation and fusion can potentially decrease approach related morbidity in select cases.

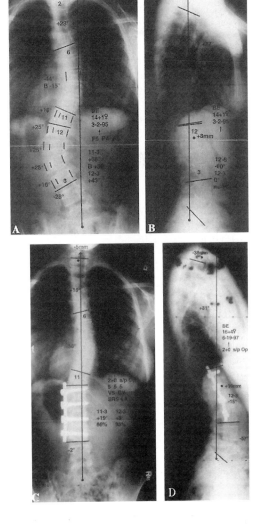

FIGURE 6. Anterior spinal instrumentation and fusion. Preoperative PA (**A**) and lateral (**B**) radiographs of a 14-year old girl with left thoracolumbar major and right thoracolumbar compensatory scoliosis. Postoperative radiographs (**C, D**) show correction following anterior spinal instrumentation and fusion. (From Asher MA: Anterior surgery for thoracolumbar and lumbar idiopathic scoliosis. Spine State Art Rev 12:706–707, 1998, with permission.)

26. When are combined anterior and posterior spinal procedures indicated for adolescent idiopathic scoliosis?

- Large stiff curves (e.g., > 75–$90°$ depending on curve flexibility and location)
- To prevent the crankshaft phenomenon (Risser stage 0 patients with open triradiate cartilages, patients prior to peak height velocity)
- To address coexistent sagittal plane deformities (e.g., excessive thoracic lordosis, hyperkyphosis)

In these situations, the anterior procedure consists of multilevel discectomy and fusion. This may be performed through an open surgical approach or through a minimally invasive thoracoscopic approach. Anterior surgery is followed by posterior segmental spinal instrumentation and fusion to provide correction of the spinal deformity.

27. What is a thoracoplasty?

Thoracoplasty is a procedure performed during a spinal instrumentation and fusion operation for scoliosis to decrease the magnitude of the convex thoracic rib prominence. The medial portions of the convex ribs are excised in order to restore symmetry to the posterior thoracic cage. The procedure may be performed from either an anterior or posterior surgical approach.

28. What potential complications are associated with scoliosis surgery?

The risks of perioperative complications have diminished with modern techniques of anesthesia, intraoperative neurophysiological monitoring, improved spinal instrumentation systems, and enhanced postoperative intensive care and pain management. However, patients must be informed of the most common complications, including but not exclusively limited to hemorrhage, infection, pseudarthrosis, instrumentation failure, trunk imbalance, risk of neurologic injury, and the possible need for future surgery.

BIBLIOGRAPHY

1. Asher MA, Burton DC: A concept of idiopathic scoliosis deformities as imperfect torsion(s). Clin Orthop Rel Res 364:11–25, 1999.
2. Bridwell KH, DeWald RL (eds): The Textbook of Spinal Surgery, 2nd ed. Philadelphia, Lippincott-Raven, 1997.
3. Collis DK, Ponsetti IV: Long-term follow-up of patients with idiopathic scoliosis not treated surgically. J Bone Joint Surg 51:425–45, 1969.
4. King HA, Moe JH, Bradford DS, Winter RB: The selection of fusion levels in thoracic idiopathic scoliosis. J Bone Joint Surg 65A:1302–1313,1983.
5. Lenke LG, Betz RR, Harms J, et al: Adolescent idiopathic scoliosis—a new classification to determine extent of spinal arthrodesis. J Bone Joint Surg 83A:1169–1181,2001.
6. Lonstein JE, Winter RB, Bradford DS, Ogilvie JW: Moe's Textbook of Scoliosis and Other Spinal Deformities, 3rd ed. Philadelphia, W.B. Saunders, 1995.
7. Lonstein JE, Carlson JM: The prediction of curve progression in untreated idiopathic scoliosis during growth. J Bone Joint Surg 66A:1061–1071,1984.
8. Mehta MH: The rib-vertebra angle in the early diagnosis between resolving and progressive infantile scoliosis. J Bone Joint Surg 54B:230–243, 1972.

43. NEUROMUSCULAR SPINAL DEFORMITIES

Steven Mardjetko, M.D.

1. Why do patients with neuromuscular diseases develop spinal deformities?

The most plausible cause of the vast majority of neuromuscular spinal deformities is spinal muscle imbalance acting in concert with gravity in a growing child. Alteration of vertebral loading patterns creates secondary changes in the vertebra and soft tissues around the spine, according to the Heuter-Volkmann principle (increased loading across an epiphyseal growth plate inhibits growth and decreased pressure tends to accelerate growth).

2. What are the different types of neuromuscular scoliosis?

The various diseases associated with neuromuscular scoliosis are categorized as neuropathic (affecting either the upper or lower motor neurons) or myopathic. Certain conditions such as myelodysplasia and spinal trauma may have both upper and lower motor neuron involvement.

Neuropathic disorders
  1. Upper motor neuron lesions
    • Cerebral palsy
    • Spinocerebellar degeneration: Friedreich's ataxia, Charcot-Marie-Tooth disease, Roussy-Levy disease
    • Syringomyelia
    • Quadriplegia secondary to spinal cord trauma or tumor
  2. Lower motor neuron lesions
    • Spinal muscular atrophy: Werdnig-Hoffman disease, Kugelberg-Welander disease
    • Poliomyelitis
    • Dysautonomia (Riley-Day syndrome)

Myopathic disorders
  1. Arthrogryposis multiplex congenita
  2. Muscular dystrophy
    • Duchenne type
    • Limb-girdle
    • Fascioscapulohumeral
  3. Fiber-type disproportion
  4. Congenital hypotonia
  5. Myotonia dystrophica

3. What is the prevalence of spinal deformities in different neuromuscular diseases?

The prevalence of spinal deformities in different neuromuscular diseases is variable: cerebral palsy (25%), myelodysplasia (60%), spinal muscular atrophy (67%), Friedreich's ataxia (80%), Duchenne muscular dystrophy (90%), and spinal cord injury before 10 years of age (100%).

4. List important differences between neuromuscular scoliosis and idiopathic scoliosis.
  • Evaluation of neuromuscular scoliosis requires assessment of the underlying disease as well as the spinal deformity. In contrast, idiopathic scoliosis is a spinal deformity occurring in otherwise normal patients.
  • Multidisciplinary evaluation is required for problems associated with the underlying neuromuscular disease (e.g., contractures, hip dislocations, seizures, malnutrition, cardiac and pulmonary disease, urinary tract dysfunction, mental retardation, pressure sores, insensate skin).
  • Neuromuscular scoliosis develops at an earlier age than idiopathic scoliosis, often before age ten.

- Neuromuscular curves tend to be longer and involve more vertebrae than idiopathic curves.
- Neuromuscular spinal deformities are more likely to progress.
- Neuromuscular curves are frequently accompanied by pelvic obliquity, which may compromise sitting ability and impair upper extremity function.
- Neuromuscular curves do not respond well to orthotic treatment.
- Spinal surgery is frequently required for neuromuscular spinal deformities.

5. How are neuromuscular spinal deformities diagnosed?

Diagnosis is based on clinical examination and confirmed with long cassette radiographs. Upright radiographs are obtained in patients who are able to stand. Patients who are able to sit without hand support are assessed in the sitting position. Patients who are unable to sit are evaluated with recumbent anteroposterior (AP) and lateral radiographs. The examiner should assess curve magnitude, curve progression, spinal balance, pelvic obliquity (if present), and curve flexibility. Spinal MRI is required if intraspinal disease (e.g., syrinx, tethered cord) is suspected. After a child is diagnosed with neuromuscular disease, the patient should have yearly examinations to assess for development of spinal deformity.

6. What radiographic features are characteristic of typical neuromuscular curves?

Neuromuscular curves are typically long, sweeping C-shaped curves that extend to the pelvic region. The curve apex is usually in the thoracolumbar or lumbar region. When secondary curves develop, they are usually unable to restore coronal balance. Significant sagittal plane deformity often accompanies the coronal plane deformity. Pelvic obliquity is common and poses a major problem because it creates an uneven sitting base.

7. What treatment options exist for managing neuromuscular scoliosis?

Regardless of the underlying neuromuscular disease, three options exist for managing neuromuscular scoliosis: observation, orthotic management, and surgical treatment with spinal instrumentation and fusion.

8. When is observation indicated?

Observation is reasonable for patients with small curves ($< 20°$), severely mentally retarded patients with large curves not associated with functional loss, and patients in whom medical comorbidities make them poor candidates for major spinal reconstructive surgery.

9. What is the role of orthotic treatment?

The role of orthotic treatment is two fold: (1) to help nonambulatory patients to sit with the use of a seating support and (2) to attempt to control spinal deformity. In most cases of neuromuscular scoliosis, a spinal orthosis will not prevent curve progression. However, orthotic treatment is valuable in slowing progression of spinal deformities until the onset of puberty and permits growth of the spine before definitive treatment with spinal instrumentation and fusion. Orthotic management is challenging in neuromuscular disorders because of poor muscle control, impaired sensation, pulmonary compromise, obesity, and difficulty with cooperating with brace wear.

10. When is surgical treatment indicated?

There is no absolute minimum age at which to consider spinal surgery. In general, operative treatment is considered when progressive curves reach 30–40° or patients develop trunk decompensation. It is not necessary to delay surgery until skeletal maturity.

11. List important preoperative considerations in evaluation of patients with neuromuscular spinal deformity.

Functional status: ambulatory function, sitting ability, hand use, mental ability, vision.

Pulmonary assessment: ask about history of upper respiratory infection or pneumonia; perform pulmonary function testing if possible.

Cardiac assessment: especially in Duchenne's muscular dystrophy, Friedreich's ataxia, myotonic dystrophy.

Nutritional status: deficits impair wound healing and increase infection risk.

Seizure disorders: require assessment by a neurologist.

Metabolic bone disease: osteopenia is common secondary to disuse, poor nutrition and anticonvulsants.

12. List the goals of surgical treatment for neuromuscular spinal deformities.

- Prevent curve progression.
- Correct spinal deformities safely.
- Obtain a solid arthrodesis.
- Balance the spine in the coronal and sagittal planes above a level pelvis.
- Correct pelvic obliquity.
- Prevent progressive respiratory compromise due to increasing spinal deformity.
- Optimize functional ability (e.g., permit the patient to sit without using the arms for trunk support).
- Decrease trunk fatigue and pain. Fatigue is associated with maintaining an upright posture in severe deformities. Pain may result from facet arthrosis or impingement of the ribs on the pelvis in severe deformities.

13. What are the basic principles of posterior spinal instrumentation and fusion for treatment of neuromuscular scoliosis?

The classic procedure for neuromuscular scoliosis is a long posterior fusion from the upper thoracic spine to the pelvis. Segmental spinal fixation consisting of sublaminar wires placed at every spinal level provides secure fixation and excellent deformity correction. Distal implant fixation is achieved by insertion of rods between the tables of the ilium along a path extending from the posterior superior iliac spine toward the anterior superior iliac spine (Galveston technique). The fixation achieved with this technique is sufficiently secure to permit mobilization of the patient without the need for a postoperative orthosis. Allograft bone is commonly used for long fusions for neuromuscular scoliosis because the ilium does not provide a sufficient amount of bone graft.

14. How does the surgeon select the appropriate distal level for spinal instrumentation and fusion?

The instrumentation and fusion should extend to the sacropelvis if the curve involves the sacrum, if there is significant pelvic obliquity, or if the patient has poor sitting balance. Ambulatory patients who lack pelvic obliquity and have mild curves that do not involve the sacrum may be considered candidates for ending the instrumentation and fusion proximal to sacropelvis to avoid potential compromise of ambulatory ability.

15. When is combined anterior and posterior surgery indicated?

1. **To enhance deformity correction.** Correction of rigid spinal deformities is improved following anterior discectomy and fusion. Indications include patients with fixed pelvic obliquity, large rigid curves with limited flexibility on bending or traction radiographs as well as significant kyphotic deformities.

2. **To enhance the fusion rate.** Indications include patients with deficient posterior elements (e.g., myelodysplasia) and adults who require a long fusion to the sacropelvis.

3. **To avoid the crankshaft phenomenon.** An important indication for skeletally immature patients in whom the presence of a posterior fusion acts as a tether to prevent elongation of the spine. As the vertebral bodies increase in height, the spine rotates out of the sagittal plane leading to a recurrent and increasing spinal curvature. Anterior fusion destroys the anterior growth plates of the vertebral bodies and prevents this phenomenon.

16. Discuss recent advances in the surgical treatment of neuromuscaular spinal deformities.

1. **Pedicle screw fixation.** Pedicle screws provide fixation across all three spinal columns and are biomechanically superior to hook or sublaminar wire fixation. Screw fixation enhances curve correction and provides a means of achieveing secure fixation in patients with congenital or acquired laminectomy defects.

2. **Iliac screw fixation.** Modular implant components facilitate linkage of longitudinal members to the ilium and eliminate the need for complex rod bends. The combination of a bicortical S1 pedicle screw and an iliac screw provides a secure foundation for correction of severe neuromuscular deformities with pelvic obliquity.

3. **Hook fixation at the proximal end of instrumentation constructs.** Use of sublaminar wires at the proximal end of instrumentation constructs has been associated with development of a proximal junctional kyphotic deformity following surgery. Use of hook fixation at the proximal end of implant constructs can decrease the incidence of this problem.

4. **Vertebrectomy/corpectomy procedures for rigid deformities.** Excision of a vertebra in the region of the apex of a severe rigid curve can enhance correction of severe spinal deformities (Fig. 1).

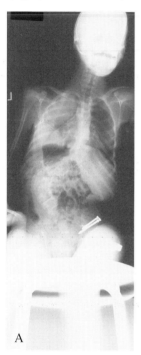 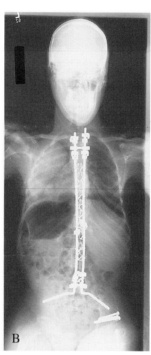 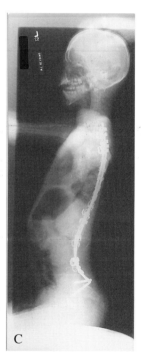

A   B   C

FIGURE 1. A, AP radiograph shows a large thoracolumbar curve with pelvic obliquity in a 12-year-old patient with cerebral palsy. Postoperative AP (**B**) and lateral (**C**) radiographs after combined anterior and posterior procedures. Anterior surgery included multilevel anterior discectomies and fusion. An apical vertebrectomy was performed to enhance deformity correction. Posterior instrumentation and fusion was performed using proximal hooks, multiple sublaminar wires, and Galveston fixation.

17. What intraoperative problems should be anticipated during spinal procedures for neuromuscluar spinal deformity?

Problems not uncommonly encountered during operations on children with neuromuscular spinal deformities include excessive blood loss, malignant hyperthermia, latex allergy, and difficulty with monitoring neurologic function .

18. What type of spinal cord monitoring is ideal in patients with neuromuscular spinal deformity?

The Stagnara wake-up test requires patient cooperation and is not an option in most patients. So-matosensory-evoked potential (SSEP) monitoring shows significant variability in patients with neuromuscular disorders, especially encephalopathies. Transcranial motor evoked potentials are contraindicated in patients with seizure disorders. The Hoppenfield clonus test can be quite misleading in this patient population because baseline deep tendon reflexes may be hyperactive. An ideal combination of spinal cord monitoring modalities is SSEP monitoring in combination with motor-evoked potentials performed by placement of electrode leads proximal to the surgical site.

19. What postoperative problems should be anticipated after spinal procedures for neuromuscular spinal deformities?

- **Pulmonary dysfunction.** Atelectasis and pneumonia are common. Postoperative ventilator support is frequently required.
- **Gastrointestinal problems.** Ileus is common. Use of hyperalimentation can be considered until adequate gastrointestinal feeding can be resumed.
- **Wound infection.** The incidence of postoperative wound infection is much higher in neuromuscular patients than in other types of spinal deformity surgery.

20. Discuss important considerations for surgical treatment of scoliosis secondary to cerebral palsy.

Cerebral palsy, the most common neuromuscular disorder, is frequently accompanied by scoliosis. Progression of scoliosis beyond 30–40° is the most common indication for surgical stabilization. Curves have been classified into two groups: group 1, which includes single or double curves in ambulatory patients with a level pelvis, and group 2, which includes lumbar or thoracolumbar curves in nonambulatory patients, typically associated with pelvic obliquity. Group 1 patients are generally treated with posterior spinal fusion and instrumentation. Fusion to the sacrum is not usually required. Group 2 patients are typically treated with fusion to the sacropelvis. If the pelvis becomes level on a traction radiograph, the deformity can be treated with a posterior spinal instrumentation and fusion from T2 to the pelvis using iliac fixation. If the deformity is rigid on the traction radiograph, combined anterior and posterior fusion is indicated.

21. What is the role of surgery for scoliosis associated with Duchenne muscular dystrophy?

Duchenne muscular dystrophy is the most common form of muscular dystrophy and is transmitted by an X-linked recessive trait. 95% of patients with this disease develop scoliosis. Patients typically become wheelchair bound by the age of 13 and develop scoliosis at this time. Because these curves progress rapidly and are associated with loss of vital capacity, surgical stabilization is advised to prevent pulmonary impairment once the curve is greater than 20°. Typically posterior spinal instrumentation and fusion are performed from T2 to the pelvis with segmental fixation, including iliac fixation. Some surgeons limit the distal extent of fusion to L5 in select patients with mild curves that are not associated with pelvic obliquity.

22. Discuss important aspects of spinal deformities associated with spinal muscular atrophy.

Spinal muscular atrophy is a group of autosomal recessive disorders characterized by degeneration of the anterior horn cells of the spinal cord resulting in trunk and proximal muscle weakness. The severity of the disease is variable. In general, the earlier the clinical onset, the worse the prognosis. Posterior spinal fusion should be performed before spinal deformities becomes severe and pulmonary function becomes compromised.

23. What curve pattern is most commonly noted in patients with Friedreich's ataxia who develop scoliosis?

Friedreich's ataxia is a spinal cerebellar degenerative disorder transmitted as an autosomal recessive genetic disease. Scoliosis develops in approximately 80% of patients. The curve pattern is similar to idiopathic scoliosis and is not usually accompanied by pelvic obliquity. Posterior spinal instrumentation and fusion are performed for curves that approach 40°. Fusion to the pelvis is rarely necessary.

24. A teenager presents with a painful 45° left thoracic curve pattern associated with thoracic kyphosis of 50°. Neurologic exam reveals asymmetric abdominal reflexes and dissociated pain and temperature loss in the extremities. What is the most likely diagnosis?

The radiographic and clinical findings are typical for syringomyelia. Syringomyelia, an abnormal cavity within the spinal cord, may lead to a spinal curvature that can be mistakenly attributed to idiopathic scoliosis. Idiopathic thoracic curves typically are not associated with pain in adolescents, are convex to the right and are associated with normal or decreased thoracic kyphosis. MRI is indicated to confirm the diagnosis. A symptomatic syrinx requires surgical treatment, which may improve neurologic deficits and prevent curve progression. Severe curves require surgical correction and fusion.

25. What is the most significant risk factor for the development of spinal deformity in a patient who sustains a traumatic complete spinal cord injury?

The age at injury is the most significant risk factor for development of spinal deformity. The incidence of spinal deformity after spinal cord injury has been reported as 100% in patients injured before 10 years of age. Various studies have reported that scoliosis developed in 97% of patients injured before the adolescent growth spurt and 50% of those injured after the growth spurt. Prophylactic bracing should be used to attempt to slow deformity progression in young patients. Surgical treatment utilizing the surgical principles for treatment of neuromuscular spinal deformities is indicated for large or progressive deformities.

26. What types of spinal deformities may occur with myelomeningocele?

Spinal deformities may be developmental (paralytic) or congenital (due to anomalous vertebra remote from the spinal bifida site). Scoliosis is common and typically associated with severe lordosis. Kyphosis may be congenital or paralytic in nature. A large, rigid kyphosis of the lumbar spine may be present at birth.

27. What underlying problems may be responsible for progressive scoliosis in a child with myelomeningocele?

Deformities and anomalies can involve the spinal canal and its contents (neural axis) and influence the behavior and management of a spinal deformity. Progressive scoliosis in a child with myelomenigocele warrants further work-up, including spinal MRI to rule out a tethered cord, syringomyelia, or decompensated hydrocephalus.

28. What is the principal factor responsible for difficulty achieving successful spinal fusion in the patient with myelomenigocele and spinal deformity?

The lack of normal posterior vertebral elements makes achieving a solid spinal fusion difficult. In general, both anterior and posterior fusion should be performed to maximize fusion success.

29. What procedure is indicated to treat congenital lumbar kyphosis in a child with spina bifida?

Kyphectomy. Indications to resect a kyphosis include skin breakdown over the kyphosis and inability of the child to use the hands due to the need to support him- or herself on the thighs. The procedure includes resection of vertebra in the region of the apex of the deformity, segmental fixation to any remaining posterior bony structures, and placement of rods as described by Heydemann and Gillespie. This technique involves placement of a rod with two 90° bends at the distal end of the rod. The most distal limb of the rod rests on the anterior sacrum. The short limb of the rod between the two 90° bends rests on the top of the sacrum. The instrumentation construct provides excellent distal fixation and permits cantilever reduction of the kyphotic deformity. Posterior skin coverage is frequently a problem in these patients. Soft tissue procedures including the use of tissue expanders or muscle flaps may be required to provide adequate coverage of the spinal implants.

BIBLIOGRAPHY

1. Bradford DS, Hu SS: Neuromuscular spinal deformity. In Lonstein JE, Winter RB, Bradford DS, Ogilvie JW (eds): Moe's Textbook of Scoliosis and Other Spinal Deforomities, 3rd ed. Philadelphia, W.B. Saunders, 1995, pp 295–322.
2. Lonstein JE: Neuromuscular spinal deformities. In Weinstein SL (ed): The Pediatric Spine: Principles and Practice. Lippincott, Philadelphia, 2001, pp 789–796.
3. Shook JF, Lubicky JP: Paralytic scoliosis. In Bridwell KH, DeWald RL (eds): The Textbook of Spinal Surgery, 2nd ed. Lippincott-Raven, Philadelphia, 1997, pp 839–880.

44. CONGENITAL SPINAL DEFORMITIES

Lawrence Karlin, M.D.

1. Define congenital scoliosis.
A lateral curvature of the spine caused by vertebral anomalies that produce a frontal plane growth asymmetry. The anomalies are present a birth, but the curvature may take years to become clinically evident.

2. What genes are thought to be responsible for the congenital spinal malformations?
Homeobox genes of the Hox class.

3. When do congenital vertebral anomalies form?
During weeks 4–6 of the embryonic period.

4. What are the two main categories of congenital scoliosis?
Defects of segmentation and defects of formation. Some congenital abnormalities cannot be placed into this classification scheme.

5. What are the common defects of segmentation?
Block vertebra, unilateral bar, and unilateral bar and hemivertebra (Fig. 1).

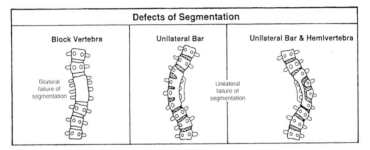

FIGURE 1. Defects of segmentation. (From McMaster MJ: Congenital scoliosis. In Weinstein SL (ed): The Pediatric Spine: Principles and Practice. New York, Raven Press, 1994, pp 227–244, with permission.

6. What are the common defects of formation?
Hemivertebra and wedge vertebra.

7. What are the types of hemivertebra?
Fully segmented, semisegmented, nonsegmented, and incarcerated (Fig. 2).

8. What is the anatomic cause of progressive deformity?
Unbalanced growth. The greater the disparity in the number of healthy growth plates between the left and right sides of the spine, the greater the deformity and the more rapidly spinal deformity develops.

9. What factors are used to prognosticate the rate of progression and ultimate deformity due to a congenital spinal anomaly?
1. The **anatomic type** helps determine the risk and rate of progression.
2. The **location** of the defect affects spinal balance and difficulty of treatment. A hemivertebra located at the lumbosacral junction causes far more spinal imbalance than one located at the mid-thoracic level. In addition, a hemiverebra at the cervicothoracic junction is more difficult to

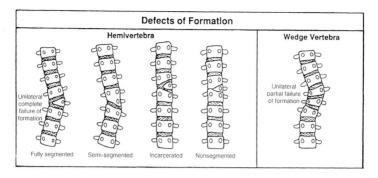

FIGURE 2. Defects of formation. (From (From McMaster MJ: Congenital scoliosis. In Weinstein SL, (ed): The Pediatric Spine: Principles and Practice. New York, Raven Press, 1994, pp 227–244, with permission.

treat surgically due to limited approach options, and timing of intervention may be altered based on this consideration.

3. The **age** of the patient determines the risk of progression. Spinal deformities are more likely to progress during times of rapid growth such as the first 2 years of life and during the adolescent growth spurt.

10. What forms of congenital scoliosis cause the most rapidly progressive deformities?

- Unilateral unsegmented bar with contralateral hemivertebra (an average of 6° progression per year)
- Unilateral unsegmented bar (an average of 5° progression per year)

11. What is the accepted initial treatment for a unilateral unsegmented bar?

Early in situ fusion is indicated. This deformity can only progress.

12. What is the risk of progression of the various types of hemivertebra?

Fully segmented. There are two extra growth plates on one side of the spine. Unbalanced growth occurs producing a scoliosis that worsens at a rate of 1–2° per year. Two fully segmented hemivertebra on the same side of the spine produce a more rapid deterioration (about 3° per year).

Semisegmented. One border is synostosed to its neighbor, producing a balanced number of growth plates on either side. The hemivertebra produces a tilting of the spine, and a slowly progressive curvature may occur.

Nonsegmented. No growth plates are associated with this type of hemivertebra, and a progressive deformity does not occur.

Incarcerated. The vertebral bodies above and below accommodate the hemivertebra, and little or no deformity is produced. The growth plates tend to be narrow with little growth potential. This form of hemivertebra causes little or no deformity.

13. What percentage of people with vertebral malformations have associated anomalies?

Sixty percent have malformations either within or outside the spine. A relatively benign vertebral abnormality may be associated with a life-threatening (but initially asymptomatic) problem. The importance of a thorough search for associated abnormalities cannot be overemphasized.

14. What common malformations are associated with congenital spinal anomalies?

- Vertebral abnormalities at another level. For example, cervical vertebral anomalies are detected in 25% of people with congenital scoliosis or kyphosis.
- Urinary tract structural abnormalities. Up to 37% of people with congenital vertebral anomalies have urinary tract anomalies, such as renal agenesis, duplication, ectopia, fusion, ureteral anomalies, and reflux.

- Intraspinal abnormalities. Up to 38% of people with congenital vertebral anomalies have intraspinal abnormalities detectable by MRI, including tethered cord, diastematomyelia, diplomyelia, and syringomyelia.
- Other associated anomalies : cranial nerve palsy (11%), upper extremity hypoplasia (10%), clubfoot (9%), dislocated hip (8%), congenital cardiac disease (7%).

15. Define diastematomyelia.

A diastematomyelia is a congenital bony or fibrocartilagenous septum in the spinal canal that impinges on or splits the neural tissue.

16. What is the incidence of diastematomyelia associated with congenital vertebral abnormalities?

5–20%.

17. What are the clinical findings in diastematomyelia?

- Cutaneous lesions, such as hair patch, dimple (55–75%)
- Anisomyelia (52–58%)
- Foot deformity usually cavus, usually unilateral (32–52%)
- Neurologic deficits (58–88%)
- Scoliosis (60–100%)

18. What radiographic findings are associated with diastematomyelia?

- Spina bifida occulta (76–94%)
- Widened interpedicular distance (94–100%)

19. What is the normal level of the conus in the pediatric population according to age?

The L2–L3 disc in the neonate and the L1–L2 disc or cephalad at 1 year and older.

20. What vertebral malformation is most often associated with an abnormality of the neural axis?

A unilateral unsegmented bar and a same-level contralateral hemivertebra. Approximately 50% of people with this vertebral abnormality have been reported to have an associated neural axis abnormality.

21. What is the VATER association?

VATER is the acronym for the association of the following congenital anomalies: **v**ertebral, **a**norectal, **t**racheo-**e**sophageal fistula, and **r**adial limb dysplasia. This acronym has now been expanded to **VACTERLS**, adding **c**ardiac and **r**enal malformations and **s**ingle umbilical artery. Trill the "**L**," and you will remember **l**ung abnormalities, another associated problem.

22. What tests should be performed to screen a patient with congenital scoliosis for renal abnormalities?

Urinalysis and renal ultrasound are sufficient.

23. When should an MRI be performed to screen for intraspinal abnormalities when a patient presents with a congenital vertebral anomaly?

Perhaps a controversial answer. A number of studies now place the incidence of associated intraspinal abnormalities in the 30% range. The standard recommendation is to perform an MRI if surgery is planned or when clinical symptoms or physicial findings are suggestive of intraspinal pathology. The author believes, as do others, that an MRI should be part of the initial evaluation of congenital scoliosis (Fig. 3). The 30% incidence is too high to ignore when clinical manifestations are frequently initially absent.

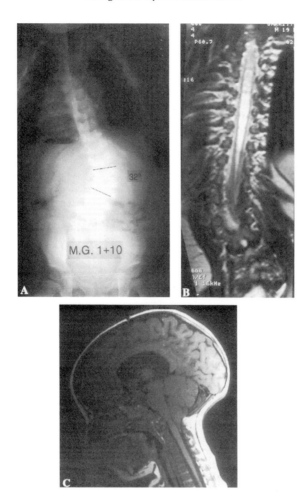

FIGURE 3. This young patient presented with a fully segmented lumbar hemivertebra. He displayed no neurologic signs or symptoms. (**A**). A screening MRI was performed and revealed a massive syrinx extending from T3 to T11. (**B**), and a Chiari I malformation and large ventricles (**C**). Neurosurgical decompression was performed on an urgent basis. In the author's opinion, all cases of congenital scoliosis warrant a screening MRI. (From Karlin LI: Congenital scoliosis. Spine State Art Rev 12:1–11, 1998, with permission.)

24. What is the accuracy of measurement of congenital spinal deformities on plain radiographs?

The abnormally shaped vertebrae make it difficult to be consistent with radiographic measurements. One study revealed an intraobserver variability of ±9.6° and an interobserver variability of ±11.8°. Another study reported an average intraobserver variance of 2.8° and an interobserver variance of 3.4°.

25. What is the role of brace treatment for congenital scoliosis?

The role is limited. Orthoses will not halt the progression of a rigid congenital structural abnormality. A brace may control a compensatory curvature or a long flexible curvature in which the rigid congenital deformity comprises a small section of the entire spinal deformity. Total contact braces may restrict chest wall development and should not be used. A Milwaukee brace (CTLSO) is preferable.

26. What are the surgical treatment options for congenital spinal deformities?

- Posterior fusion without spinal instrumentation
- Posterior fusion with spinal instrumentation
- Combined anterior and posterior fusion
- Convex growth arrest procedures
- Hemivertebra excision
- Vertebrectomy
- Combinations of the above procedures

27. In treating congenital scoliosis, what is the indication for in-situ posterior spinal arthrodesis without instrumentation?

This procedure is indicated for a small curvature that is anticipated to worsen (e.g., scoliosis due to a unilateral unsegmented bar). However, bending or crankshaft can occur with significant anterior growth. Anterior and posterior arthrodesis is indicated in the very young or when significant anterior growth (healthy anterior growth plates) is anticipated.

28. In treating congenital scoliosis, what is the indication for posterior fusion with instrumentation?

This procedure is indicated in the older child when some correction of the deformity is desired. The correction will occur not through the rigid congenital deformity but through the adjacent flexible spine segments.

29. In treating congenital scoliosis, what is the indication for convex hemiepiphyseodesis and hemiarthrodesis? What levels should be fused?

This procedure is designed to produce a gradual correction of curvatures due to hemivertebra. The prerequisites for success include a curvature with concave growth potential, limited length (5 or less vertebral bodies), limited magnitude (less than 70°), no kyphosis, and young age (less than 5 years). The entire curvature should be fused on the convex side. The benefit of the procedure is safety. The disadvantage of the procedure is the unpredicatability of final curve correction.

30. What is the indication for hemivertebra excision?

Hemivertebra excision is indicated for a fully segmented hemivertebra causing significant trunk imbalance (Fig. 4). This is a more dangerous procedure than in-situ fusion or hemiepiphyseodesis. However, it produces dramatic curve correction and maintains maximal spinal flexibility. It is the treatment of choice for a lumbosacral hemivertebra causing significant oblique takeoff. A number of surgical series using a simultaneous anterior and posterior approach for hemivertebra excision have documented excellent results with few complications.

31. What is the indication for transpedicular anterior and posterior convex hemiepiphyseodesis or transpedicular hemivertebra excision?

These procedures have been described for cases in which hemiepiphyseodesis or hemivertebra excision is appropriate but the anterior approach is difficult (e.g., the upper thoracic spine) or not desired. The anterior growth areas are accessed from a posterior approach via the pedicle.

32. Does the crankshaft phenomenon occur after the surgical treatment of congenital scoliosis?

The crankshaft phenomenon results when a scoliotic deformity previously treated by posterior arthrodesis demonstrates progressive increase in curve magnitude and rotational deformity. The cause is thought to be anterior growth tethered by the posterior fusion. This phenomenon, documented in idiopathic scoliosis, has been reported in children with congenital scoliosis treated by posterior fusion alone before age 10 years. It has not been reported when anterior and posterior arthrodesis were performed together in this population.

33. How is congenital kyphosis classified? (Fig. 5)

Type I: failure of formation
Type II: failure of segmentation
Type III: mixed anomalies

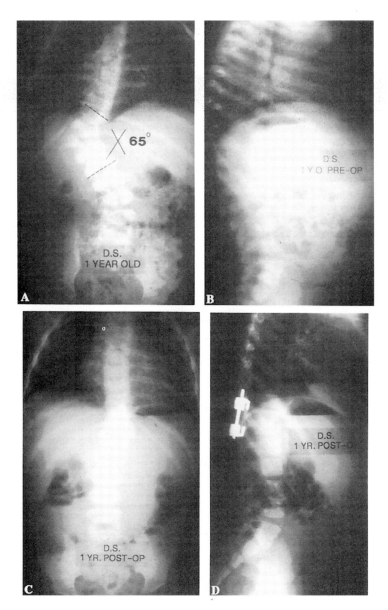

FIGURE 4. As a 1-year-old, this child had a 65° curvature produced by a single fully segmented hemiverte-bra (**A, B**). A balanced spine was produced without sacrificing growth or flexibility by hemivertebral excision (**C, D**). (Courtesy of John E. Hall, M.D.)

34. What forms of congenital kyphosis are associated with spontaneous neurologic deterioration?

Type I is associated with failure of formation and type III with mixed anomalies.

35. In congenital kyphosis when is posterior surgery alone sufficient?

Posterior surgery is reasonable in the absence of anterior neural compression, kyphosis correcting to 50° or less on supine radiographs, and age less than 5 years.

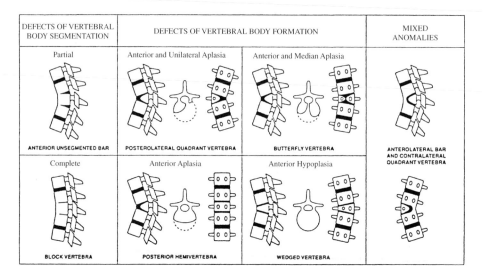

DEFECTS OF VERTEBRAL BODY SEGMENTATION	DEFECTS OF VERTEBRAL BODY FORMATION		MIXED ANOMALIES
Partial	Anterior and Unilateral Aplasia	Anterior and Median Aplasia	
ANTERIOR UNSEGMENTED BAR	**POSTEROLATERAL QUADRANT VERTEBRA**	**BUTTERFLY VERTEBRA**	**ANTEROLATERAL BAR AND CONTRALATERAL QUADRANT VERTEBRA**
Complete	Anterior Aplasia	Anterior Hypoplasia	
BLOCK VERTEBRA	**POSTERIOR HEMIVERTEBRA**	**WEDGED VERTEBRA**	

FIGURE 5. Classification of congenital kyphosis. (From McMaster MJ, Singh H: Natural history of kyphosis and kyphoscoliosis: A study of one hundred and twelve patients. J Bone Joint Surg 81A:1367–1383, 1999, with permission.)

36. What is the treatment of type I congenital kyphosis?

Arthrodesis by age 5 years. An aggressive surgical approach is indicated due to the substantial risk of neurologic deficit.

37. What is the treatment for type II congenital kyphosis?

Observation. Fusion should be performed if deformity progression is noted. The prognosis for deformity progression is greater when there is an anterolateral bar producing kyphoscoliosis than when a midline bar produces pure kyphosis.

38. What is the treatment for type III congenital kyphosis?

Arthrodesis by age 5.

BIBLIOGRAPHY

1. Andrew T, Piggot H: Growth arrest for progressive scoliosis; Combined anterior and posterior fusion of the convexity. J Bone Joint Surg 67B:193–197, 1985
2. Beals RK, Robbins JR, Rolfe B: Anomalies associated with vertebral malformations. Spine 18: 1329–1322, 1993.
3. Bradford DS, Boachie-Adjei O: One-stage anterior and posterior hemivertebra resection and arthrodesis for congenital scoliosis. J Bone Joint Surg 72A:536–540, 1990.
4. Bradford DS, Heithoff KB, Cohen M: Intraspinal abnormalities and congenital spine deformities: A radiographic and MRI study. J Pediatr Orhtop 11:36–41, 1991.
5. Callahan BV, Georgopoulos G, Eilert RE; Hemivertebra excision for congenital scoliosis. J Pediatr Orthop 17:96–99, 1997.
6. Dravaric DM, Ruderman RJ, Conrad RW, et al: Congenital scoliosis and urinary tract abnormalities: Are intravenous pylograms necessary? J Pediatr Orthop 7:441–443, 1987.
7. Facanha-Filho FA, Winter RB, Lonsein JE et al: Measurement accuracy in congenital scoliosis. J Bone Joint Surg 83A:42–45, 2001.
8. Holt DC, Winter RB, Lonstein JE., Denis F: Excision of hemivertebra and wedge resection in the treatment of congenital scoliosis. J Bone Joint Surg 77A:159–171, 1995.
9. Keller PM, Lindseth RE, DeRosa P: Progressive congenital scoliosis treatment using a transpedicular an-

terior and posterior convex hemiepiphyseodesis and hemiarthrodesis: A preliminary report. Spine 19: 1933–1939, 1994

10. King AG, MacEwen GD, Bose WJ: Transpedicular convex anterior hemiepiphyseodesis and posterior arthrodesis for progressive congenital scoliosis. Spine 17(Suppl 8): S291–S294, 1992.

11. Klemme WR, Polly DW Jr., Orchowski JR: Hemiverebra excision for congenital scoliosis in very young children. J Pediatr Orthop 21:761–764, 2001.

12. Lazar RD, Hall JE: Simultaneious anterior and posterior hemivertebra excision. Clin Orthop Rel Res 364:76–84, 1999.

13. Loder RT, Urquhart A, Steen, H, et al: Variability in Cobb angle measurements in children with Congenital scoliosis. J Bone Joint Surg 77B:768–770, 1995.

14. McMaster MJ: Congential scoliosis. In Weinstein SL (ed): The Pediatric Spine: Principles and Practice. New York, Raven Press, 1994, pp 227–244.

15. McMaster MJ, Singh H: The natural history of congenital kyphosis and kyphoscoliosis. A study of one hundred and twelve patients. J Bone Joint Surg 81A:1367–1383, 1999.

16. McMaster MJ, Singh H: The surgical management of congenital kyphosis and kyphoscoliosis. Spine 26:2146–2154, 2001.

17. Slabaugh PB, Winter RB, Lonstein JE, Moe JH: Lumbosacral hemivertebrae: A review of 24 patients, with excision in eight. Spine 5:234–244, 1980.

18. Suh SW, Sarwark JF, Vora A, Huang BK: Evaluation of congenital spine deformities for intraspinal anomalies with magnetic resonance imaging. J Pediatr Orthop 21:525–531, 2001.

19. Terek RM, Wehner J, Lubicky JP: Crankshaft phenomenon in congenital scoliosis: A preliminary report. J Pediatr Orthop 11:527–532, 1991.

20. Winter RB, Lonstein JE, Denis F: Convex growth arrest for progressive congenital scoliosis due to a hemivertebra. J Pediatr Orthop 8:633–638, 1988

21. Winter RB, Moe JH, MacEwen D, Peon-Vidales H: The Milwaukee brace in the nonoperative treatment of congenital scoliosis. Spine 1:85–96, 1976.

45. SAGITTAL PLANE DEFORMITIES IN PEDIATRIC PATIENTS

John D. Ray, M.D., Munish C. Gupta, M.D., and Theodore A. Wagner, M.D.

1. What are the common types of pediatric sagittal plane deformities?

Pediatric sagittal plane deformities include Scheuermann's kyphosis, postural round back, congenital kyphosis and lordosis, and the sagittal plane deformities associated with myelomeningocele, idiopathic scoliosis, achondroplasia, postlaminectomy kyphosis, tuberculosis, trauma, and spondylolisthesis.

2. What are Cobb angles? How are they measured?

Cobb angles define the magnitude of a curve on posteroanterior (PA) and lateral radiographs of the spine. Vertebral bodies at the top and bottom of the curve are called the end vertebrae. Cobb angles are measured from the top of the upper-end vertebra to the bottom of the lower vertebra. Curve progression is evaluated using the same end vertebra on serial radiographs. Thoracic kyphosis is measured from T2 to T12 and lumbar lordosis from L1 to S1. There is approximately 6° of error in the Cobb angle measurement.

3. What is the normal sagittal plane alignment of the cervical, thoracic, and lumbar spine?

Normal thoracic kyphosis is between 20° and 40°. Normal lumbar lordosis is between 55° and 65°, with most of the curvature between the fourth lumbar vertebra and the sacrum (Fig. 1). Cervical lordosis maintains the head over the sacrum in the sagittal plane. Thoracic kyphosis increases with age and increases at an earlier age in women than in men.

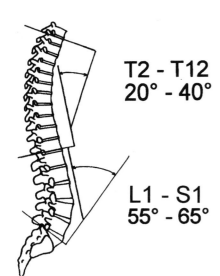

T2 - T12
20° - 40°

FIGURE 1. Normal thoracic kyphosis and lumbar lordosis.

L1 - S1
55° - 65°

4. What is the differential diagnosis in evaluating an adolescent with excessive thoracic kyphosis with or without pain?

Scheuermann's kyphosis, postural round back, fractures of the thoracic spine, infection with vertebral body collapse, congenital kyphosis, and tumor.

5. What are the subtypes of Scheuermann's kyphosis?

Type I Scheuermann's kyphosis is a rigid, angular thoracic kyphosis and has a hereditary component. Type II is located at the thoracolumbar junction, is more painful, and affects predominantly athletes and laborers. Endplate anomalies and loss of disc space height are common to both types I and II.

6. Describe the usual presentation of a patient with thoracic Scheuermann's kyphosis.

A male or female approaching the end of skeletal growth (12–15 years old) who complains of thoracic deformity and back pain. The patient has an increased angular thoracic kyphosis. A compensatory cervical lordosis brings the head forward. The angular thoracic kyphosis is accentuated on the forward-bending examination. Patients may have tight hamstrings, and 30% have mild scoliosis. Patients are not able to correct the kyphosis by active extension.

7. How does the presentation of postural (asthenic) kyphosis differ from Scheuermann's kyphosis?

The kyphosis associated with postural round back is less severe (less than 60°). The patient is able to actively correct the thoracic kyphosis and may appear more athletically active. Parents may also have some round-back deformity. Focal wedging and endplate changes are absent on the lateral radiograph.

8. Are symptoms of neural compression common in patients with Scheuermann's kyphosis?

Myelopathy and radiculopathy are very rare and more likely in adult patients. The spinal cord drapes over the focal kyphosis and is predisposed to pressure from a subsequent fracture or disc herniation.

9. What is the incidence of Scheuermann's disease?

Reports range from less than 1% to over 8% of the general population. Studies also differ on male and female predominance; near-equal male and female ratios have been reported.

10. What is included in the standard radiographic evaluation of suspected Scheuermann's disease?

Standing long cassette (36 inch) **PA** and **lateral views** of the spine are examined for excessive thoracic kyphosis, vertebral wedging, endplate changes, narrowing of the disc spaces, and scoliosis. The PA view should include the iliac apophyses and triradiate cartilage for evaluation of skeletal maturity. Arms are supported at the level of the heart so that they neither flex nor extend the spine. PA radiographs decrease the radiation exposure to the breasts and heart compared with anteroposterior views. Extension **bending radiographs** taken with the patient supine over a radiolucent wedge placed just caudal to the apex of the kyphosis are used to assess curve flexibility. Flex the hips and knees to limit the extension forces on the pelvis and distal spine and allow maximum extension through the apical kyphosis.

11. What are the accepted criteria for diagnosis of thoracic Scheuermann's disease on lateral x-ray?

The common criteria—5° of wedging of three adjacent vertebrae—was popularized by Sorenson. Total kyphosis of greater than 45°, upper and lower endplate irregularities, and apparent loss of disc space height contribute to the radiographic diagnosis. Scheuermann's kyphosis is rigid and does not correct to within normal limits with maximal extension (Fig. 2).

12. How may the radiograph differ in early and late stages of Scheuermann's disease?

Early radiographic changes may be limited to irregular endplates, narrowing of the disc spaces anteriorly, and Schmorl's nodes. Because the ring apophysis does not appear until approximately 10 years of age, the vertebral body appears rounded, and diagnosis of Scheuermann's is extremely unlikely. In skeletally mature patients, osteophytes, facet hypertrophy, and compression fractures may accentuate the spinal deformity.

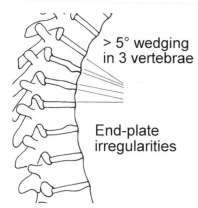

> 5° wedging
in 3 vertebrae

End-plate
irregularities

FIGURE 2. Thoracic Scheuermann's kyphosis.

13. What causes Scheuermann's disease?

The exact cause is unknown. In 1921 Holger Scheuermann associated the disorder with aseptic necrosis of the vertebral body ring apophysis. Abnormal growth plate cartilage, mechanical decompensation after endplate disc herniation (Schmorl's nodes), hormonal variation (increased growth hormone), osteoporosis, and malabsorption have been proposed as possible causes. Associations with Legg-Calvé-Perthes disease, hypovitaminosis, dystonia, dural cysts, and endocrine disorders have been described. There appears to be a familial tendency. Evidence suggests that Scheuermann's disease is autosomal dominant with high penetrance and variable expressivity; however, the genetics of this disorder are not well defined.

14. What histologic findings are reported in patients with Scheuermann's disease?

Despite the association with avascular necrosis of the ring apophysis, alteration in the growth plate cartilage without osteoporosis or necrosis of the ring apophysis has been observed. Both matrix and cells are altered. Collagen fibers are thinner and sparser. Proteoglycan content is increased.

15. Describe the natural history of Scheuermann's disease.

There is disagreement about both pain and functional limitations. Pain increases with age in some studies and decreases with age in others. Some studies suggest significant functional limitations, whereas others do not. The deformity may have profound psychosocial effects in terms of social stigma and poor self-esteem.

16. What are the indications for bracing for Scheuermann's kyphosis?

Extension bracing is appropriate for curves between 45° and 65° with two years of growth remaining and greater than 5° wedging. An apex at T9 or above requires a Milwaukee type brace. A thoracolumbar orthosis (TLSO) is used if the apex is below T9. Braces should be updated every 4–6 months to maximize correction late in the growth spurt and weaned with skeletal maturity.

17. Identify the indications for surgery for Scheuermann's kyphosis.

Painful kyphosis greater than 65° with more than 10° of local wedging resistant to 6 months of bracing may be considered for surgery. Skeletally mature patients with painful deformity unresponsive to nonoperative treatment may be considered for surgery.

18. What are the indications for isolated posterior instrumentation and fusion for Scheuermann's kyphosis?

Curves correcting to less than 50° on extension radiographs may be treated with posterior instrumentation and fusion. The instrumentation should include the entire kyphotic area proximally and extend distally to include one lordotic disc. Pedicle screws in the distal thoracic and lumbar spine provide better anchors and more powerful correction than hook fixation, especially in patients with associated scoliosis. Dual rods are secured proximally with claw hook configuration. The deformity is corrected with cantilever bending and compression force securing the rods distally with screws (Fig. 3).

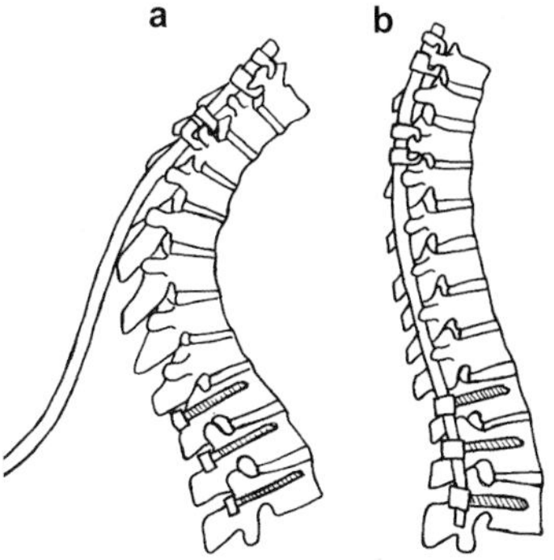

FIGURE 3. Correction of Scheuermann's kyphosis **(a)** before and **(b)** after compression.

19. When are anterior release and fusion appropriate?

Curves that do not correct to better than 50° on lateral extension radiographs are typically treated with anterior release and fusion via a transthoracic or thoracoscopic approach before performing the posterior fusion and instrumentation.

20. Define the surgery goals in terms of curve correction and balance for Scheuermann's kyphosis.

The goal is to restore normal thoracic kyphosis and lumbar lordosis while relieving pain. Approximately 50% correction is desired. Overcorrection of the deformity can lead to proximal or distal junctional kyphotic deformities, which frequently require additional surgical procedures for correction.

21. Is bracing used after surgical correction of Scheuermann's kyphosis?

It depends on surgeon preference and the bone quality of the patient.

22. What are the potential complications of surgery?

Persistent pain, residual deformity, junctional kyphotic deformity, acute or late infection, pseudarthrosis, implant failure, pulmonary complications, neurologic deficit, and the need for subsequent surgery, including implant removal, should be discussed with the patient preoperatively.

23. Describe the types of congenital kyphosis.

Type I is a defect of vertebral body formation (hemivertebra), type II is a defect of vertebral body segmentation (block vertebra or bar), and type III is a mixed or combined lesion (Fig. 4). Type 1 defects are more common and more serious because they lead to a sharp angular kyphosis that may cause paraplegia.

24. Does bracing play a role in treatment of congenital kyphosis?

No. Bracing does not maintain or correct a congenital kyphosis. Nonsurgical management does not play a role in the treatment of congenital kyphosis.

25. What surgical procedures are indicated for congenital kyphosis?

Congenital kyphosis does not respond to nonoperative treatment. Posterior in situ fusion should be considered for a young child (1–5 years old) with a kyphosis measuring less than 50°. Kyphosis greater than 50° and older children require an anterior and posterior fusion. Symptomatic neural compression at the apex of the kyphosis requires decompression. Extensive preop-

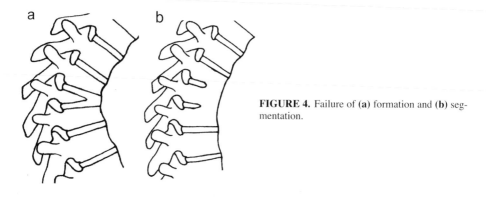

FIGURE 4. Failure of **(a)** formation and **(b)** segmentation.

erative evaluation is required, including cardiopulmonary assessment, evaluation of the genitourinary system, detailed neurologic examination, and MRI of the neural axis.

26. What is the cause of congenital lordosis?

Congenital lordosis is a rare disorder caused by failure of posterior segmentation, typically spanning multiple segments, with persistent anterior growth. The progressive thoracic lordosis causes loss of the spine–sternal distance and restriction of pulmonary function.

27. Describe the treatment for congenital lordosis.

When congenital lordosis is diagnosed early in life, surgical treatment consists of anterior spinal fusion to eliminate anterior growth potential. Patients presenting later in life require anterior and posterior spinal surgery. Anterior closing wedge osteotomies and posterior segmental spinal fixation are required. Rib resections may be required as well. Preoperative pulmonary function tests are necessary. Associated pulmonary hypertension increases mortality and may be a contraindication to surgery.

28. Is thoracic hypokyphosis commonly present in adolescent idiopathic scoliosis?

Yes. Decreased thoracic kyphosis is ubiquitous among patients with scoliosis. Thoracic lordosis is a contraindication to bracing. There is a subgroup of patients with severe hypokyphosis or actual lordosis of the thoracic spine. In patients with progressive thoracic lordosis or lordosis of –10° or more, surgical treatment should be considered, even if the coronal plane Cobb measurement is less than 40°.

29. What are the indications for surgical correction of a gibbus (severe short-segment kyphosis) associated with myelomeningocele?

Inability to maintain an acceptable sitting posture and skin breakdown over the apex of the deformity are reasons to correct the deformity surgically.

30. What is the most common sagittal plane deformity associated with achondroplasia?

Thoracolumbar kyphosis is the most common sagittal plane deformity among achondroplastic dwarfs. The kyphosis is generally evident at birth, progresses as the child begins to sit, and resolves in approximately 70% of cases with ambulation. Radiographs show anterior wedging at the apex of the deformity. Progression can lead to a focal kyphosis and possible neural compression, which may be masked by the lumbar stenosis associated with achondroplasia.

31. What are the nonoperative and surgical options for achondroplastic thoracolumbar kyphosis?

A thoracolumbar orthosis is indicated for children 3 years of age and older in whom the kyphosis does not resolve with ambulation. Anterior and posterior fusion is reserved for children with progressive deformity, thoracolumbar kyphosis greater than 50° at age greater than 5 years, or neural compromise attributed to pressure at the kyphotic region rather than lumbar stenosis. Spinal implants should not be placed into the canal because of the stenosis and lack of space in the canal.

32. What circumstances contribute to postlaminectomy kyphosis?

Laminectomies are performed on children for treatment of tumors and dysraphism. Instability after facetectomy; hypermobility associated with removal of the lamina, ligamentum flavum, and interspinous and supraspinous ligaments; and growth disturbance can contribute to postlaminectomy kyphosis. Postlaminectomy kyphosis is associated with younger patients, extensive laminectomies, and surgery in the upper thoracic and cervical spine.

33. How can postlaminectomy deformity be avoided or treated?

Maintenance of the facet joints, laminoplasty in lieu of laminectomy, and postoperative bracing help stabilize the spine. Excessive decompression or progressive deformity may require posterior fusion. If anterior release and fusion are required, care must be taken to remove the physis all the way back to the posterior longitudinal ligament.

34. How is tuberculosis of the spine uniquely associated with thoracolumbar kyphosis in children?

Among the three patterns of tuberculosis involvement, central lesions are more common in children compared with paradiscal (most common among adults) and anterior lesions. Central lesions generally involve the whole vertebral body and lead to bony collapse, vertebral plana, and kyphosis. The thoracolumbar junction is the most common location. When multiple levels are involved, healing can lead to anterior bony bridging and worsening of the kyphosis.

35. What types of fractures lead to posttraumatic kyphosis in children?

Flexion-compression, burst, and flexion-distraction (seat-belt) type injuries can cause acute kyphosis in the pediatric spine. Growth disturbances may lead to late deformity. The risk of disrupting growth potential must be considered in planning operative versus non-surgical treatment. Traumatic paralysis often results in neuromuscular kyphosis that does not respond to brace treatment. Posterior fusion is recommended for curves greater than 60°, with correction to less than 50° with extension. Curves that are more rigid may require anterior release and fusion combined with posterior spinal instrumentation and fusion.

BIBLIOGRAPHY

1. Ascani E, La Rosa G, Ascani C: Scheuermann's Kyphosis. In Weinstein SL (ed): The Pediatric Spine: Principles and Practice, 2nd ed. Philadelphia, Lippincott Williams & Wilkins, 2001, pp 413–432.
2. Fon GT, Pitt MJ, Thies AC Jr: Thoracic kyphosis: Range in normal subjects. Am J Roentgenol 134: 979–983, 1980.
3. Lindseth RE: Meylomeningocele. In Morrissey RT, Weinstein SL (eds): Lovell and Winter's Pediatric Orthopaedics, 4th ed. Philadelphia, Lippincott-Raven, 1996, pp 503–536.
4. Lowe TG: Scheuermann disease. J Bone Joint Surg 72A:940–945, 1990.
5. McMaster MJ, Singh H: The surgical management of congenital kyphosis and kyphoscoliosis. Spine 26:2146–2155, 2001.
6. Murray PM, Weinstein SL, Spratt KF: The natural history and long-term follow-up of Scheuermann kyphosis. J Bone Joint Surg 75A:236–248, 1993.
7. Warner, WC: Kyphosis. In Morrissey RT, Weinstein SL (eds): Lovell and Winter's Pediatric Orhopaedics, 4th ed. Philadelphia, Lippincott-Raven, 1996, pp 687–716.

46. SPONDYLOLYSIS AND SPONDYLOLISTHESIS IN PEDIATRIC PATIENTS

Vincent J. Devlin, M.D.

1. Define spondylolysis.

Spondylolysis is a unilateral or bilateral defect in the region of the pars interarticularis without vertebral slippage. The origin of the term is from the Greek words *spondylo* (vertebra) and *lysis* (break or defect).

2. Define spondylolisthesis.

Spondylolisthesis refers to a slippage of a portion of the spine on its underlying portion. The origin of the term is from the Greek words *spondylo* (vertebra) and *olisthesis* (movement or slippage). The slippage involves more than a single vertebra as the entire trunk moves with the slipped vertebra.

3. Define spondyloptosis.

Spondyloptosis refers to a slippage of the L5 vertebra in which the entire vertebral body of L5 is located below the top of S1. It is the most severe degree of slippage possible. Fortunately this condition is quite rare. The origin of the term is from the Greek words *spondylo* (vertebra) and *ptosis* (to fail).

4. Describe the Wiltse classification of spondylolisthesis (Fig 1).

Type 1: *Dysplastic:* associated with a congenital deficiency of the L5–S1 articulation

Type 2: *Isthmic*: associated with a lesion in the pars interarticularis.

Subtype 2A : lytic defect (stress fracture) of the pars

Subtype 2B : an elongated or attenuated pars

Subtype 2C : an acute pars fracture

Type 3: *Degenerative spondylolisthesis*: segmental instability secondary to disc degeneration and facet arthrosis and frequently accompanied by spinal stenosis.

Type 4: *Traumatic*: an acute fracture in a region of the posterior elements other than the pars (e.g., facets, pedicle, lamina).

Type 5: *Pathologic*: generalized bone disease (e.g., metabolic, neoplastic) results in attenuation of the pars and/or pedicle region.

Type 6: *Postsurgical*: after decompression of the lumbar spine.

5. Does the presence or absence of a pars defect unequivocally determine whether a spondylolisthesis is classifed as an isthmic or dysplastic type of slippage?

Not always. When a spondylolisthesis with dysplastic features increases in severity, a defect may develop in the region of the pars interarticularis that was not present when the slippage was first diagnosed. This process makes classification problematic. For this reason, many spine specialists prefer to classify spondylolisthesis into two major subgroups (developmental and acquired) based on the presence or absence of dysplasia (abnormal tissue development) at the level of spondylolisthesis. Some of the dysplastic changes that may be seen include facet tropism, deficient L5 and S1 lamina, elongation of the pars interarticularis, rounding of the dome of the sacrum, and a trapezoidal-shaped L5 vertebra. The classification of Marchetti and Bartolozzi recognizes these features and divides spondylolisthesis into two major subgroups:

Developmental	Acquired
• High dysplasia	• Traumatic
• Low dysplasia	• Degenerative
	• Post-surgical
	• Pathologic

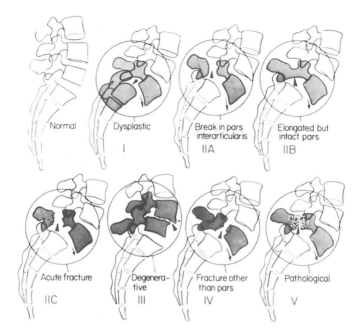

FIGURE 1. Wiltse classification of spondylolisthesis. (From Neuwirth MG: Spondylolysis and spondylolisthesis in children and adults. In Comins M, O'Leary P (eds): The Lumbar Spine. New York, Raven Press, 1987, p 258, with permission.)

6. How common are spondylolysis and spondylolisthesis?

The incidence of spondylolysis and spondylolisthesis is approximately 4% at age 6 and 6% by age 14 years; it remains constant in adulthood.

7. What causes spondylolysis and spondylolisthesis in children?

Although the exact cause remain unknown in all cases, four factors play a critical role:

1. **Biomechanics:** These conditions are not seen in patients who are nonambulatory. Upright posture and lumbar lordosis lead to stress concentration in the region of the pars interarticularis.

2. **Growth:** These conditions are never seen at birth and are most common between 7 and 10 years of age.

3. **Trauma:** Repetitive microtrauma such as the repetitive hyperextension experienced by young athletes (e.g., gymnasts, weightlifters) is considered to play a role in etiology in certain cases.

4. **Heredity:** These condition do not occur in a uniform distribution across populations. Spondylolysis and spondylolisthesis are more common in males than females and in the offspring of first-degree relatives with these conditions. The familial predisposition is greater for the dysplastic type than for the isthmic type. There is an extremely high incidence in Alaskan Eskimos (26%), but the reason is unclear.

8. When are children with spondylolysis and spondylolisthesis referred to the spine specialist for evaluation?

In some cases, spondylolysis and spondylolisthesis are diagnosed as incidental findings on lumbar or pelvic radiographs obtained for unrelated reasons in asymptomatic patients. Symptomatic patients most commonly present with low back pain, which may radiate into the buttocks and thighs. Hamstring tightness or spasm is not uncommon. Pediatric patients with spondylolisthesis occasionally present with radicular symptoms due to nerve compression at the level of the slippage. Patients with severe degrees of spondylolisthesis may present with postural deformity, scoliosis, or gait abnormality.

9. What radiographic views should be obtained to evaluate spondylolysis and spondylolisthesis?

The initial radiographic assessment should include posteroanterior (PA) and lateral lumbosacral radiographs obtained in the standing position. The standing position documents the alignment of the spine under physiologic loading. Oblique views of the lumbosacral region may be obtained to assess more closely the pars interarticularis. On the oblique view, the posterior spinal elements create a figure resembling a "Scottie dog." Spondylolysis is noted as a break in the neck of the dog. Additional useful radiographic views include flexion-extension views, supine vs. standing views, and the Ferguson view (anteroposterior [AP] view with 30° cephalad tilt).

10. What radiographic measurements are most useful for describing spondylolisthesis?

The most useful radiographic measurements for describing spondylolisthesis are the degree of slip and the slip angle (Fig. 2).

The **degree of slip** refers to the amount of translation of the superior vertebra relative to the inferior vertebra. Translation is quantified into five grades (Meyerding system): grade 1, 1–25%; grade 2, 26–50%; grade 3, 51–75%; grade 4, 76–100%; and grade 5, slippage below the anterior border of the sacrum (spondyloptosis).

The **slip angle** measures the degree of lumbosacral kyphosis. It is calculated by measuring the angle between a line perpendicular with the posterior aspect of S1 and a line parallel to either the superior or inferior endplate of L5.

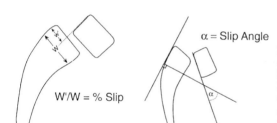

FIGURE 2. Radiographic measurements of spondylolisthesis. (From Ginsburg GM: Spondylolysis and spondylolisthesis. In Brown DE, Neumann RD (eds): Orthopedic Secrets, 2nd ed. Philadelphia, Hanley & Belfus, 1999, pp 200–204, with permission.)

11. Discuss the role of bone scan in the assessment of spondylolysis and spondylolisthesis.

A technetium bone scan is helpful when clinical findings suggest a pars defect but radiographs are negative. A bone scan is helpful in the diagnosis of a stress reaction in the pars region. This finding represents an impending pars fracture. Bone scans are helpful in distinguishing acute from chronic pars interarticularis lesions. There are two types of bone scans: planar bone scans and single-photon emission computed tomography (SPECT). SPECT is more sensitive and specific than planar bone scans for the assessment of spondylolysis.

12. What is the role of computed tomography (CT) in the assessment of spondylolysis and spondylolisthesis?

CT plays a role when a pars defect is suspected on a clinical basis but is not evident on plain radiographs. CT remains the best test for assessment of osseous detail. It is useful for preoperative planning (e.g., evaluating the lumbar pedicles before screw placement).

13. What is the role of magnetic resonance imaging (MRI) in the assessment of spondylolysis and spondylolisthesis?

The need for MRI in the assessment of pediatric spondylolysis and spondylolisthesis is rare. It is invaluable for assessment of patients with neurologic deficits. It can rule out other serious causes of back pain, such as tumor or infection. It is also valuable for assessment of lumbar intervertebral disc pathology.

14. What are the nonsurgical treatment options for an adolescent with spondylolysis or spondylolisthesis?

Asymptomatic spondylolysis discovered as an incidental radiographic finding requires no specific treatment. Treatment of symptomatic patients begins with rest, nonsteroidal anti-inflammatory medication, and activity modification. Avoidance of activities that require hyperextension of the spine is especially important. If symptoms persist, an orthosis that reduces lumbar lordosis can be prescribed.

15. When is surgery considered for spondylolysis?

Indications to consider surgical treatment include persistent or increasing pain more than 6 months in duration, persistent hamstring spasm, radiculopathy (rare), and failure of nonsurgical treatment.

16. What surgical options are advised for treatment of spondylolysis?

The surgical treatment options for spondylolysis are (1) an intertransverse fusion or (2) a direct repair of the pars interarticularis. Generally a pars repair is considered for defects between L1 and L4. An intertransverse fusion is generally considered for L5 pars defects, although pars repair remains an option at this level.

17. What are the prerequisites for successful outcome with a pars repair? How is this procedure performed?

Patients who are best suited for pars repair are less than 25 years old, have no evidence of disc or facet pathology, and have a slippage less than 2 mm. The procedure requires careful debridement of the pars pseudarthrosis and application of autogenous bone graft. Internal fixation across the pars defect is required. Fixation options include direct screw fixation (Buck technique), wire fixation (Scott technique), screw-wire fixation, or screw-hook-rod fixation (Fig. 3).

18. What clinical and radiographic factors suggest that a child with spondylolisthesis is likely to have persistent symptoms, slip progression, and spinal deformity?

Clinical factors
- Young age
- Female sex
- Presence of back pain symptoms

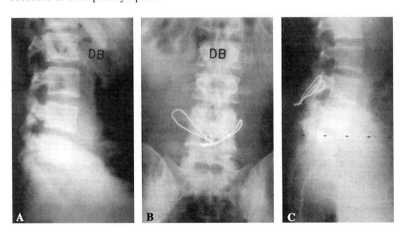

FIGURE 3. Repair of the pars interarticularis using a wiring technique and autogenous bone graft. (From Ginsburg GM: Spondylolysis and spondylolisthesis. In Brown DE, Neumann RD (eds): Orthopedic Secrets, 2nd ed. Philadelphia, Hanley & Belfus, 1999, pp 200–204, with permission.)

Radiographic factors

- Dysplastic type of spondylolisthesis
- Unstable radiographic contour(dome shaped sacrum, trapezoidal-shaped L5 vertebra)
- Instability on dynamic radiographs
- Degree of slip > 50%
- Slip angle > 40°

19. What are the indications to consider surgery for children with spondylolisthesis?

Surgical indications include intractable low back or radicular pain, progressive slippage, grade 2 or 3 slips in skeletally immature patients, patients with neurologic symptoms, gait abnormality and spinal deformity.

20. What is the procedure of choice for treatment of children with low-grade (grade 1 and 2) spondylolisthesis?

The procedure of choice is an in situ posterolateral spinal fusion (Fig. 4). The procedure can be performed through either a midline approach or a paraspinal approach. Spinal implants are not routinely used by all surgeons because of the good potential for healing of posterolateral fusions in pediatric patients with low-grade slips. Many surgeons consider pedicle fixation advantageous if a decompression is performed at the time of fusion. Traditional teaching is to perform posterolateral fusion from L5 to S1 if the slip is less than 50% and to extend fusion to L4 if the slip is greater than 50%. Use of postoperative immobilzation (brace, cast) is also controversial. To decrease motion at the L5–S1 level, an orthosis must incorporate the patient's thigh.

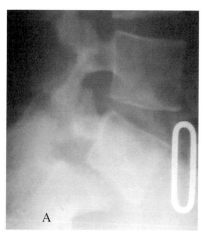
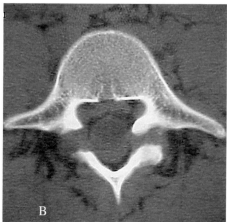
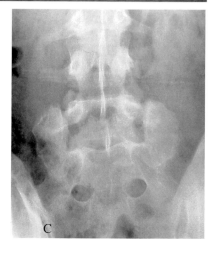

FIGURE 4. Treatment of low-grade isthmic spondylolisthesis with posterolateral in situ fusion using iliac crest autograft. **A,** Preoperative lateral radiograph. **B,** Preoperative CT. **C,** Postoperative AP radiograph showing a healed fusion.

21. What problems are associated with the treatment of high-grade (grades 3 and 4) spondylolisthesis with in situ fusion?

Problems associated with in situ fusion for patients with high-grade spondylolisthesis include progressive slippage, pseudarthrosis, persistent lumbosacral deformity, and cauda equina syndrome.

22. What type of procedure for pediatric high-grade spondylolisthesis has the highest rate of fusion?

Circumferential fusion (Fig. 5). A recent study, showed that the rate of fusion in pediatric high-grade spondylolisthesis depends on the type of fusion procedure:

Procedure	Fusion Rate (%)
Posterior fusion without spinal implants	55
Posterior fusion with spinal implants	71
Circumferential fusion with implants	100

In the circumferential fusion group, iliac screws > 60 mm in length and anterior structural grafting were used.

23. What problems are associated with spondylolisthesis reduction procedures?

Spondylolisthesis reduction procedures are technically complex and associated with numerous potential complications:

- Increased operative time compared to nonreductive techniques
- L5 nerve root injury
- Cauda equina injury
- Proximal lumbar plexus neural injury
- Sacral fixation failure

24. What are the potential advantages of spondylolisthesis reduction procedures compared with in situ fusion?

- Increased fusion rate
- Potential to correct spinal deformity
- Potential to limit fusion to a single spinal motion segment in high-grade slips
- Potential to achieve complete neural decompression
- Prevention of deformity progression
- Restoration of body posture and mechanics

25. What is the role of transfixation, decompression and transsacral interbody fusion using a fibula graft in the treatment of high grade spondylolisthesis?

Decompression, partial reduction, transvertebral screw fixation, and placement of a transsacral fibula graft are an attractive treatment option for patients with high-grade spondylolisthesis (Fig. 6). This technique permits reduction of the slip angle, which is the major component of the deformity. It minimizes the risks associated with attempting complete correction of vertebral translation (spondylolisthesis reduction) and provides a circumferential fusion through a single-stage posterior approach.[1,2,12]

26. What are the treatment options for spondyloptosis?

Fortunately, spondyloptosis is a rare condition. Treatment options include reduction of spondyloptosis and vertebral resection (Gaines procedure). The Gaines procedure (Fig. 7) is generally preferred and is performed in two stages. In the first stage, an anterior approach to the spine is performed and the L5 vertebra, L5–S1 disc, and L4–L5 discs are removed. In the second stage, the lamina and pedicles of L5 are removed to complete the L5 vertebrectomy and the L4 vertebra is placed on top of the sacrum and held in place with pedicle fixation.

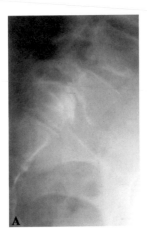
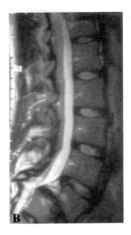
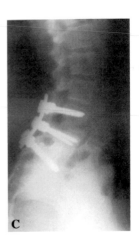

FIGURE 5. Treatment of high-grade isthmic spondylolisthesis with reduction and circumferential fusion. **A,** Preoperative radiograph, **B,** Preoperative MRI. **C,** Postoperative radiograph. Anterior column load-sharing is restored by placement of titanium mesh cages and autogenous graft. Posterior pedicle fixation and fusion restore posterior column integrity. Posterior compression negates shear forces. (From Devlin VJ, Pitt DD: The evolution of surgery of the anterior spinal column. Spine State Art Rev 12:493–528, 1998, with permission.)

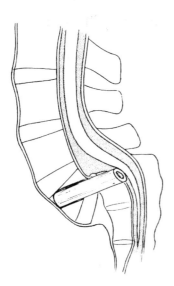
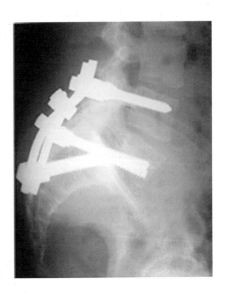

FIGURE 6. Decompression, transfixation, and transsacral interbody fusion. **Left,** A fibula graft is placed across the sacrum, L5–S1 disc and into the L5 vertebral body. (From Winter RB, Lonstein JW, Denis F, Smith MD (eds): Atlas of Spine Surgery. Philadelphia, W.B. Saunders, 1995, p 461, with permission.) **Right,** Pedicle screws are subsequently placed via the S1 pedicle from S1 into L5.

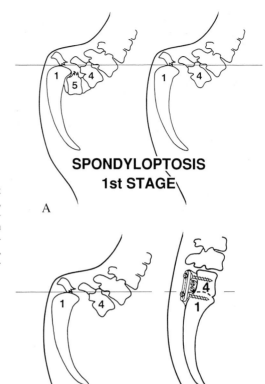

FIGURE 7. Gaines procedure. **A,** First stage. **B,** Second stage. (From Grobler LJ, Wiltse LL: Classification and nonoperative treatment of spondylolisthesis. In Fryomer JW (ed): The Adult Spine: Principles and Practice, 2nd ed. Philadelphia, Lippincott-Raven, 1997, p 1889, with permission.)

SPONDYLOPTOSIS
1st STAGE

A

SPONDYLOPTOSIS
2nd STAGE

B

BIBLIOGRAPHY

1. Abdu WA, Wilber RG, Emery SE: Pedicular transvertebral screw fixation of the lumbosacral spine in spondylolisthesis. Spine 19:710–715, 1994.
2. Boachie-Adjei O, Twee Do, Rawlins B: Partial lumbosacral kyphosis reduction, decompression and posterior lumbosacral transfixation in high grade isthmic spondylolisthesis. Spine 27:E161–E168, 2002.
3. Bradford DS, Boachie-Adjei O: Treatment of severe spondylolisthesis by anterior and posterior reduction and stabilization: A long-term follow-up study. J Bone Joint Surg 72A:1060–1066, 1990.
4. DeWald RL. Spondylolisthesis. In Bridwell KH, DeWald RL (eds): 2nd ed. Philadelphia, Lippincott-Raven, 1997, pp 1199–1210.
5. Edwards CC, Bradford DS: Controversies: Instrumented reduction of spondylolisthesis. Spine 19:1535–1537, 1994.
6. Gaines RW: The L5 vertebrectomy approach for the treatment of spondyloptosis. In Bridwell KH, DeWald RL (eds): The Textbook of Spinal Surgery, 2nd ed. Philadelphia, Lippincott-Raven, 1997, pp 1357–1370.
7. Harms J, Jeszenszky D, Stoltze D, Bohm H: True spondylolisthesis reduction and monosegmental fusion in spondylolisthesis. In Bridwell KH, DeWald RL (eds): The Textbook of Spinal Surgery, 2nd ed. Philadelphia, Lippincott-Raven, 1997, pp 1337–1348.
8. Molinari RM, Bridwell KH, Lenke LH: Complications in the surgical treatment of pediatric high-grade dysplastic spondylolisthesis. Spine 24:1701–1711, 1999.
9. Schoenecker PL: Developmental spondylolisthesis without lysis. In Bridwell KH, DeWald RL (eds): The Textbook of Spinal Surgery, 2nd ed. Philadelphia, Lippincott-Raven, 1997, pp 1255–1262.
10. Smith J, Deviren V, Berven S, et al: Clinical outcome of trans-sacral interbody fusion after partial reduction for high-grade L5–S1 spondylolisthesis. Spine 26:2227–2234, 2001.

VIII. Adult Spinal Deformities and Related Problems

---

47. ADULT IDIOPATHIC AND DEGENERATIVE SCOLIOSIS

Keith H. Bridwell, M.D.

---

1. What are the two types of adult lumbar scoliosis?

(1) Idiopathic with superimposed degenerative changes or (2) de novo/degenerative scoliosis.

2. Define degenerative or de novo scoliosis.

De novo scoliosis begins at age 40 in patients with no preexisting deformity. The deformity occurs with multilevel asymmetric disc degeneration. At various levels the discs degenerate more on one side than the other, resulting in a lumbar deformity.

3. What is the association of spinal stenosis with idiopathic scoliosis and superimposed degenerative changes?

It is uncommon to see a substantial amount of central spinal stenosis in patients who have preexisting idiopathic scoliosis with superimposed degenerative changes. It is more common to see either lateral recess stenosis or foraminal stenosis on the concavity of the distal segments.

4. Which levels are most commonly affected by spinal stenosis in patients with idiopathic scoliosis and superimposed degenerative changes in the lumbar spine?

L3–L4, L4–L5, and L5–S1. At L3–L4 stenosis may be somewhat related to the rotatory subluxation. At L4–L5, lateral recess stenosis is most common; at L5–S1, foraminal stenosis is most common. The stenosis at L4–L5 and L5–S1 is usually on the concavity of the fractional curve below.

5. What is the most common curve pattern with lumbar degenerative scoliosis?

Usually one sees a double lumbar curve pattern in which one curve, most commonly left-sided, is from T12 to L3 and the second curve is right-sided from L3 to the sacrum. At L3–L4 there is usually a rotatory subluxation, which forms the transitional segment between the two curves.

6. With adult scoliosis and foraminal stenosis at L5–S1, what nerve root is most commonly affected?

The nerve root exiting between the L5 and S1 pedicle is the L5 root. Most commonly one sees a left-sided lumbar curve from T12 to L4 and then a fractional curve from L4 to the sacrum that swings the other way. In this situation the concavity of the fractional curve is on the left side; the left L5 nerve root is the one most commonly affected.

7. What are the most common indications for surgical treatment of lumbar idiopathic scoliosis with subsequent degenerative changes?

- Progressive deformity
- Progressive pain
- Spinal claudication symptoms
- Neurologic deficit

8. What are the indications for surgical treatment in young adults with scoliosis who do not have substantial degenerative changes?

- A deformity over 50° by Cobb measurement that the patient perceives as either unacceptable or progressive
- Documented progression of the deformity
- Coronal or sagittal imbalance

9. Define neutral sagittal balance.

Sagittal balance is defined by a plumb dropped from the cervical spine. Some prefer to drop the plumb from C2, and others prefer to drop it from C7. The plumb on a standing lateral x-ray should fall through the lumbosacral disc. Falling through the lumbosacral disc is neutral balance. Falling behind it is negative sagittal balance, and falling in front of it is positive sagittal balance.

10. What is the effect of a Smith-Petersen osteotomy in the anterior, middle, and posterior column?

Smith-Petersen osteotomy opens up the anterior column, closes the middle column somewhat, and closes the posterior column (Figure 1).

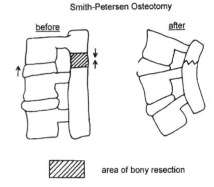

Smith-Petersen Osteotomy

before   after

area of bony resection

FIGURE 1. Smith-Petersen osteotomy. (From Booth KC, Bridwell KH, Lenke LG, et al: Complications and predictive factors for the successful treatment of flatback deformity (fixed sagittal imbalance). Spine 24: 1712–1720, 1999, with permission).

11. What is the effect of a pedicle subtraction osteotomy on the anterior, middle, and posterior column?

A pedicle subtraction osteotomy hinges on the anterior column and closes the middle and posterior column (Figure 2).

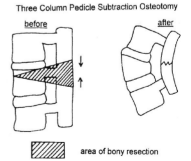

Three Column Pedicle Subtraction Osteotomy

before   after

area of bony resection

FIGURE 2. Three-column pedicle subtraction osteotomy. (From Booth KC, Bridwell KH, Lenke LG, et al: Complications and predictive factors for the successful treatment of flatback deformity (fixed sagittal imbalance). Spine 24:1712–1720, 1999, with permission.)

12. What is the most common sagittal alignment associated with progressive lumbar scoliosis?

Adults with progressive lumbar scoliosis usually have coexisting disc degeneration at all segments. The result is loss of anterior column height and thus segmental kyphosis.

13. Name four common causes for flatback syndrome or fixed sagittal imbalance syndrome.
1. Harrington instrumentation in the lumbar spine
2. Multisegment anterior compression/fusion without structural grafting
3. Progressive post-laminectomy kyphosis
4. Junctional kyphosis above a multisegment fusion

14. Name three acceptable forms of anterior structural grafting used with multisegment fusions in the lumbar spine.
1. Fresh frozen femoral rings packed with morselized autogenous bone graft.
2. Titanium mesh cages packed with autogenous bone graft.
3. Autogenous tricortical iliac bone graft. There is rarely enough bone stock, however, for more than two levels.

15. Name four surgical principles that should be accomplished in order to have a reasonable chance of getting a long fusion to the sacrum solid.
1. Segmental fixation of all segments of the lumbar spine without jumps or gaps
2. Structural grafting at L4–L5 and L5–S1
3. Negative sagittal balance
4. Four-point fixation of the sacrum and pelvis

16. What are the principal indications for surgical treatment of degenerative/de novo scoliosis?
1. Progressive deformity that is unacceptable for the patient
2. Major coronal or sagittal imbalance
3. Spinal claudication symptoms

17. List options for spinal cord monitoring in the surgical treatment of adult scoliosis.
- Stagnara wake-up test
- Somatosensory evoked potentials
- Motor evoked potentials
- Hoppenfeld clonus test

18. List complications of surgical treatment of adult scoliosis.

Pseudarthrosis	Progressive coronal deformity
Superficial wound infection	Progressive sagittal deformity
Deep wound infection	Fixed sagittal imbalance
Neurologic deficit	Increasing pain

19. How much sagittal correction is usually achieved with a pedicle subtraction osteotomy?
30–35°.

20. Does thoracic scoliosis ever progress in adulthood?
Which curves do and do not progress into adulthood is highly variable. It is generally thought that a significant percentage of curves over 50° progress into adulthood. A relatively small percentage of curves between 30° and 50° progress, and progression of thoracic curves below 30° is unlikely.

21. Is lumbar degenerative scoliosis generally progressive or nonprogressive?
This question does not have a simple answer. It is generally thought that a high percentage of degenerative scoliosis cases progress in adulthood. Degenerative scoliosis may be more inclined to progress than long-standing preexisting idiopathic scoliosis. Multiple rotatory subluxations and a relative lack of osteophyte formation seem to be predisposing factors as well.

22. **Can an adult lumbar fusion for scoliosis be stopped at L4 even in the presence of disc degeneration at L4–L5 and L5–S1?**

This issue is highly controversial. Some authors believe that the fusion can be stopped at L4 if the disc degeneration at L4–L5 and L5–S1 is not substantial. Others believe that if disc degeneration is present at these two segments, the fusion should automatically be carried to the sacrum. A middle-of-the-road philosophy is that stopping at L4 is possible and feasible only if there is no substantial deformity between L4 and the sacrum and if the disc degeneration at these two segments is "mild."

23. **List potential complications associated with an anterior approach that is performed from T12 to the sacrum.**
- Sympathectomy effect in the ipsilateral leg
- Deep venous thrombosis in association with extensive mobilization of the venous structures from L4 to the sacrum
- Bulging or diastasis of the abdominal wall postoperatively
- Retroperitoneal fibrosis

24. **Which anterior surgical approach accomplishes exposure anteriorly of all segments from T10 to the sacrum?**

The thoracoabdominal approach, which usually involves entering the chest through the 10th rib and then taking down the diaphragm and the superficial and deep abdominal muscles.

25. **For a left lumbar scoliosis, if exposure is desired from T10 to the sacrum, is it better to do the approach from the left side or the right side?**

It is generally best to approach a curve on the convexity of the curve. In most left lumbar curve patterns, the major curve has an apex between T12 and L2 and extends from T10 or T11 to L4. From L4 to the sacrum there is usually a fractional curve that extends the other way—to the right side. Generally exposure can be accomplished from the left side behind the aorta and vena cava from L10 to L5. Exposure at L5–S1 is variable from patient to patient. Sometimes it is possible to expose L5–S1 from the left side behind the bifurcation, and in other cases it is necessary to expose the L5–S1 disc beneath the bifurcation. The same skin incision can be used for both exposures.

26. **What is the effect of thoracoplasty on pulmonary function in the adult population?**

Few studies have addressed this issue. However, current literature suggests a substantial drop in pulmonary function in the first 3 months after surgery, which improves over the next 2 years. At 2 years postoperatively pulmonary function is usually close to baseline, although frequently not back to baseline. For this reason, a thoracoplasty in an adult patient who does not have exceptionally good pulmonary function may not be advisable.

27. **What is the role for parenteral hyperalimentation in adults with scoliosis?**

To date, no multicenter, randomized, prospective series has definitively answered this question. However, several articles suggest that parenteral nutrition seems to reduce complications somewhat in the adult population, particularly in patients having anterior and posterior surgery, either staged or continuous; patients with reduced protein stores preoperatively; and patients having fusions greater than 10 segments.

28. **Do long scoliosis fusions reduce back pain in the adult population?**

This question is difficult to answer definitively. Most current literature suggests that back pain is substantially improved for most patients. However, it is clear that not all patients have a reduction of pain. Furthermore, it is uncommon for back pain to be "cured" with scoliosis surgery. However, the most common outcome is substantial reduction in back pain.

29. Which is a greater problem in adult scoliosis—progression and pain with thoracic deformity or progression and pain with lumbar deformity?

One study has reported more progression with thoracic scoliosis than lumbar scoliosis in adulthood. However, most investigators have found that lumbar curves are more inclined to progress than thoracic curves. Each patient is somewhat different, and surgeons cannot always predict whether lumbar or thoracic curves will progress in adulthood.

30. For long fusions to the sacrum, which technique is currently considered the gold standard for posterior fixation at L4, L5, and the sacrum?

Currently pedicle fixation at L4, L5, and the sacrum is highly favored over hook fixation and sublaminar wire fixation. However, fixation of the sacrum is somewhat controversial. There is controversy over the best way of fixing the sacrum beyond simply the use of bicortical sacral screws.

31. With a long instrumentation to the sacrum in adults with scoliosis, if the S1 screws are inadvertently directed laterally out the ala rather than medially out the promontory and the screws perforate the anterior cortex, which nerve root is likely to be irritated?

The L5 root. The L5 root exits between the pedicle of L5 and S1 and then travels anterior to the sacral ala. If an S1 pedicle screw comes out the promontory anteriorly, it will be medial to the path of the L5 root. If it comes out laterally, it may irritate the L5 root. If the S1 pedicle screw were to perforate the medial cortex of the pedicle, it would hit the S1 nerve root. This complication (irritating the L5 root) is more likely to occur in a male patient with a narrow pelvis, in whom it is technically difficult to angle the S1 pedicle screws in a medial enough direction.

BIBLIOGRAPHY

1. Bradford DS, Tay BK, Hu SS: Adult scoliosis: Surgical indications, operative management, complications, and outcomes. Spine 24:2617–2629, 1999.
2. Bridwell KH: Osteotomies for fixed deformities in the thoracic and lumbar spine. In Bridwell KH, DeWald RL (eds): The Textbook of Spinal Surgery, 2nd ed. Philadelphia, Lippincott-Raven, 1997, pp 821–836.
3. Dickson JH, Mirkovic S, Noble PC, et al: Results of operative treatment of idiopathic scoliosis in adults. J Bone Joint Surg 77A:513–523, 1995.
4. Grubb SA, Lipscomb HJ, Conrad RW: Degenerative adult onset scoliosis. Spine 13:241–245, 1988.
5. Kostuik JP: Adult scoliosis: The lumbar spine. In Bridwell KH, DeWald RL (eds): The Textbook of Spinal Surgery, 2nd ed. Philadelphia, Lippincott-Raven, 1997, pp 733–775.
6. Weinstein SL, Ponseti IV: Curve progression in idiopathic scoliosis. J Bone Joint Surg 65A:447–455, 1983.

48. SAGITTAL PLANE DEFORMITIES IN ADULTS

John D. Ray, M.D., Munish C. Gupta, M.D. and Theodore A. Wagner, M.D.

1. Describe the normal sagittal contour of the adult spine.

In the sagittal plane , the normal spine possesses four balanced curves (Fig. 1). The kyphotic thoracic and sacral regions are balanced by the lordotic cervical and lumbar regions. In the normal state, the sagittal vertical axis (determined by dropping plumb line from the center of the C7 vertebral body) passes anterior to the thoracic spine, through the center of the L1 vertebral body, posterior to the lumbar spine, and through the lumbosacral disc. A positive sagittal vertical axis (SVA) is present when this line passes in front of the anterior aspect of S1. Negative SVA is present when this line passes behind the posterior aspect of S1.

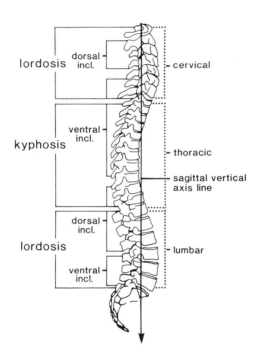

FIGURE 1. Normal sagittal alignment of the spinal column. Note the sagittal vertical axis line and the orientation of each individual vertebrae. (From DeWald RL: Revision surgery for spinal deformity, Instructional Course Lectures, Vol 41, 1992, American Academy of Orthopaedic Surgeons, Park Ride, IL, 1992, with permission.)

2. What are normal values for thoracic kyphosis, lumbar lordosis, and sagittal vertical axis in adults?

There is wide range of normal values in adults. Thoracic kyphosis (T1–T12) varies between 30° and 50°. Lumbar lordosis varies between 45° and 70°. The sagittal vertical axis ranges between 0 and −3 cm. A correlation between increasing thoracic kyphosis and lumbar lordosis tends to maintain spinal balance. In general, lumbar lordosis exceeds thoracic kyphosis by 20–30° to maintain spinal balance and normal position of the SVA

3. How does normal sagittal alignment change with age?

Aging is associated with loss of anterior spinal column height secondary to degenerative disc changes and vertebral body compression, resulting in increased thoracic kyphosis and decreased lumbar lordosis (Fig. 2). The C7 plumb line moves anterior relative to the sacrum as thoracic kyphosis (the angle between the upper end plate of T1 and the lower end plate of T12 on the lateral radiograph) increases and lumbar lordosis (from the top of L1 to the top of S1) decreases. Even asymptomatic people lean forward with age.

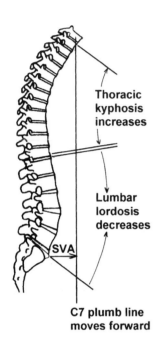

FIGURE 2. Age-related sagittal spine changes. Loss of lumbar lordosis (L1 to S1 lateral Cobb angles) and increased thoracic kyphosis (T1 to T12) lead to anterior translation of the C7 plumb line.

4. List common causes of sagittal plane spinal deformity requiring surgical treatment in the adult population.

Any adult spinal deformity sufficiently severe to require surgical treatment requires consideration of the patient's sagittal plane alignment. Degenerative disorders, fractures, scoliosis, spondylolisthesis, ankylosing spondylitis, and iatrogenic disorders are common causes of sagittal plane deformity requiring surgical treatment in the adult patient.

5. What radiographs are required for evaluation of sagittal plane alignment?

A lateral standing spine radiograph performed on a 36-inch cassette with the arms supported anteriorly allows evaluation of thoracic kyphosis, lumbar lordosis, sacral orientation and the sagittal vertical axis. Lateral flexion-extension views and supine cross table lateral hyperextension films performed over a radiolucent bolster may provide additional information about a specific spinal region.

6. Explain the biomechanical factors responsible for the development of kyphotic deformities.

The spine can be conceptualized as consisting of two columns, the anterior spinal column (vertebral bodies, intervertebral disc, and anterior and posterior longitudinal ligaments) and the posterior spinal column (facets, laminae, and associated ligaments). The anterior column resists compressive forces, whereas the posterior column resists tensile forces. Disruption of either column can lead to development of a kyphotic deformity.

7. **What terms are used to describe kyphotic deformities?**
   - **Sagittal kyphosis:** the vertebral bodies remain in the sagittal plane and angulation occurs in this plane.
   - **Short-radius kyphosis:** an acute angular kyphosis occurs over a few vertebral segments.
   - **Long-radius kyphosis:** a uniform posterior curvature develops over many segments of the spine.
   - **Flexible kyphosis:** corrects within the normal range with hyperextension.
   - **Rigid kyphosis:** deformity resists correction with hyperextension.
   - **Rotational kyphosis:** the vertebral bodies rotate out of the sagittal plane and spinal deformity develops in the sagittal, axial and frontal planes.

8. **What concepts guide the surgical treatment of kyphotic deformities?**

   The goal of surgical treatment of kyphotic deformities is to restore the function of the compromised spinal columns. The anterior spinal column is lengthened, and anterior column load sharing is restored. Integrity of the posterior spinal column is restored with spinal instrumentation, and the length of the posterior spinal column is shortened. Neural compression, if present, is relieved through either direct or indirect techniques. Lasting deformity correction is maintained by successful arthrodesis.

9. **Describe the principles of surgical treament for Scheuermann's kyphosis.**

   Scheuermann's kyphosis is a long-radius kyphotic deformity that may be either flexible or rigid. Adult deformities sufficiently severe to require surgical treatment tend to be rigid. Traditional surgical treatment consists of an anterior approach to release contracted anterior spinal column structures, including the anterior longitudinal ligament, annulus, and intervertebral disc. The disc spaces are filled with nonstructural bone graft. The deformity is corrected with posterior segmental spinal instrumentation placed above and below the apex of the kyphotic deformity. Compression forces are applied to the spine in order to shorten the posterior spinal column. Multilevel interlaminar closing wedge resections may be used to enhance correction and decrease forces on spinal implants.

10. **Describe the principles of surgical treatment for posttraumatic kyphosis.**

    Posttraumatic kyphosis is a short-radius kyphotic deformity that may be either flexible or rigid. Factors to consider in the surgical treatment of posttraumatic kyphosis include the magnitude of deformity, the presence or absence of neurologic deficit, and the stability of the anterior and posterior spinal columns. In general, isolated posterior surgical procedures are inadequate for treatment of posttraumatic kyphosis. Such procedures do not permit adequate deformity correction or adequate decompression of neural structures. Isolated anterior surgical procedures are often insufficient since the posterior osteoligamentous structures impede adequate deformity correction and restoration of normal spinal biomechanics. The most effective treatment for posttraumatic kyphotic deformity is a combined anterior and posterior procedure, which permits adequate neural decompression, deformity reduction, and stabilization.

11. **What factors are responsible for the development of kyphotic deformities in senior citizens?**

    The most common etiologies responsible for the development of kyphotic deformities in senior citizens include loss of posterior muscle and ligamentous tone, compression fractures secondary to osteoporosis, and degenerative disc changes.

12. **List some potential complications associated with osteoporotic vertebral compression fractures.**

    Potential complications associated with osteoporotic vertebral compression fractures include pain, additional vertebral compression fractures, loss of lung capacity, loss of appetite, poor nutrition, decreased mobility, and depression.

13. Discuss options for treatment of osteoporotic vertebral compression fractures.

Prevention through exercise, diet (vitamin D, calcium), and medication (bisphosphonates) is ideal. Once fractures occur, treatment options include a short period of bed rest, analgesics, and orthoses (Jewett or TLSO). Cement augmentation of compressed vertebral bodies (vertebroplasty, kyphoplasty) plays a role in acute and subacute fractures. Open surgical intervention is generally reserved for deformities associated with neurologic compromise due to the high risk of complications associated with major spinal reconstructive procedures in this population.

14. Discuss advantages and disadvantages of vertebroplasty and kyphoplasty.

Vertebroplasty is the percutaneous injection of low viscosity polymethylmethacrylate (PMMA) into a vertebral body. The cement interdigitates with the bony trabeculae to stabilize painful osteoporotic compression fractures. Improvement in pain is reported in approximately 90% of patients. Extravasation of the low-viscosity cement into the spinal canal and venous system has been associated with neural compression, embolization, and death.

Kyphoplasty involves the expansion of an inflatable (balloon) tamp in the vertebral body to create a cavity with a surrounding shell of compressed bone. This permits injection of viscous cement under low pressure and reduces the risk of cement extravasation. Balloon expansion may partially restore vertebral body height and reduce kyphotic deformity. Disadvantages of this technique include the cost of the balloon and possible fractures in adjacent vertebra due to creation of a "super-stiff" vertebral body. Pain relief achieved with this procedure is comparable with vertebroplasty

15. How is sagittal plane alignment altered in ankylosing spondylitis?

Patients with ankylosing spondylitis can develop fixed flexion deformites of the hips and spine. Patients with severe deformities are unable to look straight ahead and have extreme difficulties carrying out activities of daily living. Initial surgical treatment is generally directed at the hip joints. Total hip arthroplasty is an effective procedure in this population. Severe deformities require additional surgery with spinal osteotomy at the site of major defomity.

16. What is the effect of disc degeneration on lumbar lordosis?

Disc degeneration is associated with loss of normal lumbar lordosis, posterior rotation (extension) of the sacrum and pelvis, and anterior translation of the C7 plumb line relative to the sacrum.

17. What is "flatback deformity"?

Flatback deformity describes symptomatic loss of normal sagittal plane alignment resulting from loss of lumbar lordosis. This deformity moves the C7 plumb line and head to an anterior position relative to the sacrum.

18. What is the association between flatback deformity and Harrington distraction instrumentation for scoliosis?

Harrington instrumentation corrected the coronal plane deformity of scoliosis through the application of posterior distraction forces. This approach had the unintended consequence of decreasing the normal lordotic alignment of the lumbar region creating an iatrogenic spinal deformity.

19. List some additional causes of flatback deformity.

Flatback syndrome may occur for many reasons in addition to Harrington instrumentation for scoliosis treatment. Flatback syndrome (also termed sagittal malalignment or imbalance syndrome) may occur after lumbar fusion for degenerative spinal disorders when adequate lumbar lordosis is not restored during surgery. Transition syndrome (breakdown of spinal segments above or below a solid spinal fusion) is another frequent cause of sagittal imbalance. Autofusion of the spine as a result of Forrestier's disease (DISH) or ankylosing spondylitis may also lead to spinal imbalance. Osteoporotic compression fractures are another cause of sagittal imbalance.

20. How does loss of lumbar lordosis increase muscle fatigue?

Loss of lordosis causes anterior translation of the C7 plumb line and center of gravity, resulting in an increased flexion moment applied to the spine. The distance between the spine and the lumbar erector spinae muscles decreases, thus shortening the moment arm of the spinal extensors. The erector spinae muscles must work harder to balance the body; as a result, these muscles fatigue earlier.

21. List early and late compensatory mechanisms that attempt to accomodate for loss of lumbar lordosis.

Early compensatory mechanisms include hyperextension of adjacent mobile lumbar, thoracic and cervical segments as well as hip hyperextension. With further decompensation, knee flexion helps keep the head above the pelvis but results in quadriceps fatigue. Patients present with a "flexed-knee, flexed-hip" appearance.

22. What are the consequences of compensatory hyperextension of adjacent spinal motion segments?

Increased facet loads lead to facet and disc degeneration as well as pain. Spondylolisthesis may develop secondary to facet degeneration and /or fracture through the pars interarticularis.

23. How does operative positioning effect lumbar lordosis?

Hip flexion significantly reduces lumbar lordosis. Although hip flexion can facilitate access to the spinal canal for surgical decompression, the reduction of lumbar lordosis must be taken into account if a fusion is performed during the same procedure . Lumbar instrumentation and fusion should be performed with the hips extended to maintain and restore maximal lumbar lordosis.

24. What are the surgical options for correction of sagittal deformity in the previously unfused spine?

Posterior fusion with segmental instrumentation using appropriately contoured longitudinal members can improve sagittal alignment. More severe deformity may require anterior release and interbody fusion to restore the intervertebral disc height and segmental lordosis.

25. What are the surgical options for correction of the sagittal plane deformity in the previously fused spine?

Smith-Peterson osteotomy (resection of a posterior column wedge to achieve correction through the disc space or through a prior anterior osteotomy) and **pedicle subtraction osteotomy** (resection of a three column wedge hinging at the anterior longitudinal ligament) are powerful methods for correction sagittal deformity. Combined coronal and sagittal deformity may be corrected with a **vertebral column resection procedure.**

BIBLIOGRAPHY

1. Bernhardt M, Bridwell KH: Segmental analysis of the sagittal plane alignment of the normal thoracic and lumbar spines and thoracolumbar junction. Spine 14:717–21, 1989.
2. Gelb DE, et al: An analysis of sagittal spinal alignment in 100 asymptomatic middle and older aged volunteers. Spine 20:1351–1358, 1995.
3. Hammerberg EM, Wood KB: Sagittal profile of the elderly. J Spinal Disord Tech 16:44–50, 2003.
4. Jackson RP, McManus AC: Radiographic analysis of sagittal plane alignment and balance in standing volunteers and patients with low back pain matched for age, sex, and size. A prospective controlled clinical study. Spine 19:1611–1618, 1994.
5. Korovessis PG, et al: Reciprocal angulation of vertebral bodies in the sagittal plane in an asymptomatic Greek population. Spine 23:700–704; discussion 704–705, 1998.
6. Legaye J, et al: Pelvic incidence: a fundamental pelvic parameter for three-dimensional regulation of spinal sagittal curves. Eur Spine J 7:99–103, 1998.
7. Lieberman IH, et al: Initial outcome and efficacy of "kyphoplasty" in the treatment of painful osteoporotic vertebral compression fractures. Spine 26:1631–1638, 2001.
8. Moe JH, Denis F: The iatrogenic loss of lumbar lordosis [abstract]. Orthop Trans 1:131, 1977.
9. Vedantam R, et al: Comparison of standing sagittal spinal alignment in asymptomatic adolescents and adults. Spine 23:211–215, 1998.

49. SPONDYLOLYSIS AND SPONDYLOLISTHESIS IN ADULTS

Vincent J. Devlin, M.D.

1. Discuss similarities and differences between adult and pediatric patients with spondylolysis and spondylolisthesis in regard to classification, clinical presentation, radiographic work-up, and treatment.

Classification. The classification described by Wiltse applies to both pediatric and adult patients with spondylolisthesis. However, the degenerative type of spondylolisthesis is seen only in adult patients and is emphasized in this chapter.

Clinical presentation. In pediatric patients, back pain is the most common presenting symptom. Pain is directly related to instability at the site of spondylolysis/spondylolisthesis. Symptoms of hamstring spasm are not uncommon. Occasionally, L5 radicular pain is seen with higher-grade slips or spinal stenosis associated with dysplastic slips. Adult patients frequently present with both back and leg pain symptoms. In adult patients, symptoms may be related either to the level of spondylolisthesis or to degenerative patholgy (disc protrusion, stenosis, discogenic pain syndrome) at adjacent spinal levels. It is critical to localize precisely the pain generator in adult patients with spondylolisthesis because pain may not be related to the spondylolisthesis.

Radiographic work-up. Standing radiographs are the initial radiographic study for assessment of spondylolisthesis in both pediatric and adult patients. The degree of slip (Meyerding classification) and the slip angle are important for decision making in both patient groups. The need for additional diagnostic imaging is more common in adults to assess the cause of leg pain and the status of the lumbar discs. Magnetic resonance imaging (MRI) is the standard for evaluating neural compression in both pediatric and adult patients. Computed tomography (CT) is the method of choice for assessing osseous anatomy in both groups. Discography is occasionally used in adult patients to assess whether a particular disc is a pain generator but has little role in pediatric patients. Technetium bone scans are sometimes used in pediatric patients to assess the osseous activity related to a spondylolysis and assess its healing potential. In adult patients spondylolysis is typically inactive on bone scans, which have little value in this setting.

Surgical treatment. In pediatric patients, options for treatment of spondylolysis include either a direct pars repair or an intertransverse fusion. In adults, surgical treatment of symptomatic spondylolysis requires a fusion because the disc below the pars defect typically demonstrates degenerative changes. With respect to treatment of low grade isthmic spondylolisthesis (grade 1 and grade 2) in children, in situ posterolateral fusion is associated with a high success rate due to the excellent healing potential of pediatric patients. Adults with low-grade isthmic spondylolisthesis require more complex surgery. Adults patients require neural decompression in addition to fusion. Posterior spinal implants are commonly used in an attempt to decrease the risk of postoperative slip progression and enhance osseous union. With respect to treatment of high-grade spondylolisthesis (grade 3 and 4), a circumferential fusion provides the most reliable rate of fusion in both the pediatric and adult patient. Circumferential fusion may be performed with or without reduction of the spondylolisthesis.

2. Does isthmic spondylolisthesis progress after skeletal maturity?

Yes. Isthmic spondylolisthesis is most likely to progress during the fourth and fifth decades of life(4). Progression of slippage is associated with the development of degenerative disc changes below the level of the pars defect. The ability of the intervertebral disc to resist shear forces is compromised and progression of spondylolisthesis occurs. This explains how a pars defect which has been asymptomatic since childhood may become symptomatic in later life in the absence of precipitating trauma.

3. What nonoperative treatment options are available for adults with isthmic spondylolisthesis?

Nonoperative treatment options include nonsteroidal anti-inflammatory drugs, exercise (stretching, strengthening, flexibility), and bracing. Use of epidural injections and/or selective nerve root blocks may be considered. Weight reduction should be advised for overweight patients. Smoking should be stopped because it has been associated with back pain symptoms in adult patients and decreases the chance of successful fusion if surgery is eventually considered.

4. When is surgery considered for an adult patient with isthmic spondylolisthesis?

Surgery is infrequently required for adult patients with spondylolisthesis. General indications to consider surgical intervention for adult isthmic spondylolisthesis include:

- Failure of nonsurgical treatment for disabling back and/or leg pain
- Patients with symptomatic and radiographically unstable isthmic spondylolisthesis
- Documented slip progression to greater than grade 2 slippage
- Symptomatic grade 3 or 4 spondylolisthesis or spondyloptosis
- Symptomatic associated spinal stenosis or progressive neurologic deficit
- Cauda equina syndrome related to spondylolisthesis

5. What pattern of neural compression is most commonly associated with L5–S1 isthmic spondylolisthesis?

L5 nerve root compression is the type of neural compression most commonly associated with L5–S1 isthmic spondylolisthesis. L5 nerve root compression may occur secondary to:

- Hypertrophy of fibrocartilage at the site of the pars defect (zone 1)
- Compression in the foramenal zone (zone 2) as the L5 root is compressed between a disc bulge and the inferior aspect of the L5 pedicle
- Compression between the inferior aspect of the L5 transverse process and the superior aspect of the sacral ala (zone 3)
- Increased tension within the L5 nerve root secondary to forward displacement of the L5 vertebra.

The sacral nerve roots can become involved in high-grade isthmic spondylolisthesis as they become stretched over the L5–S1 disc and posterior aspect of the sacrum.

6. What are the surgical treatment options for L5–S1 isthmic spondylolisthesis in adult patients?

- Decompression and in situ posterolateral fusion with posterior pedicle fixation
- Decompression and posterior pedicle fixation combined with interbody fusion and reduction (partial vs. complete)
- Decompression and posterior pedicle fixation and placement of a trans-sacral interbody graft (fibula strut)

7. Define degenerative spondylolisthesis.

Degenerative spondylolisthesis is an anterior subluxation of one vertebra relative to the inferior vertebra in the presence of an intact posterior neural arch. The cause of the subluxation is degenerative changes in the intervertebral disc and posterior facet joints.

8. Who is most likely to develop degenerative spondylolisthesis?

Degenerative spondylolisthesis generally occurs in patients older than 40 years. It is more common in females (female-to-male ratio: 4:1) and more common in blacks (black-to-caucasian ratio: 3:1). The condition is more common in diabetic patients.

9. What level of the spine is most commonly involved in degenerative spondylolisthesis?

Ninety percent of cases of degenerative spondylolisthesis occur at L4–L5, and 10% of cases occur at L3–L4 or L5–S1. Degenerative spondylolisthesis is associated with sacralization of the L5 vertebra.

10. What are the common presenting symptoms of degenerative spondylolisthesis?

Symptoms include neurogenic claudication, low back pain, and radicular pain. Neurogenic claudication presents as buttock and thigh pain and cramping associated with prolonged standing or walking. Relief of these symptoms is achieved by sitting or flexion maneuvers. Patients may also report numbness, heaviness, or weakness in the lower extremities.

11. What nonspinal disorders must be ruled out during the examination of a patient with degenerative spondylolisthesis?

Degenerative arthritis of the hip joint and peripheral vascular disease. Hip joint arthrosis may cause buttock and thigh pain and can mimic symptoms of spinal stenosis. Assessment of hip joint range of motion can determine whether radiographs are needed to assess the hip joints. If both hip arthritis and degenerative spondylolisthesis are present, injection of the hip joint under fluoroscopic guidance can aid in sorting out which problem is more symptomatic. Peripheral vascular disease can also cause claudication. Assessment of lower extremity peripheral pulses is a routine part of assessment of patients with adult spinal disorders. Vascular claudication is associated with increased muscular exertion independent of trunk position. Symptoms due to vascular claudication typically occur in the distal calf and foot and are not associated with back pain.

12. What imaging studies should be obtained to assess a patient with symptoms suggestive of degenerative spondylolisthesis?

Initial studies include standing anteroposterior (AP) and lateral lumbar radiographs and lateral flexion-extension radiographs. A lumbar MRI is ordered to evaluate the spinal canal for neural compression. In patients who are unable to tolerate MRI (e.g., claustrophobia, pacemaker) and patients with associated scoliosis and spondylolisthesis, a CT-myelogram is obtained.

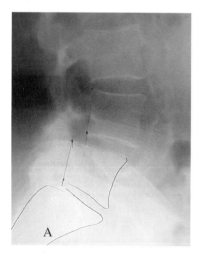
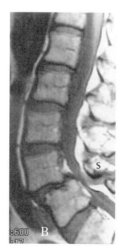
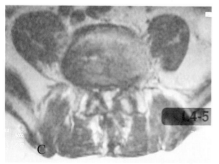

FIGURE 1. Imaging studies **A,** Standing lateral radiograph. **B,** MRI sagittal view (From Barckhausen RR, Math KR: Lumbar spine disease. In Katz DS, Math KR, Groskin SA (eds): Radiology Secrets. Philadelphia, Hanley & Belfus, 1998, with permission). **C,** MRI axial view. (*continued*)

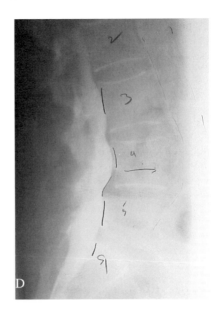

FIGURE 1. (*continued*) **D,** Myelogram.

13. What pattern of neural compression is most commonly associated with L4–L5 degenerative spondylolisthesis?

Degenerative spondylolisthsis at the L4–L5 level typically causes central spinal stenosis at the L4–L5 level. This condition is associated with subarticular (zone 1) stenosis with compromise of the L5 nerve root. The L4 nerve root is generally spared from compression unless there is severe loss of disc space height, in which case the L4 nerve root is compressed by resultant foraminal narrowing.

14. What degree of subluxation can be associated with degenerative spondylolisthesis?

In a patient who has not undergone prior spine surgery, degenerative spondylolisthesis presents with subluxations less than 50% (grade 1 or 2 slips). Further slippage is limited by the intact neural arch.

15. What are the nonsurgical treatment options for degenerative spondylolisthesis?

Options include nonsteroidal anti-inflammatory medication, physical therapy, and bracing. Physical therapy should consist of aerobic conditioning and exercises that emphasize lumbar flexion. Epiduaral injections are most likely to be effective for patients with significant lower extremity symptoms rather than for patients whose predominant symptom is back pain. Prescription of a walker may be helpful.

16. When is surgery considered for degenerative spondylolisthesis?

- Persistent or recurrent leg pain despite adequate nonsurgical management
- Progressive neurologic deficit
- Significant reduction in quality of life
- Confirmatory imaging studies consistent with the diagnosis

17. What are the surgical treatment options for degenerative spondylolisthesis?

- Decompression
- Decompression and posterior fusion without spinal instrumentation
- Decompression and posterior fusion and posterior spinal instrumentation
- Decompression and posterior fusion and posterior spinal instrumentation combined with interbody fusion

18. What is the preferred treatment for most cases of degenerative spondylolisthesis?

Multiple studies have shown that the best treatment outcomes are achieved when a decompression is combined with a posterior fusion. However, not all surgeons agree that posterior spinal instrumentation is required.

19. Describe what is involved in a typical decompression for L4–L5 degenerative spondylolisthesis. Does decompression without fusion ever have a role?

A typical decompression for L4–L5 spondylolisthesis involves removal of the inferior one-half of the lamina of L4 and the superior one-half of the lamina of L5 to decompress the central spinal canal. Next the L5 nerve roots are decompressed by removing the medial one-half of the L4–L5 facet joint and accompanying ligamentum flavum. The decompression of the L5 nerve root is continued until the L5 nerve root is mobile and a probe passes easily through the foramen. The L4 nerve root and foramen should also be checked for potential compression.

Although a posterior fusion is generally recommended for treatment of patients with degenerative spondylolisthesis and spinal stenosis, in select situations decompression without fusion can achieve a good outcome. Potential candidates for this approach are usually low-demand elderly patients. Such patients generally have a narrow L4–L5 disc space (< 2mm) and exhibit no motion on flexion-extension radiographs. They may have anterior vertebral osteophytes, which provide additional stability to the L4–L5 motion segment. Decompression in these patients should preserve at least 50% of the L4–L5 facet joints bilaterally to prevent increased listhesis post-operatively.

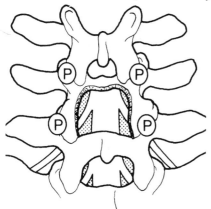

FIGURE 2. Typical decompression for L4–L5 degenerative spondylolisthesis. (From Grobler LJ, Wiltse LL: Classification, non-operative and operative treatment for spondylolisthesis. In Frymoyer JW (ed): The Adult Spine: Principles and Practice. New York, Raven Press, 1991, p 1696, with permission.)

20. Describe how a posterior fusion is performed for L4–L5 degenerative spondylolisthesis. What is the role of posterior spinal instrumentation?

After completion of the decompression, the transverse processes of L4 and L5 are carefully exposed and soft tissue is removed from the intertransverse membrane extending between the transverse processes. The transverse processes are decorticated with a curette or burr to expose the cancellous surface. Cancellous and corticocancellous bone graft from the patients's iliac crest is applied to the intertransverse region to complete the fusion procedure. If internal fixation is used, a facet fusion may also be performed. However, if no instrumentation is used, facet disruption may increase the risk of post-operative instability.

The addition of internal fixation in the form of pedicle fixation at the level of listhesis has many advantages, but its use in this disorder is not universally accepted. Pedicle fixation has been shown to increase the rate of successful fusion and decrease the risk of post-operative progressive slippage and recurrent stenosis. Use of pedicle fixation facilitates early patient mobilization following surgery and its routine use is preferred by many surgeons. Other surgeons believe that use should be limited until there is unequivocal evidence that pedicle fixation positively improves patient outcome. Noninstrumented fusion is considered reasonable in the patient with mild degenerative spondyloisthesis (< 5 mm) in whom there is no pathologic motion on flexion-extension radiographs. Most surgeons today agree that pedicle fixation should be used if > 5 mm of motion is noted on dynamic radiographs.

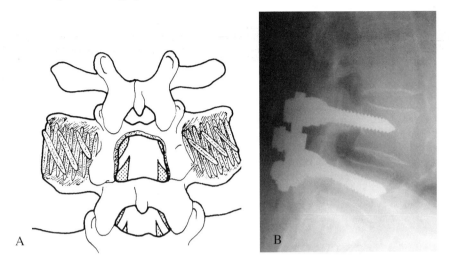

FIGURE 3. Posterolateral L4–L5 fusion. **A,** Without spinal instrumentation. (From Grobbler LJ, Wiltse LL: Classification, non-operative and operative treatment of spondylolisthesis. In Frymoyer JW (ed): The Adult Spine: Principles and Practice. New York, Raven Press, 1991, p 1696, with permission. **B,** With pedicle screw fixation.

21. When should an interbody fusion be considered for L4–L5 degenerative spondylolisthesis?

- Degenerative spondylolithesis in which the L4 and L5 vertebra are in a position of kyphosis relative to one another
- Degenerative spondylolisthesis with severe disc space narrowing associated with L4 foramenal stenosis. In this situation, addition of an interbody fusion will increase the dimensions of the neural foramen between L4 and L5 resulting in decompression of the L4 nerve root.
- Degenerative spondylolisthesis in which the required decompression has compromised the amount of available posterior bone surface available for posterior fusion. For example, if the facet joints are completely removed and/or the pars interarticularis is violated, a posterior fusion alone is less likely to heal.

BIBLIOGRAPHY

1. Booth KC, Bridwell KH, Eisenberg BA, et al: Minimum 5-year results of degeneative spondylolistheisis treated with decompression and posterior fusion. Spine 24:1721–1727, 1999.
2. Bridwell KH: Acquired degenerative spondylolisthesis without lysis. In Bridwell KH, DeWald RL (eds): The Textbook of Spinal Surgery, 2nd ed. Philadelphia, Lippincott-Raven, 1997, pp 1299–1298.
3. Fishgrund JS, Mackay M, Herkowitz HN, et al: Degenerative lumbar spondylolisthesis with spinal stenosis: A prospective randomized study comparing decompressive laminectomy and arthrodesis with and without spinal instrumentation. Spine 22:2807–2812, 1997.
4. Floman Y: Progression of lumbosacral isthmic spondylolisthesis in adults. Spine 25:342–347, 2000.
5. Mardjetko SM, Connelly PJ, Shott P: Degenerative lumbar spondylolisthesis: A meta-analysis of literature 1970–1993. Spine 19:2279S–2296S, 1994.
6. Vaccaro AR, Martyak GG, Madigan L: Adult isthmic spondylolisthesis. Orthopedics 24:1172–1179, 2001.
7. Yuan HA, Garfin SR, Dickman CA: A historical cohort study of pedicle screw fixation in thoracic, lumbar and sacral spine fusions. Spine 19: 2279S–2296S, 1994.

IX. Spinal Trauma

50. UPPER CERVICAL SPINE TRAUMA

Jens R. Chapman, M.D., Todd S. Jarosz, M.D., and Sohail K. Mirza, M.D.

1. What are the major types of injuries involving the upper cervical (occiput–C2) region?
The major types of injuries can be classified according to location:
1. Occipitocervical articulation
   - Occipital condyle fractures
   - Atlanto-occipital dislocation
2. Atlas (C1)
   - Atlas fractures
   - Transverse ligament injuries
3. Axis (C2)
   - Odontoid fractures
   - Hangman's fractures

2. How are upper cervical spine injuries diagnosed?
Any patient with a suspected cervical spine injury requires thorough evaluation. Frequently no specific symptoms or findings on physical examination strongly point to the presence of a significant osseous or ligamentous injury involving the upper cervical region. Symptoms are notoriously vague and may include headaches or suboccipital pain. Not infrequently, the patient may be unconcious following trauma. A neurologic evaluation according to the American Spinal Injury Association (ASIA) guidelines is performed. Assessment of the upper cervical spine should include evaluation of lower cranial nerve function. Most upper cervical spine injuries can be diagnosed on the lateral cervical spine radiograph. An open-mouth AP odontoid view and lateral skull radiograph should be obtained. Immobilization with a cervical collar (for stable injuries) or Gardner-Wells tong traction (for unstable injuries) should be maintained in the emergency setting. CT with sagittal and coronal plane reformatted views is usually required to assess the full magnitude of injury. MRI is indicated for patients with cervical spinal cord injury and for evaluation of suspected ligament injuries that are not evident with other imaging modalities.

3. What is the role of flexion-extension radiographs in the assessment of acute upper cervical spine injuries?
Although flexion-extension radiographs can identify instability of the atlantoaxial motion segment, they are of limited value and even potentially dangerous in the acute trauma setting. Physician supervised traction films are preferable to assess stability of the upper cervical spine.

4. How is a cervical traction test performed?
With the patient in the supine position, an image intensifier is used to obtain a baseline lateral radiographic image of the cervical spine. Traction weights are added in 5-pound increments (20-pound limit) using a head-halter or skeletal traction device (halo, Gardner-Wells tongs) as the cervical region is monitored radiographically. If distraction of more than 3 mm between the occipital condyles and atlas or between the atlas and axis occurs, the test is considered positive and is discontinued.

5. Are upper cervical spine injuries common?
Because of the fragile nature of the bony and ligamentous components of the upper cervical spine, injuries are relatively common, especially in the setting of closed head trauma. Typical in-

jury mechanisms include flexion, extension, or compressive forces applied to the head during motor vehicle accidents, falls from a height, or sporting injuries. Approximately 50% of fractures involving the atlas are accompanied by a second spine fracture. Fractures of the axis account for 27% of associated injuries; odontoid fractures account for 41%. The exact incidence of upper cervical ligamentous injuries is undetermined. Disruption of the craniocervical ligaments (Fig. 1) is reported to be the leading cause of fatal motor vehicle occupant trauma.

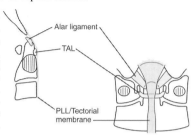

FIGURE 1. Craniocervical ligaments. The tectorial membrane is the uppermost extension of the posterior longitudinal ligament and attaches to the occipital condyles providing for stability against cranial traction and flexion forces. The alar ligaments extend from the tip of the odontoid process and attach to the anterior aspect of the foramen magnum serving as checkreins against rotation and distraction. These ligaments run from the occiput to C2 without attaching directly to C-1 which serves as a bushing. The transverse atlantal ligament (TAL) restricts translation of C1 on C2. Copyright Jens R. Chapman.

6. Are upper cervical spine injuries commonly associated with neurologic deficits?

Because of the relatively large size of the upper cervical spinal canal, neurologic deficits are relatively rare in association with upper cervical injuries. However, when upper cervical spinal cord injuries occur, they are often fatal because of injury to the respiratory and cardiac centers in the medulla and upper cervical cord. Incomplete spinal cord injuries in the upper cervical region may present as a cervicomedullary syndrome or cranial nerve injury.

OCCIPITOCERVICAL ARTICULATION

7. How are occipital condyle fractures classified?

Occipital condyle fractures typically result from a direct blow to the head or from a rapid deceleration injury. These inuries are frequently associated with C1 fractures and cranial nerve injuries. CT is used to classify these injuries into three subtypes:

Type 1: a stable comminuted fracture resulting from an axial loading injury

Type 2: a stable skull base fracture that extends into the occipital condyle

Type 3: an avulsion fracture of the condyle at the attachment of the alar ligament. This fracture type is potentially unstable and may be associated with an atlanto-occipital dislocation.

8. How are occipital condyle fractures treated?

Unilateral type 1 and 2 injuries are usually treated with a rigid cervical orthosis. Isolated type 3 avulsion injuries are managed with a halo orthosis. Type 3 injuries associated with atlanto-occipital dislocation require posterior occipitocervical fusion.

9. What is an atlanto-occipital dislocation (AOD)?

High-speed deceleration injuries may result in disruption of important craniocervical ligaments (tectorial membrane, anterior occipito-atlantal membrane, alar ligaments) resulting in craniocervical junction instability. These injuries are frequently fatal. Survivors typically present with a spinal cord injury above the C4 segment. Incomplete spinal cord injuries associated with AOD include respiratory impairment and cranial nerve injuries (cervicomedullary syndrome). Young children are the most commonly injured age group due to their relatively large head size, shallow atlanto-occipital joints and ligamentous laxity compared with adults. In the pediatric age group AOD may be the result of a "shaken baby syndrome," pedestrian vs. car injuries, or deceleration injuries in a car crash with the child immobilized in a car seat.

10. How is atlanto-occipital dislocation identified?

The most effective screening test remains the lateral cervical spine radiograph. Important radiographic parameter to assess include:

• Soft tissue swelling adjacent to the upper cervical vertebral bodies.

- Diastasis or subluxation of atlanto-occipital articulation (Fig. 2A).
- Disruption of Wackenheim's line, (which normally runs along the posterior surface of the clivus and intersects the posterior tip of the odontoid (Fig. 2B).
- An increased dens-basion interval (DBI)—the distance from the basion to the tip of the odontoid should not exceed 5 mm in adults or 10 mm in children (Fig. 2C).
- An increased Powers ratio. This ratio between the distance from the basion to the posterior arch of C1 and the distance from the opisthion to the anterior arch of C1 is usually less than 1.0. A ratio greater than 1.0 suggests an anterior dislocation of the atlanto-occipital joint.

The diagnosis of AOD is confirmed with a fine-cut CT scan and/or MRI. Occasionally a cervical traction test is necessary to confirm presence of an occult AOD.

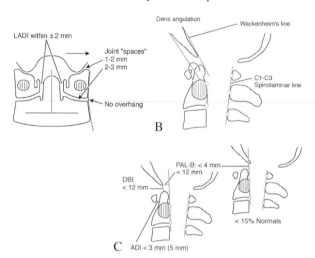

FIGURE 2. A, The lateral masses of the atlas should closely articulate with the superior articular processes of the atlas. The odontoid should be centered symmetrically between the lateral masses of the atlas. **B,** Simple reference lines, such as the one proposed by Wackenheim (extension of line from by clivus should be close to tip of odontoid process) and the spinolaminar line between the anterior laminar cortex of the C1, C2, and C3 laminae, are effective screening tools for evaluation of the upper cervical spine. **C,** The tip of the odontoid should remain in close proximity to the basion, as shown with the reference lines described by Harris. Copyright Jens R. Chapman.

11. How is an atlanto-occipital dislocation classified?

The direction of displacement of the head relative to the cervical spine can be used to differentiate anterior, vertical and posterior dislocations. However, the type of displacement in the presence of global ligamentous failure is somewhat arbitrary and can be altered by patient positioning. An alternative classification differentiates incomplete injuries that retain partial meaningful cranio-cervical ligamentous integrity (stage 1 lesions) from occult injuries (stage II) in which a rebound phenomenon lead to partial or complete deformity reduction. These injuries are easily overlooked, yet may have catastrophic consequences if left untreated. Stage III injuries show obvious craniocervical displacement (distraction or translation).

12. What is the treatment for an atlanto-occipital dislocation?

Stage I lesions are usually treated with 8–12 weeks of halo-vest immobilization. Stage II and III AOD are potentially life-threatening injuries. Emergent reduction and external immobilization attempts can be made with a halo-vest or head immobilization using a neck collar and sand bags. Definitive treatment of stage II and III lesions consists of posterior occipitocervical arthrodesis with rigid segmental spinal instrumentation. Attempts at occiput to C1 fusion are unwarranted since this treatment does not address the disrupted alar ligaments and tectorial membrane. Significant ethical challenges in terms of sustaining life-preserving support measures may arise in cases of patients with associated anoxic or traumatic brain injury.

ATLAS FRACTURES AND TRANSVERSE ATLANTAL LIGAMENT (TAL) INJURIES

13. How are C1 fractures and TAL injuries diagnosed?

Radiographs should include an open-mouth odontoid view and a lateral C1–C2 view. On the lateral view, the atlantodens interval (ADI) should be < 3 mm in adults and < 5 mm in children.

On the open-mouth view, the symmetry of the dens in relation to the adjacent lateral masses should be assessed. Any outward displacement of the lateral masses of C1 in relation to C2 should be noted. Atlantoaxial offset > 7 mm indicates C1–C2 instability and disruption of the TAL (Fig. 3). Definitive assessment is achieved with a fine-cut CT scan with reformated images. Efforts at visualizing the TAL on MRI have remained inconsistent. Isolated TAL injuries may occasionally require flexion—extension radiographs to assess for atlantoaxial instability.

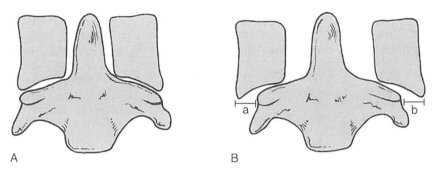

A   B

FIGURE 3. A, Lateral displacement of the C1 lateral masses of more than 7 mm indicates disruption of the transverse ligament. **B,** The sum of the displacements of the left and right sides (a+b) is used to determine the total displacement. (From Browner BD, Jupiter JB, Levine AM (eds): Skeletal Trauma. Philadelphia, W.B.Saunders, 1998, p 819, with permission.)

14. How are C1 fractures classified?

Five primary types of atlas fractures have been defined (Fig. 4):

Type 1: Transverse process fracture
Type 2: Posterior arch fracture
Type 3: Lateral mass fracture
Type 4: Anterior arch fracture
Type 5: Burst fracture (Jefferson's fracture). Burst fractures may consist of 3 or 4 parts. This injury may occur as ligamentous combination injury with TAL disruption.

Type 3, 4 and 5 fractures can be inherently stable or unstable, depending on fracture displacement and concurrent ligamentous disruption.

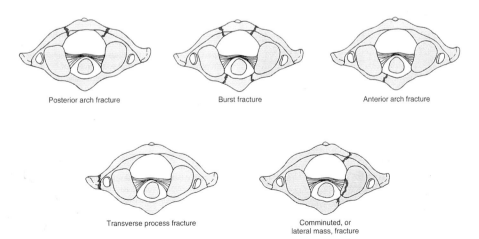

Posterior arch fracture   Burst fracture   Anterior arch fracture

Transverse process fracture   Comminuted, or lateral mass, fracture

FIGURE 4. Classification of atlas fractures. (From Browner BD, Jupiter JB, Levine AM (eds): Skeletal Trauma. Philadelphia, W.B.Saunders, 1998, p 866, with permission.)

15. How are atlas fractures treated?

Type 1 and **2** are treated with a cervical collar.

Type 3 injuries require close follow-up for potential loss of reduction and secondary collapse. Therefore, most injuries are treated with a halo-vest. If subsidence of the occipital condyle through the lateral mass of the atlas occurs, treatment options consist of closed reduction with skeletal cranial traction over a period of several weeks followed by halo immobilization or primary posterior atlantoaxial arthrodesis.

Type 4 fractures in which the odontoid has displaced through the anterior ring of the atlas are highly unstable. If atlantoaxial alignment is maintained, nonoperative treatment with a halo-vest is considered. Closed reduction and atlantoaxial arthrodesis are usually required.

Type 5 (Jefferson-type) fractures are treated based on integrity of the TAL. Disruption of the TAL is suspected if the lateral masses of C1 overhang those of C2 by the sum of 7 mm or more on the AP open-mouth radiograph (Spence's rule). TAL disruption is also present if there is translational atlantoaxial displacement of 3 mm or more in any direction. Nonoperative treatment of type 5 atlas fractures consists of fracture reduction with traction and conversion to a halo-vest after a period of days to weeks. Upon mobilization, maintenance of satisfactory alignment is checked with upright lateral and open mouth odontoid views. Surgical stabilization has been advocated based upon an unstable fracture configuration, for patients with purely ligamentous injury of the TAL or if recumbent traction or halo treatment is unsuccessful or contraindicated.

16. What are the different types of TAL injuries?

TAL injuries have been differentiated into type 1 injuries (bony avulsion) and type 2 injuries (purely ligamentous injuries).

17. How are TAL injuries treated?

Treatment options depend on the type of TAL injury. **Type 1** injuries (bony avulsion) can be successful treated with halo-vest immobilization in a significant number of patients. **Type 2** injuries (purely ligamentous injuries) are unlikely to heal with nonsurgical management and require reduction of the deformity and atlantoaxial arthrodesis.

18. What surgical techniques are used for posterior stabilization of atlas fractures and TAL injuries?

Fusion of the C1–C2 motion segment may be performed utilizing wire or cable fixation. The Gallie technique places wires under the posterior arch of C1 and around the C2 spinous process. The Brooks technique places wires under the lamina of C1 and C2. These techniques are useful for surgical treatment of isolated TAL injuries or for minimally displaced type 3 lateral mass fractures. However, in presence of a fracture through the ring of C1 neither technique is applicable. Placement of transarticular screws has been described for type 3, 4, and 5 atlas fractures. This technique requires anatomic reduction of the atlas on the axis to assure safe placement and optimal fixation of each transarticular screw. Recently, placement of lateral mass screws into the atlas and pedicle screws in the axis linked to a cervical rod on either side has been developed as an alternative to transarticular screw fixation.

AXIS FRACTURES: ODONTOID FRACTURES AND HANGMAN'S FRACTURES

19. What is the usual mechanism of injury for an odontoid fracture?

Odontoid fractures typically occur secondary to forced extension of the head and neck during a fall or collision. Associated fractures of the atlas occur in 10–15% of cases. Odontoid fractures are the most common cervical fracture in patients < 8 years of age or > 70 years of age.

20. How are odontoid fractures classified?

The Anderson and D'Alonzo classification (Fig. 5) is widely accepted and is based on the location of the fracture line:

Type 1: stable avulsion fracture occuring at the tip of the odontoid
Type 2: unstable transverse fracture involving the cortical bone of the waist of the odontoid.
Type 3: unstable fracture extending into the cancellous portion of the C2 vertebral body.

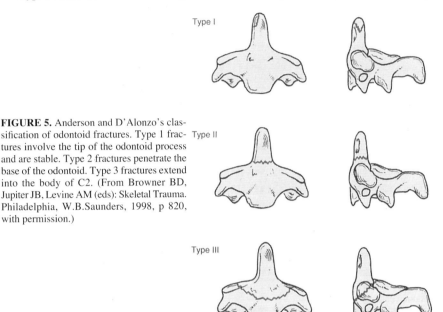

Type I

Type II

Type III

FIGURE 5. Anderson and D'Alonzo's classification of odontoid fractures. Type 1 fractures involve the tip of the odontoid process and are stable. Type 2 fractures penetrate the base of the odontoid. Type 3 fractures extend into the body of C2. (From Browner BD, Jupiter JB, Levine AM (eds): Skeletal Trauma. Philadelphia, W.B.Saunders, 1998, p 820, with permission.)

21. How are odontoid fractures treated?

Type 1 fractures are treated with a cervical collar. It is important to evaluate the cranio-cervical junction to rule out concomitant ligamentous injuries.

Type 2 fractures are associated with a high incidence of nonunion (15–85%). Risk factors associated with non-union include: initial fracture displacement > 4 mm, patient age > 50 years, posteriorly displaced fractures, angulation > 10° and inappropriate initial treatment. Treatment of type 2 fractures is based on the amount of initial fracture displacement as well as the presence of associated cervical fractures. Nondisplaced or minimally displaced fractures are treated with a halo-vest for 8–12 weeks. Maintenance of fracture reduction is checked with lateral cervical spine radiographs taken in both the recumbent and upright positions. Surgical stabilization and posterior C1–C2 fusion are performed for displaced fractures and for patients who are unable to tolerate halo treatment. Treatment with benign neglect consisting of a soft neck collar has been suggested for geriatric patients too feeble to tolerate any attempt at definitive care.

Type 3 fractures are reduced with skeletal traction as needed and externally immobilized.

22. What options exist for surgical stabilization of odontoid fractures?

Anterior screw fixation. Single or double screw fixation can be performed for patients with transverse or posterior oblique odontoid fractures. Prerequisites include a fracture that is less than 3 weeks old and a patient with reasonable bone quality.

Posterior fusion with wires or cables. For patients with an intact C1 ring, posterior wire or cable fixation can be successful. Substantial limitations to this technique include insufficient biomechanical stiffness in rotation and the possibility of undesireable C1 posterior translation.

Transarticular screw fixation. Placement of a small fragment screw from the midpoint of the inferior articular processes of C2 across the pedicle of C2 into the lateral mass of C1 provides excellent biomechanical stiffness and leads to a very high rate of bony union. Risks associated with this technique include iatrogenic injury to the vertebral artery as it passes laterally to the vertebral body of C2. Preoperative planning including CT evaluation to assess screw trajectory in relation to the vertebral artery and meticulous surgical technique are important for successful execution of this procedure.

Posterior C1–C2 rod-screw fixation. This technique utilizes lateral mass screws for C1 fixation and pedicle screws for C2 fixation. The screws are connected by rods along each side of the spine.

23. What is the usual mechanism of injury for a hangman's fracture?

The term *hangman's fracture* was orignially used to describe the C2 fracture dislocation that occurred when criminals were treated by judicial hanging. A radiographically similar injury to the second cervical vertebra occurs as a result of motor vehicle trauma and is more appropriately termed "traumatic spondylolisthesis of the axis." This fracture results in disruption of the bony bridge between the inferior and superior articular processes of the C2 segment. The fracture may be accompanied by injury to the C2–C3 disc as well as disruption of the posterior ligaments between C2 and C3. Concurrent soft tissue injuries heavily influence fracture stability and treatment.

24. How is traumatic spondylolisthesis of the axis classified?

The Effendi classification, as modified by Levine, is widely accepted (Fig. 6):

Type I injuries consist of a fracture through the neural arch with no angulation and up to 3mm of displacement

Type II fractures have both significant angulation and fracture displacement (> 3mm).

Type II-A injuries show minimal displacement but are associated with severe angulation as a result of a flexion-distraction injury mechanism. This injury may not be recognized until a radiograph is obtained in traction.

Type III injuries combine severe angulation and displacement with a unilateral or bilateral facet dislocation between C2 and C3.

There is a low incidence of spinal cord injury with type I, II, and IIA injuries but a high incidence of spinal cord injury with type III injuries.

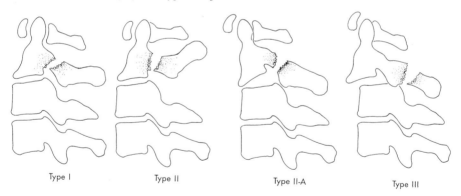

Type I   Type II   Type II-A   Type III

FIGURE 6. Types of traumatic spondylolisthesis of the axis. (From Leventhal MR: Fractures, dislocations and fracture-dislocations of the spine. In Crenshaw AH (el): Campbell's Operative Orthopaedics, 8th ed. St. Louis, Mosby 1992, pp 3517–3582, with permission.)

25. How is traumatic spondylolisthesis of the axis treated?

Treatment is based on the fracture type:

Type I injuries can be treated in a rigid neck collar.

Type II injuries are usually treated with traction followed by immobilization in a halo. If significant disruption of the C2–3 disc exists, surgical stabilization may be considered to avoid morbidity associated with prolonged traction and halo immobilization.

Type IIA injuries are usually treated by closed reduction by positioning in extension followed by halo immobilization. If significant disruption of the C2–3 disc exists, surgical stabilization is considered.

Type III injuries require surgical treatment for reduction of the facet dislocation and surgical stabilization.

26. What are the surgical treatment options for unstable traumatic spondylolisthesis of the axis?

Unstable type II and IIA fractures not amenable to treatment with a halo can be surgically stabilized by placement of C2 transpedicular screws or anterior C2–C3 plating. Type III fractures require open reduction of the facet dislocation and stabilization of the dislocation with lateral mass plates or wires. The fracture of the neural arch can be treated by placement of C2 transpedicular screws. Anterior C2–C3 plating is also an option.

BIBLIOGRAPHY

1. Anderson PA, Montesano PX: Morphology and treatment of occipital condyle fractures. Spine 13: 731–736, 1988
2. Chapman JR, Mirza SK: Upper cervical spine injuries. In Bucholz R (ed): Rockwood and Green's Fractures in Adults, 5th ed. Philadelphia, Lippincott, Williams & Wilkins, 2000.
3. Chapman JR, Bellabarba C, Newell DW, et al: Craniocervical injuries: Atlanto-occipital dissociation and occipital condyle fractures. Semin Spine Surg 13(2):90–105, 2001.
4. Chutkan NB, King AG, Harris MB: Odontoid fractures: Evaluation and management. J Am Acad Orthop Surg 5:199–204, 1997.
5. Dickman CA, Greene KA, Sonntag VK: Injuries involving the transverse atlantal ligament: classification and treatment guidelines based upon experience with 39 injuries. Neurosurgery 38:44–50, 1996.
6. Francis WR, Fielding JW, Hawkins RJ, et al: Traumatic spondylolisthesis of the axis. J Bone Joint Surg 63B:313–318, 1981.
7. Greene KA, Dickman CA, Marciano FF, et al: Acute axis fractures. Analysis of management and outcome in 340 consecutive cases. Spine 22:1843–1852, 1997.
8. Harris JH, Carson GC, Wagner LK: Radiologic diagnosis of traumatic occipitovertebral dissociation. 1: Normal occipitovertebral relationships on lateral radiographs of supine subjects. Am J Roentgenol 162:881–886, 1994.
9. Harris JH, Jr., Carson GC, Wagner LK, Kerr N: Radiologic diagnosis of traumatic occipitovertebral dissociation. 2: Comparison of three methods of detecting occipitovertebral relationships on lateral radiographs of supine subjects. Am J Roentgenol 162:887–892, 1994.
10. Levine AM, Edwards CC: Fractures of the atlas. J Bone Joint Surg 73A:680–691, 1991.

51. LOWER CERVICAL SPINE INJURIES

John Steinmann, D.O., and Lance Winter, D.O.

ANATOMY AND BIOMECHANICS

1. What motor, sensory, and reflex functions are supplied by the C5–C8 cervical nerve roots?

LEVEL	MOTOR FUNCTION	SENSORY LOCATION	REFLEX
C5	Shoulder abduction, elbow flexion	Deltoid region	Biceps reflex
C6	Wrist extension	Thumb, index finger	Brachioradialis
C7	Elbow extension, wrist flexion	Middle finger	Triceps
C8	Finger flexion	Ring, small finger	—

2. How is the neurologic level of spinal cord injury defined?

The neurologic level is defined as the most caudal level that exhibits antigravity motor function. For example, a patient with grade 5 biceps function, grade 3 wrist extensor function, and grade 1 triceps function with no motor or sensory function below this level is considered a C6 quadriplegic.

3. The subaxial cervical spine has been described as a two-column structure from a biomechanical perspective. What are the components of each column?

The cervical spine is viewed biomechanically as a two-column structure with the anterior column composed of the anterior and posterior longitudinal ligaments, vertebral body, and disc. The posterior column is composed of the pedicles, lamina, facet joints, spinous process, and interspinous ligaments.

4. Define and provide criteria for cervical instability.

White and Panjabi define spinal instability as " the loss of the ability of the spine under physiological loads to maintain its pattern of displacement so that there is no initial or additional neurological deficit, no major deformity and no incapacitating pain." They have proposed a checklist to define cervical spine instability in the traumatized patient.[5]

Checklist for the Diagnosis of Clinical Instability in the Lower Cervical Spine*

ELEMENT	POINT VALUE
Anterior elements destroyed or unable to function	2
Posterior elements destroyed or unable to function	2
Relative sagittal plane translation > 3.5 mm	2
Relative sagittal plane rotation $> 11°$	2
Positive stretch test	2
Spinal cord damage	2
Nerve root damage	1
Abnormal disc narrowing	1
Dangerous loading anticipated	1

*Total of 5 or more = unstable.

CLASSIFICATION

5. No single classification system for subaxial cervical spine injuries is universally accepted. What factors serve as the basis for the different classification systems?

The different classification systems for subaxial cervical spine injuries are based on various factors, including mechanism of injury, anatomical site of injury, radiologic description of injury, and presence/absence of neurologic deficit.

6. What is the most commonly used classification of cervical spine injuries based on mechanism of injury?

The classification of Allen and Ferguson[1] is the most widely used classification based on mechanism of injury. This classification correlates the mechanism of injury with radiographic findings and divides injuries into six groups. Each group is subdivided into stages based on the severity of injury.

Mechanistic Classification of Subaxial Cervical Spine Injuries (Allen and Ferguson)

FRACTURE TYPE	RADIOGRAPHIC SIGNS
Compression-flexion	
Stage 1	Blunting of the anterosuperior vertebral margin
Stage 2	Beaking of the anteroinferior vertebral body with decreased vertebral body height
Stage 3	Fracture of the anteroinferior vertebral body without retropulsion of fragments into the spinal canal
Stage 4	Fracture as above with retropulsion of bone into the spinal canal < 3 mm
Stage 5	Fracture with retropulsion of bone into the spinal canal > 3 mm
Vertical compression	
Stage 1	Fracture of superior or inferior vertebral endplate with cupping
Stage 2	Cupping and fracture of both endplates, minimal displacement
Stage 3	Fracture as above with significant displacement of bony fragments
Distraction-flexion	
Stage 1	Facet subluxation with divergent spinous processes
Stage 2	Unilateral facet dislocation (25% subluxation)
Stage 3	Bilateral facet dislocation (50% subluxation)
Stage 4	Bilateral facet dislocation (100% subluxation)
Compression-extension	
Stage 1	Unilateral laminar fracture without displacement
Stage 2	Bilateral laminar fractures without displacement
Stage 3	Bilateral laminar fractures without displacement with associated articular process or pedicle fractures
Stage 4	Bilateral laminar fractures with less than 100% anterior vertebral body displacement
Stage 5	Bilateral laminar fractures with more than 100% anterior vertebral body displacement
Distraction-extension	
Stage 1	Anterior ligamentous comples failure (disc space widening ± teardrop fracture)
Stage 2	Retrolisthesis of cephalad on caudad vertebral body
Lateral flexion	
Stage 1	Nondisplaced unilateral pedicle or lamina fracture with asymmetric vertebral body compression injury
Stage 2	Displaced unilateral pedicle or lamina fracture with asymmetric vertebral body compression injury

7. Provide a classification of subaxial cervical injuries that includes both mechanism of injury and anatomic site of injury.

Subaxial spine injuries can be classified into six categories according to a mechanistic anatomic classification:

- Minor compression and avulsion fractures
- Facet injuries (occult ligamentous injuries, unilateral or bilateral dislocations, facet fractures)
- Vertebral body compression fractures
- Burst fractures
- Teardrop fracture-dislocations
- Extension injuries (laminar, facet, and lateral mass fractures)

DIAGNOSIS AND MANAGEMENT

8. Describe the role of methylprednisolone in patients with spinal cord injury.

Spinal cord injury is conceptualized as occurring in stages. Following the initial mechanical injury, a secondary cellular injury cascade leads to additional cell death. In 1990 the Second National Acute Spinal Cord Injury Study (NASCIS 2) reported that patients treated with methylprednisolone within 8 hours of injury had a significantly better neurologic recovery than patients treated with placebo. However, patients treated after 8 hours from the time of injury had a worse outcome than the placebo group. This effect was attributed to complications associated with the use of high-dose steroids. Current recommendations are to administer a bolus dose of methylprednisolone (30 mg/kg body weight) over 15 minutes, followed by an infusion (5.4 mg/kg/hr). If steroid therapy is initiated within 3 hours of injury, the infusion should be continued for 24 hours. If steroid therapy is initiated between 3 and 8 hours after injury, the infusion should be continued for 48 hours if no medical contraindications exist.

9. What subaxial cervical injuries can be treated with nonsurgical management?

Stable subaxial spine injuries can be treated with nonsurgical management using a cervical orthosis (cervical collar or halo vest) for 8–12 weeks. Examples of injuries appropriate for non-surgical care include minor compression and avulsion injuries, isolated laminar fractures, lateral mass fractures without vertebral body displacement, and spinous process fractures. Careful radiographic assessment is critical during and after orthotic treatment to rule out occult spinal instability resulting in loss of spinal alignment.

10. When is emergent closed reduction of a cervical spine injury indicated?

Emergent closed reduction should be considered in all patients with cervical canal compromise and a neurologic deficit. Common fractures requiring immediate reduction include burst fractures and facet dislocations (unilateral or bilateral). In the authors' opinion, the benefits of emergent reduction of facet dislocations in neurologically impaired patients outweigh the risks of disc displacement. In patients with minor nerve root deficits or normal neurologic function, an MRI scan is appropriate before reduction.

11. When is emergent closed reduction of a cervical spine injury contraindicated?

Closed reduction via traction is usually contraindicated for patients with distractive cervical injury patterns such as complete ligamentous injuries or ankylosing spondylitis (highly unstable and difficult to reduce). Special care must be exercised with skull fractures or combative individuals. In addition, closed reduction in unconscious or anesthetized patients is dangerous and should be performed under spinal monitoring and after a disc herniation has been ruled out with MRI.

12. What data support emergent reduction of cervical fracture dislocations?

Both clinical and experimental studies have shown that the timing of the reversal of spinal cord compression correlates with the potential for neurologic recovery. The authors' experience and recent animal studies suggest that a window of opportunity (< 6 hours) exists for reversal of severe spinal cord injury if immediate reduction is performed. Personal experience includes three patients who presented within 1 hour of injury with bilateral facet dislocation and absence of motor function below the level of injury. Immediate reduction in each case led to near complete recovery of motor function. In a laboratory study, 30 beagle dogs were submitted to 50% constriction of the spinal cord, producing complete paraplegia. The dogs decompressed immediately and at one hour demonstrated significant neurologic recovery and became ambulatory. Dogs with spinal compression for 6 hours or more failed to recover.[6]

13. How is emergent closed reduction of a cervical fracture-dislocation accomplished?

The reduction is accomplished in a setting that allows constant monitoring, cervical traction, and frequent (every 3–4 min) radiographs or fluoroscopy. Use of intravenous analgesics, muscle relaxants, and nasal oxygen is recommended. Gardner Wells tongs are safe and easily applied and allow traction of up to 70% of the patient's body weight. Pin sites are prepped with betadine and anesthetized with lidocaine. Tongs are applied by inserting pins into the skull above and in line with the external auditory meatus at the proper torque. An initial weight of less than 10lb is applied to balance the head. A repeat neurologic examination and radiographic assessment are performed. This process is repeated as weight is added in 5- to 10-lb increments until either reduction occurs, deterioration in neurologic function occurs, or the disc space shows signs of overdistraction (disc height greater than 10 mm or disc space shows increased height compared to adjacent disc spaces). When reduction occurs, the head is slightly extended and weights are decreased to 20 lb.

14. What controversy is associated with closed reduction of facet dislocations?

Controversy surrounds the need to image the intervertebral disc with MRI at the level of injury prior to reduction. A significant number of facet injuries are associated with disc disruption and herniation. If the disc fragment is associated with the superiorly translated vertebra, reduction has the potential to displace disc material into the spinal canal and cause a catastrophic neural deficit. In the neurologically intact patient who is awake and cooperative, some surgeons obtain a prereduction MRI to rule out a potentially dangerous disc herniation. However, several studies have shown that immediate traction and reduction can be performed safely in alert and awake patients. When neurologic impairment exists, emergent reduction is indicated to re-establish spinal canal alignment and provide neural decompression in order to maximize the chance for neural recovery. An MRI should be obtained prior to attempting reduction in uncooperative or unconcious patients.

15. What are the indications for surgical management of subaxial cervical spine injuries?

General indications for operative intervention are (1) restoration of normal cervical alignment if this cannot be achieved with traction and closed reduction, (2) stabilization of unstable spine segments, and (3) decompression to enhance neurologic recovery. The cervical injuries that typically require surgical intervention include facet injuries, unstable ligamentous injuries, burst fractures, unstable compression fractures, and fracture dislocations. Open spine fractures, and transesophageal gunshot wounds also require surgical treatment.

16. When is emergent, urgent, and delayed surgery indicated?

The indications for **emergent surgery** include open spine fractures, transesophageal gunshot wounds involving the spine, irreducible dislocations, and neurologic deterioration in the presence of known spinal cord compression. **Urgent surgery** is indicated for nearly all other unstable cord injured patients. In support of early surgery, Krengel found that patients undergoing surgery within 24 hours showed improved neurologic outcomes compared with historical controls who were treated with delayed surgery.[7] **Delayed surgery** is appropriate for incomplete injuries without significant cord compression that demonstrate or are expected to demonstrate early recovery. An example is the patient with a central cord syndrome. This patient is best managed with the steroid protocol and observation in traction until neurologic recovery reaches a plateau. Spinal canal decompression may be considered at that time for patients with evidence of extrinsic spinal cord compression.

17. What injuries are best treated with anterior stabilization?

Anterior surgery is indicated when anterior decompression or restoration of the anterior column is required. Unstable burst fractures, traumatic disc herniations and severe extension injuries are best treated with an anterior approach (Fig. 1).

18. What injuries are best treated with posterior stabilization?

The posterior approach is indicated when the predominant pathology or instability exists within the posterior column. Hyperflexion injuries, including severe posterior ligamentous injuries as well as unilateral and bilateral facet dislocations, are best treated with a posterior approach. Extension injuries that result in an unstable isolated posterior element fracture are also

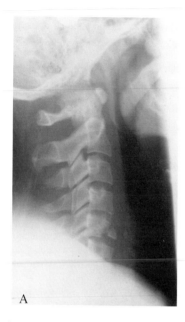

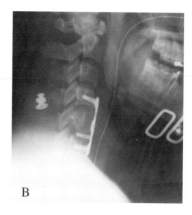

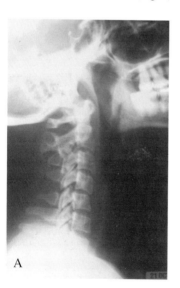

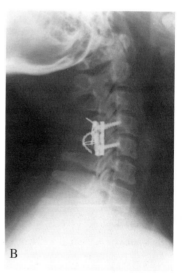

FIGURE 1. An unstable fracture of the vertebral body with associated spinal canal compromise (**A**) is best treated with decompression, fusion and stabilization via an anterior approach (**B**).

best treated with a posterior approach. When anterior stabilization is contraindicated, as in patients with tracheostomy, posterior segmental fixation with lateral mass screws has proved effective in maintaining alignment and achieving fusion in patients with spinal cord injuries secondary to anterior column fractures[5] (Fig. 2).

FIGURE 2. This C4–C5 posterior ligamentous injury with facet subluxation (**A**) is effectively stabilized by posterior C4–C5 lateral mass fixation (**B**).

19. Describe the clinical presentation of a posterior ligament injury.

Posterior ligament injury results from hyperflexion and can vary from a minor ligamentous sprain to complete ligamentous rupture with cervical instability. Examination of the conscious patient demonstrates localized tenderness. Radiographic evaluation may be normal if performed with the patient in the supine position or may show interspinous widening and localized kyphosis. MRI has the potential to demonstrate posterior ligamentous injury. Flexion and extension x-rays can demonstrate the degree of ligamentous instability but are not recommended in the acute setting (Fig. 3).

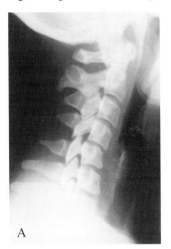
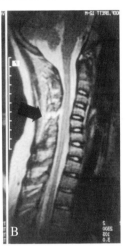

FIGURE 3. Severe posterior ligamentous injury is diagnosed based on interspinous widening and kyphosis at C4–C5 (**A**). MRI (**B**) documents the presence of posterior column ligamentous injury (arrow).

20. How does the clinical presentation of a unilateral facet dislocation differ from that of a bilateral facet dislocation?

Patients with unilateral facet dislocations will present with neck pain which may be accompanied by a mild torticollis. Although initial radiographs often miss this injury, careful inspection often shows less than 25% anterolisthesis and rotation of the spinous process. CT scan or oblique x-rays should clearly identify this injury. In a report of 24 patients with unilateral facet dislocations, 70% presented with radicuopathy, 20% presented with normal neurologic examination, and 10% presented with evidence of spinal cord injury.[7] A bilateral facet dislocation generally presents with a severe spinal cord injury, resulting in complete or incomplete tetraplegia. The lateral radiographs generally show greater than 50% subluxation (Fig. 4).

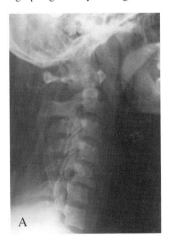
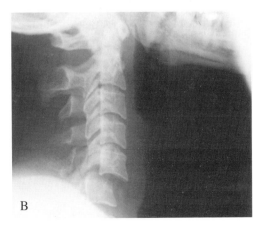

FIGURE 4. Types of cervical facet dislocation: unilateral (**A**) and bilateral (**B**).

21. Describe the clinical presentation of an ipsilateral lamina and facet fracture.

Patients with this common isolated posterior element injury often present with evidence of cervical nerve root dysfunction or dysesthesias. Plain radiographs show an asymmetry of the lateral mass on the lateral view. There is generally no evidence of increased retropharyngeal soft tissue swelling. CT scan is used to confirm the diagnosis.

22. What are the important considerations in the postoperative management of patients with spinal cord injury?

All body systems are affected by spinal cord injury. Frequent inspection and turning are necessary to prevent skin breakdown. Aggressive pulmonary toilet is necessary to help decrease risk of developing pneumonia. Neurogenic hypotension is managed with vasopressors. Prophylaxis for gastrointestinal ulceration and deep venous thrombosis is mandatory. An indwelling urinary catheter is necessary initially. Patients should be moved to a dedicated spinal cord injury rehabilitation center as soon as possible.

23. What is the prognosis for recovery in incomplete and complete cervical spinal cord injuries?

Recovery of spinal cord injury depends on the level of injury and whether the injury is complete or incomplete. In recording recovery it is helpful to use the American Spinal Injury Association motor score (see Chapter 6). Patients with complete tetraplegia show an average of a 9-point increase in motor score within the first year. This increase generally represents recovery of root function at the level of injury. Incomplete tetraplegics demonstrate an average of a 45-point increase in motor score within the first year, with 46% regaining community ambulatory status.[2]

BIBLIOGRAPHY

1. Allen BL Jr, Ferguson RL, Lehmann TR, et al: A mechanistic classification of closed, indirect fractures and dislocations of the lower cervical spine. Spine 7:1–27, 1982.
2. Anderson PA: Prognosis of spinal cord injuries. In Levine AN (ed): Orthopedic Knowledge Update—Trauma. Rosemont, IL, American Academy of Orthopedic Surgeons, 1996, pp 303–309.
3. Anderson PA: Patient assessment in spinal injury. In Levine AN (ed): Orthopedic Knowledge Update—Trauma. Rosemont, IL American Academy of Orthopedic Surgeons, 1996, pp xx–xx.
4. Bracken NB, Shephard MJ, Collins WF, et al: A randomized control trial of methylprednisolone nalolxone in the treatment of acute spinal cord injury: Results of the second national acute spinal cord injury study. N Engl J Med 322:1405–1411, 1990.
5. Brodke D, Anderson P, Newell D, et al: Anterior vs posterior stabilization of cervical spine fractures in spinal cord-injured patients. Presented at the 23rd Annual Meeting of the Cervical Spine Research Society, Santa Fe, NM, 1995.
6. Delamarter RB, Shermann J, Carr J: Pathophysiology of spinal cord damage: Recovery following immediate and delayed decompression. J Bone Joint Surg 77A:1042–1049, 1995.
7. Krengel WF, Anderson PA, Henley MB: Early stabilization and decompression for incomplete paraplegia due to a thoracic level spinal cord injury. Spine 18:2080–2087, 1993.
8. Shapiro, SA: Management of unilateral locked facet of the cervical spine. Neurosurgery 33:832–837, 1993.

52. THORACIC AND LUMBAR SPINE FRACTURES

Adam C. Crowl, M.D., D. Greg Anderson, M.D., Todd J. Albert, M.D., and Vincent J. Devlin, M.D.

1. Why is it important to assess radiographically the entire spinal axis when a significant spine fracture is identified in one region of the spine?

There is a 5–20% chance that a patient has a second fracture in a different region of the spine. Factors that increase the risk of missed spine fractures on initial evaluation include head injuries, intoxication, drug use, and multiple trauma.

2. What factors increase the risk of neurologic injury with thoracic and lumbar spine fractures?

1. High energy injuries, especially burst fractures and fracture dislocations.

2. Fractures located above the L2 level. The conus medullaris and spinal cord occupy the spinal canal in this location, and these neural elements are more prone to neurologic injury than the nerve roots of the cauda equina.

3. Define the three-column model of the spine as described by Denis (Fig. 1).

The **anterior column** is composed of the anterior longitudinal ligament, anterior half of the vertebral body and anterior half of the disc.

The **middle column** is composed of the posterior half of the vertebral body, the posterior half of the disc, and the posterior longitudinal ligament.

The **posterior column** includes the pedicles, facet joints, lamina and posterior ligament complex.

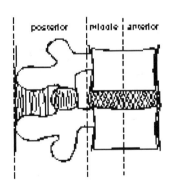

FIGURE 1.   The three-column model of the spine as described by Denis.

4. What are the six most common patterns of thoracolumbar fractures?

McAfee expanded Denis's concepts and classified thoracic and lumbar spine fractures into six patterns based on CT scan analysis:

- Compression fractures
- Stable burst fractures
- Unstable burst fractures
- Flexion-distraction injuries
- Chance fractures
- Translational injuries(fracture-dislocations)

5. What parameters are important to assess on radiographs of thoracic and lumbar fractures?

Percentage of vertebral body compression: the anterior vertebral height (B) is divided by the posterior vertebral height (A) multiplied by 100.

Sagittal malalignment: the angle (C) between the vertebral endplates above and below the injured level is determined (Cobb method). This value(regional kyphotic deformity) is compared with the normal sagittal alignment for the specific levels of the spine under evaluation.

Integrity of the posterior spinal column: findings that suggest disruption of the posterior spinal column include widening or splaying of the spinous processes or a localized kyphotic deformity of a thoracolumbar spinal segment (Fig. 2).

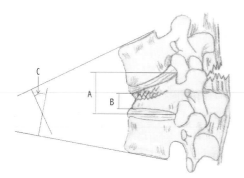

FIGURE 2. Useful radiographic parameters for assessing thoracic and lumbar fractures: percentage of vertebral body compression and regional kyphotic deformity.

6. Are plain radiographs sufficient to distinguish the six common types of thoracic and lumbar spine fractures?

No! Although anteroposterior (AP) and lateral radiographs are the best first imaging test to assess a spine fracture, a computed tomography (CT) scan must be obtained when radiographs suggest a significant thoracic or lumbar fracture. Failure to obtain a CT scan may lead to inappropriate diagnosis and treatment. Magnetic resonane imaging (MRI) is rarely needed during the initial evaluation unless the patient experiences deterioration in neurologic status.

COMPRESSION FRACTURES

7. Describe the mechanism, injury pattern, and treatment of a thoracic or lumbar compression fracture.

Compression fractures represent an isolated failure of the anterior spinal column due to a combination of flexion and axial compression loading (see Fig. 3 on following page). Because the structural stability of the spine is not compromised by this single-column injury, treatment consists of early patient mobilization. Frequently the patient is treated with immobilization in some type of orthosis (Jewett brace, thoracolumobsacral orthosis [TLSO]) until back pain resolves. Radiographic and clinical follow-up is generally carried out on a monthly basis for the first 3 months after injury.

8. What radiographic features are considered worrisome when assessing compression fractures?

- Loss of vertebral height exceeding 50% (suggests possibility of posterior ligamentous injury)
- Segmental kyphosis exceeding 20° (suggests possibility of posterior ligamentous injury)
- Multiple adjacent compression fractures (may require surgical treatment if significant kyphotic deformity occurs)

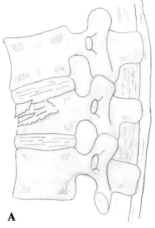

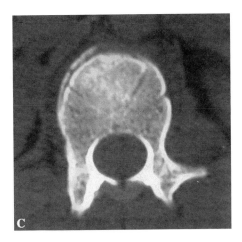

FIGURE 3.   Compression fracture. **A**, Diagrammatic respresentation. **B**, Lateral radiograph. **C**, Axial CT scan.

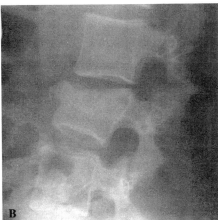

- Compression fractures that progressively collapse despite orthotic treatment. The possibility of a pathologic fracture (due to tumor or infection) should be considered.

9. Why is a compression fracture with greater than 40–50% loss of anterior vertebral body height considered "unstable"?

Because it is highly likely that an associated posterior ligament complex disruption is present. The posterior ligament complex experiences about one-third of the tensile load transmitted to the vertebral body to cause fracture. In young persons with good bone quality, the magnitude of the load required to create a compression fracture may result in tensile failure of the posterior ligamentous complex.

10. Outline the treatment of compression fractures secondary to osteoporosis.

Such fractures are usually due to low-energy trauma involving weakened bone. They are common in the elderly as well as patients on steroid therapy. Multiple fractures may occur and may lead to significant spinal deformities and/or pain. It is important to rule out pathologic fracture due to tumor infiltration (e.g., multiple myeloma, metastatic disease) or metabolic bone disease (e.g., osteomalacia). Baseline bone density studies of the spine and hip should be performed. Fracture treatment depends on severity and location of injury. Most fractures can be managed with an orthosis. Osteoporosis may be treated with exercise, hormone replacement therapy, bisphosphonate therapy, and calcitonin. Open surgical treatment with spinal canal

decompression combined with stabilization and fusion is generally reserved for fractures associated with neurologic deficit. Minimally invasive surgical procedures such as vertebroplasy and
kyphoplasty have recently been popularized for the treatment of select acute and subacute compression fractures. These procedures attempt to relieve pain by supplementing the structural integrity of the collapsed vertebral body via the injection of bone cement (PMMA).

STABLE BURST FRACTURES

11. Describe the mechanism and injury pattern associated with a stable burst fracture.
   Key features that identify a stable burst fracture (Fig. 4) include:
   • Fracture of the anterior and middle spinal columns due to compressive loading
   • No loss of posterior spinal column integrity
   • Maintanence of intact neurologic status

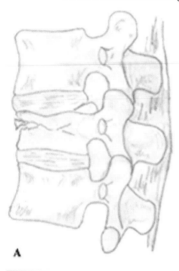

FIGURE 4.   Stable L1 burst fracture. **A,** Diagrammatic representation. **B,** Lateral radiograph. **C,** Anteroposterior radiograph. *(Figure continued on following page.)*

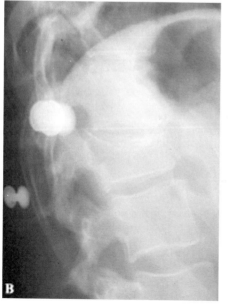

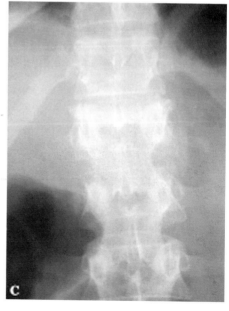

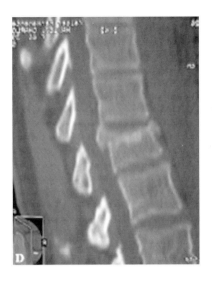

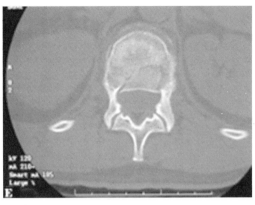

FIGURE 4. *(continued from previous page).* Stable L1 burst fracture. **D**, Sagittal view. **E**, Axial CT.

Although bone may be retropulsed into the spinal canal, the resultant compromise of the spinal canal is less than 50%. Loss of anterior column vertebral height is less than 50%. The local kyphotic deformity is generally less than 15°. Despite the possible presence of a nondisplaced vertical fracture in the lamina, the facet joints and the posterior ligaments remain intact.

12. What are the treatment options for a stable burst fracture?

Stable burst fractures are treated by nonoperative techniques. An excellent method is closed reduction and body-cast immobilization. Another commonly used method is immobilization in a TLSO. The cast or brace is generally worn for 3 months.

13. What percent of burst fractures are misdiagnosed as compression fractures on plain radiographs?

Approximately 25% of burst fractures are misdiagnosed as compression fractures if radiographs alone are evaluated. For this resason it is important to evaluate significant thoracic and lumbar spine fractures with a CT scan.

14. What radiographic criteria help to distinguish a burst fracture from a compression fracture?

Loss of posterior vertebral body height (compared with the average of the vertebrae above and below), any break in the posterior aspect of the vertebral body, or interpedicular widening on the AP view. The posterior vertebral body angle may be formed by a line drawn along the endplate and the posterior vertebral body margin. If this line forms an angle greater than 100°, the likelihood of a burst fracture is increased.

UNSTABLE BURST FRACTURES

15. Describe the mechanism and injury pattern of an unstable burst fracture.

Unstable burst fractures result from axial compression forces that disrupt all three columns of the spine. The anterior and middle columns fail in compression with retropulsion of the posterior vertebral body wall into the spinal canal. Posterior spinal column disruption permits development of a kyphotic deformity. The AP radiographs shows a widening of the distance between the pedicles at the level of fracture. The lateral radiograph shows a kyphotic deformity that may exceed 20° and is associated with loss of vertebral body height, possibly more than 50%. CT scans

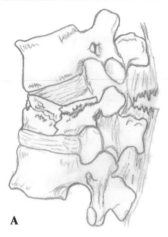

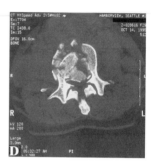

FIGURE 5. Unstable burst fracture. **A**, Diagrammatic representation. **B**, Lateral radiograph. **C**, AP radiograph. **D**, Sagittal CT view. (B–D: From Chapman JR, Mirza SK: Anterior treatment of thoracolumbar fractures. Spine State Art Rev 12:647–661, 1998, with permission.)

A

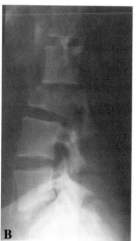

B

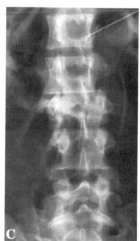

C

are used to determine the percentage of spinal canal compromise and the presence or absence of an associated laminar fracture (Fig. 5).

16. What is the major concern about a burst fracture associated with a laminar fracture?

Possible incarceration of the dura or neural elements in the fracture site with associated cerebrospinal (CSF) leakage. One study demonstrated incarceration of the dural sac in the fracture site in more than one-third of burst fractures associated with a laminar fracture .

17. What nonspinal injuries are commonly associated with burst fractures?

Calcaneus fractures, long bone fractures, and closed head injuries.

18. What are the major criteria for recommending nonsurgical treatment for burst fractures?

Burst fractures without neurologic deficit, with canal compromise less than 50%, and with less than 30° of initial kyphosis may be considered for nonsurgical treatment. Such patients require close clinical and radiographic monitoring for the potential development of neurologic deficit and progressive kyphotic deformity.

19. What are the major criteria for recommending surgical treatment for burst fractures?

Indications for surgical treatment of burst fractures are controversial and include:

- Progressive neurologic deficit
- Progressive kyphosis associated with a neural deficit
- CT evidence of spinal canal compromise associated with an incomplete neurologic deficit
- Greater than 50% loss of vertebral body height
- Kyphosis greater than 30° at the level of fracture
- Spinal canal compromise greater than 50%

20. What are the surgical goals in treating unstable burst fractures?

Decompression: spinal canal decompression is generally indicated for patients with neurologic deficits.

Realignment: spinal re-alignment is achieved through use of spinal instrumentation that can correct kyphotic deformity.

Stabilization: the combination of spinal instrumentation and spinal fusion can restore long-term stability to injured spinal segments.

21. What are the three options for decompression of spinal canal stenosis resulting from a burst fracture in a patient with a neurologic deficit?

1. **Indirect decompression.** Distraction applied to the fracture through the use of posterior spinal instrumentation has the potential to reduce the fracture and decompress the spinal canal through "ligamentotaxis." This technique is most likely to be successful if performed within the first 72 hours after the fracture occurs.

2. **Direct posterolateral decompression.** The fragments impinging on the neural elements are pushed away anteriorly to decompress the dural sac after exposure is achieved through a laminectomy or transpedicular approach. This procedure is generally performed in conjunction with a posterior spine stabilization procedure.

3. **Direct anterior decompression.** The fracture may be exposed directly through an anterior approach, and the entire vertebral body may be removed (corpectomy) to decompress the spinal canal. A bone graft is used to reconstruct the anterior spinal column. Spinal stability is restored by placement of anterior spinal instrumentation, posterior spinal instrumentation, or a combination of both anterior and posterior spinal implants.

22. What types of spinal instrumentation constructs are used for realignment and stabilization of unstable burst fractures? (see Fig. 6).

- Posterior rod and hook constructs
- Posterior rod-hook-sleeve constructs
- Posterior rod/plate and pedicle screw constructs
- Combinations of posterior spinal instrumentation and anterior structural grafting with or without anterior instrumentation
- Anterior rod and screw or plate/screw constructs

23. What are the advantages and disadvantages of using pedicle screws for treatment of thoracolumbar burst fractures?

Advantages

Fewer spine segments require instumentation and fusion.

Pedicle screws can be used with contoured rods to maintain lordosis in the lumbar spine.

Disadvantage

Short-segment pedicle screw constructs without anterior column structural support have a high rate of failure (screw breakage) in fractures with extensive vertebral body comminution.

24. Why are distraction hook/rod constructs a poor choice in the lumbar spine?

These constructs create kyphosis, which is undesireable in the normally lordotic lumbar

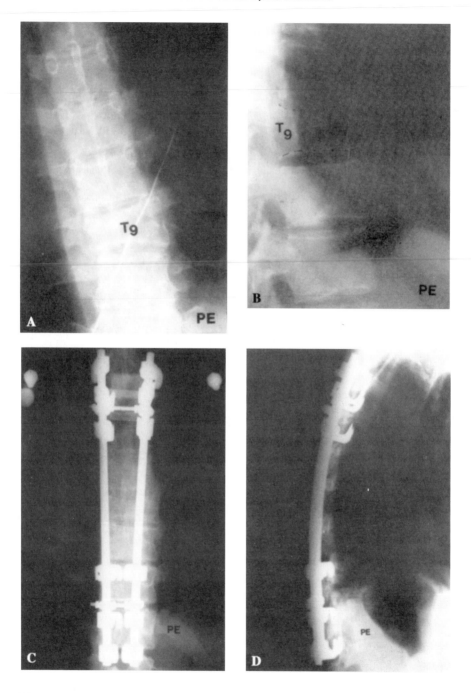

FIGURE 6. Surgical treatment options for unstable burst fractures. **A–D,** T9 burst fracture treated with posterior rod and multiple hook construct. (From Akbarnia BA: Surgical treatment of upper and thoracic spine fractures using Cotrel-Dubousset instrumentation. Spine State Art Rev 7:269–276, 1993, with permission.) *(Figure continued on following page.)*

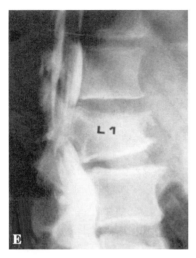

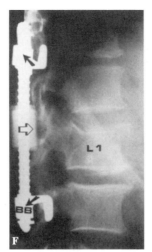

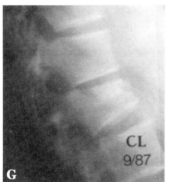

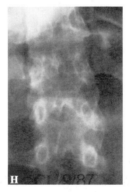

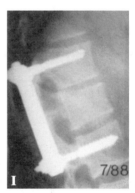

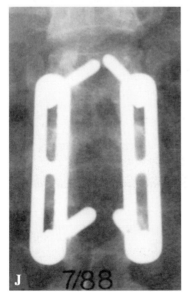

FIGURE 6 *(Continued).* Surgical treatment options for unstable burst fractures. **E** and **F**, L1 burst fracture treated with posterior rod-sleeve construct. From Edwards CC: The Edwards modular system. Spine State Art Rev 6:235–268, 1992, with permisson.) **G–J**, L1 burst fracture treated with a posterior pedicle screw construct. From Holt BT, McCormack T, Gaines RW Jr: Short-segment fusion—Anterior or posterior approach? Spine State Art Rev 7:277–285, 1993, with permission.) *(Figure continued on following page.)*

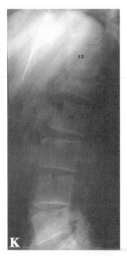

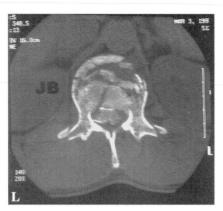

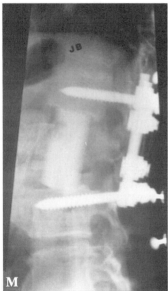

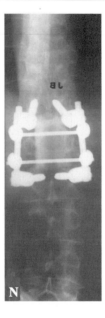

FIGURE 6. *(Continued)*. Surgical treatment options for unstable burst fractures. **K–N,** L1 burst fracture treated with posterior pedicle screw fixation followed by anterior decompression and reconstruction using structural allograft. (From Chapman JR, Mirza SK: Anterior treatment of thoracolumbar fractures. Spine State Art Rev 12:647–661, 1998, with permission.)

region. Iatrogenic loss of lumbar lordosis leads to a flat back syndrome (sagittal imbalance and back pain).

25. What are the common indications for use of an anterior approach and anterior instrumentation in a thoracolumbar burst fracture?

Indications include fractures from T11–L3, especially when an incomplete neurologic lesion with compromise of the spinal canal would benefit from direct decompression of the spinal canal. Significant kyphotic deformities in which anterior column structural grafting is indicated also respond well to an anterior approach (Fig. 7).

26. Discuss the major limitations of an anterior approach to thoracolumbar burst fractures.

Fractures above T11 or below L3 are difficult to treat with anterior instrumentation because of local anatomy. Lamina fractures noted on CT scan may need to be explored posteriorly for

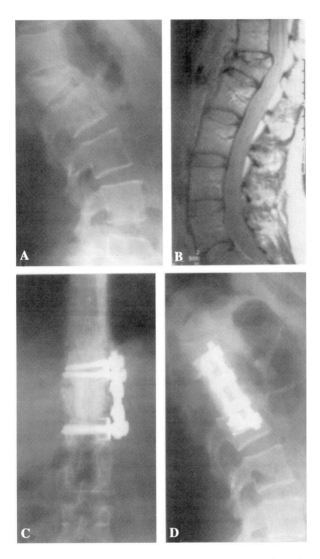

FIGURE 7. L1 burst fracture treated with corpectomy, anterior femoral allograft, and anterior rod-screw construct (Kaneda instrumentation). (From Devlin VJ, Pitt DD: The evolution of surgery of the anterior spinal column. Spine State Art Rev 12:493–527, 1998, with permission.)

potential incarceration of the dura with associated cerebrospinal fluid (CSF) leak. Care must be taken in cases with significant posterior ligament disruption and/or osteoporotic bone quality in which the strength of anterior screw fixation may not be adequate. Significant translational deformities and noncompliant/combative patients represent contraindications to anterior-only approaches. Such cases need the added stability of posterior instrumentation.

CHANCE FRACTURES

27. Describe the mechanism and injury pattern of a Chance fracture.
Chance fractures (Fig 8) generally result from a flexion injury mechanism in a lap-belt–restrained car passenger. Radiographs show the three spinal columns injured transversely due to

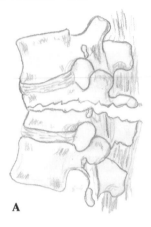

A

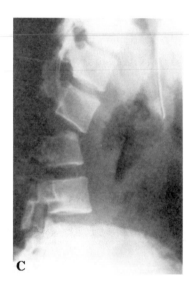

FIGURE 8. Chance fracture. **A**, Diagrammatic representation. **B**, Lateral radiograph. **C**, AP radiograph. (From Puno RM, Bhojraj SY, Glassman SD, et al: Flexion distraction injuries of the thoracolumbar and lumbar spine in the adult and pediatric patient. Spine State Art Rev 7:223–248, 1993, with permission.)

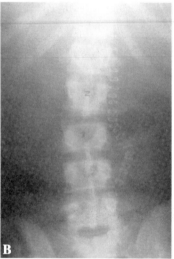

B   **C**

failure of the spinal segment in tension. The disruption of the spine may progress through bone (vertebral body, pedicle, and spinous process), soft tissue(disc, facet joint, and interspinous ligament) or a combination of bone and soft tissue structures.

28. What nonspinal injuries are commonly associated with Chance fractures?

A high incidence of intra-abdominal (bowel) injury (45%) is associated with Chance fractures.

29. What are the treatment options for a Chance fracture?

In general, patients with Chance fractures are treated with posterior spinal instrumentation and fusion (Fig. 9). Uncommonly, patients who sustain injuries entirely through bone and do not have concomitant abdominal inuries may be treated with extension casting.

FLEXION-DISTRACTION INJURIES

30. Describe the mechanism and injury pattern of a flexion-distraction injury.

Common injury mechanisms for flexion-distraction injuries include motor vehicle accidents and falls from a height. Such injuries result in tensile failure of the posterior spinal column and com-

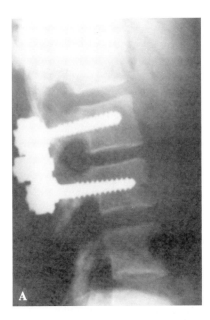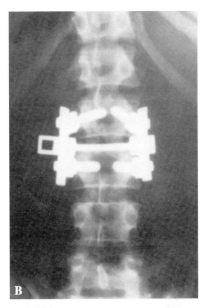

FIGURE 9. Chance fracture. **A**, Postoperative lateral radiograph. **B**, Postoperative anteroposterior radiograph. (From Puno RM, Bhojraj SY, Glassman SD, et al: Flexion distraction injuries of the thoracolumbar and lumbar spine in the adult and pediatric patient: Spine State Art Rev 7:223–248, 1993, with permission.)

pressive failure of the anterior column and possibly the middle column. Posterior column injuries include separation of the spinous processes and facet joints. The vertebral body is wedged anteriorly (see Fig. 10). Bony fragments from the middle column may be retropulsed into the spinal canal.

31. What are the treatment options for a flexion-distraction injury?
These unstable injuries are treated with posterior spinal instrumentation and posterior fusion (see Fig. 11).

TRANSLATIONAL INJURIES (FRACTURE-DISLOCATIONS)

32. Describe the mechanism and injury pattern of a translational injury (fracture-dislocation).
Fracture-dislocations result from high-energy injuries and are the most unstable type of spine fractures. The structural integrity of all three spinal colums is completely disrupted with resultant displacement of the spine in one or more planes (Fig. 12). Complete paralegia generally accompanies this type of spine fracture.

33. What are the treatment options for a translational injury (fracture-dislocation)?
These injuries are generally treated by posterior surgical procedures. Operative reduction is accompanied by posterior spinal instrumentation and fusion (Fig. 13).

GUNSHOT INJURIES OF THE SPINE

34. How does the treatment of thoracolumbar injuries due to gunshot wounds differ from other mechanisms of injury?
Gunshot injuries generally spare the ligaments and thus most injuries are "stable" with a low risk of progressive deformity despite the degree of neurologic injury. Most patients can be mobilized in

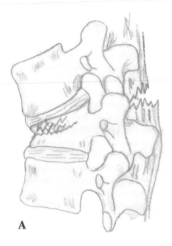

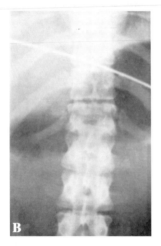

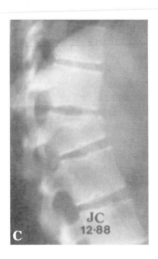

FIGURE 10. Flexion-distraction injury. **A,** Diagrammatic representation. **B,** Preoperative AP radiograph. **C,** Preoperative lateral radiograph. **D,** Preoperative CT scan. (From Holt BT, McCormack T, Gaines RW Jr: Short segment fusion: Anterior or posterior approach? Spine State Art Rev 7:277–286. 1993, with permission.)

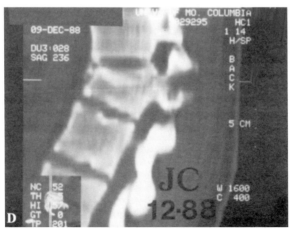

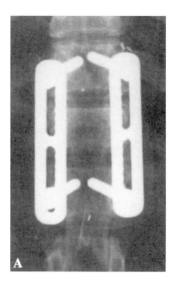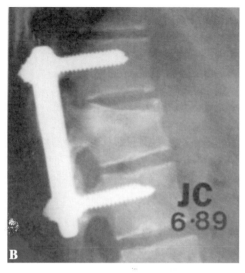

FIGURE 11. Flexion-distraction injury. **A,** Postoperative AP radiograph. **B,** Postoperative lateral radiograph. (From Holt BT, McCormack T, Gaines RW Jr: Short-segment fusion: Anterior or posterior approach? Spine State Art Rev 7:277–286, 1993, with permission.)

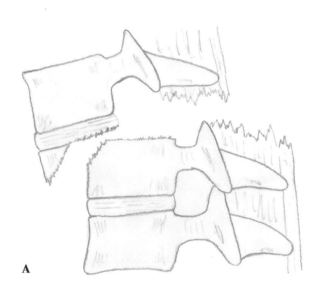

FIGURE 12. Translational injury. **A,** Diagrammatic representation. *(Figure continued on following page.)*

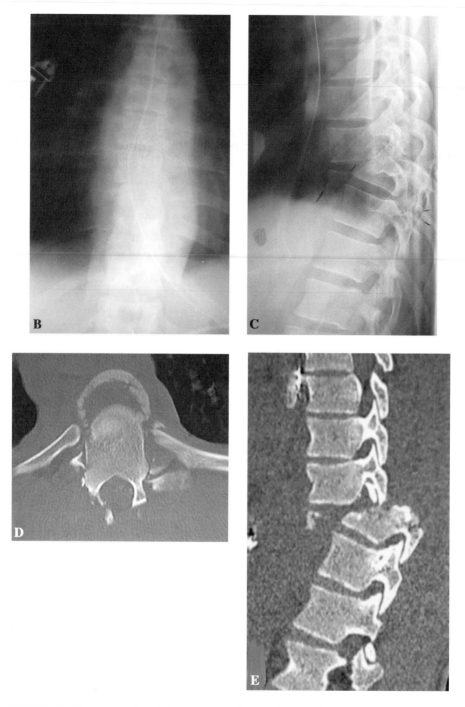

FIGURE 12. *(Continued).* Translational injury. **B**, Preoperative AP radiograph. **C**, Preoperative lateral radiograph. **D** and **E**, CT scans.

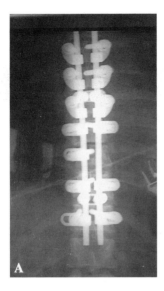 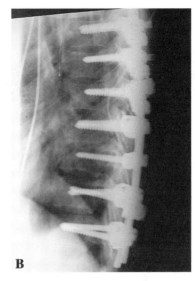

FIGURE 13. Translational injury. **A,** Postoperative anteroposterior radiograph. **B,** Postoperative lateral radiographs.

a total-contact orthosis. Indications for surgery include progressive neurologic deficit due to neural compression of bone, disc, hematoma, or bullet fragments within the spinal canal or bullets that pass through the colon bfore traversing the spine. In rare cases, multiple columns of the spine may be destroyed, requiring stabilization procedures.

BIBLIOGRAPHY

1. Akbarnia BA: Surgical treatment of upper thoracic spine fractures using Cotrel-Dubousset instrumentation. Spine State Art Rev 7:269–276, 1993.
2. Ballock RT, Mackersie R, Abitol JJ, et al: Can burst fractures be predicted from plain radiographs? J Bone Joint Surg 74B:147–150, 1992.
3. Cammisa FP, Eismont FJ, Green BA: Dural lacerations occurring with burst fractures and associated laminar fractures. J Bone Joint Surg 71A:1044, 1989.
4. Denis F: The three-column spine and its significance in the classification of acute thoracolumbar spinal injuries. Spine 8:817–831, 1983.
5. Garfin SR, Vaccaro AR: Orthopaedic Knowledge Update: Spine. Rosemont, IL, American Academy of Orthopaedic Surgeons, 1997.
6. Holt BT, McCormack T, Gaines RW: Short segment fusion- anterior or posterior approach? The load-sharing classification of spinal fractures. Spine State Art Rev 7:277–286, 1993.
7. Levine AM, Eismont FJ, Garfin SR, et al: Spine Trauma. Philadelphia, W.B. Saunders, 1998.
8. Mc Afee PC, Yuan HA, Fredrickson BE, et al: The unstable burst fracture. Spine 7:365, 1982
9. McAfee PC, Bohlman HH, Yuan HA: Anterior decompression of traumatic thoracolumbar fractures with incomplete neurologic deficits using a retroperitoneal approach. J Bone Joint Surg 63A:891, 1981
10. Puno RM, Bhojraj SY, Glassman SD, et al: Flexion-distraction injuries of the thoracolumbar and lumbar spine in adult and pediatric patients. Spine State Art Rev 7:223–240, 1993.

53. SACRAL FRACTURES

Jens R. Chapman, M.D., and Thomas A. Schildhauer, M.D.

1. What is the role of the sacrum?

The sacrum connects the lumbar spine and the left- and right-sided iliac wings by means of well-developed ligaments with little inherent bony stability. The sacrum is kyphotically aligned in the sagittal plane in a variable dimension ranging from 0° to over 90°. The sacrum distributes the torso load through the lumbar spine mainly through its S1 segment into the sacroiliac joints and from there to the hip joints.

2. Who is affected by sacral fractures?

Basically two distinct patient groups are affected by sacral fractures:

1. High-energy injury mechanisms. Patients are to be assessed and treated as polytrauma victims.
- Road traffic crashes
- Falls from a height
- Crush injuries

2. Low-impact insufficiency fractures. Patients require comprehensive metabolic and neoplasia work-up:
- Osteoporosis
- Collagen disorders
- Neoplastic disorders

3. How are sacrum fractures diagnosed?

- Patient history
- Imaging tests
- Physical examination
- Subjective symptoms
- Electrodiagnostic tests

Subjective symptoms of patients with sacrum fractures are notoriously vague and usually consist of back pain aggravated by sitting, standing, and walking. Physical examination is important and consists of inspection and palpation of the patient's back side and thorough examination of neurologic function.

4. Describe the components of the neurologic examination for patients with a sacral fracture.

Regardless of the patient's cognitive status, an evaluation consistent with the guidelines of the American Spinal Injury Association is performed. More specific to sacral fractures, anal sphincter evaluation is performed. Components of this evaluation consist of assessment for blood in the rectal vault as well as presence of the prostate in the expected position. From a neurologic perspective the assessment should include the following four components:

- Presence of spontaneous anal sphincter tone
- Maximum voluntary and sphincter contractility
- Perianal sensation to light touch and pinprick
- Presence of anal wink and bulbocavernosus reflex.

Postvoid residuals (PVR) can be used as follow-up test for patients with neurogenic bladder to assess for reinervation.

5. What imaging tests are helpful in assessing sacral fractures?

Plain radiographs
- Trauma pelvis anteroposterior view
- Pelvis inlet view
- Pelvis outlet view
- Lateral sacral view

Computed tomography (CT) scans
- Pelvic CT
- Sacral CT with sagittal and coronal reformatted views
- Three-dimensional reformations are rarely helpful.

Magnetic resonance imaging (MRI)
- Conventional imaging sequence: useful to diagnose stress fractures or assess unclear neurologic injuries.
- MRI neurography: useful to localize known root or plexus injury.

Radionuclide imaging
- Technetium 99 bone scan with single-photon emission computed tomography (SPECT): useful for insufficiency fractures.

The basic radiographic assessment starts with an anteroposterior (AP) pelvis radiograph. Because of the inclined nature of the sacrum, visualization of the sacrum is limited. Attention to subtle details, such as disruption of the foraminal lines, is important in screening for sacral fractures. If a fracture is suspected, further imaging tests should be ordered, including pelvic inlet and outlet views and a lateral sacral radiograph. If a pelvic ring fracture is suspected, a pelvic CT is ordered to assess the three-dimensional complexities of the pelvis. If a significant sacral fracture is diagnosed, a sacral CT, including sagittal and coronal reformatation, is helpful. MRI is not routinely necessary. Technetium bone scans with SPECT images are helpful in identifying insufficiency fractures of the sacrum.

6. What electrodiagnostic tests are helpful in assessing patients with sacral fractures?

- Electromyogram (EMG) of L5 and S1 innervated muscles
- Anal sphincter EMG
- Somatosensory-evoked potentials (SSEP) of tibial and peroneal nerves
- Pudendal sensory-evoked potentials (PSEP)
- Cystomyography (CMG)

PSEPs are helpful for patients with impaired cognitive status or unclear physical examination findings and suspected lumbosacral root injury. This study is useful in the assessment of the acutely injured patient. In contrast, conventional EMG is limited to assessment of the L5 and S1 roots and usually has a delay time of 3 weeks before injury-related changes are detectable. Anal sphincter EMG and CMG can diagnose lower sacral root damage but are not useful in the immediate post-injury period. CMG has been used as a follow-up study for patients with neurogenic bladder and may demonstrate bladder re-innervation.

7. Why is the diagnosis of sacral fractures frequently overlooked or delayed?

The diagnosis of sacral fractures is overlooked or delayed in 20–53% of cases. Causes for missed injuries range from vague physical symptoms and findings to difficulties in interpreting an AP pelvis radiograph for sacral abnormalities. This can be especially challenging in obese patients and in the presence of an osteopenic skeleton or osteophytes. In multiply injured patients, a challenging resuscitation setting can distract diagnostic attention from the posterior pelvic ring. A high index of suspicion on the part of the treating physician is important to avoid potential secondary damage from a missed sacral fracture.

8. What are possible consequences of a missed sacral fracture?

- Chronic pain with weightbearing
- Sacral or posterior pelvic malunion
- Secondary neurologic deficits from progressive fracture displacement and neural element impingement
- Posterior soft tissue breakdown from progressive sacral kyphosis

9. How are sacral fractures classified?

Denis has provided the most helpful general classification of sacral fractures because of its significant implications about incidence and type of associated neurologic injury. This simple classification uses the most medial fracture extension to distingush three types of fractures (Fig. 1):

- Zone 1 fractures remain lateral to the sacral foramina. This fracture type is occasionally associated with L5 root injuries.
- Zone 2 injuries extend through the sacral foramina and are associated with lumbosacral root injuries in 15 % of patients.
- Zone 3 injuries involve the central sacral spinal canal and are reported to have a 30–50% incidence of sacral root deficits resulting in bowel and bladder control deficits.

The Denis classification, however, does not address fracture stability. Any of the fracture types can be subclassified into stable and unstable variants. For Denis zone 3 fractures, Roy-Camille has provided a helpful subclassification system (Fig. 2). He differentiates simple kyphotic fractures (type 1), kyphotically and partially translated fractures (type 2), fully displaced fractures (type 3), and segmentally comminuted fractures (type 4, as described by Strange-Vognsen).

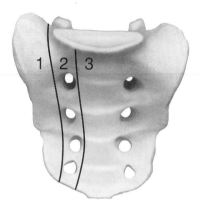

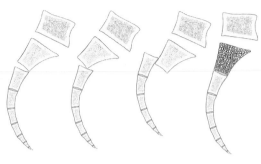

FIGURE 2. Subclassification of Denis Zone III fractures as suggested by Roy-Camille. Type 1 injuries are angulated but not translated, whereas type 2 injuries are angulated and translated. Type 3 injuries show complete translational displacement of upper and lower sacrum, whereas type 4 injuries are segmentally comminuted due to axial impaction (as suggested by Strange-Vognsen). (From Chapman JR, Mirza SK: Sacral fractures. In Fardon D, Garfin S, et al (eds): Orthopaedic Knowledge Update: Spine 2. Rosemont, IL, American Academy of Orthopaedic Surgeons, 2002, with permission.)

FIGURE 1. Three-zone system of Denis: zone I injuries remain lateral to the neuroforamina; zone II fractures involve the neuroforamina but do not involve the spinal canal; zone III injuries extend into the spinal canal.

10. What factors influences selection of treatment options for sacral fractures?

Decision-making about management of patients with sacral fractures is multifactorial. Variables include presence/absence of multiple injuries, open vs. closed fracture, associated soft tissue compromise, neurologic injury, and injury mechanism. There are no simple treatment algorithms.

11. What are the nonoperative treatment options for sacral fractures?

Stable, closed, single-system, sacral injuries without neurologic deficits are amenable to nonoperative management.
- Early, protected weightbearing
- Immobilization with unilateral or bilateral HTLSO or pantaloon spica cast
- Prolonged bed rest with recumbent skeletal traction.

12. What surgical treatment options exist for sacral fractures?

Surgical interventions can be classified as decompression procedures and procedures that provide fracture reduction and stabilization.

13. When is a surgical decompression indicated after a sacral fracture?

In presence of lumbosacral or sacral nerve deficits or sacral radicular pain, surgical decompression within 2 weeks of injury has been associated with improved outcome compared with nonsurgical management. Decompression can be accomplished directly with a dorsal midline laminotomy and foraminotomy or indirectly via fracture disimpaction or fracture reduction and stabilization.

14. What drawbacks are associated with surgical decompression of sacral fractures?

Surgical decompression may be ineffective in presence of traumatic sacral neural transsection. Approximately 35% of displaced transverse sacral fractures are associated with transsected sacral roots based on autopsy study. Unfortunately, no imaging or electrophysiologic studies can conclusively establish the presence of transsected sacral roots. Other risks associated with decompression surgery for sacral fractures include wound healing problems, persistent cerebrospinal fluid leakage, and additional fracture destabilization.

15. When is surgical stabilization of a sacral fracture indicated?

There are few strict guidelines for surgical sacral fracture stabilization. Typically, fracture displacement of 1 cm or more is considered to be consistent with fracture instability. Injuries that disrupt significant ligamentous lumbopelvic support structures usually have a poor prognosis for healing. Most patients who require surgical decompression of lumbosacral neural elements should also be considered for surgical stabilization to prevent further fracture displacement and enhance chances of neural recovery.

16. What are the options for surgical stabilization of sacral fractures?

Anterior (indirect methods)
- Symphyseal plating
- Anterior external fixation
- Retrograde superior ramus screw fixation

Posterior
- Sacroiliac screw fixation (open or closed)
- Posterior tension band plating
- Sacral alar plating (Roy -Camille technique)
- Lumbopelvic instrumentation
- Combined procedures

All sacral fractures should be evaluated in the context of its effect on pelvic ring and lumbar spine stability. Anterior pelvic ring stabilization has a supplemental role in sacral fracture stabilization, which can be achieved with anterior external fixation or symphyseal plating. Posterior pelvic ring fixation has undergone considerable evolution. Percutaneous sacroiliac screw placement has been reported to have a high success rate in the treatment of noncomplex sacral fractures. This technique allows effective indirect fracture reduction and stabilization when applied within 2–3 days from injury and has a relatively low incidence of reported complications. It is, however, limited in its biomechanical stability, especially for vertically displaced fractures and high-grade Denis zone 3 injuries. The most stable sacral fracture stabilization consists of lumbopelvic stabilization using lumbar pedicle and iliac screw fixation. This technique allows comprehensive stabilization of the sacrum through a posterior midline exposure.

17. What is the optimal time for surgical intervention for a sacral fracture?

Optimal timing of surgical intervention for sacral fractures is multifactorial. Posterior exposures usually require a posterior midline approach with the patient prone. Truly emergent open surgical decompression and stabilization of sacral fractures are rarely indicated. Because of the risk of significant blood loss, emergent surgical intervention using the open approach in the prone position is frequently postponed in favor of a delayed postprimary procedure within the first 2 weeks after injury. Additional factors to consider are presence of soft tissue deglovement (Morel-Lavalle lesion), open sacral fractures, and posterior soft tissue compromise caused by prominent bony fragments.

18. How are percutaneous sacroiliac screws placed?

Intricate knowledge of pelvic anatomy and availability of high-quality intraoperative C-arm are some of the prerequisites. Satisfactory closed reduction is achieved by means of skeletal traction or percutaneous manipulation. Radiographic anatomy should be reviewed to rule out the presence of congenital sacroiliac bony anomalies. Typically, a 7.0-mm large fragment cannulated screw system is used for unilateral or bilateral fixation. With the patient positioned supine on a fluoroscopy table, appropriate percutaneous starting points and guide-pin trajectories are determined using sacral lateral as well as inlet and outlet projections on C-arm. Intraoperative screw placement under CT guidance can be used as an imaging alternative. However, this approach is not feasible for polytraumatized patients or if intraoperative fracture manipulation is required. Screws are usually advanced over guide-wires into the vertebral body of the S1 segment. Compression screws can be used in the presence of noncomminuted fractures. Fully threaded screws are preferred for patients with comminuted zone 2 fractures.

19. How is lumbopelvic instrumentation accomplished?

The ideal instrumentation system for lumbopelvic fixation is low-profile and biomechanically stable, possess a simple connecting mechanism, and is adaptable to individual needs (Fig. 3). The instrumentation technique for lumbopelvic fixation differs significantly among various implant makers. Using side-loading implants, such as the Universal Spine System (Synthes, Paoli, PA), bilateral L5 pedicle fixation is obtained. If the S1 segment is intact, additional pedicle screws are placed into this segment. After decompression of the sacrum from the L5 segment downward, reduction of the sacral segments and the iliac wings can be accomplished with temporary threaded pins. Rods are then molded to connect from the L5 and S1 screws to the region of the posterior iliac crest overhang and the posterior sacral ala. Using the outer iliac table as an inclination guide, one or two drill holes are then placed just lateral to the rod under lateral C-arm visualization. A starting point is selected approximately 2 cm inferior to the posterior superior iliac spine and aiming toward the anterior inferior iliac spine. The thickened portion of the ilium within 2–3 cm above the sciatic notch offers the most predictable passageway for such pelvic anchoring devices. Screws of up to 130 mm in length and 8 mm in diameter have been shown to be safely anchored in the iliac wing using this technique.

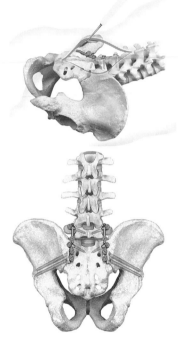

FIGURE 3. Insertion of lumbopelvic fixation. Comprehensive stabilization of the sacrum and complete decompression of the sacrum can be achieved with the insertion of long iliac screws that are attached to conventional, caudally extended lumbosacral rods.

BIBLIOGRAPHY

1. Denis F, Davis S, Comfort T: Sacral fractures: an important problem: Retrospective analysis of 236 cases. Clin Orthop 227:67–81, 1988.
2. Gibbons KJ, Soloniuk DS, Razack N: Neurogical injury and patterns of sacral fractures. J Neurosurg 72: 889–893, 1990.
3. Gunterberg B: Effects of major resection of the sacrum: Clinical studies on urogenital and anorectal function and a biomechanical study on pelvic strength. Acta Orthop Scand 162(Suppl):1–38, 1976.
4. Huittinen VM: Lumbo-sacral nerve injury in fracture of the pelvis: A postmortem radiographic and pathoanatomical study. Acta Chir Scand 429:3–43, 1972.
5. Kellam JF, McMurtry RY, Paley et al: The unstable pelvic fracture: Operative treatment. Orthop Clin North AM 18:25–41, 1987.
6. Nork S, Jones CB, Harding SP, et al: Percutaneous stabilization of U-shaped sacral fractures using iliosacral screws: Technique and early results. J Orthop Trauma 15:1236–1244, 2001.
7. Routt MLC Jr, Nork SE, Mills WJ: Percutaneous fixation of pelvic ring disruptions. Clin Orthop 375: 15–29, 2000.
8. Schildhauer TA, McCullough P, Chapman JR, Mann FA: Anatomic and radiographic considerations for placement of transiliac screws in lumbopelvic fixations. J Spinal Disord Tech 15(3):199–205, 2002.
9. Schmidek HH, Smith DA, Kristiansen TK: Sacral fractures. Neurosurgery 15:735–746, 1984.

54. PEDIATRIC SPINE TRAUMA

Ramin Bagheri, M.D., and Behrooz A. Akbarnia, M.D.

1. When does ossification of the immature vertebral body begin and in what pattern?

Primary ossification begins between 7 and 8 years of age, forming a central epiphysis and a superior and inferior growth plate, analogous to the enchondral ossification seen in long bones. By 12–15 years, the central epiphysis progressively thins, and an incomplete peripheral ring apophysis forms around the anterior and lateral portions of the vertebral body. This apophyseal ring, seen well radiographically, contributes little to the longitudinal growth of the vertebral body and is mainly responsible for the circumferential growth of the vertebral body. Longitudinal growth occurs via the superior and inferior growth plates. Final closure of the ossification centers occurs by age 21–25.

2. What is a limbus fracture? Where does it occur?

Fractures crossing the vertebral endplate in the immature spine are called limbus fractures. These fractures traverse almost exclusively through the growth zone (hypertrophic zone) of the physis, in the same pattern seen in immature long bone injuries. This region is biomechanically weak and thus susceptible to injury.

3. What are the relative strengths and weaknesses of plain radiographs, CT scan, and MRI in the detection of cervical spine injuries in children?

Plain radiographs can miss up to 50% of spinal injuries in children, typically those involving unossified tissues, such as the cartilaginous endplate. A cervical spine series consists of a lateral film (the most diagnostic view of the series), an anteroposterior film, and an open-mouth odontoid view. In a conscious and cooperative child, flexion and extension lateral films can rule out instability due to ligamentous or bony injury. If faced with equivocal films or an uncooperative child, with a mechanism of injury or physical exam that is suspicious for spinal injury, more advanced imaging is indicated. CT scan is superior for the detection of bony injuries, but one must be aware of the thickness between cuts and of the possibility of an injury in the plane of the cuts being missed. CT reconstructions can reveal such an injury. MRI is superior for the detection of soft tissue injuries that may be missed by plain films and CT scans.

4. What unique features of the pediatric cervical spine can lead to confusion during the evaluation of cervical radiographs following spine trauma?

Ten unique features of the pediatric cervical spine that can cause confusion during trauma evaluation are shown in Figure 1.

5. How does the addition of a shoulder harness to a lapbelt influence the type of spinal injury sustained by a pediatric motor vehicle passenger?

The additional of a shoulder harness to a lapbelt reduces injury to the lumbar spine by limiting the forward flexion of the thorax during impact and reducing the flexion-distraction forces on the lumbar spine. However, by restraining the thorax, a shoulder harness can increase the risk of cervical spine injuries in severe accidents. Children have a large head relative to their body length and a higher center of gravity compared with adults. During impact, the forces acting on the unrestrained head are transmitted to the cervical spine when the thorax is restrained with a shoulder harness.

6. What is the most common cervical spine injury in children?

Odontoid fractures are the most common cervical spine injuries in children, with 4 years being the mean age of injury. The injury usually occurs as an epiphyseal separation of the growth plate at the base of the odontoid. Minimally displaced fractures are difficult to diagnose on plain film, making CT scan with reconstructions and MRI important diagnostic studies.

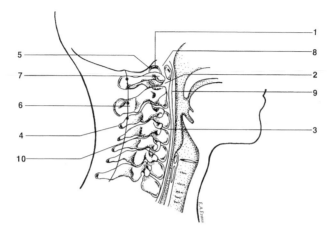

FIGURE 1. Ten unique features of the pediatric cervical spine that can cause confusion during the trauma evaluation: (1) the apical ossification center can be mistaken for a fracture; (2) the synchondrosis at the base of the odontoid can be mistaken for a fracture; (3) vertebral bodies appear rounded-off or wedged, simulating a fracture; (4) secondary centers of ossification at the tips of the spinous processes can be mistaken for a fracture; (5) the odontoid may angulate posteriorly in 4% of children; (6) C2–C3 pseudosubluxation (can be assessed with Swischuk's line); (7) the ossification center of the anterior arch of C1 may be absent in the first year of life; (8) the atlantodens interval may be as wide as 4.5 mm and still be normal; (9) the width of the prevertebral soft tissues vary widely, especially with crying, and may be mistaken for swelling; and (10) horizontal facets in young children can be mistake for a fracture. (From Flynn JM: Spine trauma in the pediatric population. Spine State Art Rev 14:249–262, 2000, with permission.)

7. What is an os odontoideum?

An os odontoideum appears as a rounded piece of bone at the apex of the odontoid with a radiolucent gap separating it from the remainder of the axis and body of C2. Many consider os odontoideum to arise from a previously unrecognized injury. Unrestricted motion following this initial fracture leads to the development of a pseudoarthrosis. Its clinical presentation may mimic an acute fracture.

8. How is an occipitoatlantal dislocation diagnosed and treated?

This is generally a catastrophic and fatal injury. The dislocation may spontaneously reduce and remain unrecognized until traction is applied to the skull. Determining the Powers ratio on a lateral plain radiograph can reveal an occipitoatlantal dislocation (Fig. 2). This ratio is calculated by dividing the distance from the basion (anterior margin of foramen magnum) to the posterior arch of the atlas by the distance from the opisthion (posterior margin of foramen magnum) to the anterior arch of the atlas. Ratios less than one are normal, whereas ratios equal to or greater than one indicate anterior occipitoatlantal dislocation. Halo immobilization is recommended as soon as this injury is recognized. Treatment consists of a posterior occipital-cervical fusion with halo vest immobilization.

9. Describe the indications for treatment of upper cervical spine instability in a patient with Down's syndrome.

The incidence of atlantoaxial instability in children with Down's syndrome varies from 9% to 22%, whereas occipitoatlantal instability occurs in up to 60% of these patients. Most cases of atlantoaxial and occipitoatlantal instability are asymptomatic. Down's syndrome patients with asymptomatic atlantoaxial and occipitoatlantal instability should undergo repeat neurologic examinations. The role of repeat radiographs is unclear. Recently, the American Academy of Pediatrics has retired its recommendation for screening radiographs in children with Down's syndrome. However, the Special Olympics continues to require radiographic studies of its participants.

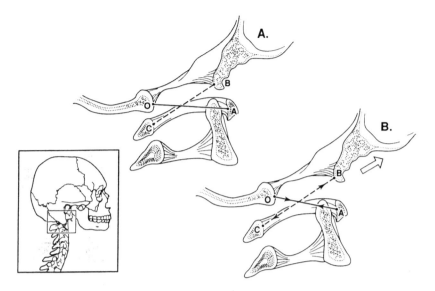

FIGURE 2. The Powers ratio is determined by means of drawing a line from the basion (B) to the posterior arch of the atlas (C) and a second line from the opisthion (O) to the anterior arch of the atlas (A). The length of the line BC is divided by the length of line OA. **A,** Values less than 0.9 are normal. **B,** A ratio greater than 1.0 suggests the diagnosis of anterior occipitoatlantal dislocation. (From Lebwohl NH, Eismont FJ: Cervical spine injuries in children. In Weinstein SL (ed). The Pediatric Spine: Principles and Practice, 2nd ed. Philadelphia, Lippincott, Williams & Wilkins, 2001, p 557, with permissions.)

The risk of catastrophic spinal cord injury during participation in organized sports is extremely low in patients with Down's syndrome in the absence of neurologic findings. Therefore, restriction placed on high-risk activities must be individualized. Patients with sudden onset or recent progression of neurologic symptoms and imaging studies confirming cord compression require immediate fusion. Controversy exists about patients with instability and minimal or chronic nonprogressive symptoms because stabilization procedures often result in minimal symptomatic improvement and are associated with an extremely high complication rate.

10. What is the appropriate treatment for a child with a Risser sign of 0 or 1 who sustains multiple compression fractures with less than 10° of deformity in each vertebra and no neurologic compromise?

Studies following these patients to skeletal maturity have shown that no treatment is necessary in such patients. Children, especially those younger than 10 years of age, have excellent healing potential and usually reconstitute lost vertebral height in the sagittal plane in mild compression fractures. Patients who are older, have more than 10° of deformity per vertebra, or have deformity in the frontal plane, usually require treatment.

11. How are flexion-distraction injuries treated in children?

Injuries confined to bone both anteriorly and posteriorly generally heal without instability if treated nonoperatively in a TLSO for 2–3 months. Bracing is usually successful if the initial kyphosis is less than 20°. Surgical treatment is indicated for:

- Unstable, purely ligamentous injuries
- Very unstable fractures that cannot be managed in a brace
- Fractures with significant kyphosis that cannot be reduced or maintained in a brace
- Fractures associated with neurologic injury

The surgical principle is to reconstitute a sufficient posterior tension band either with posterior wiring in small children or posterior compression constructs in older or larger children.

12. What are the two primary surgical indications for the treatment of pediatric burst fractures?

The first indication is partial or progressive neurologic deficit caused by canal compromise. The mere presence of bone in the canal is not a sufficient indication for surgery since bone remodeling and reabsorption occur over time. The second indication is the prevention of late kyphotic deformity. More than 25° of localized kyphosis is generally accepted as an indication for surgery.

13 How does the treatment of burst fractures differ in children and adults?

Children and adolescents have strong bone with excellent healing potential. Late kyphotic deformity is less likely in children. Combined anterior and posterior fusions, which are commonly used for highly comminuted adult burst fractures, are rarely necessary in children. Children also have greater potential to remodel bone within the spinal canal than adults. In addition, children are less likely to suffer the detrimental effects of immobilization compared to adults. Otherwise, the basic principles of adult burst fracture treatment can be applied to children and adolescents.

14. What is SCIWORA?

SCIWORA is an acronym for spinal cord injury without radiographic abnormality. The spinal column in children is more elastic than the spinal cord. It has been demonstrated that the spinal column of an infant can be stretched up to 2 inches, whereas the spinal cord can be stretched only 0.25 inches before rupturing. SCIWORA injuries occur when a traction force (such as during difficult deliveries) is applied to the spine, and accommodated by the spinal column but exceeds the elastic limits of the spinal cord. This mechanism causes a damaging stretch injury to the cord that usually results in complete tetraplegia.

15. In patients with SCIWORA injuries, what is the typical site of cord injury and what imaging studies may be helpful in diagnosis?

The typical site of injury is the cervicothoracic junction. SCIWORA is defined as an injury to the spinal cord without visible changes on plain radiographs. In the past, myelography has been used to demonstrate this injury, occasionally showing a block at the level of injury. Currently, MRI is the imaging study of choice to diagnose injury to the spinal cord and unossified tissues. Typical findings include acute hemorrhage and edema of the spinal cord.

16. What common radiographic findings are noted in a child that has sustained a spine injury as a result of child abuse?

Most of these injuries involve the vertebral bodies, with varying degrees of anterior compression. Other findings include anterior notching of the vertebral body near the superior endplate, decreased disc height caused by disc herniation as well as fracture-dislocation (Fig. 3). Injuries of the cervical region may occur but injuries to the thoracolumbar and lumbar region are more common. Although vertebral body fractures and subluxations are injuries with moderate specificity for child abuse, if a history of trauma is absent or inconsistent with these injuries, they become high-specificity lesions.

17. What are the most common clinical and imaging findings in children with limbus fractures?

Most limbus (vertebral endplate) fractures occur in the lumbar spine at the L4–L5 and L5–S1 levels. Clinical presentation is similar to that of a herniated nucleus pulposus. Most patients have symptoms of stiffness and spasm, numbness, weakness, and occasionally neurogenic claudication. Infrequently limbus fractures present with a cauda equina syndrome. Many patients have a positive Lasegue sign. Limbus fractures are difficult to visualize on plain radiographs. MRI, CT or CT-myelography can be used to confirm the diagnosis. These studies show avulsion of the apophysis, often with a small bony fragment attached.

18. What are the four types of vertebral endplate fractures? (See Fig. 4.)

Type I: Pure cartilage avulsion of the entire posterior cortical vertebral margin without attendant osseous defect.

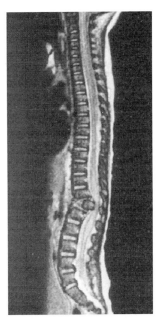

FIGURE 3. MR image of a fracture-dislocation of the spine occurring in a 10-month old infant who was the victim of child abuse. The image reveals cord compression in this patient with incomplete paraplegia. (From Akbarnia BA: Pediatric spine fractures. Orthop Clin North Am 30:531, 1999, with permission.)

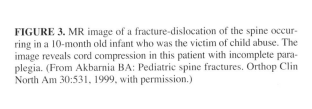

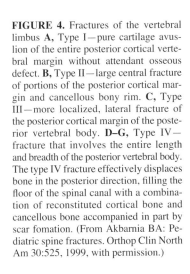

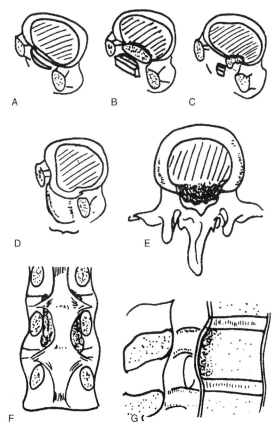

FIGURE 4. Fractures of the vertebral limbus **A,** Type I—pure cartilage avulsion of the entire posterior cortical vertebral margin without attendant osseous defect. **B,** Type II—large central fracture of portions of the posterior cortical margin and cancellous bony rim. **C,** Type III—more localized, lateral fracture of the posterior cortical margin of the posterior vertebral body. **D–G,** Type IV—fracture that involves the entire length and breadth of the posterior vertebral body. The type IV fracture effectively displaces bone in the posterior direction, filling the floor of the spinal canal with a combination of reconstituted cortical bone and cancellous bone accompanied in part by scar fomation. (From Akbarnia BA: Pediatric spine fractures. Orthop Clin North Am 30:525, 1999, with permission.)

Type II: Large central fracture of portions of the posterior cortical margin and cancellous bony rim.
Type III: More localized, lateral fracture of the posterior cortical margin of the vertebral body.
Type IV: Fracture that involves the entire length and breadth of the posterior vertebral body.

19. How would a child with a herniated disc typically present?

Children with a herniated nucleus pulposus may present with a range of physical signs, including significant back spasm and stiffness, a positive straight leg raise test, and occasionally sciatic scoliosis. Neurologic deficits are uncommon. The presentation of a central disc protrusion may be limited to back pain. The diagnosis of disc herniation in children is often delayed, because it is uncommon and typically does not significantly limit daily activity.

20. What is involved in the work-up of a child with a suspected herniated disc?

In children, a herniated nucleus pulposus is rare. One must rule out other causes of sciatica, such as a slipped vertebral apophysis, neoplasm, tethered cord, infection, spondylolisthesis, and spondylolysis. Plain radiographs, bone scan, CT scan, and MRI may be required to rule out these conditions; MRI is the procedure of choice.

21. Describe the treatment of a herniated disc in children and adolescents.

As in adults, nonoperative treatment consisting of rest, muscle relaxants, and anti-inflammatories should be attempted initially in patients without neurologic deficit. In contrast to adults, nonoperative treatment in children often fails. Surgical treatment is successful in more than 90% of cases and should be limited to a microdiscectomy that removes the herniation and decompresses the neural elements.

22. What treatment is advised for acute traumatic spondylolysis?

Treatment of traumatic spondylolysis is usually non-operative, with the defect healing in many children. Nonoperative treatment consists of immobilization with a corset or TLSO, restriction from vigorous activities, and physical therapy for stretching of the hamstring muscles and strengthening of the abdominal musculature. If nonoperative treatment fails, various surgical options exist, including posterolateral fusion or direct bony repair of the pars defect supplemented with screw or wire fixation of the spinous process.

BIBLIOGRAPHY

1. Akbarnia BA: Pediatric spine fractures. Orthop Clin North Am 30:521–536, 1999.
2. Akbarnia BA: Pediatric spine trauma. In DeWald RL (ed): Spinal Deformities—Fundamentals. Scoliosis Research Society Spine Curriculum Text,2001.
3. American Academy of Pediatrics Committee on Sports Medicine and Fitness: Atlantoaxial instability in Down syndrome: Subject review. Pediatrics 96:151–154, 1995.
4. Arlet V, Fassier F: Herniated nucleus pulposus and slipped vertebral apophysis. In Weinstein SL (ed): The Pediatric Spine: Principles and Practice, 2nd ed. Philadelphia, Lippincott Williams & Wilkins, 2001, pp 576–583.
5. Bollini G: Thoracic and lumbar spine injuries in children. In Floman Y, Farcy JC, Argenson C (eds): Thoracolumbar Spine Fractures. New York, Raven Press, 1993, pp 307–325.
6. Chambers HG, Akbarnia BA: Thoracic, lumbar, and sacral spine fractures and dislocations. In Weinstein SL (ed): The Pediatric Spine: Principles and Practice, 2nd ed. Philadelphia, Lippincott Williams & Wilkins, 2001, pp 576–583.
7. Flynn JM: Spine trauma in the pediatric population. Spine State Art Rev 14(1):249–262, 2000.
8. Lebwohl NH, Eismont FJ: Cervical spine injuries in children. In Weinstein SL (ed): The Pediatric Spine: Princips and Practice, 2nd ed. Philadelphia, Lippincott Williams & Wilkins, 2001, pp 553–566.
9. Pouliquen JC, Kassis B, Glorion C, et al: Vertebral growth after thoracic or lumbar fracture of the spine in children. J Pediatr Orthop 17(1):115–120, 1997.

55. REHABILITATION AFTER SPINAL CORD INJURY

Thomas N. Bryce, M.D., and Kristjan T. Ragnarsson, M.D.

1. Which of the following terms are currently favored to describe impairment or loss of motor and/or sensory function due to damage of neural elements within the spinal canal: (1) tetraplegia, (2) paraplegia, (3) quadriplegia, (4) quadriparesis, and/or (5) paraparesis?

Tetraplegia refers to the impairments resulting from damage to neural elements within the cervical spinal canal, whereas paraplegia refers to the impairments resulting from damage to neural elements within the thoracic, lumbar, or sacral spinal canal. As *tetra, para,* and *plegia* are of Greek origin and *quadri* is of Latin origin, to maintain uniformity in word root origins, tetraplegia is preferred over quadriplegia. Since the ASIA Impairment Scale (see question 6.) more precisely defines incomplete tetraplegia and paraplegia than the terms quadriparesis and paraparesis, their use is discouraged.

2. What is the difference between a skeletal level and a neurologic level in assessing a person with a traumatic spinal cord injury (SCI)?

The **skeletal level** is defined as the level in the spine where the greatest vertebral damage is found on radiographic examination.

The **neurologic level** is defined as the most caudal segment of the spinal cord with normal sensory and motor function bilaterally.

3. How are the motor and sensory components assessed in the determination of a neurologic level of spinal cord injury?

Motor component: a key muscle is tested from each myotome in a rostral-caudal sequence by manual muscle test and graded on a six-point scale:

0 = total paralysis, no palpable or visible contraction

1 = palpable or visible contraction

2 = active movement, full range of motion (ROM) with gravity eliminated

3 = active movement, full ROM against gravity only

4 = active movement, full ROM against resistance

5 = normal

The motor level is defined, by convention, for each side of the body by the first key caudal muscle that is graded at least 3, if all prior rostral key muscles are graded 5; the most caudal key muscle graded 5, if all prior rostral key muscles are graded 5 and the next caudal key muscle is graded 0, 1, or 2; or as the sensory level if no clinically testable key muscle meets either of the other two requirements.

Sensory component: light touch and pin sensation are tested for each dermatome and graded on a three-point scale:

0 = absent

1 = impaired (partial or altered appreciation, including hyperesthesia)

2 = normal

The sensory level is defined, by convention, for each side of the body as the most caudal dermatome graded 2, if all prior rostral dermatomes are graded 2 and the next caudal key muscle is graded 0 or 1.

4. Identify the key muscles that are tested in determining the motor level of lesion.

C5 = Elbow flexors (biceps, brachialis)

C6 = Wrist extensors (extensor carpi radialis longus and brevis)

C7 = Elbow extensors (triceps)
C8 = Finger flexors (flexor digitorum profundus) to the middle finger
T1 = Small finger abductors (abductor digiti minimi)
L2 = Hip flexors (iliopsoas)
L3 = Knee extensors (quadriceps)
L4 = Ankle dorsiflexors (tibialis anterior)
L5 = Long toe extensors (extensor hallucis longus)
S1 = Ankle plantarflexors (gastrocnemius, soleus)

5. Identify the key point for each sensory dermatome that is tested in determining the sensory level of lesion.

C2 = Occipital protuberance
C3 = Supraclavicular fossa
C4 = Top of acromioclavicular joint
C5 = Lateral side of antecubital fossa
C6 = Thumb
C7 = Middle finger
C8 = Little finger
T1 = Medial (ulnar) side of antecubital fossa
T2 = Apex of the axilla
T3 = Third intercostal space (IS)
T4 = Fourth IS (nipple line)
T5 = Fifth IS (midway between T4 and T6)
T6 = Sixth IS (level of xiphisternum)
T7 = Seventh IS (midway between T6 and T8)
T8 = Eighth IS (midway between T6 and T10)
T9 = Ninth IS (midway between T8 and T10)
T10 = Tenth IS (umbilicus)
T11 = Eleventh IS (midway between T10 and T12)
T12 = Inguinal ligament at mid-point
L1 = Half the distance between T12 and L2
L2 = Mid-anterior thigh
L3 = Medial femoral condyle
L4 = Medial malleolus
L5 = Dorsum of the foot at the third metatarsal phalangeal joint
S1 = Lateral heel
S2 = Popliteal fossa in the mid-line
S3 = Ischial tuberosity
S4–5 = Perianal area (taken as one level)

6. What is the difference between a complete and an incomplete spinal cord injury as defined by the American Spinal Injury Association (ASIA) Impairment Scale?

A = Complete. No sensory or motor function is preserved in the sacral segments S4–S5.
B = Incomplete. Sensory but not motor function is preserved below the neurologic level and includes the sacral segments S4-S5.
C = Incomplete. Motor function is preserved below the neurologic level, and more than half of key muscles below the neurologic level have a muscle grade < 3.
D = Incomplete. Motor function is preserved below the neurologic level, and at least half of key muscles below the neurologic level have a muscle grade ≥ to 3.
E = Normal. Sensory and motor function are normal.

7. What medication has been shown to improve neurologic recovery significantly if given within 8 hours of an acute SCI? What is the dose?

Methylprednisolone sodium succinate, 30mg/kg, delivered as an intravenous bolus over 15 minutes, followed by a 45-minute pause, then an infusion of 5.4 mg/kg/hour for 23 or 47 hours, beginning within 8 hours of injury, has been shown in the National Acute Spinal Cord Injury Studies (NASCIS II and III) to improve neurologic recovery significantly.

8. What findings on MRI have been shown to correlate with prognosis?

The presence of hematomyelia is associated with neurologically complete injury in approximately 90% of patients, whereas contusion and edema are associated with neurologically incomplete injury in approximately 80% of patients.

9. Identify and describe six different neurologically incomplete acute SCI syndromes.

Cruciate paralysis: damage to the anterior spinal cord at the C2 level (level of corticospinal tract decussation) with greater loss of motor function in upper extremities compared to the lower extremities, variable sensory loss, and variable cranial nerve deficits.

Central cord syndrome: damage to the central spinal cord below the C2 level with greater loss of motor function in upper extremities compared to the lower extremities with variable sensory loss, at least partial sacral sparing, and variable bowel and bladder involvement.

Anterior cord syndrome: damage to the anterior spinal cord with relative preservation of proprioception and variable loss of pain sensation, temperature sensation, and motor function.

Brown-Séquard syndrome: damage to the lateral half of the spinal cord with relative ipsilateral proprioception and motor function loss and contralateral pain and temperature sensation loss.

Conus medullaris syndrome: damage to the spinal cord at the T12–L1 level, the conus medullaris, which usually results in an areflexic bladder, bowel, and lower limbs.

Cauda equina syndrome: damage to lumbosacral nerve roots within the neural canal which results in an areflexic bladder, bowel, and lower limbs.

10. Identify six complications of SCI that may manifest within the first two days after injury.

Hypotension, bradycardia, hypothermia, hypoventilation, gastrointestinal bleeding, and ileus.

11. What causes hypotension, bradycardia, and hypothermia?

Acute cervical or upper thoracic spinal cord injuries are associated with a functional total sympathectomy with resultant loss of vasoconstrictor tone in the trunk and extremities and loss of beta-adrenergic cardiostimulation, leading to a clinical picture of hypotension with paradoxical bradycardia. The loss of sympathetic tone also leads to an inability to regulate body temperature. After it is clearly established that no visceral or extremity injury is causing occult hemorrhage and blood loss, hypotension is best treated with sympathomimetic agents.

12. What causes hypoventilation?

The innervation to the diaphragm, the major muscle responsible for inspiration, is C3–C5 ("3, 4, 5 keeps you alive"). The innervation to the internal intercostals and the abdominal muscles, the major muscles responsible for forced expiration (i.e., cough), are local thoracic and abdominal segments. Thus a cervical or thoracic spinal cord injury can affect inspiration, cough, or both depending on the level of injury.

INJURY LEVEL	RESPIRATORY SYSTEM CHANGES	MECHANICAL VENTILATION
Occiput–C2	(-) Diaphragm, (-) intercostals	Always needed
C3–C4	(+/-) Diaphragm, (-) intercostals	Often needed acutely
C5–T1	(+) Diaphragm, (-) intercostals	Only needed if there are associated pulmonary complications
T2–T12	(+) Diaphragm, (+/-) intercostals	Usually not needed

Pneumonia is the most common cause of early death for persons with tetraplegia and is often related to aspiration of stomach or oropharyngeal contents, commonly occurring at or shortly after the initial injury. Atelectasis may result from hypoexpansion of the chest due either to pain or muscle weakness or to inadequate cough predisposing to inadequate clearing of secretions.

13. What causes gastrointestinal bleeding?

Risk is increased with any physical or psychological trauma, which is exacerbated by the standard high-dose steroid protocols used after SCI.

14. What causes ileus?

Adynamic (paralytic) ileus occurs after acute SCI in 8% of cases. After its resolution, usually within 2–3 days, a bowel routine of stool softeners, stimulant laxatives, and bowel evacuants should be begun to facilitate regular timed evacuations of the bowel.

15. Name five interventions that can help prevent the development of pressure ulcers after acute SCI.

1. The length of time spent on the spine board should be minimized.
2. Patients in spinal traction should be immobilized on rotating kinetic beds.
3. Patients must be turned from side to side (30–45° from supine) every 2 hours around the clock while in bed to prevent prolonged pressure over bony prominences.
4. Bowel and bladder incontinence should be managed with timed bowel evacuations and catheter drainage of the bladder.
5. Shear pressure on the skin can be avoided by lifting rather than dragging immobile patients.

16. Justify the necessity of transferring a person with tetraplegia to a specialized SCI center.

- Overall survival rates are increased.
- Complication rates (e.g., incidence of new pressure ulcers) are decreased.
- Length of hospital stay is decreased.
- Functional gains during rehabilitation are greater.
- Home discharge is more likely.
- Rehospitalization rates are lower.

17. What is the prognosis for ambulation after traumatic spinal cord injury stratified by initial ASIA impairment scale?

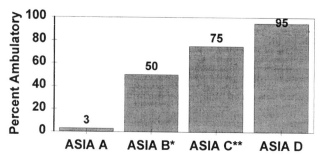

FIGURE 1. Prognosis for ambulation after traumatic spinal cord injury. * Prognosis influenced by absence or presence of pin sensation; prognosis for persons with preserved pin approaches that of the motor incomplete group. ** Prognosis influenced by age; age < 50 better.

18. What typical lower extremity motor function is required for community ambulation?

Typically, community ambulation requires bilateral grade 3 hip flexor strength and at least one knee with grade 3 knee extensor strength.

19. In a person with neurologically complete tetraplegia, what is the expected recovery of the most rostral key muscle initially found to have less than grade 3 strength?

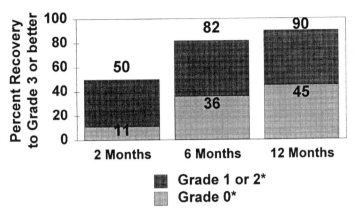

FIGURE 2. Prognosis for recovery to grade 3 or better of the most rostral key muscle with an initial grade < 3 in persons with complete tetraplegia. * Most rostral key muscle with < grade 3 strength.

20. Compare the expected patterns of muscular weakness and the expected functional outcomes for eating, bed/wheelchair transfers, and wheelchair propulsion for persons with C1–C3, C4, and C5 neurologic levels.

	C1–C3	C4	C5
Patterns of muscular weakness	Total paralysis of trunk, upper extremities, lower extremities	Paralysis of trunk, upper extremities, lower extremities; inability to cough, endurance and respiratory reserve low secondary to paralysis of intercostals	Absence of elbow extension, pronation, all wrist and hand movement. Total paralysis of trunk and lower extremities
Eating	Total assist	Total assist	Total assist for setup, then independent eating with equipment
Bed/wheelchair transfers	Total assist	Total assist	Total assist
Wheelchair propulsion	Manual: total assist Power: independent with equipment	Manual: total assist Power: independent with equipment	Manual: independent to some assist indoors on non-carpet, level surface; some to total assist outdoors Power: independent

21. Compare the expected patterns of muscular weakness and the expected functional outcomes for wheelchair propulsion and ambulation for persons with C6, C7–C8, T1–T9, and T10–L1 neurologic levels.

See table, top of next page.

	C6	C7–C8	T1–T9	T10–L1
Patterns of muscular weakness	Absence of wrist flexion, elbow extension, hand movement; total paralysis of trunk and lower extremities	Paralysis of trunk and lower extremities; limited grasp release and dexterity secondary to - partial intrinsi muscles of hand	Lower trunk paralysis; total paralysis of lower extremities	Paralysis of lower extremities
Wheelchair propulsion	Manual: independent indoors; some to total assist outdoors. Power: independent with standard arm drive on all surfaces	Manual: independent all indoor surfaces and level outoor terrain; some assist with uneven terrain	Independent	Independent
Ambulation	Standing: total assist. Ambulation: not indicated	Standing: independent to some assist in standing frame. Ambulation: not indicated	Standing: independent in standing frame. Ambulation: typically not functional	Standing: independent with equipment. Ambulation: functional, some assist to independent with knee, ankle, foot orthosis and forearm crutches or walker

22. What is spasticity? What peripheral factors can cause an exacerbation of spasticity?

Spasticity is motor disorder characterized by a velocity-dependent increase in tonic stretch reflexes (muscle tone) with exaggerated tendon jerks, resulting from hyperexcitability of the stretch reflex as one component of the upper motor neuron syndrome. **Peripheral factors** that may exacerbate spasticity include heterotopic ossification, urolithiasis, urinary tract infection, stool impaction, pressure ulcer, fracture/dislocation, and ingrown toenail.

23. Name six pathologic changes associated with late neurologic deterioration after SCI.

1. Posttraumatic cysts   3. Delayed spinal deformity   5. Residual cord compression
2. Tethering   4. Fibrosis   6. Subarachnoid cysts

24. A tetraplegic patient develops an L2–L3 destructive spinal lesion 10 years after a C5–C6 fracture-dislocation. Work-up reveals no evidence of spinal tumor or infection. What is the most likely cause of this lesion?

Neuropathic spinal arthropathy (Charcot spine). Destructive spinal lesions can develop in spinal cord-injured patients due to repetitive loads placed on the denervated spine in the course of daily activities. The most common clinical presentation is a spinal deformity. Patients may present with audible clicking or crepitus due to spinal instability, loss of sitting balance, cauda equina syndrome, nerve root compression, or obstructive uropathy. Surgical treatment is challenging and associated with a high complication rate.

BIBLIOGRAPHY

1. Bergman S, Yarkony G, Stiens S: Spinal cord injury rehabilitation: Medical complications. Arch Phys Med Rehabil 78:S53–S58, 1997.
2. Cahill D, Rechtine G: The acute complications of spinal cord injury. In Narayan R, Wilberger J, Povlishock J (eds): Neurotrauma. New York, McGraw-Hill, 1996, pp 1229–1236.
3. Devlin VJ, Ogilve JW, Transfeldt EE, et al: Surgical treatment of neuropathic spinal arthropathy. J Spinal Disorders 4:319–328, 1991.
4. Ditunno J: Rehabilitation assessment and management in the acute spinal cord injury (SCI) patient. In Narayan R, Wilberger J, Povlishock J (eds): Neurotrauma. New York, McGraw-Hill, 1996, pp 1259–1266.

5. Marino RJ, Ditunno JF, Donovan WH, et al: International standards for neurological and functional classification of spinal cord injury. Chicago, American Spinal Injury Association, 2000.

6. Piepmeier J: Late sequelae of spinal cord injury. In Narayan R, Wilberger J, Povlishock J (eds): Neurotrauma. New York, McGraw-Hill, 1996, pp 1237–1244.

7. Schaefer D, Flanders A, et al: Magnetic resonance imaging of acute spine trauma: correlation with severity of neurologic injury. ANJR 14:1090–1095, 1989.

8. Tator C: Classification of spinal cord injury based on neurological presentation. In Narayan R, Wilberger J, Povlishock J (eds): Neurotrauma. New York, McGraw-Hill, 1996, pp 1059–1073.

9. Whiteneck G, Adler C, et al: Outcomes following traumatic spinal cord injury: Clinical practice guidelines for health-care professionals. Consortium for spinal cord medicine clinical practice guidelines. Paralyzed Veterans of America, 1999.

10. Yarkony G, Formal C, Cawley M: Spinal cord injury rehabilitation: Assessment and management during acute care. Arch Phys Med Rehabil 78:S48–S52, 1997.

56. CERVICAL SPINE INJURIES IN ATHLETES

Richard Lance Snyder, M.D., Lytton A. Williams, M.D.,
and Robert G. Watkins, IV, M.D.

1. What biomechanical force is the primary cause of fracture dislocations involving the cervical spine during football?

The National Football Head and Neck Injury Registry demonstrated that most cervical fracture dislocations occurred with axial loading of the cervical spine during headfirst contact.

2. How much angulation or horizontal displacement is indicative of cervical spinal instability?

Commonly used criteria for defining instability between motion segments in the subaxial cervical region, are 11° greater angulation than an adjacent segment or 3.5-mm translation relative to an adjacent vertebra.

3. What is the "hidden flexion injury of McSweeny"?

This term refers to a purely ligamentous injury associated with three-column disruption of the spine, including injury to the posterior longitudinal ligament, facet capsule, lamina, and interspinous ligament. Such injuries can be missed on plain radiographs unless the segmental angulation (Cobb method) is measured between adjacent inferior endplates. A helpful hint is to look for a spread of the spinous process on the lateral radiograph.

4. What types of cervical stenosis affect athletes?

The same types of cervical stenosis affect athletes and the general population: (1) developmental or congenital stenosis (typified by short pedicles and decreased sagittal diameter of the spinal canal) and (2) acquired stenosis (associated with osteophytes and degeneration at the level of the disc space).

5. What is "spear tackler's spine"?

Spearing refers to contact at the crown of the head while the neck is maintained in a flexed posture. In this posture the normal cervical lordosis is no longer present, and the cervical spine is predisposed to injury. Injuries due to this mechanism have been described in football, diving, and hockey. Spear tackler's spine was defined by analysis of football players with spearing injuries and is considered to be a contraindication to participation in contact sports. Criteria for diagnosis include:
- Developmental narrowing of the cervical spinal canal
- Persistent straigtening or reversal of cervical lordosis on erect lateral cervical radiographs
- Posttraumatic radiographic changes on cervical radiographs
- History of use of spear tackling techniques during athletics

6. If a player suffers a traumatic neck injury on the athletic field, should the headgear be removed?

It is important to engage in spinal precautions and leave the headgear in place until the cervical spine can be completely evaluated. The team personnel should have a screwdriver available for removal of the facemask so that the airway is readily accessible. Immediate removal of the helmet should not be performed until the proper medical personnel are prepared for an emergency situation. Details of the methods and techniques for transportation of the spine injured patient are available at <http://www.spine.org/forms/NATA%20Prehospital%20Care.pdf.>

7. What is the most common athletic cervical neurologic injury?

"Stingers" or "burners" are the most common athletic cervical neurologic injuries. Symptoms result from injury to the brachial plexus or cervical nerve roots. Stingers have been reported to occur in up to 50% of athletes involved in contact or collision sports.

8. What is a "stinger" or "burner"?

A stinger or burner (burner syndrome) is a peripheral nerve injury associated with burning arm pain and parathesias. A stinger often presents with *unilateral* dysesthetic pain that follows a dermatomal distribution. It may be accompanied by weakness, most often in the muscle groups supplied by the C5 and C6 nerve roots (deltoid, biceps, supraspinatus, infraspinatus) on the affected side. Although pain frequently resolves spontaneously in 10–15 minutes, it is not uncommon to have trace abnormal neurologic findings for several months. *Normal, painless motion of the cervical spine* is generally present and is crucial in distinguishing a "stinger" from other types of cervical pathology, such as disc herniation or foraminal stenosis. Bilateral symptoms suggest a different etiology such as a neurapraxic injury of the spinal cord.

9. What are the likely mechanisms for a burner syndrome?

Three different mechanisms have been described:

1. Hyperextension, compression, and rotation toward the involved arm, thereby closing the neural foramen and causing a nerve root contusion. This mechanism is essentially a replication of Spurling's maneuver.

2. Lateral neck flexion associated with a shoulder depression injury, resulting in brachial plexus stretch.

3. Direct blow to the brachial plexus with resultant injury.

10. Describe a rational treatment protocol for an athlete with a stinger.

Most stingers resolve within minutes. For an athlete's first episode with only brief transitory symptoms, treatment is conservative and no special testing is required. The athlete is permitted to return to unrestricted activity after complete resolution of symptoms if a normal neurologic exam and pain-free and unrestricted cervical range of motion are present. The athlete should not be allowed to return to sports until symptoms completely subside. Further work-up is directed at patients with persistent symptoms or recurrent episodes to assess for other cervical problems, such as cervical fracture, cervical stenosis, cervical disc herniation, or cervical instability. Work-up includes cervical radiographs with physician-supervised flexion-extension views, single-photon emission computed tomography (SPECT) bone scan, cervical magnetic resonance imaging (MRI) and electromyography (EMG).

11. What is the role of EMG in assessing the athlete who experiences a stinger?

If the symptoms have not resolved by 3 weeks, it is reasonable to obtain an EMG. This test can help define the specific nerve root involved and determine the degree of injury. Results of this test may lag behind an athlete's recovery. According to Weinstein, players with demonstrable objective weakness should undergo EMG evaluation. Players who demonstrate clinical weakness and moderate fibrillation potentials on EMG are withdrawn from play. When sequential EMG studies do not reveal spontaneous, mild, or scattered postive waves with end-motor recruitment (findings consistent with reinnervation), the athlete may return to sports provided painless and unrestricted cervical range of motion and full muscle strength are present.

12. What is cervical cord neurapraxia?

Cervical cord neurapraxia with transient quadriparesis is characterized clinically by an acute transient episode of bilateral sensory and motor abnormalities. Sensory changes may include numbness, burning, tingling, or anesthesia. Motor changes may include paresis or paralysis of the arms, legs, or both. Neck pain is generally not present. An episode of cervical cord neurapraxia generally resolves in less than 10–15 minutes. The most commonly described mechanism of injury is axial compression with a component of either hyperflexion or hyperextension. This syndrome has been reported in association with developmental cervical spinal stenosis, kyphosis, congenital fusions (Klippel-Feil syndrome), cervical instability (traumatic or developmental), and intervertebral disc herniation.

13. Is transient cervical cord neurapraxia associated with with permanent neurologic injury?

Uncomplicated transient cervical cord neurapraxia is not associated with permanent neurological injury, according to Torg.

14. What is the risk of reoccurrence of transient cervical cord neurapraxia after the athlete returns to contact sports?

Studies have shown that 56% of athletes returning to contact sports experienced a recurrent episode of transient cervical cord neurapraxia. This number was higher when an athlete returned to football vs other sports.

15. Define the Torg ratio.

The Torg ratio is determined on a lateral cervical radiograph as the sagittal diameter of the spinal canal divided by the anteroposterior vertebral body diameter (Fig. 1). The sagittal diameter of the spinal canal is determined by measuring the distance between the middle of the posterior surface of the vertebral body and the nearest point on the spinolaminar line. This ratio method avoids the potential for error secondary to radiographic magnification when absolute numbers are used to determine the sagittal diameter of the cervical canal.

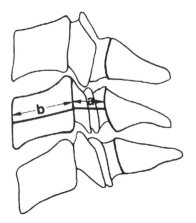

FIGURE 1. The ratio of the spinal canal to the vertebral body is the distance from the midpoint of the posterior aspect of the vertebral body to the nearest point on the corresponding spinolaminar line (*distance a*) divided by the anteroposterior width of the vertebral body (*distance b*). (From Torg JS, Pavlov H, Genuario SE, et al: Neurapraxia of the cervical spine cord with transient quadriplegia. J Bone Joint Surg 68A:1354–1370, 1986; with permission.)

16. What is the significance of the Torg ratio?

A ratio less than 0.8 suggests the presence of cervical spinal stenosis. The Torg ratio is a highly sensitive method of determining cervical stenosis (93% sensitivity) but has an extremely low positive predictive value for determining future injury (0.2%). It is not a useful screening method for determining athletic participation in contact sports and should not be used as the sole criterion for the diagnosis of cervical stenosis in an athlete. Herzog showed that, although an athlete may have the same size canal as a nonathlete, the athlete's vertebral body may be larger, thus falsely lowering the Torg ratio and implying stenosis. In addition, the Torg ratio has not been correlated with the development of permanent quadriparesis in athletes. The Torg ratio should not be used as the sole criterion in making a return-to-play decision after an episode of transient quadriplegia.

17. Besides the Torg ratio, what other factors should be considered in making a return-to-play decision for an athlete with an episode of transient quadriplegia?

Other factors that require consideration include cervical spine stability, cervical disc pathology, presence/absence of cervical degenerative changes, presence/absence of congenital stenosis, and recurrence of neurologic episodes.

18. Describe a rational treatment protocol after an episode of transient quadriparesis.

A recent review by Vaccaro et al. concluded the following:

Immediately following an episode of transient quadriparesis, the athlete should be prohibited from continuing to participate in the sport for that particular event, even if a full recovery occurs soon after the episode. A thorough history of all events leading up to and following the episode should be carefully documented. A complete onsite physical exam should be performed. Even if symptoms are momentary or resolve, a radiographic examination should be performed on a timely basis. The athlete should be considered to have a fracture until proven otherwise, especially if the patient complains of persistent or significant neck stiffness. If a neurologic deficit is present at the time of evaluation, then a cervical orthosis should be applied.[7]

19. When should an athlete be allowed to return to play?

There are no universally accepted guidelines for determining when an athlete may return to play after a cervical injury. Basic principles guiding decision-making include:
- The athlete should be symptom-free with respect to neck pain.
- Unrestricted and pain-free cervical motion should be present.
- Neurologic evaluation should be normal.
- Full muscle strength should be present.
- There should be no evidence of radiographic instability or other spinal abnormalities on advanced imaging studies.

General guidelines for return to play following cervical injury have been defined and are modified appropriately according to individual clinical factors. It is helpful to divide athletes into three general groups:
1. No contraindication to return to play
2. Relative contraindication to return to play
3. Absolute contraindication to return to play

20. Summarize guidelines for return to contact sports *without contraindication* for commonly encountered cervical spinal conditions.

The following conditions are considered to permit return to contact sports without restriction after comprehensive patient assessment:

Posttraumatic
- Healed, stable C1 or C2 fracture (treated nonoperatively) with normal cervical range of motion
- Healed stable subaxial spine fracture with no sagittal plane kyphotic deformity
- Asymptomatic clay shoveler's fracture (C7 spinous process)

Congenital
- Single-level Klippel-Feil deformity (excluding the occipital–C1 articulation) with no evidence of instability or stenosis noted on MRI
- Spinal bifida occulta
- Torg ratio less than 0.8 in an asymptomatic athlete

Degenerative
- History of cervical degenerative disc disease that has been treated successfully in the clinical setting of occasional cervical neck stiffness with no change in baseline strength profile

Postsurgical
- After anterior single-level cervical fusion (at any level), with or without instrumentation, that has healed
- After single- or multiple-level posterior cervical microlaminoforaminotomy

Other
- Prior history of 2 stingers within the same or multiple seasons. The stingers should last < 24 hours, and the athlete should have full range of cervical motion without any evidence of neurologic deficit

21. Explain what is meant by a relative contraindication to return to contact sports.

A relative contraindication to return to contact sports is defined as a condition associated with a possibility for recurrent injury despite the absence of any absolute contraindication. The athlete, family, and coach must be counseled that recurrent injury is a possibility and that the degree of risk is uncertain.

22. List commonly encountered cervical conditions that are relative contraindications to return to play.
- Previous history of transient quadriplegia or quadriparesthesia. The athlete must have full return to baseline strength and cervical range of motion with no increase in baseline cervical neck discomfort and imaging evidence of mild-to-moderate spinal stenosis.
- Three or more stingers in the same season.
- A prolonged stinger lasting more than 24 hours.
- A healed single level posterior fusion with lateral mass segmental fixation.
- A healed, stable, two-level anterior or posterior cervical fusion with or without instrumentation, excluding posterior segmental lateral mass screw fixation from C3 and below.

23. List absolute contraindications to return to contact sports.
Previous transient quadriparesis
- More than two previous episodes of transient quadriplegia or quadriparesthesia
- Clinical history or physical findings of cervical myelopathy
- Continued cervical neck discomfort or any evidence of a neurologic deficit or decreased range of motion from baseline after a cervical spine injury

Postsurgical
- History of C1–C2 cervical fusion
- Three-level spine fusion
- Status post cervical laminectomy

Soft-tissue injury or deficiencies
- Asymptomatic ligamentous laxity (i.e., greater than 11° of kyphotic deformity compared with the cephalad or caudal vertebral level)
- Radiographic evidence of C1–C2 hypermobility with an anterior dens interval of 4 mm or greater
- Radiographic evidence of a distraction-extension cervical spine injury
- Symptomatic cervical disc herniation

Other radiographic findings
1. **Plain radiography**
- Evidence of a spear-tackler's spine on radiographic analysis
- A multiple-level Klippel-Feil deformity
- Clinical or radiographic evidence of rheumatoid arthritis
- Radiographic evidence of ankylosing spondylitis or diffuse idiopathic skeletal hyperostosis
- A healed subaxial spine fracture with evidence of a kyphotic sagittal plane or coronal plane abnormality

2. **Magnetic resonance imaging**
- Presence of cervical spinal cord abnormality noted on MRI
- MRI evidence of basilar invagination
- MRI evidence of Arnold-Chiari malformation
- MRI evidence of significant residual cord encroachment after a healed stable subaxial spine fracture

3. **Computed tomography**
- C1–C2 rotatory fixation
- Occipital–C1 assimilation

BIBLIOGRAPHY

1. Clancy WG Jr, Brand RL, Bergfield JA: Upper trunk brachial plexus injuries in contact sports. Am J Sports Med 5:209–215, 1977.
2. Herzog RJ, Wiens JJ, Dillingham MF, Sontag MJ: Normal cervical spine morphometry and cervical

spinal stenosis in asymptomatic professional football players: Plain film radiography, multiplanar computed tomography, and magnetic resonance imaging. Spine 16(Suppl 6):S178–S186, 1991.

3. Levitz CL, Reilly PJ, Torg JS: The pathomechanics of chronic, recurrent cervical nerve root neurapraxia: The chronic burner syndrome. Am J Sports Med 25:73–76, 1997.
4. Torg JS, Corcoran TA, Thibault LE, et al: Cervical cord neurapraxia: Classification, pathomechanics, morbidity, and management guidelines. J Neurosurg 87:843–850, 1997.
5. Torg JS, Pavlov H, Genuario SE, et al: Neurapraxia of the cervical spinal cord with transient quadriplegia. J Bone Joint Surg Am 68A:1354–1370, 1986.
6. Torg JS, Sennett B, Pavlov H, et al: Spear tackler's spine: An entity precluding participation in tackle football and collision activities that expose the cervical spine to axial energy inputs. Am J Sports Med 21: 640–649, 1993.
7. Vaccaro AR, Watkins RG, Albert TJ, et al. Cervical spine injuries in athletes: return to play criteria. Orthopedics 24:699–705, 2001.
8. Watkins RG: Nerve injuries in football players. Clin Sports Med 5:215–246, 1986.
9. Watkins RG, Williams LA, Lin P, et al: The Spine in Sports. St. Louis, Mosby, 1996.
10. Watkins RG: Spine in sports—Criteria for return to athletic play after a cervical spine injury. Spine Line 2(4):14–16, 2001.
11. Weinstein SM: Assessment and rehabilitation of an athlete with a "stinger". A model for the management of noncatastrophic athletic cervical spine injury. Clin Sports Med 17:127–135, 1998.

57. LUMBAR SPINE INJURIES IN ATHLETES

Christopher A. Yeung, M.D., Lytton A. Williams, M.D.,
and Robert G. Watkins, IV, M.D.

1. Describe the work-up for an athlete with symptoms of low back pain with or without radiculopathy.

An accurate history and physical exam are essential. Key points to glean from the history are:
- The time of day when the pain is worse. Is the patient awakened at night by pain?
- A comparison of pain levels during activities (walking, sitting, standing).
- The type of injury and duration of low back symptoms.
- The effect of a Valsalva maneuver, coughing, and sneezing on pain.
- The percentage of back vs. leg pain (axial vs. radicular pain).
- The presence of any bowel or bladder dysfunction.

Key points to assess during the physical exam are:
- The presence of sciatic nerve tension signs.
- The presence of any neurologic deficit.
- Back and lower extremity stiffness or loss of range of motion.
- The exact location of tenderness and radiation of pain or parasthesias.
- Maneuvers that reproduce the pain, especially flexion vs. extension with or without rotation.

The diagnostic work-up must first rule out the possibility of tumor, infection, and impending neurologic crisis. If the main complaint is leg pain, plain x-rays and magnetic resonance imaging (MRI) should reveal any nerve root compression from the disc or bony structures. Electromyography (EMG) and nerve conduction velocity (NCV) studies can help differentiate a peripheral nerve lesion from a radiculopathy. A computed tomography (CT) myelogram can be added if the etiology of pain remains unclear. The work-up for back pain includes plain x-rays and single-photon emission computed tomography (SPECT) bone scan. The SPECT bone scan is a vital part of the diagnostic armamentarium in assessment of lumbar spine problems in athletes. If the SPECT scan is positive and thus suspicious for a pars fracture, a CT scan with thin cuts is ordered to evaluate the abnormal area. If the SPECT scan is negative, MRI is indicated.

2. Define spondylolysis, pars stress reaction, and spondylolisthesis.

Spondylolysis is a defect in the pars interarticularis. It may be unilateral or bilateral.

Pars stress reaction is an impending spondylolysis (microfracture) without a true pars defect. Bony healing can occur at this stage and prevent development of spondylolysis.

Spondylolisthesis is the forward slippage of one vertebra in relation to another. Isthmic spondylolisthesis refers to forward slippage in the presence of bilateral pars defects.

3. What factors are related to the development of isthmic spondylolisthesis?

Isthmic spondylolisthesis is not a true congenital disorder but does have a hereditary predisposition. A major contributing factor is repetitive microtrauma resulting in stress concentration in the region of the pars interarticularis. Repetitive hyperextension is the mechanism of injury reported in gymnasts, weightlifters, and football linemen. Repetitive flexion and rotational injuries are also contributing factors.

4. At what lumbar spinal level is isthmic spondylolisthesis most common?

L5 is the most common location. The L5–S1 level is the location where maximum stress concentration and maximum lordosis occur.

5. How prevalent is spondylolysis in athletes compared with the general population?

The prevalence is 5–7% in the general population. Studies by Rossi et al. have documented higher rates in Olympic divers (43%), wrestlers (30%), weightlifters (23%), and gymnasts (16%).

Many studies have shown increased rates in football interior linemen (15–50%). Thus, clinical suspicion in athletes should be high, especially in athletes with persistent low-grade back pain that has been unresponsive or aggravated by physical therapy or other local modalities.

6. What is the risk for progression of spondylolysis?

Only about 10% of people with spondylolysis develop spondylolisthesis. This progression most commonly occurs during the adolescent growth spurt and is more common in girls. Younger adolescents with spina bifida occulta and a dome-shaped S1 endplate have a higher propensity for slip progression.

7. How do you evaluate and treat an athlete with spondylolysis?

The spondylolysis is evaluated with standing lumbar radiographs, SPECT bone scan, CT, and possibly MRI. The treatment plan starts with rest or restriction of enough activity to relieve or improve the symptoms. This plan may require merely stopping the sport or immobilization in a lumbosacral corset. A neutral-position trunk stabilization program is initiated after a period of activity restriction and immobilization. A skilled therapist or trainer is important. Starting flexion, extension, or rotation exercises exacerbates the symptoms, whereas neutral isometric exercises are less likely to increase symptoms. Healing can occur in an early lesion and seldom in a late lesion. In patients with persistent low-back pain symptoms despite rest, immobilization, and therapy, surgery may be considered for repair of the pars interarticularis defect or in situ fusion.

Evaluation and Treatment of Spondylolysis

X-RAY STUDY	BONE SCAN	TREATMENT	LIKELIHOOD OF PARS HEALING	LENGTH OF IMMOBILIZATION	TIME OFF ATHLETICS
Negative	Unilateral pars uptake	Off athletics Trunk stabilization Wear corset	Nearly 100%	Until bone scan shows significant healing	Until bone scan shows significant healing Probably 6 months
Possible unilateral pars fracture	Bilateral pars uptake	Off athletics Trunk stabilization Wear corset	Nearly 100%	Until bone scan shows significant healing	Until bone scan shows significant healing Probably 6–9 months
Possible bilateral pars fracture	Bilateral pars uptake	Off athletics Trunk stabilization Wear corset	Fair	Until x-rays and bone scans show pars healing, or it is clear that healing will not take place	Until x-rays and bone scans show pars healing, or it is clear that healing will not take place
Definite bilateral pars fracture, appearing fresh	Still very "hot"	Off athletics Trunk stabilization Wear corset	Poor	Until x-rays and bone scans show pars healing, or it is clear that healing will not take place	Until x-rays and bone scans show pars healing, or it is clear that healing will not take place
Fracture appears old	Negative or only mildly positive	Treat symptomatically, posterior fusion, or pars repair	Poor, nearly nonexistent	May choose not to use a corset	Only until symptoms allow return

8. Can athletes with isthmic spondylolisthesis continue playing their sport?

Yes. There is a high incidence of low-grade spondylolisthesis (grades 1 and 2) in athletes. Semon and Spengler reported that 21% of football players (12 of 58) presenting with back pain had spondylolysis. In these symptomatic football players, there was no difference in time lost from sports between athletes with spondylolysis and athletes with back pain and negative findings on radiographs. Patients with high-grade spondylolisthesis (grades 3 and 4) are not likely to participate in high-level sporting activity.

9. What is the common mechanism producing vertebral endplate injury?

Axial compression.

10. What is the common mechanism producing intervertebral disc injury?

Rotation is the most common mechanism causing annular tears and herniations.

11. What is an annular tear?

The annulus fibrosus is a tough, multilayered ligamentous structure configured as concentric rings. Annular fibers are arranged in various orientations surrounding the central nucleus pulposus and connect adjacent vertebrae. Injury may cause concentric or radial tears in the annulus. Resultant inflammation may result in symptoms of spasm, back pain, and buttock and lower extremity pain. The outer annular layers are richly innervated, as is the granulation tissue that grows into the tear. This inflammatory membrane is believed to be a pain generator.

12. What nerve innervates the posterior annulus?

The sinuvertebral nerve with anastomosis through the spinal nerve and the posterior primary ramus.

13. What are the options for treatment of an annular tear?

Annular injuries are treated much like other ligamentous injuries. The first step is to control the inflammation with judicious use of anti-inflammatory medications, oral steroids, steroid injections, and ice packs. A trunk-stabilization program is started after pain and inflammation subside. This program concentrates on trunk strength, balance, coordination, flexibility, and aerobic conditioning. The vast majority of patients improve with nonoperative care. For patients with annular tears unresponsive to nonoperative care fusion surgery is a potential option. Alternative treatments such as IDET and selective endoscopic discectomy (SED) with thermal annuloplasty have been advocated as less invasive alternatives. However, more randomized trials are needed before these options can be recommended for widespread use.

14. What is the treatment of choice for athletes with herniated discs unresponsive to nonoperative treatment?

The surgical gold standard is microscopic lumbar discectomy from a posterior approach. This procedure involves making a small 2-cm skin incision, extending caudally from the midportion of the disc space. The fascia is incised, the interlaminar area is exposed by gently elevating the muscle, and a retractor is placed. A small laminotomy is often needed, depending on the size of the interlaminar area and the cephalad/caudal location of the herniation. Just enough ligamentum flavum is removed to gain access to the epidural space, protect the nerve, and remove the herniation.

Other potential surgical options include posterior endoscopic discectomy and selective endoscopic discectomy by a posterolateral/foraminal approach. Regardless of the approach, the goal in athletes, as in any patient, is to cause as little damage to the muscle and fascia as possible.

15. What is posterior endoscopic discectomy? What are its advantages and disadvantages?

Endoscopic discectomy approaches the spine from the posterior approach, thus maintaining familiar surgical anatomy. It utilizes a tubular retractor after sequential tissue dilation. An attached endoscope or microscope is used for visualization. Earlier trials with this system were hampered by technologic shortcomings with visualization, but newer systems with advanced fiberoptics have produced results that may approach microscopic lumbar discectomy. However, this procedure requires a high learning curve. It can easily be converted to an open microscopic lumbar discectomy if visualization is inadequate.

16. What is selective endoscopic discectomy (SED)?

SED involves approaching the disc via the posterolateral/foraminal approach. Utilizing triangulation techniques, a needle is flouroscopically guided into the disc in the triangular working zone. A vital dye (indigo carmine) is used with the contrast agent to perform a discogram. Sequential instruments are then inserted, including a guide wire, tissue dilator, working cannula, and the endoscope. The herniation is then visualized from inside the disc, and selective extraction of the stained, degenerated nucleus and extruded fragments is achieved via shavers, mechanical graspers, and laser ablation. A bipolar radiofrequency probe can be used for hemostasis and heating of the annular wall. The endoscope provides multichannel continuous cool saline irrigation, which helps prevent tissue overheating.

17. What is laser discectomy?

Laser (light amplification by stimulated emission of radiation) discectomy refers to the use of laser to ablate disc tissue. The two most common lasers utilized are the Ho:YAG and KTP laser. A variety of techniques utilize the laser for discectomy, but it should be emphasized that it is only an adjunctive tool, along with mechanical instruments and radiofrequency, to achieve nuclear removal.

18. What percentage of athletes return to their sport after microscopic lumbar discectomy?

In a recent study by Watkins of professional and Olympic athletes, 88% returned to their sport after microscopic lumbar discectomy.

19. What are some general recommendations for return to sport after lumbar spinal decompression procedures?

General recommendations for return to sports after spinal decompression procedures include "restoration of normal back strength, endurance, power and pain-free activity. A minimum of 6–12 weeks is allowed for healing of the annulus fibrosus to prevent recurrent disc herniation."[1]

20. What are some general recommendations for return to sport after lumbar and thoracolumbar spinal fusion procedures?

Limited data assist with decision-making for return to play after spinal fusions. According to a survey of North American Spine Society members about sports participation after spinal fusions, 80% returned to high school sports, 62% returned to collegiate sports, and only 18% returned to professional sports. Some of the criteria used to determine return to play included a solid fusion based on clinical assessment and imaging studies and full recovery as determined by near normal range of motion and normal muscular strength. Return-to-play decisions must be made on a case-by-case basis, and various factors, such as the number of levels fused, must be taken into account. For example, after a multilevel fusion, as for scoliosis or kyphosis, return to gymnastics or contact sports would not be advised because of the risk of injury due to increased stress at levels adjacent to the fusion. In contrast, after a limited fusion for spondylolysis or spondylolithesis, return to contact sports may be a consideration after the fusion has healed and a comprehensive rehabilitation program has been completed.

21. What type of rehabilitation is recommended for athletes after spinal surgery?

A neutral-position isometric trunk stabilization program is started shortly after surgery. The key is to train the muscles to support the spine and maintain a pain-free neutral position while the athlete is using the arms and legs. This program helps decrease future spine injury. The stabilization program has five levels of proficiency based on the ability of the athlete to perform the exercises.

22. Should the rehabilitation program start with flexion or extension exercises?

Neither. The authors advise starting with neutral isometric control exercises as part of the trunk stabilization program.

23. What type of aerobic activity can the athlete do after spinal surgery?

It depends. Aerobic exercise is a vital part of the trunk-stabilization rehabilitation program. The key is to diversify the aerobic conditioning to methods that are best tolerated.

24. Can the recovering athlete lift weights while recovering from spinal surgery?

Yes—after establishing good core strength and trunk stability.

25. What objective factors can guide an athlete's return to play after spinal surgery?

Return-to-play decisions are complex and must be individualized on a case-by-case basis. Factors such as patient age, type of surgery (fusion vs. decompression), radiographic factors, and type of sport activity enter into decision-making. Objective factors that can guide the physician in determining that an athlete may be ready to be considered for full return to play are as follows:

- Completion of level 5 of the trunk-stabilization program
- Completion of a course of sport-specific exercises
- Attainment of an appropriate level of aerobic conditioning for the sport
- Practicing the sport fully
- Successful slow return to the sport with some limit on minutes played
- Commitment to continue to do the level 5 stabilization exercises after return to play

BIBLIOGRAPHY

1. Brown GA, Wood KB, Garvey TA: Lumbar spine problems in athletes. In Arendt EA (ed): Orthopaedic Knowledge Update 2- Sports Medicine. American Academy of Orthopaedic Surgeons, Rosemont, IL, 1999, pp 417–427.
2. Hambly MF, Wiltse LL, Peek RD: Spondylolisthesis. In Watkins RG: The Spine In Sports. St. Louis, Mosby, 1996, pp 157–163.
3. Rossi F, Dragoni S: Lumbar spondylolysis: Occurrence in competitive athletes. J Sports Med 30:450–452, 1990.
4. Semen RL, Spengler D: Significance of lumbar spondylolysis in college football players. Spine 6:172–174, 1981.
5. Watkins RG, Williams LA: Lumbar spine injuries in athletes. In Fu FH, Stone DA (eds): Sports Injuries, 2nd ed. Philadelphia, Lippincott Williams & Wilkins, 2001, pp 988–1014.
6. Watkins RG, Williams LA, Lin PM (eds): The Spine in Sports. St Louis, Mosby, 1996.
7. Wright A, Ferree B, Tromanhauser S: Spinal fusion in the athlete. Clin Sports Med 12:599–602, 1993.
8. Yeung AT, Tsou PM: Posterolateral endoscopic excision of lumbar disc herniation: The surgical technique, outcome and complications in 307 consecutive cases. Spine 27:722–731, 2002.

X. Systemic Problems Affecting the Spinal Column

58. METABOLIC BONE DISEASES OF THE SPINE

Edward D. Simmons, M.D., M.Sc., FRCS(c), *and Yinggang Zheng*, M.D.

1. What common metabolic bone diseases cause significant problems relating to the spinal column?

Osteoporosis, osteomalacia, Paget's disease, and renal osteodystrophy are common metabolic bone diseases associated with spinal pain and spinal deformity.

2. What are two major functions of bone?

Two major bone functions are maintenance of calcium hemostasis and maintenance of skeletal integrity.

3. Describe the two major types of bone tissue.

The skeleton is composed of two types of bone tissue: cortical (compact) bone (80%) and cancellous (trabecular) bone (20%). Cortical bone provides skeletal strength and rigidity, especially under torsional and bending loads. Cancellous bone serves two major functions: resistance to compressive loads and facilitation of bone remodeling by providing a high surface area for metabolic activity.

4. Describe the composition of bone tissue.

Bone tissue is composed of cells and matrix. The cellular components of bone include osteoblasts, osteocytes, and osteoclasts. The matrix is composed of organic components (40%) and inorganic components (60%). The organic components include type 1 collagen, proteoglycans, noncollagenous matrix proteins (e.g., osteocalcin, osteonectin), and growth factors. The inorganic component, predominantly calcium hydroxyapatite [$Ca_{10}(PO_4)_6(OH)_2$], provides mineralization of the matrix and is responsible for the hardness and rigidity of bone tissue.

5. Describe the cellular components of bone tissue.

Osteoclasts develop from the hematopoietic stem cell line. These multinucleated giant cells are located in cavities along bone surfaces called Howship's lacunae and are responsible for bone resorption.

Osteoblasts develop from the pleuripotential mesenchymal stem cells of bone marrow and perform various functions, including synthesis of osteoid (unmineralized bone matrix), bone mineralization, and regulation of calcium and phosphate flux.

Osteocytes arise from osteoblasts that have undergone terminal cell division and become surrounded by mineralized bone matrix. They possess extensive cell processes that communicate with other osteocytes and osteoblasts.

6. What factors are responsible for regulation of bone mineral balance?

Bone mineral balance is tightly regulated by the interaction of vitamin D metabolites (1,25-dihydroxyvitamin D), parathyroid hormone (PTH), and calcitonin. Calcium homeostasis depends on the interaction of these factors with various organ systems, including the liver, kidney, and gastrointestinal tract as well as the thyroid and parathyroid glands.

7. Distinguish among osteoporosis, osteomalacia and osteopenia.

Osteoporosis is a metabolic bone disease characterized by a decreased amount of normally mineralized bone per unit volume, resulting in skeletal fragility and increased risk of fracture.

Osteomalacia is a metabolic bone disease characterized by delayed or impaired mineralization of bone matrix, resulting in bone fragility.

Osteopenia is a descriptive and nonspecific term for decreased radiographic bone density.

8. What are the different types of osteoporosis?

Osteoporosis has been classified into two major types: primary and secondary. **Primary osteoporosis** is further subdivided into type 1 or postmenopausal osteoporosis and type 2 or senile osteoporosis. Type 1 osteoporosis is due to estrogen deficiency and typically occurs in women 5–10 years after menopause. It predominantly affects trabecular bone and is associated with vertebral fractures, intertrochanteric hip fractures, and distal radius fractures. Type 2 osteoporosis occurs secondary to aging and calcium deficiency and is seen in both women and men after age 70 years. It affects both cortical and trabecular bone and is associated with vertebral fractures, femoral neck fractures, and pelvic fractures as well as proximal tibia and humerus fractures. **Secondary osteoporosis** occurs as a result of endocrinopathies or other disease states.

9. What are the most common causes of secondary osteoporosis?

Endocrine disorders: Cushing's disease, hypogonadism, hyperthroidism, hyperparathyroidism, diabetes mellitus.

Marrow disorders: lymphoma, multiple myeloma, metastatic disease, chronic alcohol use.

Biochemical collagen disorders: osteogenesis imperfecta, Marfan's syndrome.

Gastrointestinal disorders: malabsorption, malnutrition.

Medications: thyroid replacement, steroids, anticonvulsants, chemotherapy, aluminum antacids.

10. How can a physician determine the cause of osteoporosis?

Primary osteoporosis is a diagnosis of exclusion. The physician should perform a complete history and physical exam with attention to specific risk factors for secondary osteoporosis and osteomalacia. Laboratory tests, imaging tests, and transiliac bone biopsy may be indicated based on the history and physical examination. For example:

- To rule out local bone tumor: perform radiographs, MRI, CT, and/or bone scan.
- To rule out bone marrow abnormality: perform complete blood count with differential, erythrocyte sedimentation rate, serum protein electrophoresis, and urinary protein electrophoresis.
- To rule out endocrinopathy: assess thyroid-stimulating hormone, glucose, PTH.
- To rule out osteomalacia: assess serum calcium, phosphate, alkaline phosphatase, PTH, and 25(OH) vitamin D; consider a bone biopsy.

11. What are the risk factors for osteoporotic fractures?

The risk factors have been classified as modifiable or nonmodifiable:

Nonmodifiable risk factors

- Patient history of fracture during adulthood
- History of fracture in a first-degree relative
- Caucasian race
- Advanced age

- Female sex
- Dementia
- Poor health or frailty

Potentially modifiable risk factors

- Smoking
- Low body weight
- Estrogen deficiency (menopause before age 45, bilateral ovariectomy, prolonged pre-menopausal amenorrhea > 1 year)
- Low calcium intake
- Alcoholism
- Impaired eyesight despite correction
- Recurrent falls
- Inadequate physical activity
- Poor health or frailty

12. Summarize the major recommendations for physicians in relation to osteoporosis.

- Counsel all women about risk factors for osteoporosis, a silent disease process that is generally preventable and treatable.
- Recommend bone mineral density testing for (1) postmenopausal women with fractures, (2) postmenopausal women under age 65 with one or more additional risk factors for osteoporotic fracture, and (3) all women aged 65 and older regardless of additional risk factors.
- Advise all patients to maintain adequate dietary calcium and vitamin D intake.
- Recommend a routine of weight-bearing and muscle-strengthening exercise to reduce the risk of falls and fractures.
- Counsel patients to avoid smoking and limit alcohol intake.
- Recommend appropriate pharmacologic therapy for osteoporosis prevention and treatment. Current options include hormone replacement, alendronate, raloxifene, and calcitonin.

13. What is peak bone mass?

Peak bone mass (PBM) is defined as the highest level of bone mass achieved as a result of normal growth. Bone mineral density (BMD) increases rapidly during adolescence until peak bone mass is reached between 16 and 25 years of age. After age 30, men normally lose bone at a rate of 0.3% per year. After age 30, women normally lose bone at a rate of 0.5% per year until menopause, at which time the rate of bone loss accelerates to 2–3% per year over a 6- to 10-year period. The greater the peak bone mass achieved, the better the chance of avoiding osteoporosis later in life.

14. What are the daily recommended vitamin D and calcium requirements for different age groups?

The daily requirement of vitamin D is 400–800 units. The daily requirement for calcium (Ca) is based on patient age:

AGE GROUP	REQUIREMENT (MG OF ELEMENTAL CA/DAY)
1–10 yr	800–1000
11–25 yr	1200
26–49 yr (premenopausal)	1500
> 50 yr (postmenopausal)	1500
Pregnancy	1500
Lactation	1550–2000

15. How is BMD measured?

The most widely accepted method of determining BMD is dual-energy x-ray absorptiometry (DEXA) at the hip. BMD is reported in terms of two absolute values: T-score (units of standard deviation compared with the bone density of a healthy 30-year-old) and Z-score (units of standard deviation compared to age- and sex-matched controls). The World Health Organization has defined osteoporosis in terms of the T-score:

- Normal   Between +1 and −1 standard deviation of peak
- Osteopenia   Between −1 and −2.5 below peak
- Osteoporosis   > −2.5 standard deviations below peak
- Severe osteoporosis   > −2.5 standard deviations below peak plus fracture

The T-score can be used to predict spine fracture risk. A one-point decrease in standard deviation in T-score is associated with a 2.5 times increased risk of spine fracture. The Z-score is valuable in ruling out secondary causes of osteoporosis. Secondary causes of osteoporosis are unlikely in the presence of a normal Z-score.

16. What pharmacologic therapies are currently available for osteoporosis?

FDA-approved medications for osteoporosis prevention and treatment include:

Bisphosphonates: aledronate (Fosamax), risedronate (Actonel). These antiresorptive agents are analogs of pyrophosphates and are absorbed onto the surface of hydroxyapatite crystals in bone. They alter bone remodeling by decreasing bone resorption.

Estrogen/hormone replacement: Climara, Estrace, Premarin, Prempro. Estrogen replacement initiated after the onset of menopause is used to counteract the increased rate of bone loss noted during this period. Contraindications to estrogen use include a history of breast cancer, uterine cancer, or thromboembolism. Recent studies have raised controversy about the risks/benefits of estrogen use.

Selective estrogen receptor modulators (SERMS): raloxifene (Evista). This drugs class was developed in an attempt to provide the beneficial effects of estrogen therapy in patients unable to take estrogen due to a history of breast or uterine cancer.

Calcitonin: Miacalcin, Calcimar. Calcitonin is a peptide hormone that functions by reducing osteoclastic bone resorption. It is considered to be less effective than bisphosphonates or hormone replacement. It also provides an analgesic effect in patients with acute osteoporotic fractures. It may be administered by nasal spray or injection.

17. What pharmacologic therapies are currently under investigation for osteoporosis?

Currently available pharmacologic therapies work by decreasing bone resorption (estrogen, selective estrogen receptor modulators, bisphosphonates, calcitonin). Pharmacologic agents that increase bone formation, such as fluoride and parathyroid hormone, are under investigation for prevention and treatment of osteoporosis.

18. Describe the typical clinical presentation of a patient with spinal osteoporosis.

The clinical presentation can be quite variable. In general, patients with osteoporosis are asymptomatic until a fracture occurs. However, not all patients with spinal fractures are symptomatic, and the initial presentation may be a significant loss of height associated with development of an exaggerated thoracic kyphosis (dowager's hump). Many patients present with acute severe pain after minimal trauma. Paravertebral muscle spasm is common, and tenderness can often be elicited at the fracture site with palpation. Neurologic signs and symptoms are uncommon but may occur (senile burst fracture). Complications associated with osteoporotic vertebral fractures include postural deformity, restrictive lung disease (following thoracic fractures), abdominal dysfunction (following lumbar fractures), chronic pain, disability, and an increased mortality rate.

19. What are the treatment options for painful vertebral compression fractures?

Treatment options for painful vertebral compression fractures include bedrest, narcotic analgesics, calcitonin, and spinal orthoses. Minimally invasive injection procedures (vertebroplasty, kyphoplasty) play a role in select patients. Major open surgical procedures are reserved for patients with severe spinal deformity or neurologic deficits because of the poor surgical outcomes noted in patients with osteopenic bone and advanced age.

20. What is vertebroplasty?

Vertebroplasty is a minimally invasive procedure in which polymethylmethacrylate bone cement (PMMA) is injected with pressure into the vertebral body under fluoroscopic guidance via a bone biopsy needle using either a transpedicular or extrapedicular approach. Typically 2–5 ml of bone cement is placed per vertebral level. The procedure may be performed under local, regional, or general anesthesia. The goal of the procedure is to stabilize the spine and to decrease pain associated with compression fractures and lytic bone lesions.

21. What is kyphoplasty?

Kyphoplasty (Fig. 1) involves inserting bilateral bone tamps with balloons into the vertebral body. When inflated with visible radiocontrast medium, the bone tamp compacts the cancellous bone and reexpands the body, elevating the endplates to reduce the fracture deformity. The balloons are then deflated and removed. PMMA is then placed into the cavity created by the balloons under low pressure. Approximately 2–6 ml cement per side can be accepted at a vertebral level. The goals of kyphoplasty are spinal stabilization, pain relief, and restoration of vertebral body height.

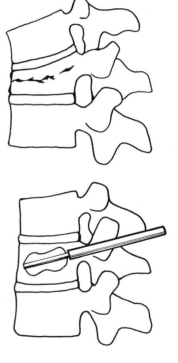

FIGURE 1. Kyphoplasty procedure. The vertebral fracture is visualized under fluoroscopic guidance **(Top).** Subsequently a trocar and balloon are inserted into the vertebral body. Inflation of the balloon restores vertebral height and creates a cavity within the vertebral body which is subsequently filled with bone cement **(Bottom).**

22. What are the indications for performing vertebroplasty or kyphoplasty?

Osteoporotic vertebral compression fractures are the most common reason to perform vertebroplasty or kyphoplasty. In addition, certain lytic vertebral body lesions (multiple myeloma, hemangiomas, metastases, benign lesions) are amenable to vertebroplasty or kyphoplasty. These procedures have also been used to augment the vertebral levels adjacent to posterior spinal instrumentation in osteoporotic patients in order to decrease the risk of adjacent level fractures.

23. What are the contraindications to performing vertebroplasty or kyphoplasty?
- Vertebral fractures associated with a high-velocity injury mechanism
- Vertebral fractures associated with retropulsed bone and/or middle column involvement
- Pain unrelated to vertebral body collapse
- Vertebral osteomyelitis in the vertebra considered for injection
- Severe vertebral collapse (vertebra plana) that makes injection technically not feasible
- Patients with coagulopathy

24. What complications have been reported in association with vertebroplasty and kyphoplasty?

Significant complications include persistent pain, nerve root injury, spinal cord compression due to cement extravasation, cement embolism, infection, hypotension secondary to bone cement monomer, and rib fractures due to patient positioning. Although these procedures are usually well tolerated, serious neurologic complications have been reported due to leakage of cement, resulting in compression of adjacent structures and necessitating emergency decompressive surgery. Concerns about such complications have led many to favor kyphoplasty over vertebroplasty because this procedure permits injection of cement under low pressure into the cavity created by the bone tamp, thereby decreasing the risk of cement extravasation.

25. What are the causes of osteomalacia?

The causes of osteomalacia are varied. To arrive at the correct diagnosis, all of the causes must considered in the course of an appropriate work-up, including:

1. Nutritional deficiency
   - Vitamin D deficiency
   - Calcium deficiency due to dietary chelators (e.g., phytates, oxalates)
   - Phosphorus deficiency (e.g., secondary to aluminum-containing antacids)
2. Gastrointestinal malabsorption
   - Intestinal disease
   - Following intestinal surgery
3. Renal tubular acidosis
4. Renal tubular defects causing renal phosphate leak (e.g., vitamin-dependent rickets, type 1 and 2; Fanconi's syndrome)
5. Renal osteodystrophy
6. Miscellaneous causes
   - Anticonvusants (induce hepatic P450 microsomal system, thereby increasing degredation of vitamin D metabolites)
   - Oncogenic
   - Heavy metal intoxication
   - Hypophosphatasia

26. Compared and contrast important findings that aid in distinguishing osteomalacia and osteoporosis.

Symptoms: Osteoporosis is generally asymptomatic until a fracture occurs. Osteomalacia is frequently associated with generalized bone pain and tenderness most commonly localized to the appendicular skeleton.

Radiographs: Osteoporosis and osteomalacia have many similar features but axial involvement predominates in osteoporosis, and appendicular findings predominate in osteomalacia. Findings consistent with osteomalacia include pseudofractures, Looser's zones, and biconcave vertebra ("codfish vertebra")

Lab tests: Lab tests are generally normal in osteoporosis. Osteomalacia is associated with decreased or normal serum calcium, low serum phosphate, increased serum alkaline phosphatase, and increased urine phosphate.

Bone biopsy: In osteoporosis a biopsy reveals a decreased quantity of normally mineralized bone. The hallmark of osteomalacia is increased width and extent of osteoid seams.

27. What is Paget's disease?

Paget's disease is named after Sir James Paget who described its clinical and pathologic aspects in 1876. Paget's disease is the second most prevalent metabolic bone disease. It has been found in up to 5% of northern European adults over the age of 55 years. However, most affected individuals are asymptomatic. The cause is unknown but is currently attributed to a slow virus infection. This disease causes focal enlargement and deformity of the skeleton. The pathologic lesion is abnormal bone remodeling. Radiographs are characteristic and show osteosclerosis with bone enlargement. The wide spectrum of clinical presentations depends on the extent and site of skeletal involvement. Paget's disease commonly affects the skull, hip joints, pelvis, and spine. Back pain in the lumbar or sacral region is common. Neurologic deficits may occur due to the compression of spinal cord or nerve roots from enlarging vertebrae. Spinal stenosis is common when the lower lumbar spine is involved. Treatment options include medication to suppress osteoclastic activity (calcitonin, etidronate, plicamycin) as well as surgical treatment for spinal stenosis, fracture, or degenerative joint disease. Approximately 1% of patients develop malignant degeneration within a focus of Paget's disease. This complication usually develops in the peripheral skeleton and rarely involves the spine.

BIBLIOGRAPHY

1. Bernstein J, Lane JM: Metabolic bone disorders of the spine. In Rothman RH, Simeone FA (eds): The Spine. 3rd ed. Philadelphia, W.B. Saunders, 1992, pp 1381–1427.
2. Buckwalter JA, Glimcher MJ, Cooper RR, et al: Bone biology. II: Formation, form, modeling, remodeling, and regulation of cell function. In Pritchard DJ (ed): Instructional Course Lectures. Rosemont, IL, American Academy of Orthopaedic Surgeons, Vol 45, 1996, pp 387–399.
3. Cosman F, Lindsay R: Thoracolumbar fractures in osteoporosis. In Floman Y, Farcy J-PC, Argenson C (eds): Thoracolumbar Spine Fractures. New York, Raven, 1993, pp 339–358.
4. Cotten A, Boutry N, Cortet B, et al: Percutaneous vertebroplasty: State of the art. Radiographics 18:311–320, 1998.
5. Garfin SR, Yuan HA, Reiley MA: New technologies in spine: Kyphoplasty and vertebroplasty for the treatment of painful osteoporotic compression fractures. Spine 26:1511–1515, 2001.
6. Hall JC, Einhorn TA: Metabolic bone disease of the adult spine. In Frymoyer JW (ed): The Adult Spine: Principles and Practice, 2nd ed. Philadelphia, Lippincott-Raven, 1997, pp 783–800.
7. Lane JM, Russell L, Khan SN: Osteoporosis. Clin Orthop 372:139–150, 2000.
8. Johnston CC Jr, Cumming SR, Lindsay R, et al: Physician's Guide to Prevention and Treatment of Osteoporosis. National Osteoporosis Foundation, Washington, DC, 1999 (www.nof.org).

59. PRIMARY SPINE TUMORS

William O. Shaffer, M.D.

1. What types of tumors arise in the spine?
Primary tumors and secondary tumors.

2. What is the difference between primary and secondary tumors of the spine?
Primary bone tumors of the spine arise de novo in the bone, cartilage, neural, or ligamentous structures of the spine. Secondary tumors grow into the spine from adjacent structures, such as a Pancoast tumor from the upper lobe of the lung, or are metastatic to the spine from distant origins. Metastatic lesions involving the spine are the most common type of spinal tumor and account for 98% of all spinal tumors.

3. What are the subtypes of primary bone tumors of the spine?
- Benign
- Intermediate
- Malignant
- Tumor-like lesions

4. What is a benign primary spine tumor?
Benign primary tumors of the spine are not aggressive. They arise in the structures of the spine and may cause pain, local symptoms, and destruction; however, they do not aggressively invade adjacent structures nor do they metastasize. Examples include:
- Osteoid osteoma
- Osteoblastoma
- Chondroma
- Chondroblastoma
- Chondrommyxoid fibroma
- Giant-cell tumor
- Hemangioma
- Lymphangioma
- Lipoma

There is a relationship between age at diagnosis and whether a tumor is benign. In patients less than 18 years, 68% of all tumors are benign. If age at presentation is greater than 18 years, more than 80% of all tumors are malignant. There is also a relationship between tumor location and whether a tumor is benign. Benign lesions tend to occur more frequently in the posterior elements (e.g., osteoblastoma, osteoid osteoma), whereas malignant lesions tend to involve the vertebral body.

5. What is an intermediate primary spinal tumor?
An intermediate tumor is one that is locally invasive but rarely metastasizes. Examples include the following:
- Aggressive osteoblastoma
- Hemangiopericytoma
- Hemangioendothelioma
- Chordoma
- Neurofibroma
- Neurilemmoma

6. What is a malignant primary spinal tumor?
A malignant tumor is locally invasive and metastasizes to other organs. It is a life-threatening tumor by its fundamental nature. Examples include:
- Osteosarcoma
- Chondrosarcoma
- Ewing's sarcoma
- Neuroectodermal tumor of bone
- Malignant lymphoma
- Myeloma
- Malignant hemangiopericytoma
- Angiosarcoma
- Fibrosarcoma
- Liposarcoma

7. What are tumor-like lesions?
A tumor-like lesion arises in bone but is not neoplastic in its cell of origin. Such lesions can cause local collapse and secondary neural injury. Examples include:
- Aneurysmal bone cyst
- Eosinophilic granuloma
- "Brown tumor" of hyperparathyroidism
- Giant-cell (reparative) granuloma

World Health Organization Classification of Bone Tumors and Tumor-like Lesions

Bone-forming tumors
1. Benign
   - Osteoma
   - Osteoid osteoma and osteoblastoma
2. Intermediate
   - Aggressive (malignant) osteoblastoma
3. Malignant (osteosarcoma)
   - Central (medullary): conventional central, telangiectatic, intraosseous well-differentiated (low-grade), round-cell
   - Surface (peripheral): parosteal, periosteal, high-grade surface

Cartilage-forming tumors
1. Benign
   - Chondroma: enchondroma, periosteal (juxtacortical)
   - Osteochondroma (osteocartilaginous exostosis): solitary, multiple hereditary
   - Chondroblastoma (epiphyseal chondroblastoma)
   - Chondromyxoid fibroma
2. Malignant
   - Chondrosarcoma
   - Juxtacortical (periosteal) chondrosarcoma
   - Mesenchymal chondrosarcoma
   - Dedifferentiated chondrosarcoma
   - Clear-cell chondrosarcoma
   - Malignant chondroblastoma

Giant-cell tumor (osteoclastoma)
Marrow tumors (round-cell tumors)
1. Ewing sarcoma of bone
2. Neuroectodermal tumor of bone
3. Malignant lymphoma of bone
4. Myeloma

Vascular tumors
1. Benign
   - Hemangioma
   - Lymphangioma
   - Glomus tumor (glomangioma)
2. Intermediate or indeterminate
   - Hemangioendothelioma (epithelioid hemangioendothelioma, histiocytoid hemangioma)
   - Hemangiopericytoma
3. Malignant
   - Angiosarcoma (malignant hemangioendothelioma, hemangiosarcoma, hemangioendotheliosarcoma)
   - Malignant (hemangiopericytoma)

Other connective tissue tumors
1. Benign
   - Benign fibrous histiocytoma
   - Lipoma
2. Intermediate
   - Desmoplastic fibroma
3. Malignant
   - Fibrosarcoma
   - Malignant fibrous histiocytoma
   - Liposarcoma
   - Malignant mesenchymoma
   - Leiomyosarcoma
   - Undifferentiated sarcoma

Other tumors
1. Chordoma
2. Adamantinoma of long bones
3. Neurilemmoma
4. Neurofibroma

Unclassified tumors
Tumor-like lesions
1. Solitary bone cyst (simple or unicameral bone cyst)
2. Aneurysmal bone cyst
3. Juxta-articular bone cyst (intraosseous ganglion)
4. Metaphyseal fibrous defect (nonossifying fibroma)
5. Eosinophilic granuloma (histiocytosis X, Langerhans cell granulomatosis)
6. Fibrous dysplasia and osteofibrous dysplasia
7. Myositis ossificans (heterotopic ossification)
8. "Brown tumor" of hyperparathyroidism
9. Intraosseous epidermoid cyst
10. Giant-cell (reparative) granuloma

From Schajowicz F, McDonald DJ: Classification of tumors and tumor lesions of the spine. Spine State Arts Rev 10:1–11, 1996 with permission.

8. What is the most common primary tumor found in the spine?

Dreghorn found 55 cases of primary axial skeleton tumors in 1,950 cases in the Leeds Tumor Registry. Chordoma was the most common tumor of the spine, and osteosarcoma was the second most common. Multiple myeloma was considered a systemic disease, and only plasmacytoma was classified as a primary bone tumor in this study. Multiple myeloma has been shown to be the most frequent tumor arising in the spine by other studies.

9. Why do primary spine tumors require classification according to an oncologic staging system?

Primary spine tumors are treated in accordance with principles of orthopedic oncology, which require assessment of tumor biology, the relation of the tumor to surrounding structures, the risk of local tumor recurrence and metastases, and the role of adjuvant therapies (e.g., embolization, radiation therapy).

10. What oncologic staging system is used to classify primary benign and malignant bone tumors?

The Enneking staging system is used to classify primary bone tumors. **Benign tumors** are classified using arabic numerals into three stages:

Stage 1: Latent lesions, which are generally asymptomatic and surrounded by a well-defined margin.

Stage 2: Active lesions, which grow slowly and are bordered by a thin capsule.

Stage 3: Aggressive lesions, which grow rapidly to invade surrounding structures.

Malignant tumors are classified using roman numerals into three stages:

Stage I: Low-grade tumors

Stage II: High-grade tumors

Stage III: Tumor of any grade with regional or distant metastases

Malignant tumors are further subdivided depending on whether the tumor is **intracompartmental (A)** or **extracompartmental (B)**.

11. How does oncologic staging guide surgical tumor treatment?

The oncologic stage of a tumor determines the surgical margin required for treatment of a specific tumor as well as the type of spine procedure required. The four types of surgical margins are:

Intracapsular: the plane of dissection is within the lesion (intracapsular) and may leave tumor at the margin of the lesion.

Marginal: the plane of dissection is within the reactive zone surrounding the tumor (extracapsular) and may leave satellite lesions beyond the reactive zone

Wide: the plane of dissection is through normal tissue beyond the reactive zone (pseudocapsule surrounding the tumor). However, "skip" lesions may persist beyond a wide surgical margin.

Radical: the plane of dissection includes removal of the tumor and the entire compartment of tumor origin. A radical margin cannot be achieved for spine tumors even if the spinal cord is sectioned above and below the lesion because the epidural space forms a continuous compartment from the skull to the sacrum.

In practice, surgical procedures performed for primary spine tumors can be considered as either curettage or en bloc excision. **Curettage** refers to the piecemeal removal of tumor and is always an intracapsular (intralesional) procedure. This type of procedure is appropriate for stage 1 and 2 benign tumors. **En bloc excision** refers to an attempt to remove the entire tumor in a single piece, together with a surrounding cuff of normal healthy tissue. The surgical specimen requires gross and microscopic assessment to determine whether the surgical margin achieved was intracapsular, marginal or wide. This type of procedure is appropriate for some stage 3 benign tumors and stage I and II malignant tumors.

12. What are the most common presenting symptoms of spinal tumors?

Pain is the most common presenting symptom. About 50–86% of patients present with local pain at the site of the tumor. Neurologic deficit is present in 55–68% of malignant tumors. Benign tumors have a 28% incidence of neurologic deficit. Pelvic girdle malignancies, including chordoma, osteosarcoma, chondrosarcoma, and malignant fibrous histiocytomas, may present with back pain and sciatica . Always remember to evaluate the pelvis if the spine appears normal or the degenerative lesion does not fit the patient's degree of pain or neurologic involvement.

13. What percentage of primary bone tumors of the spine can be diagnosed on radiographs?

Plain radiographs of the spine show 99% of primary spinal tumors. In Weinstein and McLain's study of primary spinal tumors, 81 of 82 tumors were visible on plain radiographs of the spine.

14. What work-up is required to stage a spinal lesion?
Plain radiography, MRI, CT scan with or without myelogram, technetium bone scan, and biopsy.

15. Should biopsy be performed at the same time as the CT scan?
No. A full metastatic work-up, including renal ultrasound and/or intravenous pyelogram (IVP), is needed to ensure that a renal-cell tumor is not present. If a renal-cell tumor is present, embolization of the spinal lesion should precede biopsy. If a renal-cell tumor has been excluded prior to the CT scan, needle biopsy at the time of the CT scan is permissible. Other options for biopsy include percutaneous core needle biopsy or open biopsy. The selection of the appropriate technique depends on a variety of factors, including tumor location and suspected diagnosis. Oncologic principles require that biopsy technique must minimize local contamination and permit excision of the biopsy tract if a definitive surgical resection is required.

16. What lesions require selective arteriography and embolization?
- Highly vascular lesions
- Aneurysmal bone cyst
- Angiosarcoma
- Arterial vascular malformations
- Renal-cell carcinoma metastasis
- Schwannomas or other neural-based tumors when resection requires sacrifice of the vertebral artery

17. Summarize the recommended approach to assessment of primary spinal tumors.
See Figure 1.

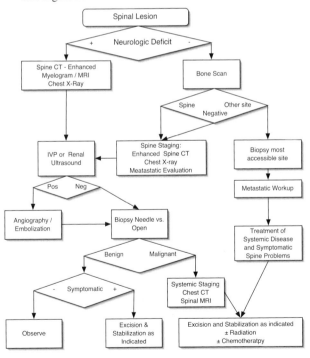

FIGURE 1. Algorithm for the evaluation of primary spine tumors (From Weinstein JN, McLain RF: Primary tumor of the spine. Spine 12:843–851, 1987, with permission.)

18. What results are expected when benign primary spine tumors are treated surgically?
Most benign primary spine tumors (e.g., osteoid osteoma, osteochondroma, Langerhans cell histiocytosis) can be adequately treated by curettage. A subset of benign lesions has either a high

rate of local recurrence or causes severe local destruction (e.g., aggressive osteoblastoma, giant-cell tumor, aneursymal bone cyst) and requires more extensive treatment. In such cases, an en bloc excision or intralesional surgery with the use of adjuvants (polymethylmethacrylate, embolization, radiation therapy) to extend the margin of the resection is considered. Overall reported success rates for surgical treatment of benign tumors range from 86% to 100%. In the Iowa study,[10] there were no deaths and 86% of patients were alive after 5 years.

19. What results are expected when malignant primary spine tumors are treated surgically?

Surgical outcomes for malignant primary spine tumors depend on the type of surgical procedure performed and the surgical margin obtained. The 5-year survival rate for curettage of primary malignant spine tumors is 0%. The Iowa study showed a 5-year survival rate of 75% with complete resection. Incomplete resection of a malignant lesion had an 18% 5-year survival rate in this study.

20. Does the presence of neurologic structures within or adjacent to a primary malignant tumor influence the choice of surgical treatment?

No. The treatment of choice is complete resection of the tumor according to oncologic surgical principles, even if nerve roots that course through the tumor must be sacrificed. Of course, nerve roots not directly in contact with the tumor should be preserved.

21. Which malignant primary spine tumors have the best survival rates?

Chondrosarcoma and solitary plasmacytoma.

22. Which malignant primary spine tumors have the worst survival rates?

Osteosarcoma and lymphoma.

23. What is the mean survival time of patients with plasmacytoma or chordoma of the spine?

Plasmacytoma and chordoma can be considered intermediate tumors of the spine with a mean survival of 7 years. Most patients with plasmacytoma develop multiple myeloma, which is fatal. Chordoma is notorious for local recurrence but rarely metastasizes.

24. Summarize Weinstein's tumor zones.

See Figure 2.

25. What extent of the resection is required for a tumor involving the spinous process?

An isolated tumor in the spinous process of a vertebral body (called a Weinstein 1B tumor) can be adequately excised by traditional laminectomy. If the lamina is involved but the tumor is benign or intermediate, again laminectomy should suffice. However, a 1B malignant tumor with invasion of the canal becomes IVB and may be unresectable.

26. What extent of resection is required for a tumor of the transverse process?

Resection of the transverse process and surrounding musculature is adequate for IIB tumors. Pedicle involvement makes the tumor IIA, requiring removal of the pedicle for benign and intermediate tumor. A malignancy of stage IIA or IIB requires the complete removal of the transverse process, facet, and pedicle to achieve an adequate resection. If the canal is involved, the tumor becomes IVB and may not be resectable.

27. What extent of resection is required for a vertebral body tumor?

A tumor arising in the center of the body can be resected by performing an anterior vertebrectomy, frequently en bloc, in zone IIIA. If the tumor involves the cortical rim of the body, adjacent soft tissue requires resection in malignant tumors. If the back wall of the vertebral body is involved, the tumor becomes a zone IVA tumor, which may not be resectable.

28. What is the WBB (Weinstein, Boriani, Biagini) surgical staging system for spinal tumors?

The WBB surgical staging system for spinal tumors attempts to correlate principles of oncologic surgery with the unique anatomy of the spine and to provide a guide for treatment. The vertebra is divided into 12 radiating zones in clockwise order. The spine is also divided into five tissue layers extending from the paravertebral extraosseous area to the dura: A, extraosseous soft tissue; B, intraosseus superficial; C, intraosseous deep; D, extraosseous extradural; E, extraosseous intradural (Fig. 3). Based on this classification, three methods for performing en bloc

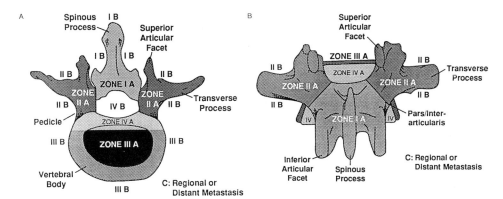

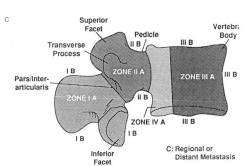

FIGURE 2. Weinstein's zones. **A,** Axial view. Zone I is composed of the spinous process, inferior articular process, and the lamina. Zone II is composed of the superior articular process, pedicle, and transverse process. Zone III is the anterior column. Zone IV is composed of the middle column and neural canal. **B,** Posterior view. **C,** Lateral view. (From Weinstein JN: Differential diagnosis and surgical treatment of primary benign and malignant neoplasms. In Frymoyer JW (ed): The Adult Spine: Principles and Practice. New York, Raven Press, 1991, pp 829–860, with permission.)

tumor excisions are defined for the thoracic and lumbar lesions: vertebrectomy, sagittal resection, and resection of the posterior arch.

29. When is a vertebrectomy indicated according to the WBB staging system?

Marginal or wide en bloc excision of the vertebral body can be performed if the tumor is confined to zones 4–8 or 5–9 (Fig. 4). In this situation, the tumor is located centrally and at least one pedicle is free from tumor. The posterior elements are removed first without entering the tumor. Subsequently the vertebral body is removed. Spinal reconstruction following tumor excision consists of an anterior allograft or structural spacer (fusion cage) combined with posterior spinal instrumentation. If the vertebral body is removed from an anterior surgical approach, anterior spinal instrumentation is typically used as well.

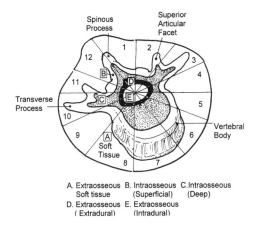

A. Extraosseous Soft tissue
B. Intraosseous (Superficial)
C. Intraosseous (Deep)
D. Extraosseous (Extradural)
E. Extraosseous (Intradural)

FIGURE 3. WBB (Weinstein, Boriani, Biagini) surgical staging system for primary spine tumors. Tumor extent is described by dividing the involved vertebra into 12 sections in a clock-face arrangement. Five tissue layers are defined, moving from the superficial paraspinal soft tissue (layer A) to the dural compartment (layer E). The longitudinal extent of the tumor is recorded according to the levels involved. (From Hart RA, Weinstein JN: Primary benign and malignant musculoskeletal tumors. Semin Spine Surg 7:288–303, 1995, with permission.)

30. When is a sagittal resection indicated according to the WBB staging system?

Sagittal resection to achieve a marginal or wide en bloc excision is indicated if tumor is confined to zones 3–5 or 8–10 (Fig. 5). In this situation, the tumor is located eccentrically in the vertebral body, pedicle, or transverse process. As in vertebrectomy, the first step is removal of the uninvolved posterior spinal structures. Then, with the patient in a lateral position, a combined anterior and posterior exposure permits the vertebra to be cut with a chisel remote from the tumor to permit en bloc excision. Spinal reconstruction is performed in a similar fashion to reconstruction following vertebrectomy.

31. When is resection of the posterior arch indicated according to the WBB staging system?

When a tumor is localized between zones 3 and 10, an en bloc excision can be achieved from a posterior approach (Fig. 6). A laminectomy is performed to expose the dural sac at the levels above and below the tumor. The pedicles are sectioned at the level of the tumor and the posterior arch is removed en bloc. The stability of the spine is restored with posterior spinal instrumentation and fusion.

32. What tumors of the spine are amenable to kyphoplasty or vertebroplasty?

Marrow-based tumors, such as multiple myeloma and plasmacytoma, and hemangiomas.

33. How is the appropriate surgical approach selected for treatment of sacral tumors?

The appropriate surgical approach for treatment of sacral tumors depends on the amount of sacral involvement. Tumors that involve only the distal portion of the sacrum (S3 and below) can be treated with a single procedure from a posterior surgical approach. Tumors that involve the S1 and S2 segments or those which involve the entire sacrum require a combined anterior and posterior resection.

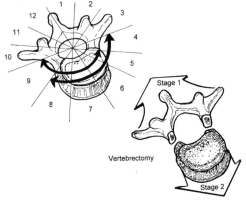

FIGURE 4. Vertebrectomy. **Left,** En bloc excision with oncologically appropriate margin for a tumor located in the vertebral body is possible if at least one pedicle is uninvolved by tumor. **Right,** A posterior approach is performed to remove the posterior spinal structures (spinous process, lamina, pedicles), transect the posterior longitudinal ligament, and separate the anterior surface of the dura from the posterior vertebral margin. An anterior approach is essential to maintain an oncologically appropriate margin if the tumor extends outside the vertebra.

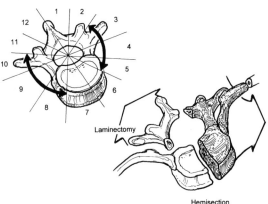

Hemisection

FIGURE 5. Sagittal resection. **Left,** En bloc excision with an oncologically appropriate margin for a tumor located eccentrically in the body, pedicle, or transverse process is possible when the tumor is confined to zones 2 to 5 or 8 to 11. **Right,** A posterior approach is performed to excise the posterior spinal structures uninvolved by tumor. A combined posterior and anterior approach is required to complete the en bloc excision safely with an oncologically appropriate margin.

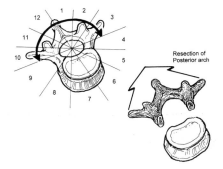

FIGURE 6. Resection of the posterior arch. **Left,** The ebloc excision of a tumor to achieve an oncologically appropriate surgical margin is possible if tumor extent is limited between zones 3 and 10. The pedicles must be uninvolved by tumor. **Right,** Surgery is performed through a posterior approach.

34. What is the relationship between the level of nerve root preservation and continence following sacral resection procedures?

If all sacral nerve roots can be preserved unilaterally, the patient will have near-normal bowel, bladder, and sexual function. If nerve root resection is required bilaterally, preservation of the S2 roots will preserve continence.

35. What vascular structures require control during the anterior approach for a complete sacrectomy?

The internal iliac vessels should be tied off during the anterior preparation for a complete sacrectomy. As the posterior resection is completed, the pelvis will hinge on the symphysis pubis. If the internal iliac vessels are not controlled, a tear of these vessels may lead to catastrophic bleeding.

36. In a complete sacrectomy, what other considerations must be taken into account during the anterior resection?

The patient is left incontinent by such a resection. Therefore, a diverting colostomy and ureterostomy should be performed during the anterior preparation. Staging the anterior preparation separately from the posterior resection should be considered.

37. How does one stabilize the spine to the pelvis after complete sacrectomy?

Spinopelvic fixation is required in this setting. Interconnection of anchors in the ilium can form a foundation that allows stabilization of the ilium to the spine and opposite ilium.

BIBLIOGRAPHY

1. Boriani S, Weinstein JN, Biagini R: Spine Update: Primary bone tumors of the spine: Terminology and surgical staging. Spine 22:1036–1044, 1997.
2. Boriani S, Biagini R, De Iuri F: Primary bone tumors of the spine: A survey of the evaluation and treatment at the Istituto Orthpedico Rizzoli. Orthopedics 18:993–1000, 1995.
3. Dreghorn CR, Newman RJ, Hardy GJ, Dickson RA: Primary tumors of the axial skeleton: Experience of the Leeds Regional Bone Tumor Registry. Spine 15:137–140, 1990.
4. Enneking WF: A system of staging of musculoskeletal neoplasms. Clin Orthop Rel Res 204:9–24,1986.
5. Malawski SK: The results of surgical treatment of primary spinal tumors. CORR 272:50–57, 1991.
6. Shaffer W: Anterior column surgery in spinal tumors. Spine State Art Rev 12:611–624, 1998.
7. Shaffer W: Revisions in spine tumor surgery. In Marguiles JY, Aebi M, Farcy JC (eds): Revision Spine Surgery. St. Louis, Mosby, 1999, pp 526–542.
8. Schajowicz F, McDonald DJ: Classification of tumors and tumor lesions of the spine. Spine State Art Rev 10:1–11, 1996.
9. Thompson RC Jr, Berg TL: Primary bone tumors of the pelvis presenting as spinal disease. Orthopedics 19:1011–1016, 1996.
10. Weinstein JN, McLain RF: Primary tumor of the spine. Spine 12:843–851, 1987.

60. METASTATIC SPINE TUMORS

Mark R. Davies, M.D., and Jeffrey C. Wang, M.D.

1. What is the most common tumor of the spine?

Metastatic lesions are the most common tumors of the spine. Metastatic lesions account for 98% of all spine lesions. Spine metastases are the most common type of skeletal metastases.

2. What percentage of spinal metastases result in spinal cord compression?

Spinal cord compression occurs in 20% of patients who have spinal metastases.

3. Which malignancies most commonly metastasize to the spine?

In descending order of frequency: breast (21%), lung (14%), prostate (7.5%), renal (5%), GI (5%), and thyroid (2.5%).

A mnemonic is useful to aid recall of the most common malignancies that metastasize to the spine: **P T B**arnum **L**oves **K**ids" (**p**rostate, **t**hyroid, **b**reast, **l**ung, **k**idney)

4. Where are metastatic spinal lesions most commonly located?

Within the vertebra, metastatic lesions first involve the vertebral body, followed by subsequent invasion of the pedicles and surrounding tissues. Within the spinal column, metastatic lesions are found most commonly in the lumbar region, less commonly in the thoracic region, and least commonly in the cervical region. Breast and lung tumors most commonly metastasize to the thoracic spine. Prostate tumors tend to metastasize to the lumbar spine, pelvis, and sacrum.

5. What are the pathways by which metastatic disease spreads to the spine?

Four potential pathways exist for spread of metastatic disease to the spinal colunm: (1) embolization through the arterial system, (2) direct extension, (3) lymphatic spread, and (4) embolization through the venous system. The most common pathway for spread of metastatic disease to the spine is thought to be through the venous system. Batson's plexus, a thin-walled system of veins that extend along the entire spinal column, provides a connection with the major organ systems most commonly involved in metastatic spinal disease.

6. What are the common presenting complaints of patients with a metastatic spinal tumors?

Eighty-four percent of patients complain of progressive and unrelenting pain. The pain is often unrelieved with rest and is worse at night. Thirty-four percent report weakness, and only 13% complain of a mass. Patients frequently report symptoms of unintended weight loss, fatigue, and anorexia.

7. Can patients with metastatic spinal tumors present with radiculopathy?

Yes. Symptomatic metastatic disease can mimic a herniated disc. However, the pain from a metastatic lesion is often progressive and does not respond well to treatment. Weakness is rarely a presenting symptom, but it can be detected in approximately 50% of all patients on initial examination.

8. What causes pain in metastatic tumors of the spine?

Many causes of pain are possible: hyperemia and edema secondary to tumor, expansion of the tumor into the periosteum of the vertebra and surrounding tissues, direct compression or invasion of nerve roots, spinal cord compression, and pathologic fractures with subsequent segmental spinal instability.

9. When are metastatic spinal tumors detectable on plain radiographs?

Most tumors of the spine are osteolytic. They are not demonstrated on plain films until more than 30% destruction of the vertebral body has occurred. An exception is prostate cancer, which tends to be blastic.

10. What radiographic signs are suggestive of a metastatic spinal lesion?

Radiographic signs suggestive of a metastatic lesion include an absent pedicle, vertebral cortical erosion/expansion, and vertebral collapse.

11. What is the "winking owl" sign?

This sign refers to the loss of one of the pedicle shadows on an anteroposterior (AP) spine radiograph. The cause for this radiographic finding is most frequently a metastatic vertebral lesion that has extended into the pedicle region and caused destruction of the pedicle.

12. What are the steps in evaluating a patient with a suspected metastatic spinal lesion?

Evaluation should occur in an organized and comprehensive fashion: (1) complete history and physical exam, (2) laboratory tests, (3) imaging assessment, and (4) biopsy.

Patient history should assess the pain pattern, sphincter control, neurologic symptoms, and pertinent factors such as smoking history.

Examination should be comprehensive and include a full neurologic assessment as well as examination of the breasts, thyroid, abdomen, and regional lymph nodes.

Laboratory studies should include routine tests such as complete blood count, erythrocyte sedimentation rate, calcium, phosphate, and alkaline phosphatase as well as special tests such as prostate-specific antigen, serum protein electrophoresis, thyroid function tests, and nutritional indices as indicated.

AP and lateral spinal radiographs are required to assess spinal alignment. Technetium total-body bone scans are helpful to survey the skeleton for metastatic lesions. Bone scans are highly sensitive but nonspecific, and their ability to detect osseous metastases depends on tumor type. Osteoblastic metastases are readily detected on bone scan, whereas osteolytic lesions such as multiple myeloma and hypernephroma may not be detectable on bone scans. In addition, bone scans cannot readily differentiate whether increased uptake is due to tumor or infection. MRI is the primary imaging study for defining the anatomic extent of metastatic spine tumors. Metastatic lesions generally demonstrate low signal intensity on T1 and high signal intensity on T2 and enhance when gadolinium contrast is administered. CT plays a role in the localization and quantification of bony vertebral destruction. If the primary tumor remains unknown, CT scans with intravenous and oral contrast should be obtained to assess the chest, abdomen and pelvis in an attempt to locate the primary tumor. Women may require mammography.

A **biopsy** should be obtained if the diagnosis remains in question at this point. CT-guided biopsy is generally preferred. Thoracic and lumbar lesions are generally approached posterolaterally, cervical lesions are approached anterolaterally, and for sacral lesions a directly posterior approach is generally used. If there is a possibility of infection, cultures should be obtained at the time of biopsy.

13. What are the options for treatment of a metastatic spinal lesion?

Treatment options include orthotic treatment, steroids, radiotherapy, chemotherapy, hormonal therapy, surgery, or a combination of these options.

14. What factors are important in determining a treatment plan for patients with a spinal metastatic lesion?

- Tumor type
- Tumor location
- Extent of spinal column involvement
- Number and distribution of metastases
- Life expectancy
- Neurologic status
- Comorbid medical conditions
- Nutritional status
- Immune status
- Patient and family wishes

15. What is the role of steroid treatment for metastatic spinal lesions?

Steroids (usually dexamethasone) play a role in the initial treatment of edema associated with neural compression prior to definitive treatment. Complications associated with use of steroids include psychosis, diabetes, infection, and GI bleeding.

16. What are the indications for radiation therapy as the primary form of treatment for metastatic spinal lesions?

Radiation therapy plays a role in the treatment of malignancies by promoting reossification of the vertebral body and reducing tumor load. Pain relief has been reported in up to 80% of patients receiving radiation. Tumors that are sensitive to radiation therapy include lung, breast, and prostate cancer as well as lymphoma. Radioresistant tumors include gastrointestinal adenocarcinoma, metastatic melanoma, thyroid carcinoma, and renal cell carcinoma. Indications for radiation therapy as the primary form of treatment for metastatic spinal lesions include:

- Radiosensitive tumors
- Stable or slowly progressive neurologic symptoms
- Spinal canal compromise secondary to soft tissue lesions
- Multilevel spinal involvement
- Preservation of spinal column stability
- Patient not a candidate for surgery due to medical comorbidities

17. What complications are associated with use of radiation therapy for metastatic spine lesions?

Complications associated with radiation therapy include neutropenia, impaired wound healing, radiation myelopathy, neoplasia, and impaired healing of bone grafts. In children, radiation therapy may lead to skeletal growth arrest, scoliosis, and neoplasia.

18. What is the role of chemotherapy in the treatment of a metastatic spinal lesion?

Chemotherapy is used in patients with documented spinal metastases, patients at risk of developing spinal metastases, and patients with spinal lesions not amenable to surgical excision. The response to chemotherapy is determined by the tumor type. Tumors that are highly sensitive to chemotherapy include small-cell carcinoma of the lung, Ewing's sarcoma, thyroid carcinoma, breast carcinoma, and neuroblastoma. Tumors that are relatively resistant to chemotherapy include adenocarcinoma of the lung and GI tract, squamous cell carcinoma of the lung, metastatic melanoma, and renal cell carcinoma.

19. What are the indications for surgical intervention for metastatic spinal lesions?

Patients who are advised to undergo surgery for metastatic lesions of the spine should be able to tolerate surgery from a medical point of view, should have adequate nutritional parameters to permit wound healing, and should have an expected lifespan greater than 3 months. Indications for surgical intervention in such patients include:

- Lack of a definitive diagnosis
- Increasing neurologic deficit despite steroid administration or during the course of radiation therapy
- Neurologic compromise at a previously irradiated level
- Spinal instability
- Radioresistant tumors
- Incapacitating pain despite orthotic treatment or radiation
- Impending pathological fracture

20. What are the relative contraindications to surgical reconstruction for patients with metastatic spinal disease?

- Widespread visceral or brain metastases
- Significant metastases in all three spinal regions

- Severe nutritional depletion
- Immunosupression
- Active infection
- Expected survival less than 3 months

21. What is the role of embolization in the treatment of metastatic spinal disease?

Embolization of spinal tumors can be used to reduce operative blood loss in hypervascular tumors such as renal cell carcinoma, thyroid carcinoma, and Ewing's sarcoma.

22. What surgical approaches have been described for treating metastatic spinal lesions?

Surgical approaches described for treatment of metastatic lesions include (1) posterior approaches, (2) anterior approaches, (3) combined anterior and posterior approaches, and (4) posterolateral approaches.

23. Why is a laminectomy usually the wrong approach for a metastatic spinal lesion?

In patients with neurologic deficit due to metastatic spinal lesions, 70% have anterior tumor pressing on the dural sac, 20% have lateral compression of the dural sac, and only 10% have posterior neural compression by tumor mass. Inadequate decompression of the anterior spinal canal is obtained by a laminectomy. Furthermore, the destabilization of the spinal column created by a laminectomy increases the risk of postoperative spinal cord compression and paraplegia due to the development of postoperative kyphotic deformity and increased spinal instability. The only indication for laminectomy as a stand-alone procedure is the relatively uncommon presentation of posterior epidural compression by metastatic tumor in a patient without anterior spinal column involvement by tumor.

24. What factors determine the choice of surgical approach for metastatic spinal lesions?

The approach to the spine depends on the location of the tumor, the presence/absence of spinal instability, and the presence/absence of neural compression/neural deficit. Because most metastases involve the vertebral body, the anterior approach is indicated to remove the affected vertebral body, decompress the dural sac, and reconstruct the anterior and middle spinal columns with an intracolumnar spacer (cage, allograft strut, methylmethacrylate), and provide anterior spinal fixation. However, if two or more vertebral bodies require removal, posterior spinal instrumentation is generally required. If the tumor involves the epidural space or posterior elements or if the patient cannot tolerate an anterior approach due to medical comorbidities, a posterior approach for decompression and stabilization provides an alternative surgical option.

25. What are the options for reconstruction of the anterior and middle spinal columns after resection of a metastatic lesion involving the vertebral body?

Options for reconstruction of the anterior aspect of the spine include bone graft (autograft or allograft), methylmethacrylate, titanium mesh cages, and carbon fiber cages. These may be used in combination with anterior spinal instrumentation (plate systems, rod systems) or posterior segmental spinal fixation.

26. A 50-year-old woman with a history of breast cancer has been treated with a right mastectomy, radiation therapy, and chemotherapy. The patient presents with a several-week history of unrelenting back pain and increasing weakness in both lower extremities. The patient remains ambulatory and has intact bowel and bladder function. The patient has normal nutritional indices and has no other major medical problems. Plain radiographs (Fig. 1), axial MRI (Fig. 2), sagittal MRI (Fig. 3), and axial CT (Fig. 4) are shown below. What treatment should be advised?

If the patient is willing to undergo surgery, this is the best treatment option. Anterior spinal cord compression is most reliably treated by an anterior surgical approach. A kyphotic deformity due to multilevel tumor involvement and pathologic fracture is most reliably treated by a combined approach with anterior and posterior spinal reconstruction. In this case, the anterior approach was used to decompress the spinal cord and place an expandable cage and bridging anterior plate. Posterior segmental spinal instrumentation was used to correct the kyphotic deformity and supplement the anterior spinal construct (Fig. 5).

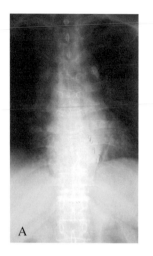
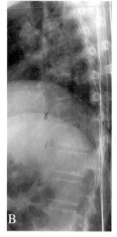

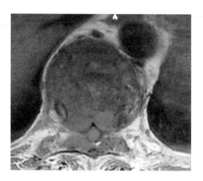

FIGURE 1

FIGURE 2

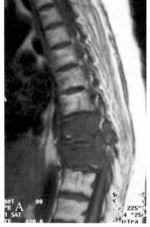
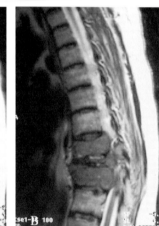
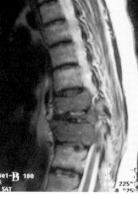

FIGURE 3

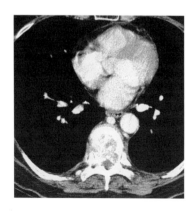

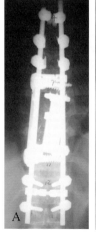
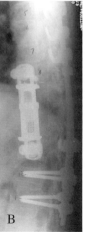

FIGURE 5

FIGURE 4

BIBLIOGRAPHY

1. Constans JP, de Divitiis E, Donzelli R: Spinal metastases with neurological manifestations. Review of 600 cases. J. Neurosurg 59:111–118, 1983.
2. Frank CJ, Brantigan JW, McGuire MH: Evaluation of patients with spinal column tumors. Spine State Art Rev 10:13–24, 1996.
3. Heller JG, Pedlow FX: Tumors of the spine. In Garfin SR, Vaccaro AR (eds): Orthopaedic Knowledge Update Spine. Rosemont, IL, American Academy of Orthopaedic Surgeons, 1997, pp 248–255.
4. McLean RF: Tumors of the spine. In Beaty JH (ed): Orthopaedic Knowledge Update 6. Rosemont, IL, American Academy of Orthopaedic Surgeons, 1999, pp 723–736.
5. Weinstein JN, McLain RF: Tumors of the spine. In Rothman RH, Simeone FA (eds): The Spine, 2nd ed. Philadelphia, W.B. Saunders, 1992, pp 1279–1318.

61. SPINAL INFECTIONS

Lance Winter, D.O., Gina Cruz, B.S., RPT, and John Steinmann, D.O.

1. What are the various methods used to classify spinal infections?
- **Host immune response:** pyogenic(bacterial agents) vs. granulatomatous (mycobacteria, fungi).
- **Anatomic location:** vertebral body, disc, epidural space, adjacent soft tissue.
- **Infectious route:** hematogenous, contiguous spread, direct implantation.
- **Host age:** pediatric vs. adult.

PYOGENIC INFECTIONS

2. Describe the three most frequent mechanisms that allow bacteria to spread to the spine.

The most common method for an organism to spread to the spine is the **hematogenous route.** Two different mechanisms for spreading have been described: a venous theory and an arteriolar theory. Batson demonstrated retrograde flow from the pelvic venous plexus to the perivertebral venous plexus via valveless veins (Batson's plexus). The arteriolar theory, demonstrated by Wiley and Trueta, implied that bacteria can become lodged in the end-arteriolar network in the vertebral endplate.

The second most common route is **contiguous spread** from an adjacent soft tissue infection or paravertebral abscess.

The third most common route is **direct implantation** via trauma, puncture, or operative procedure. The nucleus pulposus is relatively avascular, providing little or no immune response, and thus is rapidly destroyed by bacterial enzymes.

The disc is nearly always involved in pyogenic vertebral infections. In contrast, granulomatous infections typically do not involve the disc space.

3. Define the risk factors for developing pyogenic vertebral osteomyelitis.

Pyogenic vertebral osteomyelitis is most common among adolescents, elderly patients, intravenous drug abusers, patients with diabetes or renal failure, and patients who have undergone spinal surgery. Patients with rheumatoid arthritis or osteoporosis as well as patients on chronic steroid therapy are also at increased risk.

4. What is the most common pyogenic organism responsible for osteomyelitis involving the spine?

Staphylococcus aureus is the most common organism and has been identified in over 50% of cases. Gram-negative organisms (*Escherichia coli, Pseudomonas* spp., *Proteus* spp.) are associated with spinal infections following genitourinary infections or procedures. Intravenous drug abusers have a high incidence of *Pseudomonas* infections. Anaerobic infections are uncommon and typically encountered in diabetics as well as after penetrating trauma.

5. Describe the clinical presentation of pyogenic vertebral osteomyelitis.

Patients with pyogenic vertebral osteomyelitis may present with acute symptoms of fever and localized pain. However, more commonly the presentation includes vague symptoms, chronic illness, low-grade fever, and spinal pain. A delay in diagnosis is common, with 50% of patients reporting symptoms for more than 3 months before diagnosis. The most consistent symptom is back or neck pain, which is noted in > 90% of patients. Fevers are documented in approximately 50% of patients. Neurologic deficits are present in up to 17% of patients at presentation. Radicular pain occurs in < 10% of patients. Weight loss is common but occurs over a period of weeks to months. Spinal deformity may be a late presenting finding. The lumbar region is the most common site of pyogenic infection (48%), followed by the thoracic region (35%).

6. When pyogenic vertebral infection is suspected, what diagnostic tests should be obtained?

The algorithm for evaluation of a suspected spinal infection includes:

- Lab tests: complete blood count, erythrocyte sedimentation rate (ESR), C-reactive protein, blood cultures
- Imaging studies: radiographs, MRI, technetium bone scan
- Biopsy

7. Discuss the value of lab tests in the diagnosis of pyogenic vertebral infection.

The ESR is the most consistently abnormal laboratory value in vertebral osteomyelitis and is elevated in 92% of cases. C-reactive protein is also a highly sensitive test for the diagnosis of infection. However, both ESR and C-reactive protein are nonspecific studies. The leukocyte count is a less reliable indicator of vertebral osteomyelitis with elevation > 10,000 noted in only 42% of cases. Blood cultures, although helpful if positive, yield the causative organism in only 6–24% of cases.

8. What is the role of the various imaging studies in the diagnosis of pyogenic vertebral infection?

Radiographs. Positive radiographic findings are not evident for at least 4 weeks after the onset of symptoms. The earliest detectable radiographic finding is disc space narrowing, followed by localized osteopenia and finally destruction of the vertebral endplates. Radiographs are valuable to rule out other noninfectious etiologies responsible for back pain symptoms.

MRI. is the imaging modality of choice for diagnosis of vertebral infection. It provides detailed assessment of the vertebral body, disc space, spinal canal, and surrounding soft tissue not provided with any other single test. The typical findings associated with pyogenic vertebral infection are decreased signal in the vertebral body and adjacent discs on T1-weighted sequences and increased signal intensity noted in these structures on T2-weighted images. Paravertebral abscess, if present, also demonstrates increased uptake on T2-weighted images.

Radionuclide studies. Technetium-99m bone scanning is valuable in the early diagnosis of pyogenic vertebral osteomyelitis because it demonstates positive findings before the development of radiographically detectable changes. It serves as a good screening study but does not provide sufficiently detailed information to plan treatment.

CT plays a role in defining the extent of bony destruction and localization of lesions for biopsies.

9. What is the role of biopsy in the diagnosis of pyogenic infections?

In the absence of positive blood cultures, biopsy of the site of presumed vertebral osteomyelitis or discitis is essential to provide a definitive diagnosis, identify the causative organism, and guide treatment. The biopsy ideally should be performed before initiation of antibiotics. If antibiotics have been given, they should be discontinued for 3 days before the biopsy. CT-guided, closed Craig needle biopsy is safe and effective and yields the etiologic organism in 68–82% of cases. If a closed biopsy is negative after two attempts, an open biopsy can be considered.

10. What tests should be done on tissue samples from an open biopsy?

Tissue samples should be sent for Gram stain, acid-fast stain, aerobic and anaerobic cultures, and fungal and tuberculosis (TB) cultures. Bacterial cultures should be observed for at least 10 days to detect low-virulence organisms. TB cultures may take weeks to grow. Histology studies should also be done to detect neoplastic processes and to differentiate acute versus chronic infection.

11. What are the goals of treatment of pyogenic vertebral osteomyelitis?

The goals in treating vertebral osteomyelitis include early definitive diagnosis, eradication of infection, preservation of spinal stability, prevention or reversal of neurologic deficits, relief of pain, and correction of spinal deformity.

12. Describe the nonoperative treatment of pyogenic vertebral osteomyelitis.

Nonoperative treatment includes antibiotic administration, treatment of underlying disease processes, nutritional support, and spinal immobilization with an orthosis. Antibiotic selection is based on identification and sensitivity testing. Consultation with an infectious disease specialist is recommended. Intravenous antibiotics generally should be continued for 6 weeks, provided that satisfactory clinical results and reduction in ESR occur. In the setting of a broadly sensitive organism and rapid clinical resolution, intravenous antibiotics may be replaced with oral antibiotics at 4 weeks.

13. What factors suggest a successful outcome with nonoperative treatment?
- Patients younger than 60 years of age
- Patients who are immunocompetent
- Infections with *Staphylococcus aureus*
- Decreasing ESR with treatment

14. When is operative intervention indicated for the treatment of pyogenic vertebral osteomyelitis?
- Open biopsy (when closed biopsy has failed)
- Failure of medical management, as documented by persistent pain and elevated ESR
- Drainage of abscesses
- Decompression of spinal cord compression associated with neurologic deficit
- Correction of progressive or unacceptable spinal deformity
- Correction of progressive or unacceptable spinal instability

15. What are the goals of surgical management in pyogenic vertebral osteomyelitis?

Surgery should achieve complete debridement of nonviable and infected tissue, decompression of neural elements, and long-term stability through fusion (use of autogenous graft material is preferred). The surgical approach generally should include anterior debridement and grafting followed by a staged or simultaneous posterior spinal stabilization procedure (Fig. 1).

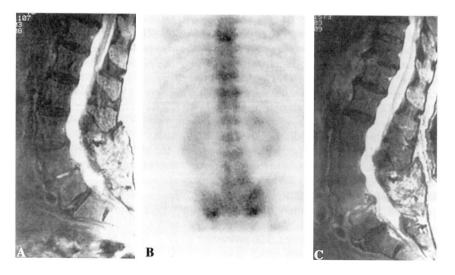

FIGURE 1. A 68-year-old woman seen in a rehabilitative hospital with a 10-week history of severe low back pain. MRI (**A**) and bone scan (**B**) from 6 weeks earlier were read as normal. Repeat MRI (**C**) and bone scan (*continued*)

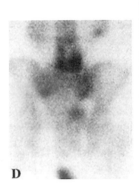
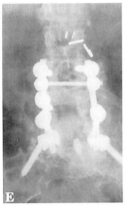
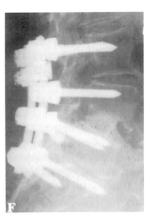

FIGURE 1. (*continued*) (**D**) revealed findings consistent with discitis/osteomyelitis at L4–L5. Anteroposterior (**E**) and lateral (**F**) radiographs after anterior debridement and fusion, followed by posterior instrumentation and fusion. (From Steinmann J: Vertebral osteomyelitis: Management considerations. Spine State Art Rev 12:628, 1998, with permission.)

16. What principles guide the selection of the appropriate surgical approach for a spinal infection?

Assessment of the location of the infection, presence/absence of abscess, extent of bone destruction, and need for stabilization are the critical decision-making factors. Posterior approaches are indicated only for posterior epidural abscesses, disc space infections below the conus with satisfactory anterior column support, and in the absence of significant paravertebral abscess. Posterior approaches in the cervical and thoracic spine, especially when anterior pathology exists, are to be condemned. Anterior approaches or combined anterior and posterior approaches are indicated in the majority of spinal infections.

17. Describe the clinical presentation of an epidural abscess.

Epidural abscess (pyogenic infectious process involving the epidural space) can result from hematogenous spread, contiguous spread, or direct inoculation. This condition is usually found in adults; risk factors include intravenous drug abuse, diabetes mellitus, prior back trauma, renal failure, and pregnancy. The majority of cases are located in the thoracic spine. The initial presentation includes localized pain and fever with elevation of the ESR and leukocyte count. Without treatment, significant neurologic deficits occur and eventually paralysis may develop.

18. What is the prognosis for neurologic recovery for a patient with an epidural abscess associated with neurologic deficit?

Significant neurologic recovery is observed in patients with mild neurologic deficits or paralysis of less than 36 hours' duration who undergo surgical intervention. Complete paralysis of greater than 36–48 hours duration has not shown recovery. The death rate associated with epidural abscess has been reported as 12%.

19. What operative approach is recommended for epidural abscess?

The surgical approach is determined by the location of the epidural abscess. An abscess located posteriorly and extending over multiple levels is best treated by a posterior laminectomy, taking care to preserve the facet joints. An abscess located anteriorly and associated with vertebral osteomyelitis is most directly treated with an anterior surgical approach. If an abscess involves both the anterior and posterior epidural space, an anterior and posterior approach combined with spinal stabilization using posterior instrumentation is recommended.

20. Is nonoperative management of an epidural abscess ever indicated?

An epidural abscess should be considered a medical and surgical emergency. The combination of surgical and antibiotic treatment is considered the standard of care. Nonoperative management is considered only in patients who are extremely high-risk surgical candidates and in patients with an established complete neurologic deficit for greater than 72 hours.

21. Describe the presentation and management of a child with discitis.

The presentation of childhood discitis is highly variable. Spinal infection should be considered when children present with back pain, refusal to bear weight, or a flexed position of the spine. Children may also complain of nonspecific abdominal pain. Infants are more likely to become systemically ill, whereas nonspecific findings are more common in children over the age of 5 years. Less than 50% present with fever. After several weeks radiographs may demonstrate disc space narrowing, which is the earliest detectable radiographic finding. Endplate erosions, bony destruction, and paravertebral soft-tissue swelling may occur later. The ESR is usually elevated. Blood cultures are usually negative, and the leukocyte count is usually normal. Initial treatment includes bedrest, immobilzation, and administration of an antistaphlococcal antibiotic (initially parenteral but may be changed to oral medication after resolution of symptoms). Treatment failure or abscess formation requires biopsy and/or surgical intervention.

TUBERCULOSIS

22. What are the risk factors for contracting tuberculosis of the spine?

Certain factors define the high-risk population and should raise suspicion. Patients from countries with a high incidence of tuberculosis, such as Southeast Asia, South America, and Russia, are considered high-risk. Patients who live in confinement with others, such as homeless centers and prisons, are also at risk. Elderly adults, chronic alcoholics, patients with AIDS, and patients with a family member or a household contact with tuberculosis are additional high risk groups.

23. Describe the presentation of a patient with a tuberculous spinal infection.

The presentation is highly variable. Mild back pain is the most common symptom. Patients with tuberculous infections may present with malaise, fevers, night sweats, and weight loss. In addition, chronic infections may result in cutaneous sinuses, neurologic deficits (in up to 40% of patients) and kyphotic deformities.

24. Discuss the value of lab tests in the diagnosis of tuberculous vertebral infection.

The leukocyte count may be normal or mildly elevated. The ESR is mildly elevated (typically < 50) but may be normal in up to 25% of cases. Although the purified protein derivative skin test (PPD) may detect active infection or past exposure, this test is unreliable because false-negative results may occur in malnourished and immunocompromised patients. Anergy panel testing should be included for this reason. Urine cultures, sputum specimens, and gastric washings may be helpful for diagnosis if the primary source is unknown. The most reliable test for diagnosis is CT-guided biopsy.

25. What is the value of imaging studies in the diagnosis of tuberculous vertebral infection?

Radiographs. A clue to diagnosis is the presence of extensive vertebral destruction out of proportion to the amount of pain. Typically the intervertebral discs are preserved in the early stages of this disease. Chest radiographs can be useful in demonstrating pulmonary involvement.

Radionuclide studies are not helpful because of the high false-negative rate in TB.

MRI is the imaging modality of choice for diagnosis of spinal tuberculosis.

CT plays a role in defining the extent of bony destruction and localization for biopsies.

26. What are the three patterns of spinal involvement associated with tuberculosis?

The three patterns of spinal involvement are peridiscal, central, and anterior. The most common form, **peridiscal**, occurs adjacent to the vertebral endplate and spreads around a single intervertebral disk as the abscess material tracks beneath the anterior longitudinal ligament. The intervertebral disk is usually spared in distinct contrast to pyogenic infections. **Central** involvement occurs in the middle of the vertebral body and eventually leads to vertebral collapse and kyphotic deformity. This pattern of involvement can be mistaken for a tumor. **Anterior** infections begin beneath the anterior longitudinal ligament, causing scalloping of the anterior vertebral bodies, and extends over multiple levels.

27. Discuss the nonsurgical and surgical treatment of spinal tubeculosis.

Chemotherapy (four drug regimen, for a minimum of 6 month duration includes isoniazid, rifampin, pyrazinamide, and ethambutol) and brace immobilization are the intial treatment except in patients presenting with neurologic deficit or progressive deformity. The indications for surgery and the principles of surgical reconstruction are similar to those advised for pyogenic spinal infections.

NONTUBERCULOUS GRANULOMATOUS SPINAL INFECTIONS

28. Which organisms are associated with nontuberulous granulomatous spinal infections?

Atypical mycobacteria (*Actinomyces, Nocardia,* and *Brucella* spp.) as well as fungal infections (coccidioidomycosis, blastomycosis, cryptomycosis, candidiasis, aspergilliosis) are potential pathogens. Immunocompromised patients are at high risk for developing infections with atypical mycobacteria. Fungal infections can occur following use of broad-spectrum antibiotics in combination with central venous catheters for parenteral nutrition. Sarcoidosis can involve the spine and cause lytic, granulomatous lesions and should be included in the differential diagnosis.

29. What treatment is advised for nontuberculous granulomatous spinal infections?

Basic principles of treatment include correction of host factors, antimicrobial drug therapy, and surgical treatment following the general principles for treatment of spinal infections.

30. Describe the presentation of coccidioidomycosis of the spine.

The patient with spinal coccidioidomycosis typically presents with a low-grade fever and an abscess with a draining sinus. Imaging findings include a paraspinal mass and multiple vertebral lesions with sparing of the disc spaces in combination with involvement of the ribs and posterior spinal elements.

BIBLIOGRAPHY

1. Crawford AH, Kucharzyk DW, Ruda R, Smitherman HC Jr: Diskitis in children. Clin Orthop 266:70–79, 1991.
2. Currier BL, Eismont FJ: Infections of the spine. In Rothman RH. Simeone FA (eds): The Spine, 4th ed. Philadelphia, W.B. Saunders, 1999, pp 1207–1258.
3. Doub HP, Badgley CE: The roentgen signs of tuberculosis of the vertebral body. Am J Roentgenol 27:827–837, 1932.
4. Greenspan A: Orthopedic Radiology: a Practical Approach. Philadelphia, Lippincott Williams & Wilkins, 2000, pp 744–766.
5. Slucky AV, Eismont FJ: Spinal infections. In Bridwell KH, DeWald RL (eds): The Textbook of Spinal Surgery, 2nd ed. Philadelphia, Lippincott-Raven, 1997, pp 2141–2183.
6. Steinmann J: Vertebral osteomyelitis: Management considerations. Spine State Art Rev 12:625–638, 1998.
7. Tay BK, Deckey J, Hu SS: Spinal infections. J Am Acad Orthop Surg 10:188–197, 2002.
8. Torda AJ, Gottlieb T, Bradbury R: Pyogenic vertebral osteomyelitis: Analysis of 20 cases and review. Clin Infect Dis 20:320–328, 1995.
9. Wood GW. Infections of Spine. In Canele XX (ed): Campbell's Operative Orthopeadics, 9th ed, vol. 3. St. Louis, Mosby 1998, pp 3094–3106.

62. RHEUMATOID ARTHRITIS

Ronald Moskovich, M.D., FRCS

1. What is rheumatoid arthritis? How does it manifest?

Rheumatoid arthritis (RA) is an immunologically mediated systemic disorder of uncertain cause; it primarily affects the smaller diarthrodial joints of the appendicular skeleton in a symmetrical fashion. Spinal involvement is usually isolated to the cervical spine. Systemic manifestations of the disease include hematologic, pulmonary, neurologic, and cardiovascular disorders.

2. What is the differential diagnosis of RA of the cervical spine?

- Seronegative spondyloarthropathies (often behave in a similar fashion to rheumatoid arthritis and can be distinguished only by serologic testing)
- Psoriatic spondyloarthritis (usually manifests as premature degenerative disk disease in the cervical spine and is rarely associated with instability)
- Systemic lupus erythematosus (may also affect the vertebral column)
- Ankylosing spondylitis (results in progressive ankylosis of the entire spine with maintenance of disk height and marginal calcification, producing a typical radiological appearance of a "bamboo" spine)
- Reiter's syndrome and spondyloarthritis associated with inflammatory bowel disease (rarely involve the cervical spine)

3. How does rheumatoid arthritis affect the spine?

- Rheumatoid synovitis may result in erosion and subluxation of the facet joints.
- The synovial joints around the dens are similarly affected, leading to erosion of the dens and progressive damage of the transverse and accessory atlantoaxial ligaments, which results in atlantoaxial subluxation (AAS).
- Secondarily, the disks in the subaxial spine (below C2, the axis vertebra) degenerate, which may result in subluxation of the joints and/or ankylosis.

4. How commonly does rheumatoid arthritis affect the spine?

- Seropositive rheumatoid arthritis affects 0.8% of the adult population in Europe and 0.8% of the white adult population in North America.
- Between 5% and 73% develop AAS 2–10 years after the clinical diagnosis is made.
- About 20% develop symptomatic subaxial disease.

5. How is rheumatoid arthritis diagnosed?

- Clinical evaluation and exclusion of other disease processes
- Elevated erythrocyte sedimentation rate ($\geq$ 30 mm in the first hour) and low-grade anemia
- Rheumatoid factor (positive in 70–80% of patients)
- Antinuclear antibody (ANA) factor (positive in 20–60% of patients)
- Synovial fluid analysis (nonspecific or inflammatory)

6. What types of atlantoaxial subluxation occur?

- Anterior (most common)
- Lateral
- Vertical, also described as cranial settling (up to 75% after 25 years of rheumatoid arthritis)
- Posterior (associated with erosion or fracture of the dens)
- Rotary

7. What types of subaxial involvement may occur?

- Subluxations
- Anterior soft tissue masses
- Thickened yellow ligaments
- Ankylosis
- Osteophytes
- Bone collapse
- Kyphosis

8. What is the *staircase phenomenon*?

Multiple subaxial subluxations giving the appearance of a staircase on a lateral radiograph of the cervical spine (Fig. 1).

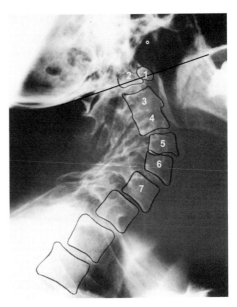

FIGURE 1. Lateral cervical radiograph of a rheumatoid patient (the cervical vertebrae are numbered). Note (1) vertical atlantoaxial subluxation with proximity of the base of the dens (C2) to McGregor's line and the paradoxically small atlantodens interval (ADI), the space between the anterior ring of C1 and the dens; (2) C3–C4 ankylosis; and (3) multilevel subluxations giving rise to the "staircase" appearance.

9. What is the natural history of rheumatoid atlantoaxial subluxation?

- 33–50% of patients develop AAS within 5 years of diagnosis of rheumatoid arthritis.
- 2–10% of patients with AAS develop myelopathy over the next 10 years.
- Once diagnosed with myelopathy, 50% die within 1 year.

10. What symptoms and clinical findings may occur?

- Pain (neck pain, occipital neuralgia, facial and ear pain)
- Lhermitte's sign (electric shock-like sensation in the limbs and trunk when the neck is flexed)
- Symptoms and signs of myelopathy

11. List typical symptoms and signs of myelopathy.

- Loss of endurance
- Gait disturbance
- Loss of dexterity
- Paresthesia
- Change in walking ability
- Bowel and bladder dysfunction
- Weakness
- Spasticity
- Loss of proprioception
- Brisk reflexes
- Babinski sign
- Hoffman sign

12. What are some of the pitfalls in evaluating neurologic status in rheumatoid patients?

1. Chronic polyarthritis and deformity interfere with motor and reflex testing. For example, the Babinski response may be absent in patients with severe forefoot deformity, hallux valgus, or ankylosis of the joints. Similarly, reflex jerks and the Hoffmann reflex may be difficult to elicit.

2. Patients may have had operations to ankylose joints, the subsequent fusion of which can interfere with muscle and reflex testing.

3. Muscle atrophy is common in chronic deforming arthritis and may not be due to neural compression.

4. Root symptoms may be confused with nerve entrapment and polyneuropathy.

13. How is the American Rheumatologic Association (Steinbrocker) Classification of Functional Capacity scored?

Class I: complete ability to carry on all usual duties without handicap.

Class II: adequate for normal activities despite a handicap of discomfort or limited motion at one or more joints.

Class III: limited only to few or none of the duties of usual occupation or self-care.

Class IV: incapacitated, largely or wholly bedridden or confined to a wheelchair; little or no self-care.

14. How is the Ranawat Class of Neurologic Function scored?

Class 1: no neural deficit.

Class 2: subjective weakness with hyperreflexia and dysesthesia.

Class 3: objective findings of weakness and long-tract signs.

Class 3A: able to walk.

Class 3B: quadriparetic and not ambulatory.

15. Which radiologic measurements are useful to evaluate atlantoaxial stability?

- **Anterior atlantodental or atlantodens interval (ADI).** This measurement is generally the inverse of the space available for the cord (SAC) but becomes unreliable if vertical subluxation occurs.
- **SAC or posterior atlantodental interval.** This measurement may have prognostic significance for spinal cord compression.
- **Redlund-Johnell measurement,** or the distance between McGregor's line and the lower endplate of the C2 vertebra. A distance less than 34 mm in men or 29 mm in women is defined as vertical subluxation. Vertical subluxation is usually diagnosed when the top of the dens lies significantly above McGregor's palato-occipital line or when it is situated above the level of the foramen magnum. However, visualization is often difficult due to the overlapping shadows. Erosion of the dens also limits the usefulness of this technique, but the landmarks used for the Redlund-Johnell measurement are usually easy to see (Fig. 2).

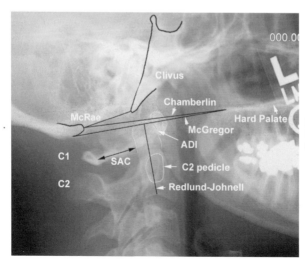

FIGURE 2. Radiologic landmarks and lines in the occipitocervical region.

16. What neuroimaging techniques are used to evaluate the spine in RA?
- Myelography and postmyelogram CT scan: to evaluate the combined effects of bone and soft tissues on the neuraxis in flexion and extension
- Magnetic resonance imaging (MRI): noninvasive imaging with excellent visualization of soft tissues and neural structures, but dynamic studies are difficult to perform (Fig. 3).
- Dynamic stand-up MRI: exciting new technology that allows acquisition of flexion and extension views noninvasively.

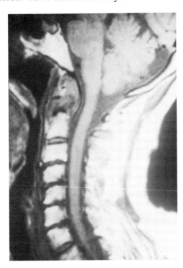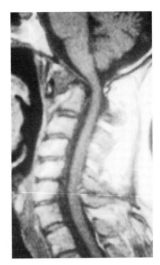

FIGURE 3. Extension (**left**) and flexion (**right**) sagittal MRIs demonstrating exuberant pannus with dens destruction and severe atlantoaxial instability. The high-grade subluxation and its effect on the craniocervical junction may have been missed if the flexion view had been omitted. These images were acquired using standard MRI equipment.

17. What are the indications for surgical treatment of rheumatoid atlantoaxial subluxation?
- Spinal cord compression
- Severe neck symptoms
- Marked subluxation
- Surgical stabilization for AAS greater than 6 mm has been recommended in rheumatoid patients who are otherwise well to prevent progressive instability

A combination of two factors below indicates surgical intervention:
- Cervical myelopathy (clinical signs)
- Delayed central motor latency (motor evoked potentials [MEPs])
- Spinal cord diameter less than 6 mm in neutral or flexed position (MRI)
- Spinal canal diameter less than 10 mm in flexed position (MRI)
- Inflammatory tissue behind the dens greater than 10 mm
- Increasing C1–C2 instability (atlantodens interval more than 10 mm)
- Cranial migration distance less than 31 mm

18. Describe operative techniques to treat a rheumatoid patient with reducible atlantoaxial subluxation.
- Transarticular screw fixation with supplemental posterior wiring and autograft is the most reliable technique (Fig 4).
- C1 lateral mass screws and C2 pedicle screws and rods permit direct reduction and provide superior fixation for more complex cases; cancellous autograft bone should also be used.

- Interlaminar (Halifax) clamps with structural autograft is a reasonable alternative (Fig. 5).
- Posterior Brooks or Gallie wiring with autograft has a relatively high failure rate due to poor control of rotation and translation. Supplemental halo-vest use may increase the success rate. More extensive procedures may be necessary if the bone quality is poor,

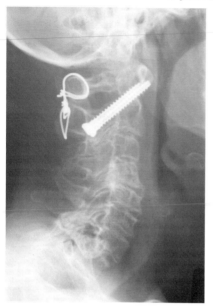

FIGURE 4. Posterior atlantoaxial fusion for rheumatoid atlantoaxial subluxation, 4 years postoperatively (63-year-old patient). Transarticular screws and modified Gallie wiring were used with autograft. The subaxial disks have progressively settled; the C7–T1 spondylolisthesis has remained stable.

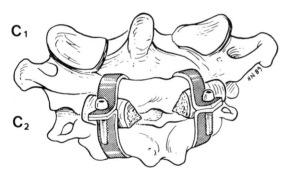

FIGURE 5. Diagram of a skeletonized atlantoaxial motion segment viewed from its posterior aspect. The method of application of the interlaminar clamps can be seen. The bone grafts lie under the clamps and help lock the posterior structures tightly together, providing immediate stability. (From Moskovich R, and Crockard HA. Atlantoaxial arthrodesis using interlaminar clamps: An improved technique. Spine 17:261–267, 1992, with permission)

19. Describe the management of a 75-year-old patient with atlantoaxial and subaxial disease, myelopathy, and poor bone quality.

- Occipitocervical fixation using a contoured Hartshill-Ransford loop and sublaminar wires without bone grafting is a well-validated technique with a high success rate and low morbidity (Fig. 6).
- Occipitocervical fixation with plates and screws to spread out the load is another viable technique, but good bone stock for screw purchase and iliac crest bone harvest are required.

20. Describe the management of an elderly Ranawat IIIb patient who is bed-bound or has severe spinal cord atrophy.

The prognosis for surgical management is poor. Supportive management rather than an operation may be preferable.

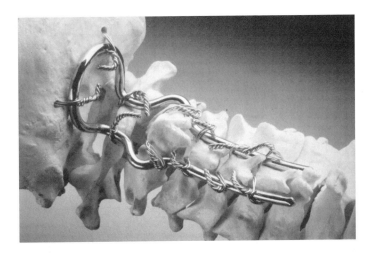

FIGURE 6. A Hartshill-Ransford loop wired into place on a skeleton model. The cranial loop is attached to the occiput using wires which pass through paired full-thickness burr holes. The wires are not passed around the foramen magnum. The loop is prebent to conform to the posterior craniocervical angle and may be adjusted intraoperatively. The limbs of the loop are attached via sublaminar wires at each level. Note how the C2 laminar wires are tightened below the flare of the loop, which serves to maintain distraction between the occiput and the C2 vertebra. (From Moskovich R, Crockard HA, Shott S, Ransford AO: Occipitocervical stabilization for myelopathy in patients with rheumatoid arthritis. Implications of not bone grafting. J Bone Joint Surg 82A:349–365, 2000, with permission.)

21. What is the fate of periodontal rheumatoid pannus after atlantoaxial arthrodesis?

A solid fusion usually results in reduction of pannus.

22. Under what circumstances should transoral resection of the dens be performed?

- Anterior neuraxial compression
- If satisfactory reduction of the subluxation cannot be obtained in a patient with a severe neurologic deficit
- Basilar invagination associated with the Chiari malformation
- Marked vertical subluxation with cervicomedullary compression
- When the pannus itself results in severe cord compression

23. What airway management techniques are used when transoral surgery is performed on a rheumatoid patient?

- Nasotracheal intubation (commonly)
- Tracheostomy (rarely)
- Elective postoperative intubation for 24 to 48 hours to allow pharyngeal swelling to resolve

24. List complications of bed rest and prolonged skull traction for rhematoid vertical atlantoaxial subluxation.

- Pressure sores
- Deep venous thrombosis and pulmonary embolism
- Kidney stones and other problems of prolonged recumbency such as osteoporosis and muscle wasting
- Failure to reduce vertical AAS

25. Is there evidence that cervical collars protect patients with cervical subluxation?

No.

26. How should the spine be operatively stabilized after anterior diskectomy and interbody arthrodesis for subaxial subluxation with cord compression?
  • Anterior plate fixation
  • Concomitant posterior fixation should be strongly considered, because this pathology generally occurs in patients with long-standing rheumatoid arthritis in whom bone quality is usually poor.

BIBLIOGRAPHY

1. Casey A, Crockard HA, Bland JM, et al: Surgery on the rheumatoid cervical spine for the bed-bound, non-ambulant myelopathic patient—too much, too late? Lancet 347:1004–1007, 1996.
2. Crockard HA, Calder I, Ransford AO: One-stage transoral decompression and posterior fixation in rheumatoid atlanto-axial subluxation. J Bone Joint Surg 72B:682–685, 1990.
3. Crockard HA, Moskovich R, Ashraf J: Upper cervical stabilisation: Front, back or sides? J Neurol Neurosurg Psychiatry 52:1464, 1989.
4. Dvorak J, Grob D, Baumgartner H, et al: Functional evaluation of the spinal cord by magnetic resonance imaging in patients with rheumatoid arthritis and instability of upper cervical spine. Spine 14:1057–1064, 1989.
5. Konttinen YT, Santavirta S, Kauppi M, Moskovich R: The Rheumatoid Cervical Spine. Curr Opin Rhematol 3:429–440, 1991.
6. Moskovich R, and Crockard HA. Atlantoaxial arthrodesis using interlaminar clamps. An improved technique. Spine, 17:261–267, 1992.
7. Moskovich R: Atlanto-axial Instability. Spine State Art Rev 8:531–549, 1994.
8. Moskovich R, Crockard HA, Shott S, Ransford AO: Occipitocervical stabilization for myelopathy in patients with rheumatoid arthritis: Implications of not bone grafting. J Bone Joint Surg 82A:349–365, 2000.

63. ANKYLOSING SPONDYLITIS

Edward D. Simmons, M.D., and Yinggang Zheng, M.D.

1. Define ankylosing spondylitis.

Ankylosing spondylitis (AS) is a seronegative inflammatory arthritis of the spine of unknown etiology. It presents in the early stages with an inflammatory arthritic pain that typically involves the sacroiliac joints initially and later the other spinal regions. Initially, range of motion is normal or mildly limited. However, as the disease progresses, ossification of the spine occurs. The spine may eventually fuse in a kyphotic position. AS may affect the lumbar, thoracic, and cervical spinal regions; it may also affect the hip joints.

2. What is the incidence of AS?

AS affects about 0.2–0.3% of the U.S. population at any given time. It is more common in males than females.

3. What criteria are used to diagnose AS?

- Pain and stiffness beginning in the sacroiliac joints with subsequent spread to the lumbar, thoracic, and cervical regions.
- Limitation of spinal motion in the coronal and sagittal planes.
- Decreased chest expansion relative to normative values for age and sex.
- Radiographic evidence of arthritic changes in the sacroiliac joints is considered the hallmark for diagnosis of AS. Additional radiographic findings include ossification of the spinal ligaments and squaring of the lumbar vertebrae.
- Spinal deformity may result from loss of normal cervical and lumbar lordosis as well as increased thoracic kyphosis. Severe kyphotic or flexion deformity of the spine may result. The disease may also affect the hip joints.
- HLA-B27 antigen test is positive in 90% of patients.

4. Is AS the same as rheumatoid arthritis?

No. AS is a different disease and has a different serology. Rheumatoid arthritis is more common in women and tends to affect the joints of the appendicular skeleton. Ankylosing spondylitis is more common in men and usually affects the axial skeleton and hip joints.

5. Can instability of the cervical spine occur in patients with AS?

Despite the fact that AS results in ossification of the cervical region, spinal instability may still occur. Ossification may stiffen the lower cervical region but spare the upper cervical spine. This process may result in increased stress concentration at the craniocervical junction and lead to instability. In addition, inflammation may result in attritional effects on the transverse ligament due to hyperemia at its bony attachments. As these changes progress, atlantoaxial subluxation and dislocation may occur.

6. What is ankylosing spondylodiscitis?

The typical inflammatory process of AS results in erosion and sclerosis of bone adjacent to the sacroiliac joints. Occasionally, erosive sclerotic changes may involve the intervertebral disc and adjacent bone; this process is termed *spondylodiscitis*. This type of lesion is reported in 5–23% of patients and occurs most commonly in the lower thoracic spine. Currently spondylodiscitis is believed to arise from a chronic nonunited fracture rather than from extension of a localized inflammatory process. Treatment consists of posterior spinal instrumentation and fusion. Supplemental anterior column bone grafting may be indicated. Spinal stenosis may develop at the level of spondylodiscitis. When stenosis is present, spinal decompression is required in combination with spinal stabilization and fusion.

447

7. What are the indications for spinal osteotomy in patients with AS?

Cervical spine osteotomy is indicated for fixed flexion deformity of the cervical region. In the most severe case, a "chin-on-chest" deformity is present. Cervical deformities impair the ability to maintain a forward gaze, cause difficulty with personal hygiene, and lead to swallowing difficulty. Because cervical osteotomy is a high-risk procedure, patients should have an earnest desire to accept the risks and rehabilitative measures required for surgical correction.

Kyphotic deformity of the thoracic spine in AS does not usually reach proportions that require surgical correction. Combined anterior and posterior approaches are necessary in rare cases that require surgical correction. The diaphragm must not be violated because patients breathe solely with the diaphragm due to absence of motion through the costovertebral joints.

Osteotomy of the lumbar spine is commonly done for AS patients with fixed flexion deformities due to lumbar hypolordosis or lumbar kyphosis.

8. What are the contraindications for spinal osteotomy in patients with AS?

Contraindications include patients who are not suitable candidates for medical reasons and patients with less severe deformities. Severe osteopenia is also a relative contraindication. Patients with fixed flexion deformities of the hip joints secondary to hip arthrosis should be considered for total hip replacement before an osteotomy procedure is done.

9. What are the advantages of spinal osteotomy in patients with AS?

Spinal osteotomy can be performed as single-stage posterior procedure in the lumbar and cervical region. It allows a high degree of correction in a relatively safe manner. The results of spinal osteotomy procedures can be highly gratifying in terms of overall improvement in functional status and quality of life.

10. What are the disadvantages of spinal osteotomy in patients with AS?

The disadvantages of the procedure are related to potential surgical complications and morbidity. Many patients with AS have concomitant medical illnesses, including cardiac problems, and must undergo thorough preoperative medical risk assessment. Major neurologic deficits are relatively infrequent but obviously are a major problem when they occur.

11. How does the surgeon determine how much correction is needed when performing a cervical or lumbar osteotomy?

The angle between the chin–brow line and a vertical line (the chin–brow line to vertical angle) is measured. A long cassette lateral spinal radiograph is obtained with the patient standing with the hips and knees extended and the neck in its neutral or fixed position. Based on this angle, the size of the wedge removed during osteotomy is determined (Fig. 1).

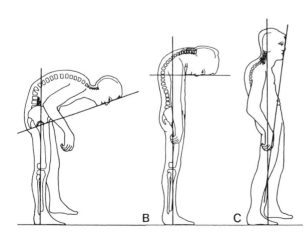

FIGURE 1. The chin–brow to vertical angle is used to measure the degree of flexion deformity of the spine in ankylosing spondylitis. **A,** For thoracolumbar deformity. **B,** For cervical deformity. **C,** For postoperative assessment. The chin–brow to vertical angle is the angle between a line connecting the brow to the chin and a vertical line with the patient standing with the hips and knees extended and the neck in a fixed or neutral position. (From Simmons ED Jr, Simmons EH: Ankylosing spondylitis. Spine State Art Rev 8:589–604, 1994, with permission.)

12. Is a cervical spine fracture a common cause of flexion deformity in patients with AS?

Yes. Sudden cervical pain after minor trauma (e.g., car accident) requires the physician to rule out a fracture in patients with AS. Late flexion deformity of cervical spine may result from a nondiagnosed fracture that heals in a displaced position. The site of injury is usually in the lower cervical spine or at the cervicothoracic junction. The fracture is generally a transversely oriented shear-type fracture. This injury may not be obvious on plain radiographs, and tomographic studies or computed tomography (CT) scans are required for diagnosis. An epidural hematoma may occur and consitutes a surgical emergency in this population.

13. What treatment is recommended for a cervical fracture in a patient with AS?

When such a fracture is recognized, a halo should be applied. Traction to restore the alignment of the head and the neck to its *prefracture position* may be used. If the head was in a previously flexed position, realignment with traction into a neutral position may cause severe neurologic injury. When the appropriate alignment has been obtained, the patient should be immobilized in a halo vest or a well-molded halo cast for 4 months. A high union rate is associated with this protocol. If pseudarthrosis develops, cervical fusion can be performed.

14. What is the preferred level for a cervical osteotomy?

The osteotomy should be carried out at the C7–T1 level. The osteotomy should be centered over the posterior arch of C7. This site is below the entry point of the vertebral arteries, which typically enter at the foramen transversarium at C6. The spinal canal at C7–T1 is relatively capacious, and the cervical spinal cord and the eighth cervical nerve roots have reasonable flexibility. Injury to the C8 nerve root would cause less disability than injury to other cervical nerve roots.

15. What imaging studies should be obtained before a cervical osteotomy?

Cervical radiographs (anteroposterior [AP] lateral, lateral flexion-extension, and swimmer's views) should be obtained. These radiographs outline the shape and size of the spinous processes of C6, C7, and T1, allowing them to be more readily recognized at surgery. Flexion and extension lateral radiographs rule out the presence of instability at the craniocervical junction. A CT scan centered at the C7–T1 level should be obtained preoperatively to assess the spinal deformity. This scan also assesses the size of the spinal canal at the proposed site of osteotomy and identifies areas of spinal stenosis requiring decompression. Magnetic resonance imaging (MRI) may be considered for complex cases.

16. Are the halo vest and skull traction useful during a cervical osteotomy procedure?

Yes. A halo vest is applied to the patient preoperatively, and a 9-pound traction weight is applied in direct line with the patient's neck to stabilize the head throughout the procedure.

17. What special considerations should be given to patient positioning and anesthesia for cervical osteotomy procedures in AS?

The operation is carried out under local anesthesia, with the patient awake in the sitting position using a dental chair. This protocol allows active spinal cord monitoring and immediate assessment of vital functions and neurologic status. Intravenous sedation may be used in conjunction with local anesthesia. Routine monitoring of vital signs, pulse oximetry, carbon dioxide, and systemic blood gases is performed. A Doppler device is fixed to the patient's chest to detect air embolism. The anesthetist may administer oxygen to the patient during the procedure by a face mask or nasal catheter. The patient is allowed to listen to music throughout the procedure and may converse with the anesthetist.

18. What is the extent of spinal decompression advised before to completion of a cervical osteotomy?

The entire posterior arch of C7 with the inferior portion of C6 and the superior portion of T1 is removed. The eighth cervical nerve roots are identified at the C7–T1 neuroforamen and are widely decompressed through the lateral recess, removing the overlying bone at the foramen (Fig. 2). The cervical pedicles need to be undercut with Kerrisons to allow ample room for the eighth cervical nerve roots when the osteotomy site is closed. The amount of bone to be resected is carefully assessed preoperatively and intraoperatively to avoid compression of the nerve roots during closure of the osteotomy. The residual portions of the laminae of C6 and T1 must be carefully beveled and undercut to avoid any impingement or kinking of the spinal cord on closure of the osteotomy site.

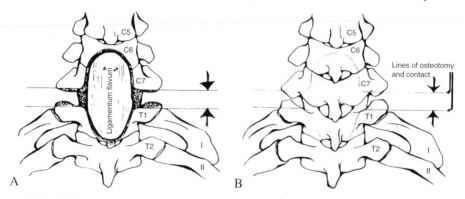

FIGURE 2. Outline of area of bony resection for a cervical osteotomy. The lines of resection of the laterally fused facet joints are beveled slightly away from each other, extending posteriorly so that the two surfaces will be parallel and in apposition following correction. The pedicles must be undercut to avoid impingement on the C8 nerve roots. The midline resection is beveled on its deep surface above and below to avoid impingement against the dura following extension correction. (From Simmons ED Jr, Simmons EH: Ankylosing spondylitis. Spine State Art Rev 8:589–604, 1994, with permission.)

19. How is closure of a cervical osteotomy performed?

After adequate removal of bone, the osteotomy is completed (osteoclasis). The patient is given an intravenous dosage of short-acting barbiturate, usually brevital sodium or sodium pentathol. The surgeon grasps the halo and brings the neck into an extended position. This maneuver closes the osteotomy posteriorly as osteoclasis occurs anteriorly. An audible snap and sensation of osteoclasis are noted. The lateral masses should be well approximated. With the surgeon holding the patient's head in the corrected position, the assistants attach the vest to the halo.

20. How is bone grafting of the cervicothoracic region performed after closure of the cervical osteotomy?

The posterior elements of the spine are decorticated at the C7–T1 area and autogenous bone graft is packed on each side over the decorticated areas. The local bone removed from the posterior decompression is used as bone graft.

21. Are there any "secrets" to facilitate closure of the posterior incision after cervical osteotomy?

Before closure of the osteotomy site, it is often helpful to place the deep sutures, which are somewhat difficult to insert after closure of the osteotomy. The wound is then closed in layers, and sterile dressings are applied. The posterior uprights are connected to the halo and secured.

22. Describe the postoperative regimen after cervical osteotomy.

The awake patient is helped to stand and walk to a circle electric bed that is in a vertical position. The bed can be then tilted to the horizontal position, and the patient is transported to the surgical intensive care unit. When the patient is sufficiently mobile to transfer, a regular bed can be substituted for the circle electric bed. The patient is instructed to leave the vest and halo in place for 4 months. When the vest and halo are removed, lateral tomography centered at C7–T1 is necessary to evaluate radiographic union. Further bracing with a sternal occipital mandibular immobilization (SOMI) brace can be carried out for an additional 2 months.

23. What are the pitfalls and complications of a cervical osteotomy?

Potential pitfalls include osteotomy at the wrong level. If osteotomy is performed proximal to C7, injury to the vertebral arteries may occur. If osteotomy is performed below C7–T1, little or no correction is obtained. Radiographic confirmation is always necessary to prevent this pitfall. Other pitfalls include inadequate or excessive removal of bone, resulting in too little or too great correction.

Neurologic injuries may occur. The dura may infold in the region of the osteotomy and result in kinking of the spinal cord. If this problem is noted, the dura can be carefully opened to relieve compression. Most C8 nerve root problems resolve as long as they are partial. Some postoperative distraction through the halo vest can be carried out if C8 nerve root compression is noted.

Other potential complications include air embolism because surgery is performed in the sitting position. A Doppler monitor with sound amplification is fixed to the patient's chest preoperatively and monitored during the procedure. To prevent embolus, the wound should be filled with irrigation fluid and wet sponges.

24. What different types of lumbar osteotomies are used to treat spinal flexion deformities in patients with AS?

Two types of lumbar osteotomies may be used: (1) Smith-Peterson type (removal of a V-shaped wedge of bone from the posterior spinal column) or (2) Thomasen type (removal of bone from all three spinal columns through a posterior approach by a combination of laminectomy, pedicle resection, and posterior decancellation of the vertebral body). The Smith-Peterson type of osteotomy is preferred by the authors for AS. (See Chapter 47 for description of osteotomy types.)

25. What is the preferred level for performing a Smith-Peterson lumbar osteotomy?

The preferred level for osteotomy is the L3–L4 level. The posterior elements are removed with the apex of the osteotomy at the L3–L4 disc space. The L3–L4 level is located at the normal center of lumbar lordosis, below the termination of the conus medullaris. The spinal canal area is relatively capacious at this level. These factors decrease the neurologic risk of an osteotomy procedure at L3–L4 compared with osteotomy at proximal spinal levels, where the presence of the distal spinal cord and conus within the spinal canal increases the risk of neurologic injury. A CT scan should be obtained to evaluate the spinal canal preoperatively and to assess for spinal stenosis.

26. How is the patient positioned during a lumbar osteotomy procedure?

The lumbar spine osteotomy is performed with the patient in the prone position. The patient must be carefully positioned on the operating table in a flexed knee–chest position. Use of an Andrews table may be helpful. Such patients have fixed ankylosed spines, and undue pressure in any one particular area must be avoided. The thoracic chest support must often be elevated considerably to accommodate patients on the operating table. The procedure is done under spinal cord monitoring. A wake-up test can also be used if necessary.

27. How does the surgeon expose and decompress the spine in preparation for a Smith-Peterson lumbar osteotomy?

Exposure. Radiographic confirmation of the level of osteotomy is necessary because the posterior bony landmarks are indistinct. As the interspinous ligaments are usually ossified, the osteotomy can be initiated with a large bone cutter. Bone and spinous processes are removed in a V-shaped fashion. The laminae are thinned out with Leksell rongeurs, and the bone is saved for use as autogenous bone graft. A high-powered burr can also be used. However, exclusive use of a burr decreases the amount of bone that can be saved for subsequent grafting.

Decompression. The precise amount of bone requiring removal posteriorly is calculated to arrive at the amount of correction desired. The entire L4 lamina is removed along with a portion of the L3 and L5 laminae. The laminae are undercut in order to bevel their undersurfaces and prevent impingement during closure of the osteotomy. It is necessary to remove the entire superior L4 facet and widely expose and undercut the L3–L4 neuroforamina to prevent neural impingement during closure of the osteotomy (Fig. 3). The pedicles also must be undercut, removing the superior edge of the L4 pedicle and inferior edge of the L3 pedicle, again to allow adequate room for the nerve roots during the extension correction of the spine. On closure of the osteotomy by osteoclasis of the spine anteriorly, the lateral masses should meet with good bone surface contact.

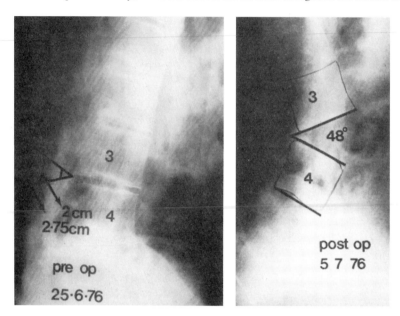

FIGURE 3. Left, Lateral preoperative lumbar radiograph showing the angle of correction and amount of bone to be resected. Removal of 2 cm of bone is required on each side at the level of the fused posterior joints, 2.5 cm at the level of the laminae, and 5 cm at the level of the tips of the fused spinous processes. **Right,** Postoperative lateral radiograph showing angle of correction obtained after closure of resected defect posteriorly with anterior osteoclasis through the L3–L4 disc space. (From Simmons ED Jr, Simmons EH: Ankylosing spondylitis. Spine State Art Rev 8:589–604, 1994, with permission.)

28. What spinal instrumentation is most commonly used when a lumbar osteotomy procedure is performed?

Pedicle screw fixation is the preferred method of fixation after osteotomy because pedicle screws permit control of all three spinal columns. After decompression, pedicle screws should be inserted in L1, L2, L3, L5, and S1. It is not usually possible to have screws in L4 because they will impinge on the L3 screws after closure of the osteotomy.

29. How is closure (osteoclasis) of a Smith-Peterson lumbar osteotomy performed?

Osteoclasis is carried out by extending the foot-end of the operating table, thereby bringing the hips and thighs into an extended position. Additional pressure can also be applied manually by pushing downwards at the L3–L4 level and creating a fulcrum around which osteoclasis may occur. As the anterior spinal column is disrupted, the lateral edges of the posterior column osteotomy come together in extension. Anterior column disruption can be detected by manual palpation and may be accompanied by an audible snap. The lower extremities and hips are kept in an extended position, preferably with the knees flexed to avoid tension on the lumbar nerve roots. Rods are then cut and contoured to the appropriate length and shape and connected to the pedicle screws.

30. What are the potential complications of a Smith-Peterson lumbar osteotomy?

Potential complications specific to this procedure include neurologic deficit, instrumentation-related problems, insufficient or excessive deformity correction, and gastrointestinal difficulties.

Neurologic injury may result from neural impingement during osteotomy closure or intraspinal hematoma. Instrumentation-related problems may result from poor screw purchase in osteopenic bone or difficulty with implant insertion due to distortion of normal anatomic landmarks. Removal of too little or too much bone posteriorly can result in too little or too great a correction. Asymmetric bone removal may lead to postoperative imbalance in the coronal plane. Careful preoperative planning is necessary to determine the amount of correction desired and the appropriate amount of bone removal. Gastrointestinal problems can be minimized by leaving a nasogastric tube in place for several days until intestinal motility has returned. Failure to do so may result in emesis and aspiration due to the patient's inability to rotate the neck and clear the airway.

BIBLIOGRAPHY

1. Calin A: Ankylosing spondylitis. In Kelly WN, Harris ED, Ruddy S, Sledge CB (eds): Textbook of Rheumatology. Philadelphia, W.B. Saunders, 1981, p 1017.
2. Simmons EH, Fielding JW: Atlanto-axial arthrodesis. J Bone Joint Surg 49A:1022, 1967.
3. Simmons EH: Surgery of the spine in ankylosing spondylitis and rheumatoid arthritis. In Chapman M (ed): Operative Orthopaedics, vol. 3. Philadelphia, J.B. Lippincott, 1988, p 2077.
4. Simmons EH: Kyphotic deformity of the spine in ankylosing spondylitis. Clin Orthop 128:65, 1977.
5. Simmons EH: Alternatives in surgical stabilization of the upper cervical spine. In Charles HT (ed): Early Management of Acute Spinal Cord Injury. New York, Raven Press, 1982, pp 393–434.
6. Simmons EH: Ankylosing spondylitis and rheumatoid arthritis. In Lauren CA, et al (eds): An Atlas of Orthopaedic Surgery. Chicago, Year Book, 1989, pp 502–528.
7. Simmons ED, Simmons EH. Ankylosing spondylitis. In Farcy JPC (ed): Complex Spinal Deformities. Philadelphia, Hanley & Belfus, 1994, pp 589–603.
8. Simmons ED, Capicotto PN: Clinical cervical deformity and postlaminectomy kyphosis. In White AH, Schofferman JA (eds): Spine Care. St. Louis, Mosby, 1995, pp 1633–1650.
9. Urist MR: Osteotomy of the cervical spine: Report of a case of ankylosing rheumatoid spondylitis. J Bone Joint Surg 40A:833–843, 1958.

XI. Emerging Technology

64. MINIMALLY INVASIVE SPINE SURGERY

Baron S. Lonner, M.D.

1. List the basic principles of minimally invasive spine surgery (MISS).
- Small incisions
- Use of an endoscope and light source
- Minimal disruption of musculature compared to standard open approaches
- Decreased blood loss compared with open procedures
- Rapid postoperative recovery
- Maximal preservation of structure and function of the spine

The term *minimally invasive* is frequently used but potentially misleading. Spinal procedures remain "maximally invasive" but are performed through smaller skin incisions. In spine surgery, as with most other invasive procedures, less is more as long as surgical goals are fully met.

2. Are the goals of MISS different from standard open procedures?
No. The surgeon must be able to achieve the same surgical goals with MISS techniques as with traditional open surgical procedures:
- Adequate neural decompression
- Stabilization and arthrodesis
- Spinal balance and correction of deformity
- Relief of back and/or leg pain

3. List applications of MISS using an anterior surgical approach.
- Laparoscopic lumbar interbody fusion
- Lumbar interbody fusion via a minilaparotomy approach
- Anterior thoracic discectomy and fusion with or without instrumentation via a thoracoscopic approach

4. List applications of MISS using a posterior surgical approach.
- Traditional microdiscectomy
- Microendoscopic discectomy
- Percutaneous discectomy
- Laser discectomy
- Intradiscal electrothermy (IDET)
- Lumbar arthrodesis (posterolateral fusion with instrumentation, minimally invasive PLIF or TLIF)
- Vertebroplasty/kyphoplasty

5. How does the use of endoscopes enhance visualization during MISS?
- Provides focused intense illumination
- Provides magnification of surgical field
- Use of multiple portals and angled lenses allows extensive field of view without large incision

6. What are the indications for microendoscopic discectomy?

They are the same as for traditional microdiscectomy. At present, none of the alternative techniques have been shown to equal or improve upon the excellent results achieved with traditional microdiscectomy.

7. List proposed selection criteria for percutaneous or laser discectomy.

Percutaneous or laser discectomy techniques have not shown results equivalent or superior to traditional microdiscectomy. Advocates of percutaneous and laser techniques consider their use for the following indications:
- Patients with leg and/or back pain refractory to non-operative therapy
- Contained disc prolapse or bulge
- Patients in whom disc height is at least partially preserved

8. What are the characteristics of the ideal potential candidate for an IDET procedure?

The role of this procedure in the treatment of back pain is not fully defined. Proposed criteria for patient selection include:
- Chronic back pain with or without leg pain
- Absence of neurological deficit
- Pain refractory to nonoperative management
- Imaging evidence of disc abnormality (dessication, annular tear, contained bulge)
- Discogenic pain confirmed by discography
- Absence of significant spinal stenosis or spinal instability

9. List potential indications for thoracoscopic spinal surgery.
- Biopsy
- Treatment of symptomatic thoracic disc herniation
- Anterior release and fusion for spinal deformities (rigid scoliosis > 70°, kyphosis that does not correct below 55° on hyperextension radiographs)
- Prevention of crankshaft phenomenon in patients with pediatric spinal deformities (Risser stage 0 or 1 maturity, age < 10 years, open triradiate cartilage)
- Anterior fusion and instrumentation for flexible thoracic adolescent idiopathic scoliosis (40–70°) with hypokyphosis or normal kyphosis
- Internal thoracoplasty for large rib prominences associated with scoliosis

10. What are the potential advantages of thoracoscopic spinal fusion and instrumentation compared with traditional open thoracotomy approaches for treatment of idiopathic scoliosis?
- Diminished blood loss
- Decreased postoperative pain
- Improved cosmesis due to small incisions
- Diminished length of hospital stay

11. What are the disadvantages of thoracoscopic spinal instrumentation and fusion compared with traditional open thoracotomy approaches for treatment of idiopathic scoliosis?
- Significant learning curve
- Additional equipment required
- Need for postoperative brace
- Potentially decreased rate of fusion and less curve correction

12. List potential complications of thoracoscopic spinal decompression, fusion, and instrumentation.
- Dural tear
- Direct spinal cord injury

- Pulmonary complications (pneumothorax, hemothorax, mucous plug, pneumonia)
- Intercostal neuralgia
- Vessel injury (segmentals, azygous vein, aorta)
- Pseudarthrosis
- Implant misplacement

13. What neural structures are routinely encountered in the thoracoscopic operative field?
- Sympathetic chain
- Greater and lesser splanchnic nerves
- Vagus nerve
- Phrenic nerve
- Intercostals nerves (internal thoracoplasty)

14. What are the two types of approaches for laparoscopic lumbar interbody fusion?
Carbon dioxide gas insufflation technique and balloon-assisted gasless approach.

15. What are the major disadvantages of laparoscopic spinal surgery in comparison with open techniques?
- Steep learning curve
- Potential for lengthier operative time
- Increased complication rate
- Need for general surgeon to assist with surgical approach

16. What are the major potential complications of the laparoscopic approach for lumbar interbody fusion?
- Common iliac vein tear
- Retrograde ejaculation in men as a result of disruption of the sympathetic plexus at the sacral promontory
- Bowel injury
- Ureteral or kidney injury

17. Why are mini-open laparotomy approaches preferred by many surgeons for lumbar interbody fusion?
Mini-open laparotomy approaches offer similar advantages compared with laparoscopic techniques while avoiding many of the challenges inherent in laparoscopic surgery. Mini-open techniques are routinely accomplished through a single small incision and generally require shorter operative times. These procedures are associated with a low complication rate and allow relatively rapid patient recovery.

18. True or false: Minimally invasive approaches have become the gold standard for exposure of the thoracic and lumbar spine.
False. These applications are evolving and certainly hold promise for improved outcome compared with existing proven techniques. Long term follow-up and critical analysis of results are necessary to determine the role of these techniques in the spine surgeon's armamentarium.

19. List the indications for vertebroplasty or kyphoplasty for thoracic and lumbar spinal fractures.
- Acute or subacute vertebral compression fracture
- One or two level involvement
- Absence of neural element impingement
- Absence of spinal instability pattern or high energy injury

20. What are the major potential complications of vertebroplasty or kyphoplasty?
- Cement extravasation causing spinal cord, nerve root, or anterior visceral injury
- Adjacent segment compression fractures due to stress transfer
- Hemodynamic instability as a result of methylmethacrylate polymer reaction

21. What steps should a surgeon take to overcome the learning curve and maximize patient safety when learning MISS techniques?

- Attend courses
- Study the anatomy, indications, and potential complications of MISS
- Practice in animal and cadaver labs
- Visit experienced surgeons currently performing these procedures
- Perform cases with an experienced surgeon, if posssible
- Develop a game plan for addressing intraoperative problems
- Maintain competence in MISS techniques through adequate surgical case volume
- Perform a critical analysis of personal surgical outcomes

22. List ways in which the morbidity of bone-grafting procedures can be minimized.

- Harvest iliac crest or other sites through small cortical windows that are replaced after cancellous bone is harvested
- Use structural allograft for anterior structural grafts instead of iliac autograft
- Use bone graft substitutes or extenders

23. List several bone graft substitutes or extenders.

- Allograft
- Demineralized bone matrix (gel, putty, sheets)
- Calcium phosphates
- Ceramics
- Coralline hydroxyapatite
- Marrow aspirate
- Osteoinductive factors (platelet–rich plasma, BMP-2, OP-1)

BIBLIOGRAPHY

1. Boden SD: Biology of lumbar spine fusion and use of bone graft substitutes: Present, future, and next generation. Tissue Eng 6:383–399, 2000.
2. Landreneau RJ, Hazelrigg SR, Mack MJ, et al: Postoperative pain-related morbidity: Video-assisted thoracoscopy versus thoracotomy. Ann Thor Surg 56:1285–1289, 1993.
3. Lane JM, et al: Minimally invasive options for the treatment of osteoporotic compression fractures. Orthop Clin North Am 33:431–438, 2002.
4. Mathews HH: Transforaminal endoscopic microdiscectomy. Neurosurg Clin North Am 7:59–63, 1996.
5. McAfee PC, Regan JR, Zdeblick T, et al: The incidence of complications in endoscopic anterior thoracolumbar spinal reconstructive surgery. A prospective multicenter study comprising the first 100 consecutive cases. Spine 20:1624–1632, 1995.
6. Newton PO, Shea KG, Granlund KF: Defining the pediatric spinal thoracoscopy learning curve: Sixty-five consecutive cases. Spine 25:1028–1035, 2000.
7. Picetti GD, Ertl JP, Bueff HU: Endoscopic instrumentation, correction, and fusion of idiopathic scoliosis. Spine J 1:190–197, 2001.
8. Regan JJ, McAfee PC, Mack MJ (eds): Atlas of Endoscopic Spine Surgery. St. Louis, Quality Medical Publishing, 1995.
9. Saal JA, Saal JS: Management of chronic discogenic low back pain with a thermal intradiscal catheter. Spine 25:382–387, 2000.

65. ARTIFICIAL DISC REPLACEMENT

Iris Yaron, M.D., Michael G. Neuwirth, M.D., and Fabien D. Bitan, M.D.

1. What is the function of the lumbar spine?

According to Bogduk, "the lumbar spine is designed to provide axial rigidity to the lower trunk, to sustain axial compression loads exerted from the trunk and upper limbs, and to permit *certain* movements between trunk and pelvis."[2]

2. Name the articulations that comprise a spinal motion segment.

The motion segment or functional spinal unit consists of two adjacent vertebrae and the interconnecting soft tissue, devoid of musculature. The spinal motion segment has three articulations— the intervertebral disc and two posterior facet joints.

3. Explain the function of the lumbar facet joints.

The facet joints provide a posterior articulation between adjacent vertebrae and limit mobility of the motion segment. The sagittal shape of the facet joints limits rotation, and the facet capsules limit distraction.

4. What are the two components of an intervetebral disc?

Nucleus pulposus and annulus fibrosus.

5. Explain the function of the intervertebral disc.

The intervertebral disc is responsible for transmission and attenuation of complex compressive, torsional, and bending forces to which the trunk is subjected. Compressive and bending forces are resisted hydrostatic pressure within the gel-like nucleus. Torsional forces are primarily resisted by annular fibers. The nucleus moves dorsally with flexion and ventrally with extension. The kinematics of lumbar motion are complex, and the center of rotation is constantly changing as the lumbar spine moves.

6. Describe the relationship between the intervertebral disc and the posterior facet joints.

According to Gries et al., "Biomechanical and histologic studies have highlighted the close functional relationship between lumbar discs and their associated facet joints, and it is conceivable that their degenerative changes are interdependent."[5] According to Haher et al., "It has been reported that facet arthrosis and degeneration never occur without the presence of adjacent disc degeneration. This suggests that intact discs protect the facets from severe loading and degeneration."[6]

7. Where does normal load transfer occur within the intervertebral space?

Through the nucleus pulposus to the central endplates, which bulge into the adjacent vertebral bodies. With degeneration of the disc, compressive loads are transferred through the annulus to the periphery of the endplates

8. Describe the changes that occur during degeneration of an intervertebral disc

During the degenerative disc process, changes occur in the nucleus and annulus. In the nucleus, a decrease in the content of mucopolysaccharides and proteoglycans impairs the ability of the nucleus to bind water. The ability of the nucleus to bear axial loads is impaired, resulting in abnormal loading of the motion segment. The annular fibers are subjected to abnormal stress and injury. Because the annulus is innervated by pain fibers, abnormal loading of the motion segment may lead to back pain symptoms.

9. Explain what is meant by the degenerative cascade.

The spectrum of degenerative changes in the functional spinal unit can be divided into three phases. In phase 1, the degenerative phase, early disc degeneration results in alteration of the load-carrying capacity of the motion segment. Annular tears may cause back pain, and disc herniations may result in radicular symptoms. In phase 2, the instability phase, degenerative disc changes progress, leading to facet subluxation, abnormal facet loading, facet degeneration, segmental instability, and occasionally lateral spinal stenosis. In phase 3, the stabilization phase, the body attempts to restore spinal stability through bony hypertrophy and osteophyte formation. This process is imperfect and may result in symptomatic spinal stenosis, degenerative spondylolisthesis, and degenerative scoliosis. The term *spondylosis* refers to any lesion of the spine resulting from degenerative changes.

10. What are the limitations of current surgical treatment for degenerative spinal problems?
   Current spinal procedures (discectomy, laminectomy, fusion) do not restore normal spinal function. Procedures for neural decompression (discectomy, laminectomy) violate the integrity of the three-joint complex and may increase segmental spinal instability. This instability may lead to pain and require additional surgical procedures, such as fusion. Spinal fusion procedures increase stress at adjacent spinal levels and may accelerate the degenerative process and lead to adjacent level instability and spinal stenosis. Furthermore, fusion procedures may generate the need for additonal procedures, such as implant removal. In addition, bone graft harvest for fusion procedures is accompanied by a myriad of problems, including chronic bone graft donor site pain.

11. What are the major goals of disc replacement surgery?
   - Maintain and/or restore normal segmental spinal motion
   - Prevent or alleviate back pain associated with the degenerative cascade
   - Restoration of disc space height
   - Indirect decompression of foraminal stenosis
   - Restoration of segmental lordosis and global sagittal balance
   - Protection of adjacent spinal levels from iatrogenically accelerated degeneration

12. What criteria are used for selecting appropriate candidates for disc replacement surgery?
   General indications for disc replacement surgery include:
   - Patients with back and leg pain not responsive to appropriate nonsurgical treatment.
   - Symptomatic one- or two-level disc degenerative changes with disc space collapse
   - Symptomatic early stage degenerative disc changes identified by magnetic resonance imaging (MRI) and/or discogram, provided no facet arthritis is present.
   - Patients without prior history of back surgery at the affected level.
   Qualifications for selecting appropriate surgical candidates include:
   - Previous discectomy or laminectomy are not absolute contraindications, providing the facets have been respected.
   - Absence of major spinal stenosis other than foraminal stenosis.
   - Absence of significant osteoporosis, infection, or instability, such as spondylolisthesis.
   - Patients with recurrent disc herniation at the same intervertebral level who otherwise would be candidates for fusion may potentially be candidates for disc arthroplasty. In this setting, careful evaluation of the following is required:
     1. How large was the previous facetectomy?
     2. Is there an extruded fragment in the canal that would be difficult to access?
     3. Is facet arthritis present?

13. What are the major contraindications for disc replacement?
   - Significant spinal deformity
   - Facet joint arthrosis (degree to which this is a contraindication remains undefined)
   - Spinal stenosis other than foraminal stenosis due to disc space collapse at the target level
   - Spinal instability (e.g., spondylolisthesis)
   - Altered posterior elements secondary to prior surgery (e.g., laminectomy, facetectomy) or congenital bony anomalies
   - Infection

- Metabolic bone diseases (osteoporosis, osteomalacia)
- Pain related to severe scarring after previous spinal surgery
- Poorly motivated patient

14. What are the different types of lumbar disc replacement?

In total disc replacement the entire nucleus pulposus is replaced, and most of the annulus, with the exception of the peripheral part, is removed. In nucleus replacement the annulus remains intact, and a gel-like substance is inserted into the space formerly occupied by the nucleus pulposus.

15. What are the components of a commonly used lumbar total disc replacement prosthesis?

Two endplates made of cobalt-chromium alloy are attached to the vertebral endplates by means of anchoring teeth along their border (Fig. 1). A polyethylene-sliding core is placed between these endplates to allow near-physiologic segmental movement. These components are supplied in various sizes to better match the different space that is available for each individual patient (modular prosthesis). Positioning of the disc components is performed intraoperatively under fluoroscopic guidance so that optimal placement in the frontal and saggital planes is achieved. In addition, proper tensioning of the soft tissues is important for ideal functioning of the components.

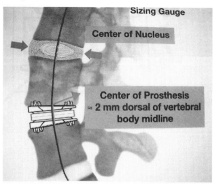

FIGURE 1. The Charite III disc.

16. What is the optimal placement of the prosthesis in the intervertebral space?

First, the degenerated disc tissue has to be excised in its entirety with sparing of the subchondral bone. Then, under fluoroscopic guidance, the prosthesis is placed exactly in the midline in the frontal plane and as posterior as possible in the sagittal plane without entering the spinal canal (Fig. 2).

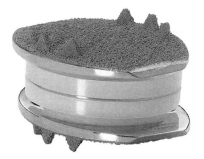
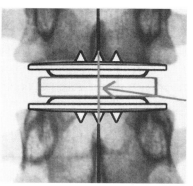

Sizing Gauge

Center of Nucleus

Center of Prosthesis
≈ 2 mm dorsal of vertebral
body midline

FIGURE 2. Optimal positioning of the prosthesis in the intervertebral space.

17. List the requisite design criteria for a lumbar disc prosthesis.

- Endurance. Most disc replacement patients are young, and longevity of the prosthesis is a major consideration.
- Biocompatibility of the materials

- Recreation of normal disc geometry
- Relatively normal kinematics and dynamics
- Constraints to motion to avoid instability of the motion segment or dislocation of the prosthesis. The optimal degree of constraint is still controversial. The different prostheses on the market have varying degrees of constaints. Studies are ongoing in the U.S. to determine the pros and cons of these products.
- Fixation to bone that is both immediate and long-term

18. What types of segmental motions are permitted by available artificial disc prostheses?
- Lateral bending
- Flexion and extension
- Rotation (which is limited by competent facet joints)

19. Describe the desirable properties of material for use in an artifical disc.

In addition to biocompatibility, a significant concern when designing an articulating implant is the volume of wear particles generated. Therefore, the materials selected should have high wear-resistant properties in the articulating surface. Wear complications with disc replacements have been suspected due to the decreased height of some polyethylene inserts. However, over the past 15 years no bony destruction comparable to the osteolysis noted with hip and knee prostheses has been reported with artificial discs. The absence of synovial tissue in the anterior compartment of the spine may account for this finding.

20. What is the most common surgical approach for a lumbar intervertebral disc replacement?

The most commonly used approached is the anterior retroperitoneal approach. The transperitoneal approach is reserved for patients with prior surgery through the retroperitoneal space to avoid the need for mobilization of blood vessels surrounded by scar tissue.

21. What complications may be associated with lumbar disc replacement procedures?
- Abdominal wall hematomas
- Vascular injury
- Dural tears
- Nerve injury
- Sexual dysfunction in males (mostly retrograde ejaculation)
- Migration or dislocation of the prosthesis
- Malpositioning of the prosthesis, resulting in development of asymmetric facet arthritis secondary to asymmetric loading of the facet joints. This complication can result from insufficient exposure of the disc (Fig. 3).

22. What factors lead to failure following intervertebral disc replacement?
- Posterior facet arthritis
- Osteoporosis
- Structural deformities
- Secondary facet pain

23. Review the advantages and disadvantages of artificial disc replacement.
Advantages:
- Preserves spinal motion
- Restores disc space height
- Provides indirect decompression of foraminal stenosis
- May prevent progression of the degenerative cascade (Fig. 4)

Disadvantages:
- Risks inherent in an anterior approach to the spine
- Results may deteriorate if facet degeneration or pain results
- Because of the innovative nature of this procedure, relatively short follow-up is available.

BIBLIOGRAPHY

1. Bao QB, Yuan HA: Prosthetic disc replacement: The future? Clin Orthop 394:139–145, 2002.
2. Bogduk N: The artificial disc. In Churchill Clinical Anatomy of the Lumbar Spine and Sacrum, 3rd ed. Edinburgh, Livingstone, 1997.

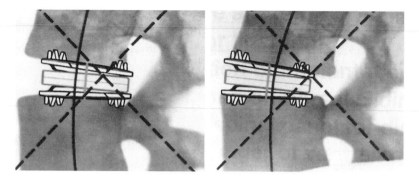

FIGURE 3. Malpositioning of the prosthesis. The figure on the right illustrates a prosthesis that is placed too far anteriorly; the figure on the left shows a prosthesis that is too far posterior and encroaches the spinal canal.

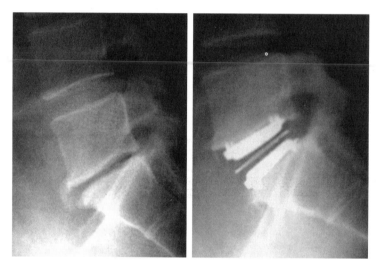

FIGURE 4. The radiograph on the left shows the decrease in disc space height and degeneration that is typically seen in phase 1 of the degenerative cascade. The postoperative radiograph shows the artificial disc replacement with restoration of disc space height and sagittal alignment.

3. Buttner-Janz K, Schellnack K, Zippel H, et al: Experience and results with the SB Charite lumbar intervertebral endoprosthesis. Klin Med 43(20):3–7, 1988.
4. Dooris AP, Goel VK, Grosland NM, et al: Load-sharing between anterior and posterior elements in a lumbar motion segment implanted with an artificial disc. Spine 26(6):E122–E129, 2001.
5. Gries NC, Berlemann U, Moore RJ, et al: Early histologic changes in lower lumbar discs and facet joints and their correlation. Eur Spine J 9:23–29, 2000.
6. Haher TR, et al: The role of the lumbar facet joints in spinal stability. Identification of alternative paths of loading. Spine 19:2667–2670, 1994.
7. Keller TS, Hanson TH, Abram AC, et al: Regional variations in the compressive properties of lumbar vertebral trabeculae—effects of disc degeneration. Spine 14:1012–1019, 1989.
8. Langrana NA, Lee CK, Vuono-Hawkins M: Artificial intervertebral disc prosthesis. In Bridwell K, DeWald R (eds): The Textbook of Spinal Surgery, 2nd ed. Philadelphia, Lippincott-Raven, 1997, pp 2267–2274.
9. Lemaire JP, Skalli W, Lavaste F, et al: Intervertebral disc prosthesis, results and prospects for the years 2000. Clin Orthop Rel Res 337:64–76, 1997.
10. Thierry JD: Lumbosacral disc prosthesis. In Margulis JY (ed): Lumbosacral and Spinopelvic Fixation. Philadelphia, Lippincott-Raven, 1996, pp 881–887.

66. BONE GRAFTS AND BONE GRAFT SUBSTITUTES

Munish C. Gupta, M.D.

1. What graft materials are currently available for use in spinal fusion procedures?
- Autograft
- Allograft
- Demineralized bone matrix (DBM)
- Ceramics
- Composite grafts (synthetic scaffold combined with biologic elements to stimulate fusion)
- Bone morphogenetic proteins

2. Define autograft, allograft, and xenograft.

Autograft: bone harvested from the patient undergoing the spinal fusion.

Allograft: bone harvested in a sterile manner from cadaver donors. This bone is preserved and processed for use in other patients.

Xenograft: bone harvested from different species such as cows or pigs. Xenograft bone is not used in humans.

3. What three properties should be provided by the ideal bone graft material for spinal fusion?

1. **Osteoinduction.** The graft should contain growth factors (noncollagenous bone matrix proteins) that can induce osteoblasts precursors to differentiate into mature bone forming cells.

2. **Osteoconduction.** The graft should provide a framework or scaffold (bone mineral and collagen) onto which new bone can form.

3. **Osteogenesis.** The graft should contain viable progenitor stem cells that can form new bone matrix and remodel bone as needed.

4. Compare the properties of present bone graft materials in relation to an ideal bone graft material.

GRAFT	PROPERTIES	EXAMPLES
Autograft	Osteogenic, osteoconductive, osteoinductive	Iliac crest, fibula, rib
Allograft	Osteoconductive, weakly osteo-inductive	Structural: femur, fibula Nonstructural: morselized femoral head
Demineralized bone matrix	Osteoinductive, osteoconductive	Grafton, Opteform, Dynagraft, Osteofil, DBX
Ceramics	Osteoconductive	Hydroxyapatite, tricalcium phosphate
Composite grafts	Osteoinductive, osteoconductive	Ultraporous beta-tricalcium phosphate (Vitoss) combined with bone marrow aspirate
Bone morphogenetic proteins	Osteoinductive	rhBMP-2, rhBMP-7

5. What properties make autograft an ideal choice for spinal fusion?

Autograft has all of the necessary properties for achieving a spinal fusion; it is osteoinductive, osteoconductive, and osteogenic.

6. What are the drawbacks of using autograft for spinal fusions?
- Supply of autograft is limited. This is a problem in revision spinal surgery after prior bone graft harvest or when fusion of multiple levels is necessary.

- Increased operative time and a second incision are required to obtain bone graft.
- Iatrogenic complications can occur secondary to graft procurement. Bone graft site pain, infection, hematoma, lumbar hernia, sciatic nerve injury, pelvic fracture, and superior gluteal artery injury are a few examples.

7. What are the two available methods for preserving allograft bone grafts?

Allograft bone is harvested under sterile conditions and preserved by freezing or freeze-drying. These methods reduce imunogenicity and permit extended storage. Allograft bone is available either as a nonstructural graft (corticocancellous chips) or as a structural graft (e.g., femoral rings, tricortical wedges, fibular shaft, tibial or femoral shaft, machine contoured threaded dowels).

8. What is the risk of disease transmission with allograft bone graft?

The risk of disease transmission with allograft bone is extremely low. Donors are screened for a history of medical problems, and serologic tests are performed to identify HIV, hepatitis B and hepatitis C. According to a 1995 report, 3 million allografts were used since the identification of the HIV virus with only two documented cases of HIV transmission. Both cases occurred when a single donor was not properly screened. Bone allografts have a much lower incidence of disease transmission than blood transfusions.

9. Compare the advantages and disadvantages of freeze-dried and fresh-frozen allograft bone.

- Freeze-dried allograft bone can be stored at room temperature, whereas fresh frozen grafts require storage in a −70° C freezer.
- As a result of processing, fresh-frozen allograft bone contains more viable osteoinductive factors than freeze-dried allograft.
- Freeze-dried bone that is gamma-radiated has less chance of transmitting infection than fresh-frozen bone.
- Freeze-dried bone is brittle if not hydrated adequately. Fresh-frozen bone can be thawed and consequently used more quickly than freeze dried bone.

10. Give three examples of how allograft is used successfully in spinal fusion procedures.

1. Fibular allograft used to reconstruct the anterior spinal column after cervical corpectomy.

2. Femoral ring allografts with autograft placed inside the medullary canal are used for lumbar interbody fusions.

3. Nonstructural allograft (corticocancellous chips) is used in lengthy posterior spinal fusions for neuromuscular scoliosis in pediatric patients.

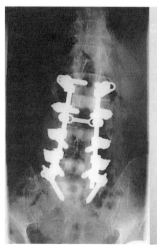 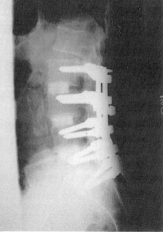

FIGURE 1. Allograft femoral rings packed with autograft cancellous bone are used with a high rate of success for intradiscal fusion.

11. How does allograft incorporate into a spinal fusion mass?

The method of incorporation into a fusion mass depends on the type of allograft bone graft. Allograft cortical bone can take years to incorporate fully because it is remodeled by creeping substitution. Osteoclasts resorb the allograft, and osteoblasts form new bone as the graft is revascularized. Corticocancellous bone is incorporated more rapidly because bone apposition on existing bony trabeculae is the primary mode of incorporation.

12. What are the advantages of allograft bone in spinal fusion procedures?

Allograft can supplement autograft when autograft alone is not sufficient. Allograft fibula and femoral cortical shaft can provide greater structural support than autograft iliac crest wedges or cancellous chips.

13. What are the disadvantages of allograft bone in spinal fusion procedures?

Allograft bone weakens as it undergoes remodeling. Allograft, in rare instances, can transmit infections. In some countries allograft bone is not allowed to be used on cultural, religious, or ethical grounds (e.g. Japan). Lastly, the expense involved in processing, preserving, and storing allograft can make it difficult to obtain.

14. What is demineralized bone matrix (DBM)?

DBM is an osteoconductive scaffold produced by acid extraction of banked bone. It possesses no structural strength. Its consitituents include noncollagenous proteins, osteoinductive growth factors, and type 1 collagen. DBM is more osteoinductive than allograft bone because the demineralization process makes growth factors (bone morphogenetic proteins) more accessible. Preclinical data support the use of DBM as a bone-graft extender but not as a bone-graft substitute in posterior spinal fusion procedures performed with autograft bone. Few studies address its efficacy in anterior spinal fusion procedures.

15. What is the role of ceramics in spinal fusion procedures?

Ceramic materials (calcium phosphate, calcium sulfate, natural coral ceramics) have been evaluated in animal and human studies. Data support the role of ceramics in osteoconduction. In the future, ceramics may play a role as part of a composite graft composed of a ceramic "delivery vehicle" for osteoinductive bone growth factors.

16. What are bone morphogenetic proteins?

Bone morphogenetic proteins (BMPs) are part of a larger transforming growth factor beta superfamily that contains 30 such related proteins. These proteins are cytokines that can induce bone formation. They were first identified as the active osteoinductive fraction of DBM. Molecular cloning techniques permitted subsequent identification and characterization of these proteins. Using genetically modified cell lines, recombinant BMP has been produced. Recombinant human bone morphogenetic protein-2 (rhBMP-2) is presently available for clinical use in anterior lumbar interbody fusion. RhBMP-7, also called recombinant human osteogenic protein-1 (rhOP-1), is expected to be available in the near future.

17. How do BMPs signal for bone formation on a cellular level?

BMPs bind to BMP receptors on the cell surface. There are five type I and seven type II receptors. These receptors are serine/threonine protein kinases that phosphorylate and activate proteins called Smads (term derived from merging Sma and Mad, which are cytoplasmic proteins activated by BMP in different species).

18. What can interfere with action of BMPs?

BMP-binding proteins (inhibin, lefty 1, lefty 2) bind to BMPs themselves and prevent attachment to BMP receptors. In addition, BMP antagonists (Dan, chordin, noggin) bind to BMP receptors, thus preventing BMPs from attaching to their receptors.

19. What happens after the BMPs bind to their receptors?

Once BMPs bind to the receptors, the receptors phosphorylate intracellular substrates known as Smads. There are three kinds of Smads:

1. Receptor-regulated Smads (R-Smads)
2. Common mediator Smads (co-Smads)
3. Inhibitory Smads (I-Smads)

Multiple Smads are present in each group. The Smads and other non-Smad pathways interact with various proteins in the nucleus to initiate transcription of BMP specific genes.

20. What is the difference between rhBMP use in humans and nonhuman primates compared with species such as rabbits and dogs?

Humans and nonhuman primates require higher dosages of rhBMP and take longer for fusion to occur compared with rabbits and dogs. For example, rabbits achieve fusion in 4 weeks compared with 6 months for nonhuman primates.

21. Describe the potential advantages of using rhBMP-2 or rhBMP-7 for spinal fusion.

- Obviates the need for autograft
- Provides a higher rate of successful fusion
- Accelerates the fusion process (e.g., a structural bone graft such as allograft bone dowel is incorporated more quickly)

22. Describe potential disadvantages or concerns with use of rhBMP-2 or rhBMP-7 for spinal fusions.

- Possibility of bone formation in ectopic sites separate from the area of intended fusion (e.g., within the spinal canal)
- Expense
- Incomplete knowledge about optimal dose, carrier, and long-term follow-up of the procedure in humans

23. In what form are rhBMPs used in spinal fusions?

RhBMPs are usually used in combination with a carrier.

24. Describe the role of the carrier.

A carrier is a substance that serves as a delivery vehicle for the osteoinductive protein.

25. What carrier matrices have been used to deliver rhBMPs?

- Collagen: sponge or putty form
- Polymers: polylactide-co-glycolide (PLGA)
- Organic matrices: cortical allograft and demineralized bone matrix
- Inorganic matrices: tricalcium phosphate or hydroxyapatite

26. Are carriers equally effective when used for anterior and posterior fusion procedures?

No. Certain carriers are optimal for use in anterior compared with posterior fusion sites. Anterior interbody fusion can be successfully achieved with a compatible collagen sponge protected by a structural support such as a bone dowel or titanium cage. In a posterolateral spinal fusion, a noncompressible matrix such as a combination of tricalcium phosphate and hydroxyapatite is more effective.

27. What are the two major methods of gene therapy used to enhance spinal fusion in experimental studies?

1. **In vivo:** the vector carrying the genetic material is placed in the site of fusion.
2. **Ex vivo:** the marrow cells or other cells are transfected in a culture and introduced into the spine fusion site.

28. What are the potential advantages and disadvantages of gene therapy over rhBMP for spinal fusions?

Advantage: Gene therapy has the postential to deliver a sustained production of osteoinductive proteins compared with a one-time dose of rhBMP, which disappears from the surgical site within 72 hours.

Disadvantage: An immune response from the host may block any therapeutic benefit. Ineffective transfer of genetic material and insufficient production of osteoinductive factors may occur.

29. What is the most common vector used for gene therapy?

Both retroviruses and adenoviruses have been used. However, adenoviruses are the most common vectors for gene therapy.

30. What prevents the adenovirus from replicating again and again at a gene therapy site?

Unlike retroviruses, which integrate into the target cell genome and consequently become expressed during every replication cycle, adenoviruses act in an epichromosomal fashion. Therefore, the genetic material is not passed on to subsequent generations.

BIBLIOGRAPHY

1. An HS, Lynch K, Toth J: Prospective comparison of autograft vs. allograft for adult posterolateral lumbar spine fusion: Differences among freeze-dried, frozen, and mixed grafts. J Spin Disord 8:131–135, 1995.
2. Davy DT: Biomechanical issues in bone transplantation. Orthop Clin North Am 30:553–564,1999.
3. Goldberg VM, Stevenson S: Natural history of autografts and allografts. Clin Orthop 225:7–16, 1987.
4. McKay B, Sandhu HS: Use of recombinant human bone morphogenetic protein-2 in spinal fusion applications. Spine 27(16S): S66–S85, 2002.
5. Miyazono K, Kusanagi K, Inoue H: Divergence and convergence of TGF-β/BMP signaling. J Cell Physiol 187:265–276, 2001.
6. Reddi AH: Bone morphogenetic proteins: From basic science to clinical applications. J Bone Joint Surg 83A (Suppl 1–1): S1–S6, 2001.
7. Scaduto AA, Lieberman JR: Gene therapy for osteoinduction. Orthop Clin North Am 30:625–634, 1999.
8. Stevenson S: Biology of bone grafts. Orthop Clin North Amer 30:543–552, 1999.
9. Suh DY, Boden SD, Louis-Ugbo J, et al: Delivery of recombinant human bone morphogenetic protein-2 using a compression-resistant matrix in posterolateral spine fusion in the rabbit and in the non-human primate. Spine 27:353–360, 2000.
10. Younger EM, Chapman MW: Morbidity at bone graft donor sites. J Orthop Trauma 3(3): 192–195, 1989.

XII. General Issues

67. ASSESSMENT OF OUTCOMES AFTER SPINE SURGERY

Reginald Q. Knight, M.D., and Stephen M. Hansen, M.D.

1. What are clinical outcomes?

Clinical outcomes are an assessment of how patients respond to the interventions recommended by physicians. Interventions can take the form of surgical or nonsurgical modalities. Outcomes can be obtained from the physician, patient, or payor point of view. The data points recorded include items that one is quite accustomed to retrieving, such as surgical demographics (e.g., estimated blood loss, operative time, curve reduction, or complications). In addition, such data are correlated with functional changes in patients who have undergone treatment For example, do patients require less pain medication? Move better in the community? Require fewer adaptive aids?

2. What types of data should be collected?

The type of data collected depends largely on one's interest and role as physician, patient, or payor. Are data analyzed to assess response to a given therapy, or is the focus resource utilization during an episode of care? In most cases it is best to retrieve as much information as possible at multiple time intervals, including preintervention and postintervention time frames. Data are categorized to allow comparison of like patient groups (e.g., age, sex, disease entity, procedure, co-morbidity, complications).

3. What factors have stimulated current interest in outcomes research?

- Increasing health care costs
- Variation in clinical practice and utilization of health care resources
- Deficiencies identified in the current medical literature that fail to provide solid evidence about the theraputic efficacy of medical care

4. How is outcomes research defined?

Outcomes research has been defined as enhanced clinical research that places an emphasis on patient-based outcomes in contrast to process measures.

5. Give examples of patient-based outcomes.

Patient-based outcomes include data such as pain, functional status, and satisfaction with care rendered. Patient measures are subjective assessments that measure the results of care as perceived by the patient.

6. Give examples of process measures.

Process measures include objective data such as radiographic results, curve correction, fusion rate, or range of motion.

7. What is an instrument?

An instrument is a method for collecting patient-based outcome data via a high-quality questionnaire. An instrument requires extensive testing and validation prior to clinical use. It provides a source of standardized and comparable data. It permits useful and valid comparisons of different treatment methods.

8. What are the two main types of outcome instruments?

The two main types of outcome instruments are general status instruments and disease-specific instruments.

9. Explain what is meant by a general status outcome instrument.

A general status outcome instrument (also termed a global instrument) attempts to assess the overall functional status of a patient after a medical or surgical intervention. The most commonly used instrument in this category is the SF-36. This instrument collects information on eight scales (domains): (1) physical function, (2) role limitation secondary to physical health problems, (3) bodily pain, (4) social function, (5) general mental health, (6) role limitation due to emotional problems, (7) vitality, and (8) general health perception.

10. Explain what is meant by a disease-specific instrument. Give examples of such instruments currently used to assess patients after spinal surgery.

A disease-specific outcome instrument collects data from patients with a specific disease after a specific medical or surgical intervention. Disease-specific outcome instruments used to assess patients with spinal disorders include:

- Scoliosis Research Society Instrument (SRS-22): evaluates outcomes after surgery for adolescent idiopathic scoliosis.
- Oswestry Disability Questionnaire, North American Spine Society (NASS) Instrument, and the Musculoskeletal Outcomes Data Evaluation and Management System (MODEMS): evaluate adult spine patients after various interventions.

11. How is the quality of an outcome instrument determined?

Instruments have been scientifically tested to determine their reliability, validity, and sensitivity. Outcome date is considered reliable when the measurement is reproducible with low levels of random error. An instrument is considered valid if it measures what it is intended to measure. An instrument is sensitive if it has the ability to measure change over time.

12. Can computer software facilitate gathering, organizing, and interpreting outcome data?

Current technology allows the use of computers with most instruments. If not available directly from the developer of the instrument, data entry may be used to format one's own system for ease of data acquisition and analysis. Computerized instruments designate a numerical value to patient symptoms. It is important to realize that each subjective or objective finding does not necessarily carry the same numerical weight. Any changes in the developers' numerical assignment may invalidate one's data.

13. Can patients participate directly in the recording of outcome data?

If the goal is measurement of patient function, primary data obtained directly from the patient are very important. Such data are less valid if obtained through an intermediary. Primary data directly from the patient do not have the same potential for bias with respect to the interpreter or researcher. Nonfunctional outcome data may be obtained from the patient record.

14. Can the Internet play a role in data collection?

As institutions become more sophisticated, the Internet may play a larger role in patient-physician communication and data exchange. It is possible to have the information presented to the patient on a secure web page for completion and analysis. One potential weakness of this modality is the inability to confirm the actual source of the data entered.

15. What additional technologies exist to aid in collection of data?

Imagination and financial constraint are the limits to use of present technology. Office scanners, touch screen data entry, and voice-activated retrieval offer additional options for data collection. Classic print media remain the most frequently used method for collecting data due primarily to cost constraints and familiarity.

16. How can measurement of clinical outcomes improve daily practice patterns?

Information gained from assessing clinical outcome studies can lead to the establishment of clinical pathways. Clinical pathways may be instituted in a formal fashion or adapted on an individual practice basis. When patients are not following the expected postoperative course, adjustments in care can be made. As a result, information provided to patients preoperatively has more credibility because it has been gathered from other patients who have undergone similar treatment. Properly acquired outcome data can aid in the justification of treatment options and provide valuable data for improvement and standardization of care. This reduction in variability may have a positive impact on reduction of clinical errors related to patient care.

17. Are clinical outcomes important only for academic practices?

Clinical outcomes are important for all practice types—academic or private, group or individual. Improved patient care, reduction in variability of practice patterns, and development of clinical pathways are positive results of prospective outcome analysis.

18. Will gathering outcome data influence patient referral patterns?

We are not aware of any direct data that confirm this assumption. However, the ability to gather, analyze, and improve patient care via outcome data should be seen as a positive endeavor by the medical and patient community. In this situation, it is reasonable to anticipate that one's practice should ultimately benefit.

19. Can gathering clinical outcome data change a patient's perception of one's practice?

Patient satisfaction studies support the idea that time spent with the patient is reflected in an improved rating. The nature of the outcome data-gathering process requires that members of your office interact with the patient. It is important, therefore, that the members of your patient care team assigned to this task take it as a positive duty.

20. Are reimbursements currently tied to clinical outcomes?

At present reimbursement is not tied to clinical outcome. In the future, government agencies and local insurers may require a certain level of patient satisfaction or functional improvement as a means of inclusion on care panels. Functional outcome and patient satisfaction data are currently used as a marketing tool (e.g., total joint replacement or cardiac statistics) in some competitive hospital markets.

21. Is there evidence to prove that gathering clinical outcomes is cost-effective?

The direct costs in material and time are major deterrents to widespread application of functional outcome analysis. Until patients and insurers require physicians to provide practice-specific data, little incentive will exist to expend the required resources. At present it is probably not cost-effective for every practice to study every procedure it performs. However, simple measures of patient satisfaction and periodic assessment of the functional outcome related to its most common procedures may prove beneficial to a practice and its patients.

22. Can gathering clinical outcome data become a legal liability for a practitioner?

Material gathered via this process remains subject to patient confidentiality. Various states may have different regulations with respect to disclosure of such data. Despite these issues, practices that are actively involved in patient assessment can use this process as a positive indicator of improved patient care.

BIBLIOGRAPHY

1. Deyo RA, Andersson G, Bombardier C, et al: Outcome measures for studying patients with low back pain. Spine 19(Suppl 18):2032s–2036s, 1994.
2. Eddy DM: Clinical decision making: From theory to practice. Designing a practice policy: Standards, guidelines, and options. JAMA 263:3077–3084, 1990.
3. Haher TR, Gorup JM, Shin TM, et al: Results of the Scoliosis Research Society Instrument for Evaluation of Surgical Outcome in Adolescent Idiopathic Scoliosis. A multicenter study of 244 patients. Spine 24(14):1435–1440, 1999.
4. Hyams AL: Practice guidelines and malpractice litigation: A two-way street. Ann Intern Med 122:450–455, 1995.
5. Keller RB: The methods of outcomes research. Curr Opin Orthop 5:86–89, 1994.
6. Keller RB: Outcomes research in orthopaedics. J Am Acad Orthop Surg 1(3):122–129, 1993.
7. Wong DA: Developing treatment guidelines. In Mayer T, Gatchel R, Polatin P (eds): Occupational Musculoskeletal Disorders: Functions, Outcomes, and Evidence. Philadelphia, Lippincott Williams & Wilkins, 2000, pp 721–727.

68. MEDICAL–LEGAL ISSUES IN SPINE CARE

Jeffrey R. Erickson, B.S., J.D.

1. What are the essential elements to a medical malpractice action?
- Creation of the physician-patient relationship.
- Breech of duty on part of the physician as to that relationship.
- Causation
- Damages

2. What is the legal definition of standard of care?

A physician must possess the degree of learning and skill ordinarily possessed by reputable physicians and exercise that skill and learning in a manner consistent with reputable and prudent physicians in the same or similar localities under similar circumstances.

3. Does standard of care mean average ability or average care?

The standard of care with regard to negligence is whether the physician possess and exercises the minimal common learning and skill of other physicians of reputable standing.

4. Are specialists held in the same standard?

Specialists are held not only to a minimal common skill of physicians in general but also to the minimal common skill of reputable physicians in their field.

5. How does the outcome of a surgical case influence the determination of liability?

The law is clear that medical perfection is not required as it pertains to physician liability. A physician is not necessarily negligent because he or she makes errors in judgment or because his or her efforts prove unsuccessful. The physician is negligent if the failure in judgment or lack of success is secondary to his or her failure to possess the requisite skill and knowledge of like practitioners and the failure to exercise that skill.

6. Is there a legal accommodation for "schools of thought" for different medical procedures?

As long as a "reasonable minority" of physicians practice a particular alternative, the defendant physician is entitled to be judged according to the tenets of the school that he or she professes to follow. However, practices that are considered "state of the art" may be deemed as experimental or untested by reputable experts.

7. In what circumstance is an expert not necessary to prove a plaintiff's case?

Only simple medical questions within the common knowledge of laymen may be resolved without conclusive expert testimony. Hence, expert evidence may not be necessary to resolve straightforward cases such as failure to x-ray a traumatic injury, administration of an anesthetic agent with an unsterile needle, or leaving foreign objects in a wound after an operation.

8. How does the concept of causation play into a medical malpractice matter?

A jury is instructed by the court to consider whether the actions of a physician are the actual cause of injury. The jury is told that the care or act must be a "substantial factor" in bringing about the injury claimed by the plaintiff. Although the term *substantial* is not generally defined, it is distinguished from causes that are "insignificant, trivial, or negligible." In general, the substantial factor must be more likely than not, or to a reasonable medical probability, the injury-producing factor.

9. What happens if the plaintiff has a preexisting injury or condition that is exacerbated by the alleged negligence of the defendant physician?

Although there may be more than one cause to an injury, if the physician's conduct is a "substantial factor" as determined by the jury, the physician cannot escape liability only because there is another concurrent cause.

10. How does a patient's noncompliance with a physician's directives or advice influence medical malpractice litigation?

Only when the patient's injury is attributable solely to the negligent failure of the patient to follow his or her doctor's instructions or advice can the physician be found not negligent. This is a difficult standard for the defense to prove. The concept of contributory negligence serves only to reduce the damages awarded to the patient by the jury and is not considered in the analysis of whether the doctor violated the standard of care. For example, if the jury finds that the total damages are $100,000 and that the plaintiff was 30% negligent or responsible for causing damages, the award is reduced to $70,000.

11. What are the essential elements of defense of a surgeon?

In any case dealing with a surgical complication, certain elements must be proved by the defense. Although it is correct that the defense is under no legal obligation to prove anything, this notion lacks practicality. The defense should be prepared to show:

1. The indications for surgery were proper and reasonable.
2. The appropriate informed consent was obtained prior to surgery.
3. There was no surgical or technical mishap.
4. When the complication presented, it was addressed in a timely manner in order to prevent further harm.

It is also beneficial if the defense can present an alternative argument about how the complication developed that differs from the allegation made by the plaintiff.

12. What consideration should be made in terms of indications for the surgery?

Considerations that should be discussed in detail before recommending surgery include:

- The degree to which surgical intervention would be beneficial to the patient
- The success/failure of prior nonoperative treatment
- The patient's potential comorbidities that may work against a good surgical result.

13. What role does a physician's judgment play in litigation?

An undesirable outcome cannot be the basis to argue retrospectively that a physician erred and therefore must have been negligent. In fact, the jury is instructed that an error in medical judgment is not considered in a vacuum but must be weighed in terms of the professional standard of care. In certain circumstances there is more than one recognized method of treatment and no single method is used exclusively and uniformly by all practitioners of good standing. A physician is not negligent if, in exercising his or her best judgment, he or she selects one of the approved methods that later turns out to be a wrong choice or a choice not favored by certain other practitioners.

14. How is judgment deemed reasonable?

Reasonable judgment is determined by expert witnesses who establish the community standard. Judgment must be reasonable and based on reasonable data. Therefore, a good rule of thumb is that when a physician's decision is based on empirical data in the patient's chart, his or her professional judgment must be consistent with the realities of that data.

15. What are the essential elements of informed consent?

The physician must explain the following:

- The nature of treatment
- The risks and possible complications

- Expected benefits or effects of the treatments
- Alternatives to the treatment and their risks and benefits

16. What is considered standard in a discussion of risks and possible complications?

The law couches this standard in terms of materiality. A physician must communicate material information, which he or she knows or should know would be regarded as significant by a reasonable person in the patient's position when deciding to accept or reject a recommended medical procedure. The physician likewise has a duty to express in lay terms the reasonably likely complications that follow a procedure. A complication that is remote is not ordinarily required to be included in the surgeon's consent discussion.

17. What should be included in a discussion of expected benefits or effects of a proposed treatment?

Discussion should be material, factual, and, most importantly, realistic. Frequently, discussion of the physician's experience with like patients allows the patient to form some idea of the range of possible benefit that he or she can expect from a particular procedure.

18. What needs to be included in a discussion of treatment alternatives and their risks and benefits?

The question often arises as to whether a physician has a duty to tell the patient of alternatives that they either do not practice or do not necessarily favor. The short answer to this question is "yes." A litany of all possible treatments is not required by the physician. However, discussion of the two or three specific schools of thought that may exist about any given situation is part of the consent.

There also may be situations in which the physician would recommend against a particular procedure (sometimes called the doctrine of informed refusal of consent). The court has made the law clear in this regard. If a patient indicates that he or she is going to decline a test or treatment, the doctor has the additional duty of advising about all material risks of which a reasonable person would want to be informed before deciding *not* to undergo the procedure.

Therefore, it is sometimes necessary to have a frank and directed discussion in which the patient is told that the choice not to pursue the recommended treatment or therapy poses a significant potential detriment to his or her health. A brief, factual, and nonexculpatory note to this effect should also be included in the chart.

19. Are there any exceptions to the general rule of consent?

In emergent cases, treatment may proceed without the patient's consent. However, many elements must exist for this option to be viable. For instance, the law sometimes implies consent if several factors exist. Generally, it is considered that a medical emergency exists when:

1. Immediate services are required for the alleviation of severe pain;
2. Immediate diagnostic studies of unforeseen medical conditions are necessary; or
3. The physician in his or her best judgment feels that a condition will lead to serious bodily harm or death if not diagnosed and treated.

Nonetheless, once those goals have been met, further consent is required for additional procedures. In other words, once the emergent circumstances have dissipated, the general rules regarding consent are in full force and effect.

20. What issues of consent are linked to competency of the patient?

If there is insufficient time to inform the patient fully because of emergent circumstances or if the patient is unconscious, a physician may proceed without informed consent. If a person is legally incapable of giving informed consent and the physician has a reasonable belief that the procedure needs to be undertaken immediately, then he or she may also proceed. Similarly, if consent is obtained from a family member, the family member should be competent.

However, obtaining consent from the patient or another person legally capable of consenting should be weighed against the likelihood that a delay in treatment will result in severe disability, continuation of severe pain, or death. If delay does not jeopardize the condition of the patient in these regards, treatment must be delayed.

21. What duty does the surgeon have in term of requesting consultation?

There is no legal requirement that a physician seek consultation. At times, however, hospital facility guidelines or protocols necessitate consultation for specific procedures (e.g., determination of brain death, administration of tissue plasminogen activator in acute stroke patients). It is generally considered a matter of discretion for the treating physician to determine whether a consultation is advisable or emergent.

22. What are the duties of the consulting spinal surgeon?

First, if a physician is called for consultation, the consulting physician should document his or her opinion in the patient's medical record. If the consulting surgeon determines that radiographic studies, blood work, or other consultations are necessary and recommends them in the note, it is a risky policy to assume that either the emergency department physician or the primary care provider (depending on the circumstances of the consultation) will follow through with these recommendations. The consulting physician should follow through.

23. What medical-legal issues often arise in relation to spinal surgery and the treatment of spinal diseases?

One of the most common issues involves the evaluation and treatment of compression of the spinal cord and nerve roots. Issues center on delay in diagnosis of pathology causing symptoms and/or timing of surgical intervention. The typical case centers on a delay in properly assessing and treating the spinal pathology. Cases of cauda equina or spinal cord compression may present with a mixed bag of signs and symptoms. Timing is an essential consideration. For example, some schools of thought state that in cauda equina cases the standard of care is to intervene within 24 hours of the onset of loss of bowel or bladder control or in the presence of other focal neurologic signs. The physician needs to be aware that as time passes, more information will become available. There is likely to be more documentation in the chart about the patient's complaints and status for which he or she will be held responsible.

24. What legal issues may arise with spinal implants such as pedicle screws?

Because medical devices such as spinal implants are often carefully monitored by the Food and Drug Administration (FDA) and other advisory panels, a physician must be knowledgeable about the role of these organizations. The FDA does not have the legal authority to regulate the practice of medicine. However, after passage of the Medical Device Amendments of 1976, the FDA was granted authority to evaluate medical devices before they can be marketed. The FDA classifies medical devices into three categories based on the degree of regulation that the FDA deems necessary to provide a reasonable degree of assurance about device safety and efficacy:

Class 1 device: the least restrictive category. Only general control standards are required, such as registration and listing of the product with the FDA, filing of a Premarket Notification or 510[k] application, filing reports documenting device marketing experience, and adherence to good manufacturing standards.

Class 2 device: a more restrictive category in which the safety of the device cannot be ensured only on the basis of general control standards. Special controls (e.g., laboratory testing) are required in addition to general controls.

Class 3 device: the most restrictive category. Class 3 devices are considered to be entirely new or newly designed. Data about their safety and efficacy are considered to be insufficient.

To be approved by the FDA, class 2 and 3 devices must file one of two types of documents: (1) Premarket Notification or 510[k] or (2) Premarket Approval Application. Unapproved devices can be made available under an Investigational Device Exemption (IDE), in which a limited number of devices can be used for a clinical investigation during the processing of the Premarket Notification or Premarket Approval Application. In addition, courts have now indicated that "a physician is free to use a medical device for off label purpose if, in the physician's best medical judgment, he or she believes that the use of the device will benefit the patient."

25. What is the current status of pedicle fixation according to the FDA?

On August 26, 1998 the FDA reclassified pedicle screws from class 3 to class 2 devices for certain spinal disorders. This change reflected the presentation of sufficient evidence demonstrating the safety and efficacy of pedicle screw systems intended to provide immobilization and stabilization of the spine as an adjunct to fusion in the treatment of acute and chronic instability or defomity of the thoracic, lumbar, and sacral spinal regions. This reclassification specifically applied to degenerative spondylolisthesis with objective evidence of neurologic impairment, fractures, dislocations, scoliosis, kyphosis, spinal tumors, and pseudarthrosis. This reclassification did not apply to use in the cervical spine or pediatric population.

BIBLIOGRAPHY

1. Benett CR, Bendo JA: Lumbar pedicle fixation: An update. Spine State Art Rev 13:313–327, 1999.
2. Garfin SR: North American Spine Society Memorandum, August 6, 1998.
3. Garfin SR, Yuan HA: Food and Drug Administration regulation of spinal implant fixation devices. Clin Orthop 335:32–38, 1997.
4. Mishra N, Yahiro M, Morrey BF: The Food and Drug Administration's regulation of orthopedic devices. J Bone Joint Surg 76A: 919–922, 1994.
5. Schultz WB. Orthopedic devices: Classification and reclassification of pedicle screw spinal systems. Fed Reg 63(143):400025–400041, 1998.

69. SPINE CARE AND THE INTERNET

Sylvia Devlin, B.S., Information Systems

1. What benefits may be realized by patients who use the Internet to obtain information relating to spinal disorders?

- Ability to locate information relating to nearly any spine topic rapidly.
- Well-informed patients are better able to participate in their health care decision-making.
- Patient office visits and treatment interventions are facilitated by improved understanding of spine health care issues.

2. What problems are commonly encountered when patients use the Internet to obtain information relating to spinal disorders?

- Information overload.
- Information obtained may include misinformation, commercially biased information, or data that do not apply to the patient's specific problem.
- Lack of direction. An Internet search on a general search engine can lead virtually anywhere. General search engines may lead to sites ranging from professional societies, universities, spine clinics, spinal device manufacturers, patient advocacy groups, and news media to non-medically related areas.

3. Describe steps that patients can take to minimize the most common problems encountered in attempting to research their own spinal problems.

1. Clarify your goal to focus your Internet search. Are you looking for information about a symptom (e.g., low back pain) or information about a specific condition that is responsible for low back pain symptoms (e.g., L5–S1 spondlylolisthesis)? Are you looking for information to assist in confirming a diagnosis, or is your goal to analyze various treatment options for a specific condition?

2. Do not rely on a single Internet site for information. Obtain information from multiple sites of varying types, including professional societies, government agencies, universities, medical practices, and nonprofit groups.

3. Look for information that is supported by published medical research in peer-reviewed journals or by links to other reputable sites.

4. Avoid sites that feature testimonials, product sales, advertising, or "secret cures."

5. Avoid sites that offer diagnosis and treatment without a complete medical history and physical examination.

6. Discuss your Internet search results with your personal physician.

4. How can one judge whether the information obtained on the Internet is reliable?

The Health Summit Working Group, available at <http://hitiweb.mitretek.org/docs/policy.html>, selected, defined, ranked, and evaluated seven major criteria for assessing the quality of Internet health information:

1. **Credibility:** The site will include the source, currency, relevance/utility, and editorial review process related to how the information was gathered.

2. **Content:** Look for accuracy and completeness as well as an appropriate disclaimer.

3. **Disclosure:** Communicates to the user what the purpose of the site is.

4. **Links:** Connections to other external sites that are assessed according to selection, architecture, content, and back linkages.

5. **Design:** Takes into consideration how user-friendly the site is by evaluating accessibility, logical organization, and internal search capability.

6. **Interactivity:** Contains a means for users to exchange information as well as feedback opportunities for the user to offer comments, concerns, or criticisms.

7. **Caveats:** Inform the user what the purpose of the site is; that is, whether it is to market products and services or to provide informational content.

5. How can a patient avoid some of the problems associated with using general search engines to access medical information?

Two simple steps to improve one's Internet experience include:

1. Learn more about how to use the Internet's search capabilities. For example, The Medical Library Association, available at <http://www.mlanet.org>, provides a user guide and lists top consumer health sites.

2. Become familiar with a health-focused search engine. For example, <http://www.vitalseek.com> is a health-focused search engine that allows the user to filter health information according to a wide range of criteria.

6. What is a reliable Internet site that provides access to spine-related information from U.S. governmental agencies?

The National Institutes of Health and related governmental agencies provide a wealth of information at <http://www.medlineplus.gov>. At this site overviews relating to diagnosis and treatment of various spinal disorders are provided as well as links to various directories and organizations. Noteworthy are the links to ongoing clinical trials and to MEDLINE, the National Library of Medicine's database. The links on this portal have been screened by the National Institute of Health to help the lay public locate reliable information on the web. A Spanish language version is available.

7. List professional societies that are recognized as credible and nonbiased sources of information relating to spinal disorders and that are valuable for both patients and physicians.

- North American Spine Society at <http://www.spine.org/>
- American Academy of Orthopaedic Surgeons at <http://www.aaos.org/>
- American Association of Neurological Surgeons at <http://www.neurosurgery.org/>
- Cervical Spine Research Society at <http://www.csrs.org/>
- American Spinal Injury Association at <http://www.asia-spinalinjury.org/>
- Scoliosis Research Society at <http://www.srs.org/>
- American Academy of Physical Medicine and Rehabilitation at <http://www.aapmr.org/>

8. List several Internet sites associated with major U.S. universities that provide comprehensive information relating to spinal disorders.

- The Mayo Foundation for Medical Education and Research at <http://www.mayoclinic.com>
- The Cleveland Clinic Spine Center at <http://Clevelandclinic.org>
- University of Iowa–The Children's Virtual Hospital at <http://www.vh.org/pediatric>
- Mount Sinai–NYU Health–Orthospine at <http://www.orthospine.com/>

9. List commercially supported Internet sites that provide potentially useful patient-oriented information relating to spinal disorders.

- Spine universe at <http://spineuniverse.com> provides information about a diverse range of spinal conditions, including a comprehensive list of treatment options as well as a physician locator.
- All about back pain at <http://www.allaboutbackpain.com> is owned by DePuyAcromed and provides wide-ranging information about the diagnosis and treatment of neck pain, low back pain, and scoliosis.

- Spine health at <http://www.spine-health.com>. Interdisciplinary spine specialists provide a wide range of information for spine patients.

10. What Internet sites may be of potential value to patients diagnosed with scoliosis or kyphosis?
- Scoliosis Research Society at <http://www.srs.org/>. An extensive patient library section provides information about various types of spinal deformities. See "In Depth Review of Scoliosis: Introduction" at <http://www.srs.org/htm/library/review/review01.htm>.
- National Scoliosis Foundation at <http://scoliosis.org>. Extensive educational resources for patients, including brochures, video, and local support groups.
- American Academy of Orthopaedic Surgeons at <http://www.aaos.org/>. Educational material relating to diagnosis and treatment of scoliosis. See "What is Scoliosis?" at <http://orthoinfo.aaos.org/brochure/thr_report.cfm?Thread_ID=14&topcategory=Spine>.
- Children's Virtual Hospital. See "Questions Often Asked about Scoliosis" at <http://www.vh.org/Patients/IHB/Ortho/Peds/Scoliosis/Questions/Scoliosis.html>.
- Ask NOAH at <http://www.noah-health.org/english/illness/orthop/scoliosis.html>.
- <Scoliosis-world.com> offers wide-ranging coverage of various aspects of scoliosis.
- <http://iScoliosis.com> features treatment using implants from device manufacturer Sofamor Danek.

11. What sites are of potential value for patients with lumbar spine disorders?
- Back Pain at <http://www.nlm.nih.gov/medlineplus/backpain.html>.
- "Back Pain Exercises" and "Low Back Pain" as well as various other helpful topics are available at <http://orthoinfo.aaos.org/category.cfm?topcategory=Spine>.
- Lower Back Pain at <http://www.familydoctor.org/healthfacts/117/>.
- North American Spine Society for Spine Patients at <http://www.spine.org/fsp.cfm>.
- Back pain: mechanical at <http://emedicine.com/emerg/topic50.htm>.
- <http://backpain.com> features treatment using implants from device manufacturer Sofamor Danek.

12. What are some sites of potential value for patients with cervical spine disorders?
- Herniated Cervical Disc at <http://www.spine.org/articles/herniatedcervdisc.cfm>.
- <http://spineuniverse.com>.
- American Academy of Orthopaedic Surgeons at <http://www.aaos.org/>.
- <http://neckreference.com> features treatment using implants from device manufacturer Sofamor Danek.

13. What sites are of potential value to patients with osteoporosis?
- National Osteoporosis Foundation at <http://www.nof.org>. This nonprofit voluntary health organization is a good starting point for information about osteoporosis.
- National Institutes of Health Osteoporosis and Related Bone Diseases-National Resource Center at <http://www.osteo.org/bone_health_info.htm>. This site provides useful fact sheets about a variety of bone diseases, including osteoporosis, Paget's disease, osteogenesis imperfecta, myeloma, and fibrous dysplasia.
- Kyphon at <http://www.kyhon.com> provides information from the device manufacturer about treatment of compression fractures using balloons and bone cement.

14. What sites are recommend for patients interested in applying complementary and alternative treatments for spinal disorders?
- American Academy of Orthopaedic Surgeons at <http://www.aaos.org/>. See the Wellness section or directly access this area at <http://www3.aaso.org/courses/cam/camtoc.htm>.

- The National Center for Complementary and Alternative Medicine at <http://nccam.nih.gov/health/>.
- The National Institutes of Health's Office of Dietary Supplements at <http://dietary-supplements.info.nih.gov>.
- American Association of Medical Acupuncture at <http://www.medicalacupuncture.org>.

15. Can patients use the Internet to locate a spine specialist?

Yes. However, caution is necessary when the Internet is used for this purpose. Many sites list spine specialists based on information submitted by the physician. Information is not verified, and payment of a registration fee is the criterion for listing on many sites. Patients are advised to check that practitioners are board-certified and in good standing with national, state, and local medical societies and licensing boards. It is important that a spine specialist devote the majority of his or her practice to spinal disorders.

16. How can a physician use the Internet to enhance their practice?

1. Obtain and interchange professional information.
2. Provide real-time remote diagnosis (telemedicine).
3. Obtain continuing medical education (CME) credits.
4. Communicate with colleagues.
5. Communicate with patients by scheduling appointments or authorizing prescription refills.
6. Provide patient forms that can be downloaded and completed prior to an office visit.
7. Use electronic medical records (EMRs) to eliminate redundancy by having the physician enter patient information one time.

17. What is HIPAA? How will it affect medical practice?

The Health Insurance Portability and Accountability Act (HIPPA) is a collection of security guidelines working toward the secure collection, transmission, and storage of patient data. HIPAA is a result of the information age and is scheduled to become effective in April 2003. The security risks faced by health care organizations are both similar to and different from those of other businesses. As with other businesses, IT infrastructures, networks, servers, and desktop PCs share risks that include identity theft and network hijacking. Differentiating health care from other businesses are the sensitive data being stored and the public embarrassment and loss of credibility if such sensitive data were released. One of the biggest challenges is the transmittal of e-mail that contains individual-identifiable health care information.

Practical authentication also raises concerns. Many health care professionals complain that there are too many passwords to remember for the various applications used at medical centers. Biometrics would be ideal, but cost-benefit analysis shows this to be an extreme measure to take; passwords will suffice for the time being. Patient confidentiality has been practiced, but the information age has brought about easier access to the patient data. Electronically shared data make diagnosis a lot faster. HIPAA will make information sharing more difficult, and physicians are concerned about its impact on patient care. Educating health care professionals in the need to ensure confidentiality and security will be paramount in successfully exercising HIPAA standards.

18. What are some critical issues regarding medical consultation over the Internet?

If a physician provides medical advice via the Internet, awareness of issues beyond the immediate doctor-physician relationship is critical. State laws vary as they apply to physicians who provide medical information within a state as well as across state lines. Confidentiality and integrity of electronically transmitted patient information must be assured. The relevant issues and regulations are presently evolving and can be reviewed through sites such as The Office for the Advancement of Telehealth at <http://telehealth.hrsa.gov/links.htm>.

BIBLIOGRAPHY

1. Butler L, Foster FE: Back pain online: A cross-sectional survey of the quality of Web-based information on low back pain. Spine 28:395–401, 2003.
2. Crocco AG, Villasis-Keever M, Jadad AR: Analysis of cases of harm associated with use of health information on the Internet. JAMA 287:2869–2871, 2002.
3. Li L, Irvin E, Guzman J, et al: Surfing for back pain patients: The nature and quality of back pain information on the Internet. Spine 26:545–557, 2001.
4. Marietti C: HIPPA. Healthcare Informatics 19(1):55–60, 2002.
5. Silberg WM, Lundberg GD, Musacchio RA: Assessing, controlling and assuring the quality of medical information on the Internet. JAMA 277:1244–1245, 1997.

INDEX

Page numbers in **boldface type** indicate complete chapters.